AF560293

Indian Traditional Animal Husbandry and Ethnoveterinary Science

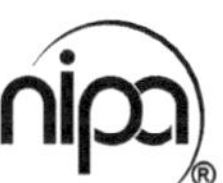

NIPA® GENX ELECTRONIC RESOURCES & SOLUTIONS P. LTD.
New Delhi-110 034

About the Editors

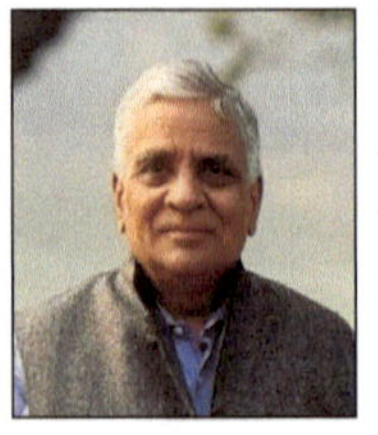

Dr D. Swarup, MVSc, PhD (Veterinary Medicine), is a distinguished veterinary scientist with over 34 years of service in the Indian Council of Agricultural Research (ICAR), internationally recognized for his pioneering contributions to ethnoveterinary medicine (EVM) and herbal veterinary therapeutics. He successfully led eight major research programs, notably serving as the veterinary lead for the World Bank-funded ICAR-NATP Mission Mode project on Indigenous Technical Knowledge and as National Coordinator and Principal Investigator of ICAR's Ad-hoc Scheme and Outreach Program on EVM. His work has rich contribution to the scientific validation and integration of traditional herbal practices into mainstream veterinary healthcare. Dr. Swarup has significantly advanced the development of herbal veterinary formulations, contributing to three patents for novel antimicrobial agents and a herbal preparation for managing fluorosis in animals. With over 200 scientific publications and numerous awards and honours—including the ICAR- Hariom Ashram Trust Award and IHRS National Gold Medal for Research in Herbal Veterinary Medicine—he has also served on several high-level expert committees such as the National Advisory Committee for Animal Husbandry and Dairying, and CPCSEA (Government of India), and was the President of the Indian Society for Veterinary Medicine. His contributions have been instrumental in shaping national policy, promoting research, and fostering sustainable animal health practices grounded in traditional knowledge systems.

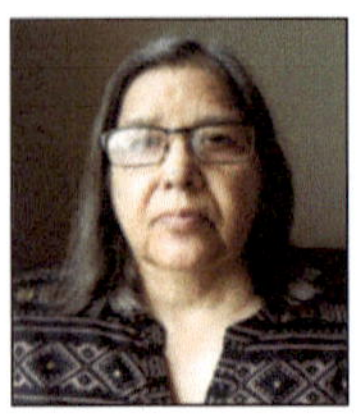

Dr Aruna T. Kumar is a distinguished expert in animal husbandry and agricultural mass communication, with MSc (Animal Nutrition, GBPUAT, Pantnagar), PhD from CCS University, Meerut (thesis -*Animal Husbandry in Ancient Indian Literature—Implications for Modern Science* published by LAP, Germany) and a postgraduate diploma in Mass Communication from Bhartiya Vidya Bhavan, New Delhi. With over three decades of service at the Indian Council of Agricultural Research (ICAR), including as Chief Editor (English), she played a pivotal role in modernizing agricultural and veterinary publishing and strengthening scientific communication through research journals, handbooks, and academic textbooks. A prolific editor and consultant, she has contributed to key projects, viz., NATP, NAIP and FFP of ICAR, edited India's top-ranking *The Indian Journal of Animal Sciences* (1984–2020); publications from FAO, ILRI, CIMMYT, TAAS; and currently serves as Consultant Editor with NIPA. Her editorial leadership includes developing e-publishing systems, conducting editorial trainings, and aligning book acquisitions with Agricultural Education Division, ICAR. Her work reflects a unique blend of subject matter expertise in animal sciences and exceptional editorial acumen in agricultural communication.

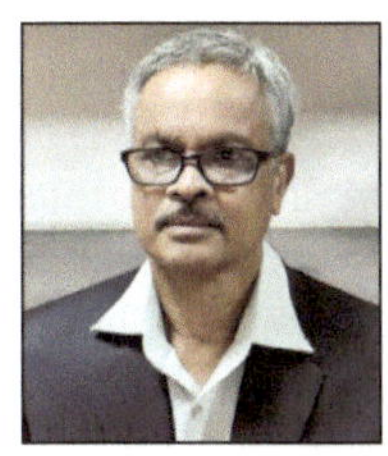

Dr S. Dey MVSc, PhD (Veterinary Medicine), currently serving as Professor and Head of Clinical Veterinary Medicine at Bihar Veterinary College, is a distinguished researcher with over three decades of contribution to ethnoveterinary science and herbal medicine. His work focuses on bridging traditional knowledge with modern scientific approaches, particularly in validating the efficacy and safety of medicinal herbs used in Indian traditional animal healthcare systems. He has served in key positions within ICAR, including as Principal Scientist and Acting Head, Division of Medicine at ICAR-IVRI, and as National Coordinator of the ICAR Network Programme on Ethnoveterinary Medicine. His research has led to the development of four herbal technologies and a patented formulation for combating fluoride toxicity. His interdisciplinary work has identified bioactive phytochemicals that offer therapeutic potential for disorders affecting the pancreas, kidneys, cardiovascular system, and skin. Dr Dey has authored over 119 research papers in international journals, four technical manuals, two book chapters, and is also a contributory author to a book on Ethnoveterinary Science and Indian Traditional Animal Husbandry. He has delivered 21 international presentations and guided 18 Master's and 11 Doctoral students in research on medicinal plants and herbal therapeutics.

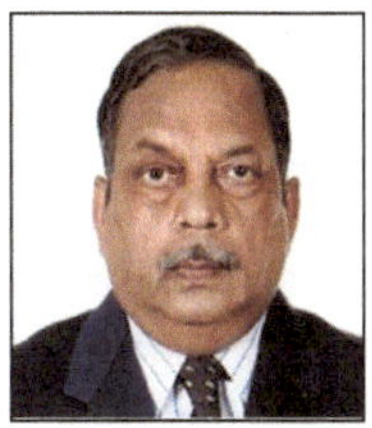

Dr R. Somvanshi, MVSc, PhD (Veterinary Pathology), FRCVS (Sweden), Diplomat, ICVP, is a distinguished Veterinary Pathologist whose pioneering contributions have significantly advanced the understanding of animal diseases and the history of veterinary science in India. With over four decades of rich experience in animal disease research, diagnosis, and postgraduate teaching, he has held prestigious positions including Joint Director, CADRAD (Acting), Head of the Division of Pathology, ICAR-National Fellow, ICAR-Emeritus Scientist and ICAR-Emeritus Professor at IVRI. Dr Somvanshi is widely recognized for his extensive scholarly work on the evolution of veterinary medicine and animal husbandry in ancient India, having authored several books and articles on the subject. He played a pivotal role in organizing the NAVS First Conference on Veterinary Medicine in Ancient India, and was instrumental in establishing the National Museum of Veterinary and Animal Sciences at IVRI. Dr Somvanshi received over two dozen national awards, including the DST Dr Meghnad Saha Award (thrice), ICAR Dr Rajendra Prasad Award (twice), UP Government S&T Vigyan Ratna Award and the IAVP Dr N.C. Jain Lifetime Achievement Award, along with fellowships from five national scientific societies. He also served as elected President of Indian Association of Veterinary Pathologists.

About Other Contributors

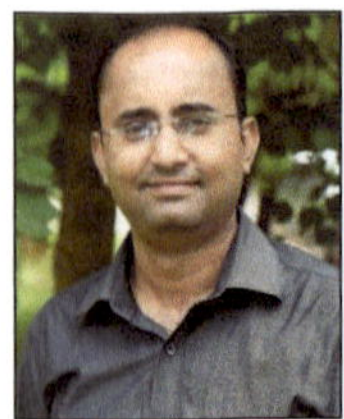

Dr S.K. Kumar, BAMS, MD (*Dravyaguna*), PGDCR, PGDOH, is the Medical Director at the School of Ancient Wisdom's Ayurveda Hospital in Bengaluru, with over 20 years of experience in Ayurveda spanning clinical practice, research, and academics. Currently pursuing a PhD, he specializes in Veterinary Ayurveda, *Vrikshayurveda,* and Panchakarma therapies, and has guided 27 postgraduate diploma students. A prolific contributor to the field, he has authored 18 research papers, four books, and three book chapters, and presented at over 30 national and international forums. Dr Kumar is a visiting faculty at the University of Trans-Disciplinary Health, Sciences and Technology (TDU), a consultant to dairy and pharma sectors, and a member of global bodies like the World Ayurveda Foundation and the Romanian Ayurveda Academy. He has delivered international lectures across eight countries, conducted research on ethnoveterinary medicine and antimicrobial resistance, and received a CCRAS grant for his postgraduate thesis. Fluent in four languages, he is passionate about Ayurvedic research, and traditional knowledge systems.

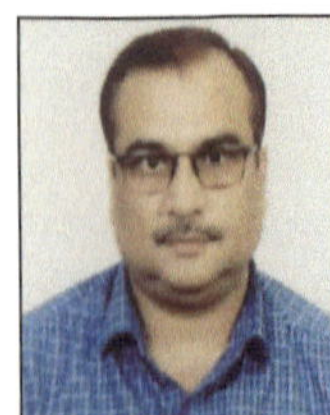

Dr P. Tripathi, MSc, PhD (Agronomy) is a Principal Scientist (Agronomy) at the ICAR–Indian Institute of Soil Science (IISS), Bhopal. He holds a PhD in Agronomy, with his doctoral research focused on *"Residue Management Studies in Wheat–Rice System."* Prior to his tenure at IISS, he served at the ICAR–Central Institute for Research on Goats (CIRG), Makhdoom, where he was actively involved in research on fodder crops, silvi-pastoral systems, and the establishment of herbal and multi-purpose plant gardens in rugged and marginal soils—experience that directly contributes to his expertise in medicinal and aromatic plant cultivation and herbal garden development. At present, Dr Tripathi is engaged in research on conservation agriculture and natural resource management, with continued interest in sustainable land use, plant-soil interactions, and integrated cropping systems. He has published over 45 research papers in national and international journals and has guided seven M.Sc. (Ag.) students in their thesis research. His broad agronomic expertise and practical experience in land rehabilitation and plant-based systems make him a valuable contributor to projects involving thematic herbal gardens and biodiversity conservation.

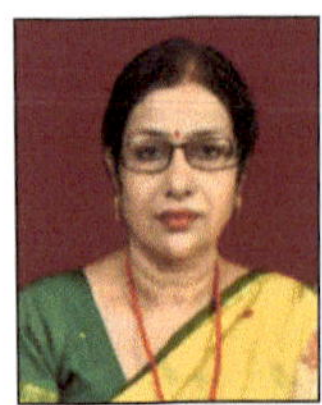

Dr Ananya Dan, MSc, PhD (Organic chemistry) earned her PhD from the University of Calcutta, India, in 2001. With nine years of post-doctoral research experience, she has published over 27 research articles in high-impact, peer-reviewed journals. She has presented her work at numerous national and international scientific forums and conferences. Her research primarily focuses on phytochemistry, with a particular emphasis on activity-guided isolation and purification of secondary plant metabolites. Her work aims to counteract the harmful effects of toxic heavy metals and address the multisystemic complications of diabetes. The majority of her research projects have been funded by the Council of Scientific and Industrial Research (CSIR), India. Throughout her academic and research career, Dr Dan has received several awards and research grants in recognition of her contributions to science. She is a life member of the Indian Science Congress.

Indian Traditional Animal Husbandry and Ethnoveterinary Science

Domestication History and Herbal Approaches to Animal Healthcare

D. Swarup
Aruna T. Kumar
S. Dey
R. Somvanshi

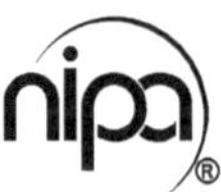

NIPA® GENX ELECTRONIC RESOURCES & SOLUTIONS P. LTD.
New Delhi-110 034

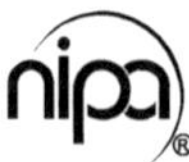

NIPA• GENX ELECTRONIC
RESOURCES & SOLUTIONS P. LTD.

101,103, Vikas Surya Plaza, CU Block
L.S.C.Market, Pitam Pura, New Delhi-110 034
Ph : +91 11 4386 0225, 9717133558, 9540816132
E-mail: newindiapublishingagency@gmail.com
Website: www. niparesources.com

Print ISBN: 978-93-58879-03-2

ebook ISBN: 978-93-5887-799-1

Composed and Designed by NIPA®.

Foreword

Animal husbandry has been an intrinsic part of Indian civilization since antiquity and continues to play a pivotal role in the country's agrarian economy. Blessed with rich livestock biodiversity, India's diverse agro-climatic zones nurture a wide array of indigenous breeds that are well-adapted to local conditions. Today, the livestock sector contributes significantly to national food security, rural livelihoods, and socio-economic resilience—especially in the face of agricultural uncertainty brought on by climate extremes and other natural calamities. India boasts the world's largest livestock population, with over 535 million animals, and ranks as the leading milk producer globally. The dairy sector alone contributes approximately 6% to the national economy, supporting nearly 25 million people. Livestock rearing provides livelihood to over two-thirds of rural households and contributes up to 29% of the agricultural and allied sector output. It accounts for 16% of the income of smallholder farmers and about 14% of income across all farming categories, while also generating around 8.8% of total employment. For India's rural population—comprising nearly 75% of the country's demographic—livestock remains a dependable source of income, nutrition, manure, fuel, and draught power, making it a viable and sustainable pathway to poverty alleviation. With increasing consumer awareness around food safety, traceability, and organic production, India enjoys a comparative advantage in livestock production due to its low unit cost in products such as milk, bovine meat, pork, and eggs. However, challenges remain—particularly in animal health, welfare, and the sustainability of veterinary practices. These concerns necessitate a closer look at India's rich legacy of traditional animal healthcare, which finds its roots in the Vedas and other ancient texts.

India's veterinary heritage is as old as its civilization. The philosophy of *Sarve Santu Niramaya* ('May all be free from disease') underscores the holistic worldview of ancient Indian medicine, including veterinary care. The science of Mrig Ayurveda (animal Ayurveda), referenced in the Rig Veda, Atharva Veda, and epics like the Puranas, showcases a sophisticated understanding of animal ailments and their treatment through herbs, dietary management, and holistic therapies. The Ashwini Kumaras, revered as divine physicians, are credited with profound knowledge of veterinary and human medicine alike. Archaeological evidence from the Indus–Saraswati civilization (ca. 2500 BCE) points to an organized practice of animal domestication and healthcare, with further elaboration found in Buddhist texts, the Arthaśāstra of Kautilya, and linguistic treatises of scholars like Pāṇini. These ancient works not only describe animal disease management but also illustrate the societal reverence for livestock—where even kings and warriors were expected to be well-versed in veterinary knowledge, considering the strategic and economic significance of animals.

Today, this traditional wisdom presents viable alternatives to address modern veterinary concerns such as antimicrobial resistance, chemical residues in animal products, and the overuse of antibiotics. Herbal remedies rooted in Ayurveda offer dual benefits: effective treatment and reduced risk of adverse side effects. The integration of validated traditional practices into contemporary veterinary systems can enhance both animal welfare and public health. In this context, the present volume—Indian Traditional Animal Husbandry and Ethnoveterinary Science: Domestication History and Herbal Approaches to Animal Healthcare, edited by Drs. D. Swarup, Aruna T. Kumar, S. Dey, and R. Somvanshi—is both timely and valuable. Comprising twelve meticulously crafted chapters, the book begins with a comprehensive account of the domestication history of animals and presents the current status of domestic species in India, followed by detailed documentation of traditional animal husbandry practices and indigenous ethno-knowledge systems. It then explores early veterinary practices, the concept of zoopharmacognosy, and the development of a rich ethnoveterinary Materia medica. The narrative further delves into evidence-based evaluations of traditional veterinary remedies, a systematic overview of Ayurvedic veterinary principles, and discussions on phytopharmacology, scientific validation, and herbal drug development. A concluding section focuses on the design and significance of herbal gardens for veterinary and educational use.

The book organizes scattered yet precious knowledge—both classical and community-based—and situates it within a modern scientific framework. It effectively bridges tradition with innovation, offering insights relevant to practitioners, researchers, and policymakers alike. Importantly, it highlights the role of veterinarians of the future, who must adopt more non-invasive, eco-friendly, and cost-effective practices. A deeper understanding of local ecosystems, animal breeds, and herbal resources will be essential in maintaining low-cost livestock production while ensuring food safety and public health under the One Health paradigm.

This well-researched and accessibly written volume is a commendable scholarly contribution that documents centuries of experiential knowledge while demonstrating its continued relevance in the modern era. The editors have undertaken the formidable task of synthesizing vast cultural and scientific domains with clarity and precision. I extend my heartfelt congratulations to the editors and authors for this remarkable effort and recommend this book to all stakeholders invested in sustainable animal healthcare and agricultural development.

Mahashivaratri
February 15, 2026
Noida, Uttar Pradesh, India

Dr K.M.L. Pathak
Former Vice Chancellor
UP Pt Deen Dayal Upadhyaya Pashu Chikitsa Vigyan Vishwavidyalaya
Evam Go-Anusandhan Sansthan (DUVASU), Mathura
Former Deputy Director General (Animal Sciences)
Indian Council of Agricultural Research, New Delhi

Preface

The domestication of animals stands as one of the most transformative milestones in human history. It marked the transition from foraging to farming, laying the foundations for settled life, the rise of civilizations, and the evolution of complex socio-cultural and ecological systems. At the heart of this process were early Human–Animal Interactions (HAI) and Human–Animal Relationships (HAR), which not only gave rise to animal husbandry but also to indigenous systems of animal care and healing.

This book, *Indian Traditional Animal Husbandry and Ethnoveterinary Science: Domestication History and Herbal Approaches to Animal Healthcare*, brings together interdisciplinary perspectives to explore the ancient roots, cultural contexts, and scientific relevance of traditional animal management and veterinary practices in India. Beginning with a global overview of animal domestication and the Neolithic revolution, the book sets the stage for understanding how animal husbandry emerged as both a survival strategy and a civilizational cornerstone. Subsequent chapters delve into India's long and diverse history of animal husbandry—from the Indus Valley Civilization and Vedic period to medieval and contemporary rural systems. Animal welfare and care have been integral to Indian cultural and spiritual life, as reflected in the principle of *Ahimsa* found in Vedic literature, the Ramayana, the Mahabharata, and Buddhist and Jain traditions. In modern times, the Constitution of India also upholds these values by emphasizing animal welfare and environmental conservation. Article 21 guarantees the right to life and personal liberty, while Article 51A (g) – described by the Hon'ble Supreme Court of India as the Magna Carta of animal rights in India–places a fundamental duty on every citizen to protect and improve the natural environment and to show compassion toward all living creatures.

A major focus of the book is the rich tradition of Indigenous Traditional Knowledge (ITK) and Ethnoveterinary Medicine (EVM), which encompasses time-honoured animal healing practices using herbs, minerals, and behavioural therapies. These include herbal, mineral, herbo-mineral, and ethnozoological remedies—as well as the emerging science of zoopharmacognosy, the roots of which can be traced to ancient Indian scriptures. Many of these traditional practices have undergone scientific validation and are increasingly being adopted in modern veterinary care. The volume also provides a comprehensive overview of Ayurveda-based animal healthcare (Pashu Ayurveda), highlighting its origin, core principles, and continued relevance. The contributions of renowned ancient scholars such as Shalihotra, Nakul, Palkapya, Jayadatta, Charaka, Sushruta, Jivaka, and Vagbhata are discussed, along with practical applications of Ayurvedic formulations in current livestock management. Notably, ancient Indian texts also reflect early ideas that resonate with today's concepts of reverse pharmacology, animal-assisted therapy, and One Health. In addition, the book addresses phytopharmacology, the scientific validation of herbal therapies, herbal drug development, and the design and utility of herbal gardens for therapeutic, educational, and conservation purposes.

To support visual learning and enhance reader engagement, the chapters are richly illustrated with colourful photographs that capture the cultural, socioeconomic, and ritual significance of domestic animals in Indian life—from village festivals and farming practices to temple rituals. Detailed images of medicinal plants and herbal gardens offer inspiration and practical guidance for those involved in ethnobotany, herbal healthcare, and biodiversity conservation.

This volume is primarily intended for students and scholars in veterinary and animal sciences, ethnobotany, rural development, and complementary medicine, as well as for veterinary practitioners, traditional knowledge holders, policy makers, and researchers interested in sustainable animal welfare and healthcare systems. It promotes an appreciation of India's rich cultural and ecological heritage, and encourages the integration of traditional wisdom with scientific inquiry to support sustainable, evidence-based veterinary practices.

We are deeply honoured that Dr KML Pathak, former Vice-Chancellor of DUVASU and Deputy Director General (Animal Sciences) at the Indian Council of Agricultural Research, graciously agreed to write the Foreword to this volume. His endorsement adds great value to the book, and we are truly grateful for his support.

The authors gratefully acknowledge the generous contributions of colleagues and institutions who provided valuable photographs and illustrations featured throughout this volume. Select images from public domain platforms—such as Wikimedia Commons and the World History Encyclopedia—have also been included, with appropriate credit in the relevant chapters. In addition, digital repositories such as the Vedic Heritage Portal (https://vedicheritage.gov.in), e-Samhita - National Institute of Indian Medical Heritage, Wisdom Library (https://www.wisdomlib.org), and the Internet Archive (https://archive.org) proved invaluable for accessing classical texts and rare books on India's heritage. Google Scholar served as a key resource for academic and research articles, while platforms like Wikipedia (https://www.wikipedia.org/) and Encyclopaedia Britannica (https://www.britannica.com) helped in contextualising and cross-referencing information.

English translations of Rig Veda, Atharva Veda, Yajur Veda and Arthashastra by esteemed scholars H.H. Wilson, R.T.H. Griffith, T.R. Sharma, and R. Shamasastry have been invaluable for tracing historical insights, particularly regarding ancient knowledge on animal husbandry and welfare. We gratefully acknowledge their pioneering contributions.

This book would not have been possible without the encouragement and committed support of our publishers—Shri Sumit Jain and the team led by Mr. Raj Kumar at NIPA—whose enthusiasm helped transform our vision into reality. We also extend our heartfelt appreciation to our family members for their unwavering support and encouragement, which enabled us to bring this work to completion. Finally, we invoke the timeless wisdom of ancient Indian thought, seeking harmony between humans, animals, and nature, and the protection of all forms of existence. As expressed in the Īśopaniṣad (Verse 1):

īśāvāsyam idaṁ sarvaṁ yat kiñca jagatyāṁ jagat;
tena tyaktena bhuñjīthā mā gṛdhaḥ kasya svid dhanam.

'The entire universe, both animate and inanimate, is pervaded by the Supreme. Therefore, one should enjoy life through renunciation, accepting only what is allotted as one's share, and not coveting the possessions of others.'

Mahashivaratri **The Editors**
15 February 2026

Contents

1

Human-Animal Interactions and Animal Domestication

D. Swarup

God had given men reason by which they could find out things for themselves, but He had given animals knowledge which did not depend on reason, and which was much prompter and more perfect in its way, and by which they had often saved the lives of men.

(Black Beauty: The Autobiography of a Horse:Anna Sewell, 1820 -1878)

Introduction

Association between man and animals involves rich, intricate, and dynamic interactions and relationships spanning over millennia of the evolutionary history of modern man (*Homo sapiens*). Men shared the world with an array of other animals and perhaps interacted with them in diverse manners in different roles as food competitors, hunters, herders, protectors, chaperones, healers, admirers, and even worshippers. The primeval relationship between man and animals was more that of a predator and prey and as the competitors for food. The early men hunted and killed other animals or chased them away from carcasses to get food to satisfy their hunger. Over time, human-animal interactions and relationships changed beyond the predator, competitor, and prey to the new diverse inter-species relationships and bonding as animals came to play new roles (Mithen 1999).

Apart from being the source of food, fur, fibre, hide, and other utility products for man, the animals have served as the means of animal power for agriculture, transport, and war, and companionship, social security, amusement, and symbol of power, authority, and wealth throughout the history of mankind. Animals also find a prominent place in mythology, cosmology, kin relations, religious beliefs, music, literature, and other different cultural manifestations of mankind's social organizations. Archaeologists are increasingly recognizing now that human-animal relations in the past were constituted in complex ways that go beyond the utilitarian mode in many ancient societies. Animals were the essential components of the total social phenomenon and were not animals at all; they were persons (Alves 2012, Hill 2013). This chapter briefly covers salient features of human-animal interactions and relationships including the domestication of animals, changing perception of man towards animals, animal-assisted intervention and benefits to humans, animal welfare, and the sociocultural influence of human-animal interactions during the long history of their coexistence

Human-Animal Interactions

Human-Animal-Interactions (HAI) are defined differently by different authors varying with the category of animals and the context in which these are studied. Types of human-animal interaction include affiliative interactions (e.g., pet ownership), animal-assisted interventions, and service animals (Thayer and Stevens 2019). Broadly, HAI is 'the relationship between humans and animals, whether it is for work, companionship, sport, or any other purpose' (Khandai and Shrivastava 2023). In the context of companion animals, HAI is 'mutual and dynamic interactions between people and animals and how these interactions may affect physical and psychological health and well-being' (Griffin *et al.* 2011). Regardless of varying definitions, HAI is a rapidly growing subject explored by the recent discipline of anthrozoology.

Human Animal Studies and Anthrozoology

Human-animal studies (HAS), Animal studies, and anthrozoology are often used synonymously. More specifically, Anthrozoology is the scientific study of human-animal interaction and human-animal bonds. It is truly an interdisciplinary and multidisciplinary subject placed between the sciences and the humanities and overlaps many other related disciplines of biological sciences. HAS is comparatively a broader term used to refer to the study of the interactions and relationship between human and non-human animals. HAS explores the space that animals occupy in the human social and cultural worlds and the interactions humans have with animals. These studies are valuable to understanding the social, cultural, economic, and traditional roles played by animals as well as for animal management and conservation. Animal Studies are defined as 'the scientific study of or medical use of, nonhuman animals, as in research' (DeMello 2012). The term 'animal study' is preferably used for HAS in humanities. Anthrozoology is commonly used in natural science (Hosey and Melfi 2019).

Anthrozoology Approaches: A variety of approaches comprising ethological, psychological, anthropological, sociological, historical, ethnographical, economic, legal, and philosophical collectively constitute anthrozoology (Hosey and Melfi 2019, DeMello 2012), as such anthropologists can be from diverse subjects like veterinary science, zoology, ethology philosophy, sociology, psychology, and history. Ethnozoology, another branch of ethnobiology deals with different ways of interactions, both past and present between human cultures and animals, and the knowledge concerning animals accumulated by human societies, as well as their significance to those people and their uses (Alves 2012). Anthrozoology focuses on relationships between humans and animals at the level of species; and ethnozoology studies various bonds between people, ethnic groups, and animals (Vorobiev 2018).

Human-Animal Relationships (HARs) and Human-Animal Bonds (HABs): These are the consequences of HAI. HAR involves a series of interactions over time between two individuals (man and animal) who are recognizable to or familiar with each other. HAR. may vary in quality from good to bad and can be reflected in the form of positivity (e.g., friendly contact, play) or negativity (e.g., aggression), or neutral depending upon the net quality of the interactions which make up the history of that HAR. HAB is defined as a mutually beneficial and dynamic relationship between people and animals, which is influenced by behaviours that are essential to the health and well-being of both. This includes but is not limited to, emotional, psychological, and physical interactions of people, animals, and the environment. Particularly good HARs can be regarded as Human–Animal Bonds (HABs) if they are reciprocal and promote the well-being of both partners (Hosey and Melfi 2014, Hosey *et al.* 2018).

Changing Ways of Human-Animal Interactions

All human societies have coexisted to a certain degree with animals and interacted with almost all global species of animals at some point in time, and in a variety of ways, depending on the types of animals, the environmental conditions, the evolutionary phase of mankind, and socio-cultural milieu, and the individual or collective attitude of people towards animals. A single species of animal can be used in different ways for different purposes in different societies and at different times. The long history of the human relationship with other animals that dates back several millennia is differentiated into three stages- the pre-domestic era of hunter-gatherer culture when people did not perceive a difference between themselves and other animals; a domestic era marked by the development of beliefs in the difference between man and other animals and superiority of humans; and finally, the post-domestic era, where most of the population have little direct experience of animals, particularly the food animals (Bulliet 2005). At the beginning of the pre-domestic era, there were only two categories of animals- humans and other persons (non-human animals). The domestic era beginning from the Neolithic Agricultural Revolution and the evolution of ancient cultures added more categories of animals to human societies like farm animals, war and sport animals, captive wild animals, and those used for ritual and religious purposes. Today people interact in different ways with different varieties of animals classified in five broad categories based on their roles in modern societies for example, **companion animals, agricultural** or **farm animals, laboratory animals, zoo animals,** and **wild animals** (Hosey and Melfi, 2014). In general, the interactions between humans and animals are not only limited to utilitarian and economic contexts but also include sociocultural constructs and relationships and bonds involving the mutual well-being of either party.

Hunter-Gatherer Culture and Early Foragers

Hunter-gatherer culture refers to an original way of human subsistence based on hunting wild animals, fishing, and foraging (hence foragers) for other edible commodities like wild vegetables and fruits, fungi, insects, and honey with no domesticated plants or domestic animals, except the dog. The forager way of life is also the most enduring successful competitive adaptation covering 90 % of the history of mankind and many communities across the world still use the foraging lifestyle (Lee and Daly 1999). Besides hunting, gathering– food items from local sources, flints, wood, bamboo, bones, ivory, and skin– was a primary activity of foragers (Harari 2015 p 54-55). It is suggested that *Homo sapiens* have lived as foragers for the most extended period. Before the emergence of hunter-gatherer cultures, the early humans relied primarily on the practice of scavenging animal remains that predators left behind.

Most hunter-gatherers lived in small bands of several dozen to several hundred. Although the foragers fed themselves on a variety of items, meat, and fish were the primary sources of protein, and during the transition period between 80 and 70 millennia ago, some hunter-gatherers invented a series of new skills, strategies, and technologies, and specialized tools such as nets for fishing and trapping small animals, hooks, bone harpoons, projectiles, and spears that characterized hunting and fishing- the two oldest activities of mankind (Sahrhage and Lundbeck 1992,

Alves 2012, Fagan 2017). These specialized skills and sophisticated technologies enabled hunters to catch small animals efficiently, and even to hunt mega-herbivores such as elephants, mammoths, mastodons, bison, and rhinoceros. A team of researchers has reported that Gravettian people, who inhabited regions stretching from Spain to southern Russia approximately 29,000 to 22,000 years ago, may have been the earliest known practitioners of net hunting. They used nets, rather than speed and might, to capture vast numbers of hares, foxes, and other mammals (Pringle 1997).

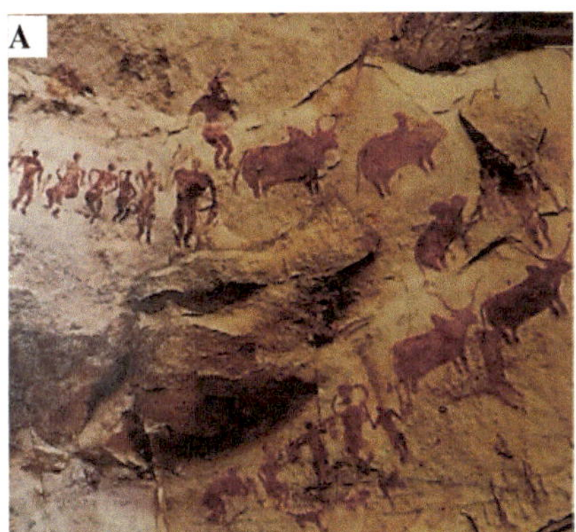

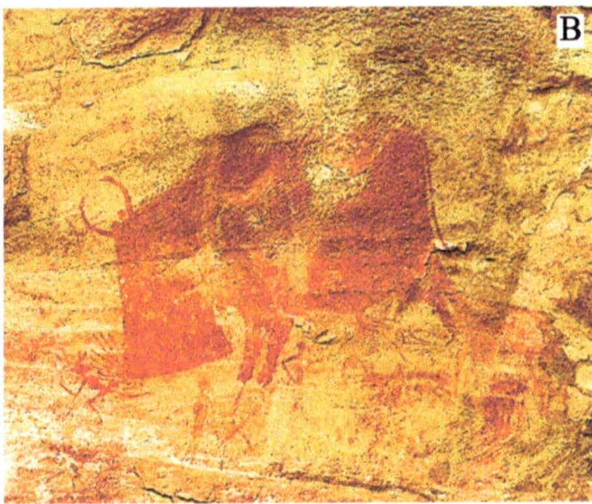

***Fig. 1.1.** Glimpses of hunter-gatherer life in Mesolithic paintings. (A) Scene of hunting and festivities in the rock shelters of the Kaimur Hills in Bihar (Photo source: Author) and (B) Bhimbetka rock shelter painting depicting a wild beast chasing a human, while other people stand nearby (Photo courtesy of Dr. Meenakshi Dubey- Pathak).*

Supported by advanced technologies, zooarchaeological studies from many Paleolithic sites throughout Asia, Europe, Africa, and the Levant indicate that Proboscidean hunting was popular among ancient foragers, and advanced hunting weapons like light throwing spears, thrusting spears, and projectiles made of mammoth ivory were used for hunting elephants and mammoth (Agam and Barkai, 2018). The Proboscideans were not only the source of the vast quantity of meat, a crucial requirement to feed the expanding group sizes, but also that of tasty and nutritionally valuable fat to supply omega-3 fatty acids in the diet of ancient foragers (Guil-Guerrero *et al.*2018). Mammoths also provided warm fur, as well as bones and valuable ivory used for manufacturing various artifacts, hunting tools, decorative objects like beads, and material for dwelling construction for Mammoth-Culture people (Harari 2015, Agam and Barkai 2018). Not only for food items, but the Hunter-Gatherers also foraged for knowledge, which was important to maximize their efficiency in searching for food. It is theorized that early hominids made mental maps of their territories, which enabled them to predict where food items like carcasses or fruits might be found easily (Blumenschine and Cavallo 1992). Hunter-gatherers ought to know the growth and availability of each plant, the habit and habitat of each animal including fish, and the topography of their terrain. It was also vital for the early foragers to understand which plant is suitable to eat and how to defend themselves from snakebites or hungry lions; how to lay traps to catch a rabbit and how to keep their excess food for dry season. They mastered the surrounding world of animals, plants, and objects as well as the internal world of their own body. Most researchers agree that these ancient foragers were animists, who believed that no barriers exist between man and other living and non-living beings. They hunted animals basically for meat but believed in communicating directly to their prey and if the hunt succeeded the hunter would ask the dead animal to forgive him (Harari 2015). Perhaps such belief amongst early foragers laid the foundation for the empathetic attitude of humans toward other animals.

Domestication of Animals: Beginning of New HAI

Domestication of animals is a complex and multistage process of a prompt, artificial, and intensive selection of wild animals spanning over a long period of several millennia. The process itself was a result of natural and cultural evolution. The animal species, which were ultimately domesticated, possessed specific behavioural and physical traits and humans selected and bred them for specific reasons like large or small size, or to produce fine wool, fur, or hair or more meat (DeMello 2012). A broad, biologically centred definition describes domestication as an evolutionary process that arises from mutualistic ecological interaction, in which one species (the domesticator) constructs an environment where it actively manages both the survival and reproduction of another species (the domesticate) to provide the former with resources and/or services. This definition, synthesized from other available definitions for the domestication of plants and animals, includes fitness and adaptation for interacting organisms within the mutualistic relationship, leading to the evolution of favourable traits to ensure stable association between the two mutual partners across the generations (Purugganan 2022).

Wild and Domestic Animals

There is no clear biological separation between wild and domestic animal species. Biologically, domestication is a separation of a domestic sub-population from the original wild population of the same species and must therefore be seen both as an anthropogenic and a biological process (Uerpmann and Uerpmann 2017). Domestic animals have evolved from small groups of individuals of their respective wild forms. Under human influence, they gradually became reproductively isolated from their progenitor forms and adapted to the unique ecological conditions imposed by humans. In some cases, they have developed considerable population sizes (Sánchez-Villagra 2022). Certain traits favoured domestication initially. According to DeMello (2012) most of the fourteen truly domesticated large animal species possessed favourable behavioural and physical traits like, flexibility in diet and a tendency towards scavenging, sexual promiscuity and rapid maturity rate, reasonable size, calm disposition, ability to live in a group, and hierarchical social life. On the contrary, ferocity (zebras, rhinos, hippos), apex position on food chains (tigers, lions, and other carnivores), picky diet (pandas and koalas), slow growth (elephants), territoriality and solitary habits (deer, antelope), reclusive breeding or elaborate courtship (cheetahs) and tendency to panic (gazelles) are some of the traits, which were found unsuitable for domestication. Further, a domestic animal must have something to offer to humans such as food, clothing, companionship or to work as beasts of burden (DeMello 2012). In general, domestication is an endless process and domestic species, particularly livestock species, are still evolving today owing to changes in technology and husbandry practices, which themselves are evolving thus constantly improving a domesticated animal species both phenotypically and genetically leading to the evolution of high performance-industrial breeds (Teletchea 2019).

There is a basic agreement that the domestication of animals ushered in an era of novel forms of human-animal relationships and intensification of human-animal relationships and bonding both from ecological and socio-economic points of view (Vigne 2015). Domestication is described as the ultimate phase of intensification. HAI progressing through continuum phases -anthropophilic stage, commensalism, control in the wild, control of captive animals, extensive breeding, intensive breeding and ultimately pet keeping (Vigne 2011). A domesticated animal must be owned and controlled by humans in a human-cultural environment, creating a profoundly different human-animal relationship that is completely different from non-agricultural societies (DeMello 2012).

Pathways of Domestication

It is widely accepted that humans have domesticated around 40 animal species primarily as resources for food, and subsequently to get secondary utility products like hide, wool, skin, and/or to provide valuable services as a companion or draught animals. Considering the shared phases of intensification between different groups of domestic taxa, anthrozoologists have proposed three main pathways to domestication: (i) commensal pathway, (ii) prey pathway, and (iii) directed pathway (Zeder 2012, Irving-Pease *et al.* 2019). Dog (*Canis familiaris*), cat (*Felis catus*), and chicken (*Gallus domesticus)* followed the commensal pathway. These animals were perhaps attracted to human waste to enter anthropogenic surroundings and in due course developed partnerships with men. Sheep (*Ovis aries*), goat (*Capra hircus*), or cattle (*Bos taurus*), the main livestock species, which were hunted by man for several thousand years, were likely domesticated through prey pathway, possibly to enhance the yield or predictability of meat, hide and wool. In the directed pathway, humans deliberately selected certain animal species including the horse (*Equus caballus*), donkey (*Equus asinus*), and dromedary (*Camelus dromedarius*) for domestication (Zeder 2012, Larson and Fuller 2014, Teletchea

2019). Under this pathway, humans applied their prior experience of directed breeding of already domesticated animals, understanding to capture wild animals, and intentionally bringing them under increasing levels of human control. The species that followed the commensal or prey pathways tended to possess more traits suitable for appropriate candidates for domestication; whereas those on directed pathways were not likely to possess many key pre-adaptive behavioural traits favourable for domestication. Another category of animals is tame captive, in which animals are brought under human control for specific reasons, for example, elephants are tamed for draught purposes, and cheetahs and eagles were used as hunting aids. Although tame animals are not bred in captivity; they qualify in some ways, as domesticates since their movement, feeding, and protection are mainly controlled by the man in a sustained, multigenerational relationship (Zeder 2012).

Domestication of Dog: The First Animal Companion

Archaeozoological investigations suggest that domestication of wolf (*Canis lupus*)- the first animal and the only large canid ever domesticated by humans, eventually led to the origin of Paleolithic dogs (*Canis lupus familiaris*). The domestication of dogs occurred in two phases: the first phase – domestication of gray wolves to primary dogs, and the second phase – subsequent morphological and behavioural changes suitable for a mutual relationship, intensification of HAR and evolution of emotional bonding between the two different species, global dispersal and genetic diversification leading to indigenous dogs into various modern breeds.

The process and ways of domestication of wolves are not precisely understood and remain controversial. A self-domestication hypothesis for the domestication of wolves proposes an initial stage marked by the opening of an ecological niche during the last glacial period that facilitated novel and sustained associations between humans and wolves. Perhaps wastes generated by humans attracted some adult wolf populations providing a novel feeding ecology that was most profitably exploited by wolves (*Canis lupus*) with the least fear of humans. Subpopulations of wolves likely became synanthropic, benefiting from life nearby or in human environments before experiencing waves of selection for phenotypes that gradually favoured stronger bonding with humans (Wang *et al.* 2016, Herbeck *et al.* 2022).

According to the human initiated domestication hypothesis, wild wolf pups were captured and brought to the Upper Paleolithic campsites by male hunters where women and children nurtured and interacted with the pups. The breeding was selected for behaviour and only the most docile adopted pups were allowed to mate. After several generations of selection for docile behaviour, primitive dogs evolved. The selection for friendly behaviour among the captive canids that led to the development of a reciprocal relationship could have been repeated several times. Gender and age of the human caretakers conceivably played an important role at the start of this process (Germonpré *et al.* 2021).

Apart from playmate and company, the adoption of wolf pups by hunter-gatherer societies also provided easy access to products like fur, meat/brain for ritual consumption and could have been a first stepping stone on the path to wolf domestication (Germonpré *et al.* 2018, Sánchez-Villagra 2022).

There is another hypothesis that discards both self-domestication and human-initiated processes and advocates a coevolutionary relationship way of wolf-domestication. In this relationship, which was probably initiated by the wolves and to which humans responded cooperatively, each species influenced the other to the point that eventually these two species evolved into contemporary humans and the closest non-human companion (domestic wolves). During the early stage of the coevolutionary relationship, both species likely exhibited profound behavioural changes with few observable physical changes. The physical changes due to human-directed selective breeding for the behavioural trait (Pierotti and Fogg 2017), became apparent only during the later stages. Regardless of the difference in opinions on some basic aspects, the domestication of wolves was a landmark event in the history of mankind that eventually culminated in the origin of the domestic dog, the first non-human animal companion of man sharing the life of humans for the longest time with a positive relationship. The relationship and emotional bonding between man and dog is one of the most defining symbiotic relationships in the history of humanity that has ever existed. Hachikō, an Akita dog from Japan, is a famous symbol of loyalty and the deep bond between humans and dogs. After his owner, Prof. Hidesaburō Ueno, died unexpectedly, Hachikō continued to wait at Shibuya train station every day for nine years, hoping for his return. He continued to do so until his own death on March 8, 1935, from cancer and filariasis. Hachikō's remains rest beside his owner Professor Ueno in Minato, Tokyo. A bronze statue of Ueno reuniting with Hachikō was unveiled at the University of Tokyo on March 9, 2015 (Hidesaburō Ueno - Wikipedia, accessed on 17-07-2024).

The second phase of the domestication process of dogs was marked by the evolution of novel forms of interspecies cooperation and social relationships between humans and dogs. Ethological research has underlined a common biological basis between the parent-infant relationship and the positive human-dog relationship, notably through the secretion of oxytocin (Jeannin 2018). A recent study suggested a critical role of oxytocin and other physiological responses in both stages of domestication; in the initial stage attenuating fear and stress associated with interspecies contact, and in the later stage evolution of affiliative social behaviour, social engagement, and cooperation with humans (Herbeck *et al.* 2022). Finally, there are many neuronal similarities on the neuronal level between men and dogs, which partly explain the effectiveness of human-dog communication. Humans have also adapted to their life companions in the very same way, for example, by modulating their verbal communication (Jeannin 2018).

The scientific community is divided over the exact time, place, and frequency of the domestication of dogs. Till recently, most archaeologists believed that the dog was first domesticated around 15,000 years ago. This date is being challenged based on modern zooarchaeological findings. The ancient dog-wolf split constituted the first step in the domestication of wolves and their evolution into domestic dogs (Wang *et al.* 2016). Mitochondrial DNA (mt DNA) analysis of zooarchaeological samples suggests that this split could have occurred more than 100,000 years ago and that humans may have been living with dogs for a much longer time than we think (DeMello 2012). Genome sequencing from a worldwide collection of dogs indicated an ancient origin of domestic dogs in Southern East Asia 33, 000 years ago (Wang *et al.* 2016). Domesticated dog skulls dating to about 31,700 years before present (BP) and skeletons dating to 26,000 BP have been found in archaeological sites in Europe indicating the possible existence of domestic dogs earlier than 30 millennia BP (DeMello 2012). Current scientific information indicates that the domestication of dogs took place independently at different places and times in Eastern and Western Eurasia from distinct wolf populations between 20,000 and 41,000s BP and 11, 000 and 16,000 BP (Treves and Bonacic 2016, Zhang *et al.* 2020b, Perri *et al.* 2021).

Population genetics studies point to the tandem movement of humans and dogs resulting in the divergence of lineage and dispersal of dogs alongside people in different parts of the world, for example, American dogs were not derived from North American wolves, but form a monophyletic lineage that likely originated in Siberia and dispersed into the Americas alongside people (Perri *et al.* 2021). Sequencing of ancient and modern canid mitochondrial and nuclear genomes and analyses of the nuclear data indicated that all dogs represent a genetically homogeneous group that possesses varying degrees of ancestry from three major ancestral lineages: a western Eurasian lineage -mostly found in European, Indian, and African dogs; an East Asian lineage e.g., dingoes; and an Arctic lineage e.g., huskies and ancient American dogs (Ní Leathlobhair *et al.* 2018).

Today we have 360 recognized breeds of dogs worldwide (World Canine Organisation: Fédération Cynologique Internationale: FCI), categorized as sporting, hound, terrier, herding, working, non-sporting, and toy breed according to their role in human society. Dogs are not only the most popular companion animal in the modern world, but they are also employed in many more roles such as guarding dogs, tracking missing persons, digging underground, and tracing toxic substances, as police dogs for detecting drugs and explosives and as therapy animal to encourage patients towards recovery, a guide for blind animals, and as laboratory animals. German Shepherds and Bloodhounds breeds have much more sense of smell than others and are more appropriate as police dogs. The short-nosed breed Pugs are engaged in tracking. Collie puppies are known to herd children, ducklings, and each other. The Maremma or *Kuvasz* or Rottweiler are bred to guard flocks. Guarding and Tarriers to chase the rodents. American and English Cocker Spaniel, Brittany, Golden Retriever, Labrador Retriever, and Ponter are some of the selected sports breeds. Purebred dogs, especially Beagle, a Hound breed, is also used as a laboratory animal in biomedical research and for safety testing and pharmacological studies of drugs and novel chemical substances intended for human use. Historically, a stray mongrel or mixed breed dog named Laika from the streets of Moscow was sent abroad to Sputnik 2 in 1957 to learn the effects of space flight on a living being. It was one of the first animals in space and the first to orbit the Earth. The test animal died of overheating on the craft's fourth orbit, but provided scientists with some of the first data on the biological effects of spaceflight. The experiment sparked a debate and protests from animal rights groups. However, in Russia Laika was memorialised in the form of a statue and plaque at Star city, and in the form of a monument, unveiled in 2008, where she poised atop a space rocket (https://en.wikipedia.org/wiki/Laika, accessed on 12.03. 2024). In recognition of their love, loyalty, companionship, and immense services to modern societies, the International Dog Day, established in 2004 by animal advocate and behaviourist Colleen Paige, is observed every year on August 26 in several countries.

Table 1.1. Origin of major livestock species

Common (Scientific Name)	Main Potential Wild Ancestor	Probable Place and Approximate Time of Domestication	References
Sheep (*Ovis aries*)	Mouflon (*O. orientalis*), Urial (*Ovis orientalis*)	Fertile Crescent (Upper Euphrates Basin / Anatolia); ca.10,500 BP	Teletchea (2019), Fuks and Marom (2021)
Goat *(Capra hircus)*	Bezoars (*C. aegagrus*)	Fertile Crescent; ca.10,000 BP	Naderi *et al.* (2008), Amills *et al.* (2017)
Cattle *(Bos taurus)*	Aurochs (*B. primigenius primigenius*)	Fertile Crescent; ca.10,000 BP	Pitt *et al.* (2019)
Humped cattle *(Bos indicus)*	Asian Aurochs sub-species (*B. pri. namadicus)*	Lower Indus Valley; ca. 8,500 BP	Pitt *et al.* (2019)
Pig (*Sus domesticus*)	Wild boar (*S. scrofa*)	Fertile Crescent, China; ca. 9,000 BP	Ramos-Onsins *et al.* (2014)
Horse (*Equus caballus*)	From wild horse (*E. ferus*/ *E. przewalski ?*)	Western Eurasian steppes (Kazakhstan &Turkmenistan); ca. 5,500 BP	Teletchea (2019), Atsenova *et al.* (2022)
Asian water buffalo (*Bubalus bubalis*)	Wild Asian water buffalo (*Bubalus arnee)*	Indian subcontinent (river buffalo), China/ Indochina border (Swamp buffalo); ca. 4,300 BP	Zhang *et al.* (2020)

Continued

Table 1.1. (Concluded)

Common (Scientific Name)	**Main Potential Wild Ancestor**	**Probable Place and Approximate Time of Domestication**	**References**
Donkey *(Equus asinus)*	African wild ass (*Equus africanus*)	North East Africa; 3,500-6,000 BP	Marshall *et al.* (2014)
Dromedary camel (*Camelus dromedarius*)	Wild dromedaries (*C. dromedarius*)	Arabian Peninsula; 3,000-4,000 BP	Burger *et al.* (2019)
Bactrian camel (*C. bactrianus*)	Wild camel *(C. ferus*)	NE Iran or Kazakistan and Mongolia; 3,000-6,000 BP	Burger *et al.* (2019)
Alpaca (*Vicugna pacos* also *Lama pacos)*	*V. vicugna*	Central Andes; 6,000 BP	Goñalons (2008)
Llama (Lama *glama*)	*L. guanicoe*	Central / South-Central Andes; 4,600-3,000 BP	
Mithun *(Bos frontalis*)	Multiple origin; wild Gaur *(B. gaurus)* for Indian sp	Hilly region of NE India, China, Bangladesh, Myanmar; ca. 8,000 BP	Prabhu *et al.* (2019)
Reindeer (*Rangifer tarandus)*	*R. tarandus*	Eurasia (North Western Siberia); >2,000 BP	Anderson *et al.* (2019), Losey *et. al.* (2021)
Yak (*Bos grunniens*)	Wild yak hybridization with *B. taurus*	Tibetan plateau; end of 4th millennia BCE	Jacques *et al.* (2021)

The Neolithic Revolution, and The First Herders

The Neolithic Revolution, also known as the First Agricultural Revolution is the most vital phase of mankind. Archaeological data indicate that in the Holocene geological epoch around 12 millennia ago, certain Hunter-Gatherer populations underwent dramatic transformations mainly linked to a change in their lifestyle to sedentary culture by adopting farming practices beginning with the domestication of plants and animals, primarily to improve, control, and secure their food supply. The process, known as Neolithization, is characterized by a slow but drastic techno-economic shift from hunting-gathering practices to food production farming practices and strategies, laying the foundation for strong demographic transitions such as urbanization, the birth of empires, industrialization, and, more recently the globalization (Vigne 2011).

Box 1.1. Why Neolithization

The question that –Why did prehistoric human cultures across the world change their beliefs, their techno-economic practices, and their social organization? – is difficult to address. Possibly, several factors such as climate, biogeography, environment, demography, techno-economic practices, diet and health, social structure, and mentality might have induced Neolithization. For example, in the Middle East, possibly the demographic growth due to three millennia of sedentism combined with the more predictable Holocene climate would have increased both the hierarchy and the specialization of society, creating mental and social conditions necessary for animal appropriation. These appropriations might have been further stimulated by the social prestige of animal ownership, by the quest for new foods such as milk, and/ or by the buffering effect of domestic animals for easing the seasonal irregularities of subsistence ultimately leading to the final adoption of husbandry as the main socio-economic mode of animal resources procurement (Vigne 2015).

Neolithization lasted for many centuries during which domestication of farm animals took place independently at different times or simultaneously in different parts of the world giving rise to Herder Culture and practices of animal husbandry. The initial stage of domestication consisted of capturing, controlling, and taming wild ancestors of ungulates and their acclimatization in an anthropogenic environment, followed by stock-keeping and selective breeding, feeding, and management of domesticates (animal farming). Pastoral nomadism to increase territories for production facilitated the spread of herder culture to other parts of the world. Most archaeological data indicate that the Fertile Crescent a region stretching north from the southern Levant through eastern Anatolia and northern Mesopotamia, then east into the Zagros Mountains on the border of modern-day Iran and Iraq formed the cradle of Neolithization with evidence of the earliest cultivation and stock-keeping (Broushaki *et al.* 2016) This is the region where four of the five major farm animals–sheep, goats, pigs, and cattle–were domesticated between ca.11,000 BP and ca. 9,000 BP. The fifth major farm animal, the horse was domesticated almost 5 millennia after the birth of the Four Neolithic farm animals. Other nine important farm animals were domesticated from their ancestors in different regions of the world at different times (Table 1) completing the list of the 14 valuable big domestic mammals of the world (Vigne 2011, Teletchea 2019).

Domestication of animals has been associated with the invention of several animal management, feeding, breeding, and animal healthcare practices leading to the evolution of modern multidisciplinary subjects of veterinary sciences and animal husbandry. A brief account of some important features of domestication of major farm animals, including avian species, and their socio-economic impact in the past and modern world synthesized from the published scientific literature is presented in this chapter.

Sheep and Goats: The First Farm Animals: Irrespective of the initial ways and purposes for their domestication, farm animals acquired momentous significance in human society due to their multipurpose utilization. The sheep and goats were the first agricultural animals domesticated by the man (Fig. 1.2). The wild ancestors of domestic sheep (*Ovis aries*) are mouflon (*Ovis musimon*) and the urial (*Ovis orientalis*), and that of domestic goat (*Capra hircus*) is bezoar (*Capra aegagrus*). Most archaeological investigations suggest the Fertile Crescent as the centre of the domestication of sheep and goats that took place 10–12 millennia ago (Teletchea 2019, Fuks and Marom 2021). Sheep and goats were first domesticated for access to meat and were the major food source for ancient human societies for centuries after their domestication. However, over time the requirement of antemortem or secondary products such as milk, fibre, and wool from these animals increased throughout the Neolithic region, leading to a Secondary Product Revolution marked by demand-driven pastoral production practices in the early societies. Scientific studies provide ample evidence that sheep and goats played different but probably complementary roles in animal production and economic systems of ancient societies significantly contributing to the advancement of human civilizations. Along with cattle and pigs, these two earliest farm animals make up the key animal components of the Neolithic package, which subsequently spread throughout the globe from the centre of their origin (Helmer *et al.* 2007, Fukes and Marom 2021).

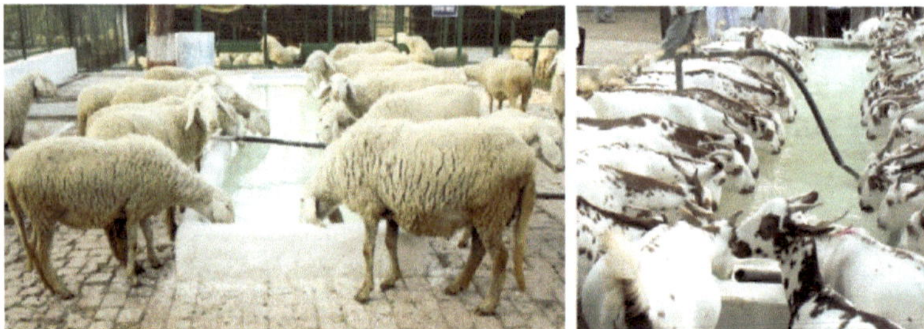

Fig. 1.2. Sheep (left) and goats (right), housed at the ICAR-CIRG farms. The two species represent the earliest domesticated livestock, retaining significant value within the global livestock production system. Collectively, they constitute the most abundant and widely dispersed ruminant livestock worldwide (Photo source: ICAR-CIRG).

A changing pattern of sheep and goat production and husbandry strategies post-Neolithization (8700–2000 BCE) is reported based on archaeozoological and ethnological investigations from the Ancient Near East. Goat management strategies remained more conservative and static and were primarily aimed at small-scale production of meat, milk, and hair from the early Neolithic period onwards without much change. On the contrary, the sheep production system and husbandry practices changed significantly over time. Sheep became the dominant livestock and herding practices and management strategies focused on fleece and milk -the two sought-after products (Helmer *et al.* 2007). Larger herds of sheep were used to produce wealth through the production of mutton, milk, and wool, the primary role of goats seems to have been to provide subsistence security and to hedge against the uncertainties of valuable but potentially vulnerable sheep herds (Arbuckle *et al.* 2009). Sheep were probably more profitable in the well-watered plain areas and being a source of precious wool became an asset and sign of prosperity for ancient human societies (Coulthard 2020).

Sequencing of early Neolithic genomes has revealed that farming and animal herding spread from the Fertile Crescent into surrounding regions, including Anatolia and, later, Europe, southern Asia, and parts of Arabia and North Africa around 10,000 BP (Broushaki *et al.* 2016). Tracking of the long-term globalization of animals and plant cultigens, concerning production intensity, geographic diffusion, and diversity has revealed a high degree of interdependence between specialized pastoralists and farmers. A different type of diversity contributing to agropastoral buffering capacity involved the set of trade-offs between sheep and wheat vis-à-vis their respective counterparts, goats, and barley. For example, changes under domestication to seasonal cyclicity in reproduction, involving flowering time adaptations for wheat and multiple lambing seasons in sheep, were key to their global diffusion. Both sheep and goats provided meat, milk, and hides; both wheat and barley provided kernels for food and fodder, as well as chaff and straw for fodder, kindling, building, and other crafts (Fukes and Marom 2021).

The post-domestication dispersal of sheep and goats was followed by a population expansion across the world, especially in Asia and Africa. Together these two species are the most abundant and widely distributed ruminant livestock around the world today with over 2.46 billion headcounts comprising 1.32 billion sheep and 1.14 billion goats as estimated in 2022 (https://www.fao.org/faostat/en/#data/QCL, accessed on 18-01-2024). Sheep and goats have been bred intensively to optimize the production of meat, milk, fat, wool, fibre, hair, or hide and draught purposes creating over 800-1,400 distinct breeds of sheep, and 500-600 breeds of goats globally, classified based on primary use (Teletchea 2019). Many of these breeds are also considered dual-purpose or multipurpose breeds. Other than the recognized breeds, there are several local populations of sheep and goats, which are not managed via phenotypic standardization, herd book registration, and controlled reproduction. These might have not figured in the recognized list of breeds.

Sheep and goats are important culturally in many societies in the world. They are adaptable to harsh environments and are the better choice for animals in arid and extreme humidity. More importantly, both species are easy to manage with minimum financial risk and faster return on investment. They are often considered as insurance against crop failure. Besides, ready sources of milk and meat, sheep and goats serve as currency and urgent sources of cash in various sociocultural contexts such as weddings, funerals, and festive gatherings, especially in rural societies of developing economies. The two species are also used in sacrificial rituals and socio-religious ceremonies, which are still prevalent in many cultures world over. Overall, these small ruminants remain a vital component of the modern global livestock production system. According to FAO, sheep and goats together produced ~16.64 million tonnes of meat, ~3.25 million tonnes of raw hide and skin, ~2.93 million tonnes of milk, 0.833 million tonnes of fat >3.08 million tonnes of edible offal, besides contributing to over 1.75 million tonnes of shorn wool annually in 2022 (https://www.fao.org/faostat/en/#data/QCL, accessed on 18-01-2024). The Changthangi goat, an indigenous breed in the Himalayan region, produces Pashmina or Cashmere fibre, regarded as one of the best, extravagant, and costliest fibrous strands on the planet. The word Pashmina is originates from the Persian word *pashm* meaning 'soft gold', and often regarded as the king of fibres. It is well known for its fineness, warmth, softness, desirable aesthetic value, elegance, and timelessness in fashion. It is the most luxurious fibre, commanding a higher price and is softer than superfine merino wool of the same diameter (Sofi *et al.* 2018, Singh *et al.* 2023).

In addition to their formidable contribution to the global livestock production system, sheep and goats have been used as laboratory animals in biomedical research, and to produce biologicals. Although equines continue to be the conventional source of plasma-derived antivenoms, sheep are increasingly recognized as advantageous owing to their strong humoral immune response, cost-effective maintenance, and ease of handling, immunization, and plasma collection. The cloning of an adult sheep in 1996 using its somatic cells instead of its gametes at the Roslin Institute in Scotland is one of the most important scientific events of the last century. The offspring generated from the cloning was named Dolly. It was described as the most extraordinary creature ever born by Ian Wilmut, the scientist whose team succeeded in cloning it (Franklin 2002). The production of Dolly had unanticipated consequences. One of these unanticipated effects was that the boundaries between animal and human health blurred and new professional spaces emerged. Dolly- the sheep transformed from a tool for livestock improvement into a universal symbol of the new cloning (García-Sancho 2015)

Cattle: The First Big Farm Animal: Cattle are the first big mammal domesticated by humans from a more challenging wild animal — the large and dangerous wild ox or aurochs (*Bos primigenius*) via the prey pathway. The origin of domestic cattle and their management have attracted immense scholarly interest for decades. The domestication of cattle was thought to have occurred on two or three occasions. Archaeological and genomic evidence suggest that two species of domestic cattle *B. taurus* and *B. indicus* originated from two divergent aurochs populations.

Taurine cattle (*Bos taurus)* were domesticated from aurochs (*Bos primigenius*) in the Fertile Crescent in the middle of the 11th millennium BP; whereas indicine cattle (*Bos indicus*) were domesticated from the humped Asian subspecies of aurochs (*Bos p. namadicus*) in lower Indus valley ca. 8,500 years BP. The two species shared the aurochs (*Bos primigenius*) as a common ancestor ca. 250,000 years ago (Pitt *et al.* 2019, Teletchea 2019). A large number of seals from Lothal, Surkotada in Gujarat, and Kalibangan in Rajasthan show an animal resembling *Bos primigenius* (Randhawa 1980 Vol I p. 185). A third independent domestication event, leading to the origin of African taurine cattle (*B. p. primigenius)* from African aurochs, thought to have occurred in the Western Deserts of Egypt about 8,000–9,000 BP is hypothesized based on zooarchaeological remains recovered in the late twentieth century (Stock and Gifford-Gonzalez 2013). However, the hypothesis is not supported by modern genetic studies and remains disputed. Scholars argue that African cattle are hybrids that possess both a European (taurine) mitochondrial signal and an Asian (indicine) Y-chromosome signature (Hanotte *et al.* 2002). While neither mtDNA nor autosomal DNA diversity supports a scenario with multiple domestication events in *B. taurus*, the Y-chromosomal data indicated a scenario of secondary introductions of local wild aurochs into the domestic gene pool (Stock and Gifford-Gonzalez 2013). Analysis of bovine SNP array (~54,000 loci) data across 3,196 individuals representing 180 taurine and indicine populations, revealed that local African cattle possessed high levels of shared genetic variation with Asian indicine cattle due to their recent divergence, and with African taurine cattle through relatively recent gene flow. Disapproving the hypothesis of the third centre of cattle domestication, the study concluded that both taurine and indicine cattle hybridized with local aurochs in Africa naturally or possibly local farmers mixed them with African aurochs to restock their herds leading to the origin of African taurus (Pitt *et al.* 2019).

Now extinct, the aurochs were one of the largest herbivores of the Holocene period. During the Pleistocene and Holocene, aurochs were distributed in a vast geographical area that ranged from the Atlantic to the Pacific coasts and from the northern tundra to India and Africa. Fossil remains showed that male aurochs were as tall as 1.8 m at the shoulder—roughly a quarter taller than a Holstein cow—and may have weighed a metric ton. Aurochs bulls had nearly 130 cm long and 20 cm thick menacing horns (Stokstad 2015). Indian aurochs *Bos primigenius namadicus*, the ancestors of Zebu cattle, roamed throughout the Indian subcontinent from Baluchistan, the Indus Valley, and Ganges Valley to South India. They were slightly different and relatively smaller in size but had long horns than their Eurasian counterparts. Indian aurochs disappeared before the 13th Century (https://en.wikipedia.org/wiki/Indian_aurochs) and the Eurasian aurochs (*Bos primigenius primigenius*) got extinct about 400 years ago in 1627. However, aurochs' genes persist in living breeds of their progeny domestic cattle (Stokstad 2015).

Most likely, people first lured the wild ancestors of cattle with food and captured orphaned aurochs' calves individually using advanced hunting strategies and technology of that time. Those adapted well to the human environment would have been bred with other docile cattle to gradually produce a more desirable domesticated breed. Over time, humans were able to achieve smaller aurochs with smaller horns, suitable for herding-a long process that must have been the work of settled farmers, not nomads. Sequencing of ancient and modern mitochondrial DNA suggested that as few as 80 female aurochs could have initially been involved in the domestication process (Bollongino *et al.* 2012). Archaeological pieces of evidence from the earliest levels of the Neolithic village of Çatalhöyük, in the Fertile Crescent suggested that aurochs were subject to forms of management including penning, foddering, and selective culling, and that human-aurochs relationships of hunting slowly shifted into management, which in combination with population isolation, eventually transformed aurochs into cattle (Arbuckle and Kassebaum 2021).

Following domestication, cattle accompanied human migrations leading to their rapid dispersal and extensive gene flow among different groups of domestic cattle (taurine, indicine, or mixed origin) over Asia, Africa, Europe, and lately in the New World. Taurine cattle dispersed rapidly northwest from the Fertile Crescent through Turkey into the Balkans and northern Italy, either following a Mediterranean coastline or a route partially along the Danube River, reaching Southeastern Europe (8,800 BP), Southern Italy (8,500 BP), Central Europe (8,000 BP) and Northern Europe with cheese being made as early as 7,000-8,000 BP (Scanes 2018). It may have also migrated along the northern coast of Africa, eventually crossing into the Iberian Peninsula, and mixing with local cattle. Genetic studies demonstrate that taurine cattle did interbreed with the native European aurochs, but only the male calves (traced on the Y chromosome) of aurochs were kept, perhaps because they could improve the herd's size or resistance to disease without affecting milk yields. mtDNA tracing suggested that all the milch cows probably descended from mothers who had come from Anatolia. Wild aurochs cows were probably relatively poor milk producers and might have been temperamentally difficult to milk. As such, Neolithic European farmers ensured that all cows were born of long-domesticated mothers. They also allowed crossbreeding with native wild bulls in some cases to obtain larger domestic bulls (Anthony 2007). During the last four centuries, cattle crossed the Atlantic and reached New World with human emigrants following four major routes (i) from Spain and North Africa to the Caribbean, (ii) from Portugal to São Paulo (Sao Vicente), marked by arrival of the first cattle in Brazil, (ii) northern Europe to North America (as well as Australia), and (iv) introduction of zebu from India to Brazil (Ajmone-Marsan *et al.* 2010).

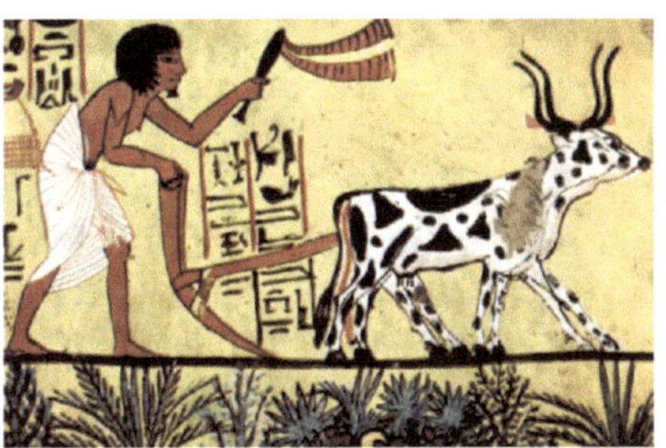
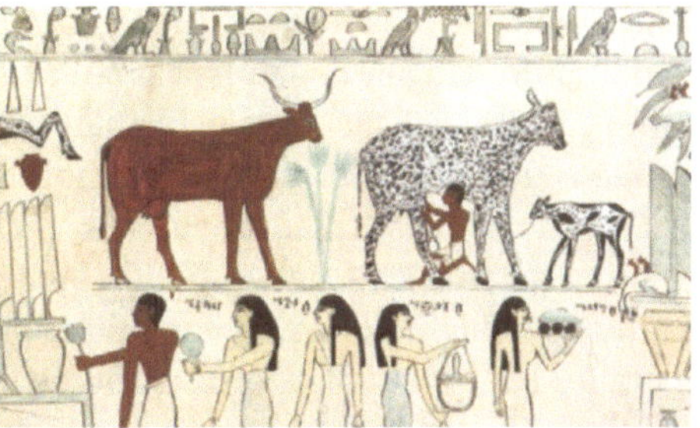

Fig. 1.3. Ancient Egyptian farmers used cattle as draft power in agriculture, as well as a valuable source of secondary products such as milk (Photo source: Courtesy of World History Encyclopedia:https://www.worldhistory.org/image/112/plowing-egyptian-farmer/,accessed on 16-08-2023, and https://www.worldhistory.org/image/2887/early-domestication-of-cattle/, accessed on 12-11-2023).

The indicine cattle also dispersed far beyond their domestication centre in the Indus Valley, reaching China and much of South-East Asia (Pitt *et al.* 2019). Meta-analysis of different microsatellite datasets also revealed taurine-zebu admixture over Europe, southwest Asia, and Africa indicating that two species fully interbreed after domestication. At the onset of the current geological age- the Meghalayan, a rapid and widespread introgression of *Bos indicus*, from the Indus Valley occurred throughout the South-West and Central Asia. The process of the westward migration of zebu cattle was likely stimulated by climate change due to widespread drought around ca.4,200 BP that lasted for almost two centuries. Zebu (*B. indicus*) cattle are adapted to arid and tropical regions of the world, and cattle herders throughout southwest and central Asia used arid-adapted zebu bulls for selective breeding to enhance the survival of their local cattle herds. Mitochondrial DNA stasis supports this male-driven introgression. This human-mediated migration of zebu-derived genetics, represented the start of a global *B. indicus* genome diaspora that has continued through millennia, altering tropical herding on each continent (Verdugo *et al.* 2019). Introgression of indicine cattle from the Indian subcontinent into East African cattle occurred for the second time in the second half of the eighth century (Decker *et al.* 2014). Scientists have also indicated the possibility of zebu cattle crossing with other species in some areas of the world, including the yak (*Bos grunniens*) in Nepal or banteng (*Bos javanicus*) in Southeast Asia and Indonesia following their dispersion in Southeast Asia (Groeneveld *et al.* 2010). In the last 150 years, zebu cattle reached the Americas and Oceania, where they contributed to the prosperity of emerging economies (Utsunomiya *et al.* 2019) and the development of several new breeds, notably including Brahman (USA, Australia, Brazil) and Nelore, Gir, Tabapuã, Guzerá, Indubrasil, and Sindi (Brazil).

Cattle were invaluable resources for the transition of human society from nomadic hunter-gatherers to sedentary farming communities throughout much of Europe,

Asia, and Africa (Pitt *et al.* 2019). In the beginning, cattle were exploited for beef and raised like sheep and goats, but soon they became the major source of milk, meat, and hides, and a valuable part of religious ceremonies. Zooarchaeological studies indicated the existence of cattle farming in Anatolia as early as 6000 BCE (Thrusfield 2018). The prehistoric Saharan African people practiced dairying during the fifth millennium BCE (Dunne *et al.* 2012). Powerful bulls were used to provide draught power for agriculture and transport. A yoke dating to the Cardial culture (ca. 6400 BCE – ca. 5500 BCE) indicates some early experimentation with cattle traction, and there is zooarchaeological evidence of cattle regularly pulling heavy weights in the Near East from the Pottery Neolithic (Klimscha 2017). Ancient Egyptian hieroglyphic images (Fig. 1.3) portray the use of cattle for ploughing as early as 1200 BCE (Scanes 2018).

The Neolithic cattle were smaller than aurochs and continued to decrease in size until the Middle Ages. Domestic cattle adapted to variable environments ranging from green pastures to deserts and developed a large variety of visible phenotypes such as the emergence of short-horned and even hornless (polled) cattle. By selection, cattle also regained their size, although modern bulls are still smaller than the huge aurochs bulls (Ajmone-Marsan *et al.* 2010). It is suggested that the management of cattle must have preceded changes in phenotype and likely emerged a millennium or earlier across a wide geographic region including much of the northern and southern Levant (Arbuckle and Kassebaum 2021). Dispersal and adaptation of cattle to diverse environments along with considerable variation in their appearance and performance are reflected in the development of hundreds of specialized breeds evolved especially during the last few centuries through the application of the principle of mating the best with the best is a winning strategy (Ajmone-Marsan *et al.* 2010). Globally, there were over 1.5 billion cattle in 2021. Over 1,000 cattle breeds from around the globe were defined and catalogued by different scholars (Felius 2007, Porter 2020). An encyclopaedia on breeds of cattle has arranged different breeds geographically into 16 groups: six European groups, four Asian groups, four African groups, one American group, and one group covering modern breeds of the Americas, Australia, and New Zealand and the genus *Bison* (Felius 2007).

Phenotypically, Indian cattle (zebu) are recognized by their hump, large ears, and excess skin. They are rustic, resistant to tick parasites, and capable of bearing the hot and humid climates of the tropics. These economically important traits have been naturally selected for millennia and played a major role in the evolution of *B. indicus* cattle, which together with their sister subspecies *Bos taurus*, have contributed to important socioeconomic changes that have shaped modern civilizations (Utsunomiya *et al.* 2019). Zebu cattle were introduced to Brazil for the first time in 1875 through multiple imports of 6,262 animals of Indian origin. The country is now regarded as the second homeland for Zebu cattle. It is estimated that 80 % of the 12 million cattle, registered in Brazil until 2012, were pure or crossbred Zebu animals belonging to Nellore (85 %), Gir (4 %), Tabapuã (3.8 %), Guzerá (3.5 %), Brahman (2.1 %), Indubrasil (0.7 %), and Sindi (0.2 %) breeds (Santana Jr. *et al.* 2016). About 20 % of the genes present in the Brazilian Nellore cattle were from the six Ongole bulls (Golias, Godhavari, Karvadi, Kurupathy, Mahal, Taj, and Rastã), which are regarded as the genetic base of the Nellore breed in Brazil (Vozzi *et al.* 2006).

There are two distinct different types of Brahman cattle in the US: the Red Brahman and the Gray Brahman, which are developed from different breeds of Indian cattle (Sanders 1980). The US imported four Indian cattle (*Bos indicus*) breeds (Ongole, Krishna, Gir, and Gujarat) from India between 1854 and 1926 for crossbreeding with local cattle (*Bos taurus*) to create the Brahman cattle (Koufariotis *et al.* 2018). Brahman bulls were imported for the first time in 1933 from the US for crossbreeding with Australian *B. taurus* cattle to develop a beef breed that could withstand the harsh conditions of the region. Presently, Brahman (*Bos indicus*), is the most prevalent breed of cattle in much of northern Australia due to their stress resistance and ability to perform better than *Bos taurus* cattle in harsh conditions as well as their resistance to ticks and worms (Frisch *et al.* 2000, Schatz *et al.* 2020). Apart from well-defined breeds, many non-descript local cattle populations also exist in the world.

Beef and milk are the two most widely consumed and commercialized livestock products, and cattle is the single most widely distributed livestock species in the world with an estimated 1.55 billion headcount in 2022 (https://www.fao.org/faostat/en/#data/QCL, accessed on 18-01-2024). Approaches to enhance beef and milk production are responsible for the evolution of well-organized modern beef and dairy industries contributing to socioeconomic development all over the world. Most of the modern cattle breeds are, therefore, developed by focusing on economically important traits and enhancing efficiency to produce milk and beef. Feed efficiency is becoming a popular trait for genomic selection not only for economic reasons but also to reduce environmental footprints. Advanced genomic tools are applied to produce cattle with superior ability for both thermal adaptation and food production to meet the challenge of global climate change. The latest scientific advancements in genetics, animal nutrition, health, and husbandry practices have provided the impetus to create sustainable food systems including milk and beef production. For example, farmers in the USA produced 26.2 billion pounds of beef in 2017 with a 53% smaller herd than that would have been required to produce the same amount of beef in 1975 (Mateescu 2020). During the past 100 years, implementation of genomic selection approaches and modern husbandry practices such as permanent unique identification (animal ID) that includes pedigree information, routine recording of performance traits, widespread use of AI, and development of state-of-the-art statistical models and evaluation systems have led to increasing genetic gains in traits of economic importance for dairy cattle. The resulting improvement in production efficiency allows dairy products to be produced with fewer cattle, thereby reducing adverse environmental impacts and conserving natural resources (Norman 2010). Although draught cattle breeds are losing utility for farm operations like ploughing and transport owing to mechanization, they remain an important resource for agricultural works. In many livestock settings, the cattle husbandry is still primarily for draught purposes with beef or milk as a secondary product leading to the existence of sizeable populations of draught and dual-purpose cattle breeds.

Asian Buffalo: The Second Domesticated Bovine: Belonging to the Bubalina group of family *Bovidae*, the Asian buffalo includes three species: *Bubalus depressicornis* or Anoa in Indonesia, *Bubalus mindorensis* in the Philippines, and *Bubalus bubalis* the Indian domestic water buffalo (Borghese and Mazzi 2005). There are two distinct types (river and swamp) of domestic buffalo, which have descended from different wild Asian water buffalo (*Bubalus arnee*) populations that diverged some 900 kyr BP and then evolved in separate geographical regions, assumed to have been separated by Patkai, Barail, and Arkan-Yoma Mountain range of Myanmar (Zhang *et al.* 2020, https://crib.icar.gov.in >history). The river and swamp domestic buffaloes also differ in morphological and behavioural traits and have different karyotypes, purposes, and geographical distributions.

Morphologically river buffaloes are black in body colour with generally curved horns. These are mostly selected as dairy animals with several recognized breeds spread across the Indian subcontinent and west to the Balkans and Italy. River buffaloes prefer clear water and like to wallow in rivers, canals, and ponds. The swamp buffalo has a consistent phenotype and is considered as one type, even if many breeds are recognized within it (Minervino *et al.* 2020). They are usually dark grey with white chevrons (one or two white stripes on the throat), socks, and the tip of the tail, and have relatively massive horns growing straight backward and outward and curbed on tips. Swamp buffaloes are primarily used as draught animal providing power for ploughing and transport, with meat production as a secondary consideration. They are distributed in wide areas from eastern India, through southeastern Asia, Indonesia to eastern China. The two types are genetically distinct and their chromosome number also differ, river buffaloes have 50 chromosomes and swamp buffaloes possess 48 chromosomes, due to the fusion of chromosomes 4p and 9 (Zhang *et al.* 2020). The two subspecies are interfertile with their progeny containing 49 chromosomes. Owing to these distinct characteristics, scholars have proposed two distinct subspecies *Bubalus bubalis bubalis* for river buffalo and *Bubalus bubalis carabanesis* for water buffalo (Kumar *et al.* 2007).

Archaeological and genetic studies indicated the domestication of the river buffalo in the western region of the Indian subcontinent around 6,300 years BP (Kumar *et al.* 2007, Nagarajan *et al.* 2015), and that of the swamp buffalo in the China/Indochina border region around 3-7 Kyr BP. Seals depicting buffalo were recovered from Indus civilization. One of these seals shows a buffalo with long horns resembling that of wild buffalo from Assam. This evidence indicated that the Punjab and Sind are the home of the early domestication of buffalo (Randhawa1980). The two types of buffaloes though domesticated independently, descended from buffalo from the wild water buffalo *(B. arnee)*, which was distributed in marshes and jungles in eastern India, Sri Lanka, and Southeast Asia until the beginning of the 19th century. It is hypothesized that the wild Asian buffalo originated in the mainland of Southeast Asia and spread north toward China and west toward the Indian subcontinent, where the river type was probably domesticated (Wang *et al.* 2017). The wild buffalo is a very large animal reaching a height of up to 200 cm and a weight of up to 1,000 kg, either a grey-black, dark grey, or dark brown body colour with large horns (Zava *et al.* 2020).

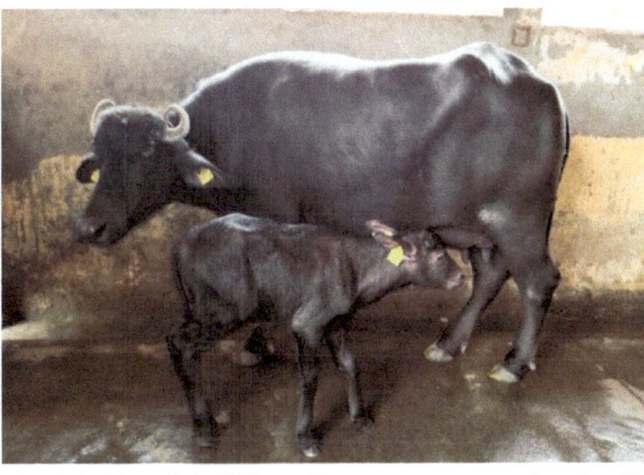

Fig. 1.4. *Murrah buffalo is the most represented and well-known dairy breed of the world (Photo source: ICAR-CIRB, courtesy of Dr. Naveen Kumar).*

Following domestication, the two types of buffaloes migrated to other parts of the world. The river buffalo dispersed westward from its domestication centre as far as Egypt, the Balkans, and Italy by the 7th century CE. Archaeological evidence, mtDNA, and SNP data indicated that a series of migration events occurred at different times and geographical scales. The two independent migration events that are compatible with the observed population differences are proposed as – one that took the proto-Mediterranean gene pool through the Balkans to Italy, and another that spread the proto-Middle Eastern gene pool toward Mesopotamia and the Caspian Sea, followed later by expansion to Turkey and Egypt (Nagarajan *et al.* 2015, Colli *et al.* 2018, Zhang *et al.* 2020). It is widely accepted that domestic river buffaloes were in use for various agricultural operations before 2500 BCE in Mesopotamia during the period of the Akkadian dynasty and in the Indus Valley civilization of the Indian subcontinent extending to Harappa, Mohenjo-Daro, and some parts of Gujarat, Rajasthan, and Haryana (https://crib.icar.gov.in >history). The swamp buffalo spread south through peninsular Malaysia to the islands of Indonesia (Sumatra, Java, and Sulawesi), north/northeast into central China, and then through an eastern island route via Taiwan to the Philippines and Borneo. Probably introduced from southeast Asian areas bordering China, the domestic water buffaloes were present in China by the time of the Shang dynasty (ca. 1766–1123 BCE) or even earlier (Zhang *et al.* 2020). More recently, buffaloes were introduced to other continents of the world. They arrived in Australia's Northern Territory between 1826 and 1866; the South Americas, around the end of the 19th century, and North America in the late 20th century. In South America, Brazil has the highest number of buffaloes, mainly introduced through importations from India and Italy. In Venezuela and Colombia, riverine buffaloes were imported from Trinidad, and Swamp buffaloes from Australia. In the United States, buffaloes have been raised since 1975, first for meat production in marshy lowlands of Florida, and in fields of Louisiana, Texas, and Arkansas, and subsequently for dairy productions initially in California and then in Vermont and other States (Zava 2012).

Currently, domestic buffaloes inhabit 77 countries across five continents. Among the 123 buffalo breeds worldwide, 90 are found in Asia alone, comprising primarily local breeds, while only 15 are transboundary breeds (Minervino *et al.* 2020). According to the FAO, the estimated global buffalo population reached approximately 205.14 million in 2022. Most of this population resides in Asia, accounting for 201.14 million, with substantial numbers also present in South America (2.08 million) and Africa (1.41 million). In terms of production, global buffalo output in 2022 has been estimated over 143.573178 million tonnes of raw milk, 69.034 tonnes of meat, 1.409 million tonnes of raw hides and skins, and 1.17 million tonnes of edible offal. (https://www.fao.org/faostat/en/#data/QCL, accessed on 18-01-2024).

The buffalo is known for its efficient conversion of feed, displaying remarkable adaptability to various environments characterized by distinct topographies, climates, and vegetation. It serves as a vital animal resource, providing draught power, milk, and/or meat, and finds utility as a sport animal and for riding in numerous regions (Minervino *et al.* 2020). In comparison to cow milk, buffalo milk boasts higher levels of fat and protein, ranging from 6–9% and 4–5%, respectively, as opposed to 3.4% and 3.5%. Additionally, it contains approximately 30% more solid content. River buffalo milk is exceptionally well-suited for cheese production, notably for the traditional "mozzarella" cheese originating from Italy, which can be exclusively prepared from river buffalo milk (Zhang *et al.* 2020, Minervino *et al.* 2020). The consumption of buffalo meat has been on the rise in numerous countries such as Italy, Cambodia, Indonesia, the Philippines, Thailand, and Vietnam (Zhang *et al.* 2020). Buffalo-raising systems are gaining prominence as a viable production and commercial option in tropical regions. They are increasingly recognized as superior to conventional species breeding, particularly when employing the dual-purpose model (Bertoni *et al.* 2021). It is noted that a significant number of people rely on domestic buffalo for their livelihoods more than any other domestic animal. Consequently, this species holds substantial potential in global livestock production, serving as a vital source of high-quality animal protein to meet the needs of the expanding human population (Zhang *et al.* 2020).

Pig: The First Domesticated Monogastric Farm Animal: The domestication of the pig (*Sus domesticus*) is one of the critical events in the history of human agricultural civilization. Amongst all the farm animals, pigs are the most efficient convertor of poor-quality feedstuffs including household garbage and agricultural wastes into pork — a valuable edible animal protein. Pigs also possess several characteristics that differentiate them from other livestock species. They are omnivorous and multiparous (give birth in litters). They are curious and intelligent, and able to adapt their behaviours when faced with different social and environmental conditions (Price and Hongo 2020). Because of their better adaptability and generalized omnivorous habit, pigs may have a wider range of possible relationships with humans than any other species (Albarella *et al.* 2006). Genetic and archaeological studies indicated that domestication of pig (*Sus domestica*) occurred independently at least in two locations: East Anatolia (Near East) and China. Pigs were first domesticated in Anatolia around 10,500 BP and then in China around 8,000 BP (Groenen 2016, Zhang *et al.* 2022). Pig domestication happened in Western Europe about 5-6 Kyr BP either through introgression using local wild sows for breeding for repeated generations or domestication of wild boars. The possibility of separate domestication pathways of one population in India and three wild boar populations indigenous to Peninsular Southeast Asia is also speculated. However, these cryptic domestication processes in India and Southeast Asia are currently based only on genetic data (Larson *et al.* 2010).

Sus scrofa (wild boar) is widely accepted as the wild ancestor of domestic pigs (*Sus scrofa domestica*) based on mitochondrial genotyping. Multiple *Sus* species comprising the bearded pig *S. barbatus*, the warty pigs *S. celebensis,* and *S. verrucosus,* and wild *S. scrofa* originated roughly 4 million years ago in the Island of Southeast Asia (Bosse 2018). The island structure in this region probably promoted speciation, and except for *S. scrofa*, all species of the genus exist naturally only in Southeast Asia and the islands of Southeast Asia (Price and Hongo 2020). *S. scrofa*, colonized almost the entire Eurasian mainland and part of North Africa. The widespread and opportunistic nature of this species probably contributed to the fact that it is the only pig species that was successfully domesticated (Bosse 2018).

The pathway of domestication for pigs is less clear. Recognizing the complexity of the domestication process of pigs due to their multifaceted behavioural and ecological flexibility of pigs and wild boar (*S. scrofa*), researchers have proposed several pathways to pig domestication. Pigs were hunted for food as such their domestication followed the prey pathway, or since pigs were capable of readily consuming human waste and converting it to productive protein, commensalism between humans and pigs evolved leading to their domestication (Larson and Fuller

2014). The commensal pathway is also supported by scientific evidence suggesting that evolution from wild boars to domestic pigs was a gradual phenomenon involving an extended era of commensalism and domestication spanning over many generations. A review of scientific information on the archaeology of pig domestication in Eurasia indicated that pigs followed a combined pathway to domestication, wherein wild boars were first attracted to permanent human settlements, their garbage, and their cultivated foods in the early Holocene and subsequently hunter-gatherers began to practice game management and eventually herd management of populations of wild boar. Likely, commensal, and managed populations regularly interbred, swapping genes and epigenetic traits. It is argued that the domestication process arose from relationships initiated both by humans (management) and wild boar themselves (commensalism) adding even greater complexity to the issue of intentionality in the process of domestication (Price and Hongo 2020). The scenario that has emerged from analysis of pig mitochondrial genomes and more recently from whole-genome sequence data is that this domestication process was very diffused, taking many millennia and involving repeated admixture and gene flow from wild boars into the domesticated populations. Therefore, pig domestication should not be considered as a series of fixed events that happened some 10,000 years ago but as a gradual process, in which both animal and human played their part. Wild boars might have been initially attracted to human settlements as an easy way of accessing food, and it is only after millennia that humans might have started to keep pigs as a truly domesticated species (Groenen 2016).

After initial domestication, pigs accompanied early farmers and spread to different parts from the centres of their origin. From East Anatolia, pigs spread across the Middle and Near East and westward into Europe. The movement of domestic pigs from western Anatolia into Europe is consistent with recent aDNA studies of human remains that support a demic diffusion model of the initial Central European Neolithic. Most probably, early domestic pigs in Europe must have been introduced from Anatolia by the mid-6th millennium BCE before spreading to the Paris basin by the early 4th millennium BCE. Once domestic pigs set out from southeastern Anatolia but possessing the western Anatolian Y1 haplotype arrived in Europe, they acquired European wild boar genetic signatures and lost the Y1 haplotype through admixture between introduced pigs and European wild boar. As a result, European wild boar mtDNA lineages replaced Near Eastern/ Anatolian mtDNA signatures in Europe and subsequently replaced indigenous domestic pig lineages in Anatolia. By the 5th century CE, European domestic pig haplotypes had completely replaced the endemic lineages possibly coinciding with the widespread demographic and societal changes that occurred during the Anatolian Bronze and Iron Ages (Ottoni *et al.* 2013).

Genetic studies have demonstrated that the modern Chinese domestic pigs are the direct descendants of the first domestic pigs in this region and that the most common modern domestic haplotypes found in pig populations in Central China are also the most common Asian haplotypes in the pigs across East Asia, in Australian feral pigs, and in modern European as well as in American pigs. It is argued that Neolithic expansions of agricultural populations into different geographical regions of Southeast Asia could have brought domestic pigs from Central China with them, including Austronesian speakers through Island Southeast Asia and parts of the mainland coastal regions. Pacific Clade is indigenous to peninsular Southeast Asia. However, no modern domestic pigs possessing Pacific Clade haplotypes have yet been found in mainland Asia indicating the likelihood of the replacement of native pigs by the pigs introduced from Central China (Larson *et al.* 2010). Hybridization between domesticated pigs of different origins and recurrent gene flow between wild and domestic pigs contributed to the presence of common genetic signatures in pig populations in many parts of the world. Admixture studies indicated that Asian pigs contributed to 35 % of the European pig genome (Groenen 2016).

European and Asian domesticated pigs have been geographically isolated for over a million years because they have distinct wild origins. Therefore, they genetically resemble local wild boars more than domestic pigs from different geographic origins. Also, the traits selected as well as how animals were kept, strongly differed in Europe and Asia resulting in highly different domesticated pigs between Europe and Asia. While European pigs were roaming freely in forested areas in the surroundings, Asian pigs were kept near humans, and often integrated into their settlements (Bosse 2018). However, during the Industrial Revolution in Europe in the 18th century, European farmers deliberately hybridized their local stock with Asian pigs to improve their stock in such a way that pigs had to become adapted to living in small(er) enclosures, be more prolific and gain weight more rapidly resulting in introgression of Asian genetic material into Asian haplotypes into European pigs (Larson *et al.* 2010, Bosse 2018).

Pigs are widely distributed across the world contributing substantially to the total global livestock production. Pigs are raised in a variety of systems, ranging from backyard to intensive systems, with different levels of technical development and diverse feed sources (Lassaletta *et al.* 2019). Local husbandry and breeding techniques have created an enormous diversification of pig breeds. There are more than 978.97 million swine/pigs globally as estimated in 2022 (https://www.fao.org/faostat/en/#data/QCL, accessed on 18-01-2024), and more than 730 pig breeds or lines. Of these breeds, 2/3 are in China and Europe. More than 270 pig breeds are endangered or critically endangered, whereas 58 breeds are 'transboundary' breeds occurring in more than one country. Five international transboundary breeds viz. Large white (117 countries), Duroc (93 countries), Landrace (91 countries), Hampshire (54 countries), and Pietrain (35 countries) dominate the global pig production system (Teletchea 2019). Driven by the rising demand for livestock products, specialization, automation, production and trade of cheap feedstuffs, market liberalization, cheap energy, and improved technologies in genetics and feeding strategies, pig production has increased manyfold over the last five decades (Lassaletta *et al.* 2019). Global pig production in 2022 included 122.58 million tonnes of meat with bones, 8.01 million tonnes of edible offal and 1.11 million tonnes fat in 2022 (https://www.fao.org/faostat/en/#data/QCL, accessed on 18-01-2024). Pig production is expected to rise further during the coming decades due to growing urbanization and demand for quality food.

Domestication of Horse: Beginning of a Glorious Age of the Horse Culture: Throughout the history of mankind, people and scientists have been fascinated by the horse. Though the question of how the equine species evolved is still somewhat debatable as many subspecies developed over time, there is no debate about the major contributions this animal has made to the development of the world (Beaver 2019). The horse is a thread that connects history, mythology, art, literature, folklore, and popular belief over several millennia since its domestication. 'From horse we may learn not only about the horse itself but also about animals in general, indeed about ourselves and life as a whole', said George Gaylord Simpson, one of the most influential paleontologists of the twentieth century.

Now extinct, *Equus ferus* from central Asia was the wild ancestor of the domestic horse *Equus caballus* (Marshall *et al.* 2014). Genomic and archaeological shreds of evidence such as corralling, manure management, mare's milk residue in ceramics, morphological changes in metacarpal bones and size of horses provide strong evidence of domestication and husbandry of horse in the Eneolithic Botai culture in Northern Kazakhstan around 5,600–5,000 BP (Levine 2005, Olsen 2006, Klecel and Martyniuk 2021, Atsenova *et al.* 2022). Although the evidence for the Botai horse domestication is strong, recent studies on ancient genomics, however, indicate that the Botai culture contributed very little (between 2.0% and 3.8%) to the genetic makeup of all the modern domestic horses dated from ca. 4,000 years to the present. The Botai lineage is instead related to Przewalski horses (*Equus przewalskii*) thought to be the feral descendants of early domestic horses herded at ancient Botai culture and not truly wild early horses. The lower Volga-Don region is especially pinpointed as the homeland of modern domestic horses (Librado *et al.* 2021). The lineage of modern domestic horses dispersed outside their core region, first reaching Anatolia, the lower Danube, Bohemia, and Central Asia by approximately ca.2200–2000 BCE, and then soon afterward to Western Europe and Mongolia, ultimately replacing all local populations by around ca.1500 – 1000 BCE (Marshall *et al.* 2014). It appears that the complex process of horse domestication took place many times in the Eurasian steppes within at least two different cultures (Klecel and Martyniuk 2021), and involved continuous genetic restocking from the wild horse (*Equus ferus*), in a sex-biased manner, mostly from mares. The ancient DNA studies have also shown that the domestication process was quite dynamic and uneven through space and time, as particular human groups selected different phenotypic traits (Librado *et al.* 2016).

The horse was the last of the five most common livestock species (sheep, goat, cattle, and pig) domesticated, but its role in shaping ancient civilizations cannot be underestimated. In the beginning, horses were domesticated most probably by people who regraded them as a cheap source of winter meat, enabling them to survive the steppe winter when cattle and sheep needed to be supplied with water and fodder. By 4500 BCE, in addition to a source of meat, peri-domesticated horses were also ridden and milked in the Eurasian steppes (Anthony and Brown 2011). It is not clear how people learned to ride the horse. Probably after familiarization with horses as domesticated animals, and after a relatively docile male bloodline was established, someone used a particularly submissive horse for a fun ride. Soon riding found its first serious use in the management of herds of domesticated cattle, sheep, and horses (Anthony 2007).

The utility of horses in the war and transport in the modern world has diminished considerably, the horse however remains a valuable livestock and companion animal with diverse uses. It is a crucial asset to agriculture in many countries. There were over 111.28 million horses worldwide in 2022 (https://www.fao.org/faostat/en/#data/QCL, accessed on 18-01-2024). These are used for work, food, sports and for biomedical purposes including therapy animals. Owing to their strength and endurance, horses are well-suited for heavy work and employed to carry heavy loads or to perform other heavy work such as ploughing, pulling loaded carts, and carrying goods. Horses remain an important means of land transport particularly in hilly tracts and remote rural areas. Meat of horses is not a preferred choice of food in many countries, but it continues to provide high-quality protein for people around the world including Asia, Europe, and South America (Beaver 2019). In 2022, more than 775.54 million tonnes meat and 99,084 tonnes edible offal were produced by horses and other equines globally in 2022 (https://www.fao.org/faostat/en/#data/QCL, accessed on 18-01-2024).

Milk of mares has been consumed for thousands of years in the Eurasian steppe, and is an important source of vitamins and other nutrients for the modern Kazakh, Kyrgyz, Bashkir, Mongol, Yakut, and other Eurasian steppes peoples. The fermented milk of the mare, known as *Koumiss,* in Kazakh, or *airag*, in the Mongolian language or as *kumis* or *koumiss* in the international literature, is a popular traditional drink (Olsen 2006, Kondybayev *et al.* 2021). Horse raw milk is rich in whey protein, polyunsaturated fatty acids, and vitamin C. Both fermented and raw forms of horse milk are reported to possess therapeutic properties including antituberculosis and anti-atherosclerosis properties. The risk of microbial infections due to consumption of equine milk is relatively less as it contains fewer pathogens as compared to cow milk. Horse milk is also reported safe for children allergic to cow milk protein (CMPA) and for immunocompromised or debilitated people

(Kondybayev *et al.* 2021). Nutritional and health-promoting properties of horse milk have renewed interest towards horse and donkey breeding to produce milk for health benefits, which could contribute to the rural eco-sustainable development of the micro-economies of those areas threatened by marginalization. Equine dairy enterprise is developing in China, Mongolia, Kazakhstan, Kyrgyzstan, and many European countries (Miraglia *et al.* 2020). In France, Germany and Italy mare milk is used as a nutritional substitute for children allergic to cow milk (Kondybayev *et al.* 2021).

Horses are unique animals with incredible capacity for athletic performance as biomechanics and many other physical characteristics allow them to perform a wide variety of events (Reed 2022). They shine today in sports and recreation as never before and thrill people with their speed and stamina in races (Hendricks 2007). Horse racing is among the most popular and increasingly lucrative global industries worth several crores. Several equestrian events ranging from horse racing and vaulting to polo are part of the Olympics and other multi-sports competitions. For many people, horses are trusted pets, and companion animals for leisure activities such as riding and hiking. They are also frequently used for producing biologics and therapeutics such as hormones, antibodies, and immune serum (Manteca Vilanova *et al.* 2021). The human health benefits of horses have been known since ancient times. The first known study published in 1870 provided evidence of the positive benefits of horse riding on balance, posture, and muscle control in individuals with disabilities. The development of modern-day equine-assisted activities and therapies (EAT) gained impetus in the 20th century with the physical effects of EAT on individuals with cerebral palsy as the most documented area of research (Berg and Causey 2014). Equine-assisted therapy is a treatment that has rehabilitation goals and includes equine activities and/or equine environments. It includes a variety of activities divided into therapeutic horseback riding and hippotherapy. Metanalysis of randomized clinical trials identified highly significant positive effects of EAT on exercise tolerance and the quality of life of people with disabilities and moderately significant effects on mobility, interpersonal interactions, and relationships (Prieto *et al.* 2022).

Human-driven management, through selection for favourable traits and use of animals for various tasks beyond the range of normal behaviour, has dramatically influenced the recent history of domestic horses, developing multiple breeds around the world with a wide range of phenotypic peculiarities to meet a specific need, or highlight a specific appearance or gait (Librado *et al.* 2016, Beaver 2019). For example, Thoroughbred, Quarter Horse, and Arabian racing breeds of horses were developed for specific purposes. Paso-Finos, Tennessee Walking horses and Missouri Fox trotters have specialized gait (Beaver 2019). Domestic horses exhibit remarkable variation in coat colouration, including the bay or bay-dun wild-type phenotypes, other basic colours like chestnut and black, as well as dilution such as cream and silver, and spotting patterns like leopard complex, tobiano, and sabino (Librado *et al.* 2016). Interestingly, correlations have been observed between tamability and increased variation in coat colour, as well as between certain behavioural traits and allele distribution at coat-colour loci in several species, including horses; however, the precise molecular mechanisms linking behavioural and colour phenotypes have yet to be elucidated (Klecel and Martyniuk 2021). Over 618 local breeds of horses exist worldwide. Also, there are populations of free-ranging and semi-free-ranging horses throughout the world, representing unique breeds in some areas, or as genetic hybrids in others. The largest number of free-ranging horses-Brumbies is in Australia followed by Mongolian horses in China and Mustangs in the USA (Beaver 2019). However, a significant part of equine genetic diversity is currently endangered; 87 horse breeds are already extinct, and among the remaining almost a quarter are categorized as at risk. After the extinction of the Tarpan horse in 1909, which populated Eastern Europe a few centuries ago, the only surviving wild relative of the horse is the endangered Przewalski's horse (Librado *et al.* 2016). The population structure of horses is characterized by high interbreed and low interbreed genetic diversity due to commonly practised inbreeding and line-breeding in the modern horse industry (Librado *et al.* 2016, Beaver 2019).

Domestication of Donkey (*Equus asinus*): The domestic donkey is the oldest-known pack animal that has played an important role as a beast of burden in many civilizations since 4000 BCE. It is also one of the two members of the multi-subspecies genus *Equus* (the other being the horse) and is the only ungulate domesticated solely in Africa. Archaeological and genetic findings support that domestic donkey originated most likely in northeastern Africa via a directed pathway from their wild ancestors-African wild asses (*Equus africanus*), primarily to serve as a transport animal under the arid environments of the region around ca. 6,000–3,500 BP (Marshall *et al.* 2014). Genetic studies of donkeys have revealed two distinct mitochondrial DNA (mtDNA) haplotypes, indicating two distinct domestication events. Analysis of ancient archaeological and historical museum samples suggests that donkeys of clade 1, which have a long history in the Sahara, originated from the Nubian wild asses (*Equus africanus africanus*), that were crossed with domestic donkeys over a long period by introducing several maternal haplotypes from the wild asses; the gene flow of this clade is continuous (Wang *et al.* 2022). Extinct Atlas wild ass (*Equus africanus atlanticus*), endemic to northern Africa, or another undescribed subspecies that potentially ranged outside of Africa is suggested as the ancestor of clade 2 donkeys (Todd *et al.* 2022).

Domestication of the donkey was possibly driven by the response of pastoralists and other societies in Northeastern Africa to the desertification of the Sahara (Beja-Periera *et al.* 2004). Apart from being the source of meat and milk, cattle were used for transport also in ancient Northeastern Africa. However, as desert conditions began to develop and the climate became drier, pastoralists needed to move more frequently to sustain themselves. Cattle are not an ideal form of transport under arid conditions, as they require substantial watering at least every other day. On the other hand, pastoralists might have found that wild asses, which were hunted in the region, were well adapted to hot and harsh environments, and required less water because they do not ruminate. Asses could digest coarse grasses, have labile metabolic rates, and have numerous water-sparing mechanisms. Thus, they possessed distinct advantages over cattle as domesticates for transport during times of increasingly unpredictable rainfall and desertification (Kimura *et al.* 2013).

Upon domestication, donkeys were principally used for traction and transportation. Donkeys enhanced the exchange of transport of goods by making it easier and cheaper to transport commodities over both long and short distances, which resulted in enhanced intra- and inter-regional exchange of goods and the movement of people (Greenfield *et al.* 2018). Other than cattle, these beasts of burden allowed a flourishing of long-distance exchange networks that connected the ancient Near East to central and southern Asia to Egypt, Anatolia, and the Mediterranean coastal ports. The donkey became progressively valuable and spread to Asia (ca. 2600 BCE), Europe (ca. 2800 BCE), and other parts of the world over the centuries (Todd *et al.* 2022, Wang *et al.* 2022).

The introduction of the domestic donkey to the Near East at the end of the 4th and beginning of the early 3rd millennium BCE dramatically changed the nature of transportation of people and goods in early complex societies (Greenfield *et al.* 2018). A new class of merchants emerged and donkey caravans were formed to specialize in the transportation of goods leading to the spread of donkeys as a totem associated with worship among merchants and herders, who occupied specialized positions in the growing complexity of the social structure of urban societies (Wang *et al.* 2022). Donkeys were sacrificed to the gods across the Fertile Crescent and were associated with kingship in this part of the world. They were ridden long before the arrival of horses in the Near East. Christ entered Jerusalem on the back of a donkey on a Palm Sunday (Mitchell 2018). Recovery of a bit along with a sacrificed domestic donkey (*Equus asinus*) skeleton from an Early Bronze Age (ca. 2800–2600 BCE) deposits at Telleṣ-Ṣâfi/Gath, Israel provides the earliest evidence for the use of a bit among the domestic equids and suggests that bit on donkeys was used early to mid-

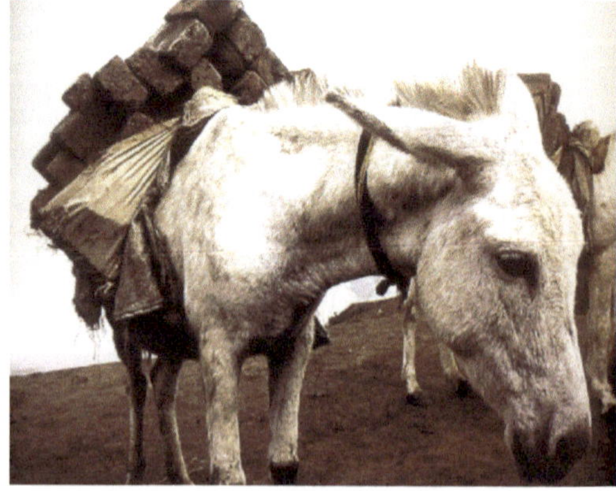

Fig. 1.5. *The donkey continues to serve as the primary beast of burden and a vital mode of transportation in numerous regions across the modern world (Photo by the Author).*

3rd millennium BCE long before the appearance of horses in the ancient Near East (Greenfield *et al.* 2018). Carts driven by donkeys were the appropriate transport for the royalties and kings. The famous Standard of Ur shows donkeys or onagers (Asiatic wild ass *Equus hemionus)* pulling royal carts (Mitchell 2018). Improved donkeys were bred by Romans to produce mules essential for their military power and economy (Todd *et al.* 2022). Along with their hybrid offspring mule, donkeys formed a core technology for moving goods at both local and international levels, especially in the areas of rugged and mountainous terrain. They transported agricultural products throughout the Mediterranean basin, the Middle East, and beyond, tin and wool for Bronze-Age merchants between Assyria and Anatolia, and supplies for the Roman army (Michell 2018).

Box 1.2. Donkey Milk: A Valuable Animal Product

Donkey milk has been utilized for nutritional, cosmetic, and medicinal purposes since antiquity, and today it is making a strong resurgence as a functional food for human nutrition in the third millennium. Modern research has substantiated its potential biological properties, including antioxidant, anti-inflammatory, antibacterial, and immune-enhancing effects, as well as its nutraceutical properties.

Donkey milk also regulates gut microflora, with a higher lactoferrin content compared to cow milk, making it suitable for infants with cow milk protein allergy. Commercially, donkey milk finds its primary use in the production of cheese, chocolates, ice creams, cheddar, and other products. During the COVID-19 pandemic, consumption of donkey milk increased due to its recognized biological properties. Recognized by the Food and Agriculture Organization (FAO) as a balanced diet due to its richness in dietary energy and proteins, donkey milk has gained significance. The global market for donkey milk was valued at USD 23.2 million in 2021 and is projected to grow at a compounded annual growth rate of 9.9% between 2022 and 2028. Increasing awareness of skincare products and the growing demand for powdered jenny milk worldwide are expected to drive market growth, particularly in countries like China and India. This growth may consequently reinforce the need for well-organized dairy donkey farming.

(Source:https://www.grandviewresearch.com/industry-analysis/donkey-milk-market-report Accessed on 9-10-2023)

Donkey milk also occupied a prominent place in ancient times. It was used to feed newborns through toy-shaped bottles. Hippocrates (460 – 370 BCE), Pliny the Elder (23 – 79 CE), and French Naturalist Georges-Louis Leclerc (1707–1788) mention the virtues of donkey milk including health benefits. It was also a favoured cosmetic. Cleopatra (69 BCE –30 BCE), the queen of the Ptolemaic Kingdom of Egypt; Messalina, the wife of Roman Emperor Claudius (10 BCE – 54 CE); Poppea (30 – 65 CE), the second wife of Roman Emperor Nero and

Pauline, sister of Napolean Bonaparte used donkey milk as cosmetics (Bertino *et al.* 2022). Donkeys remain a critical resource for the subsistence of millions of the poor in the world today. They serve as the main beast of burden and source of transportation (Fig. 1.5), especially in the regions where horses cannot easily survive or where extreme poverty prevents locals from owning horses (https://www.britannica.com/animal/donkey, accessed 29-09-2023). Donkeys are particularly suited for transport in mountainous and arid environments, and mules and donkey carts are important means of public transport and income generation, especially in rural areas. Recently, the donkey milk has generated considerable interest for its use as a functional food. During the 19th century, some European countries started to use donkey milk regularly in maternity hospitals and to feed infants and until the beginning of the 20th century marketed it for the feeding of orphan infants, unhealthy children, ill people, and the elderly. Consequently, the donkey farms were set up in Italy, France, Belgium, Switzerland, and Germany (Aspri *et al.* 2017). Donkey hide has been extensively used to produce *ejiao*, a gelatine utilized in traditional Chinese medicine. However, the donkey is the most affected livestock species by industrialization, depopulation of rural districts, and mechanization of agriculture leading to a substantial population decline during the 20th century (Camillo *et al.* 2018). In 2022, global populations of donkeys (asses) and production of meat were 53.033 million and 104,304 tonnes, respectively (https://www.fao.org/faostat/en/#data/QCL, accessed on 18-01-2024).

There is a growing interest in the utility of donkeys beyond their traditional role. Possible new roles of donkeys include milk and meat production, animal-assisted therapies (onotherapy), landscape and soil maintenance, donkeys as livestock guardians, and donkeys for ecotourism and leisure (Camillo *et al.* 2018, Seyiti and Kelimu, 2021). Production of milk is the most promising new role for donkeys. Donkey milk possesses unique functional properties consisting of antimicrobial, immunomodulation, antioxidant, and hypo-allergenic activities and its nutritional properties are comparable to human milk (Aspri *et al.* 2017). Already donkey meat is recognized as a nutritive food for humans. It contains good-quality proteins, vitamins, and minerals. Donkey farming for meat, and milk is becoming an important industry in many countries. Further, the selective feeding behaviour of donkeys encourages the growth of endangered species of plants and insects. Donkeys are also being used as controllers of grass growth in regions where soils are too fragile. The survival of donkey breeds and the possibility of an increase in the number of these animals depend on the economic interest in the donkey and its products (Camillo *et al.* 2018). In general, the donkey industry in the world, especially in countries like China, is developing rapidly, and donkey farming is transforming gradually from the family farming model to large-scale, intensive, and integrated industrial operations (Wang *et al.* 2022).

Domestication of Camel: The camel, known as the 'ship of desert', is a pseudo-ruminant belonging to order Artiodactyla (even footed ungulates) and family *Camelidae*. The ancestors of camel migrated from America in the late Tertiary period and evolved in different parts of the world. Ancestors of Old-world camels reached Eurasia via the Bering land bridge around 6.5–7.5 millennia ago, and those of New World camels entered South America around 3 millennia ago (El-Agamy, 2006, Burger *et al.* 2019). At present the family *Camillidae* comprises two genera and seven extant species. The genus *Camelus* includes three species of Afro-Asian or Old-world camels–the one-humped Arabian or dromedary camel (*Camelus dromedarius*) and the two-humped or Bactrian camel (*C. bactrianus),* and the wild Bactrian camel (*C. ferus*) under tribe Camelini. Genus *Lama* consists four species of the new world camelids llama (*L. glama*), alpaca *(Vicugna pacos* or *L pacos*), guanacos (*L. guanicoe*) and vicuñas *(V. vicugna*) in the tribe Lamini (Burger *et al.* 2019, Jemmet *et al.* 2023). Domestication of Old-world camels happened in two different locations via a directed pathway.

Archaeological, pictorial, and genetic evidence suggested that Bactrian camels were domesticated from wild Bactrian camel (*C. ferus*) during the late fourth and early third millennium BCE in northeastern Iran, and the adjacent Kopet Dagh foothills in southwestern Turkmenistan–part of the historical region Bactria–and spread to the Central Asian countries including Mongolia, China, Kazakhstan, northeastern Afghanistan, Russia, Crimea and Uzbekistan (Burger *et al.* 2019, Khomeiri and Yam 2015). Wild Bactrian camels are categorized as critically endangered species by the International Union for Conservation of Nature (ICUN) as their number and range are severely reduced with only four locations worldwide: three in China and one in Mongolia are left as the last home for these wild camels (Burger *et al.* 2019). The Bactrian camels have been an important pack animal in inner Asia since ancient times. They are the largest land mammals in their native range and are exceptionally adept at withstanding wide variations in temperature ranging from freezing cold in the winter to extremely hot temperatures in summer, and the harsh conditions of limited vegetation and water sources.

Dromedary camels were probably domesticated in the late second millennium (1800- 1100 BCE) in the Arabian Peninsula from now-extinct wild dromedaries. However, mitochondrial, nuclear, and ancient DNA analyses of a global dataset of modern individuals and up to 7000-year-old wild dromedary samples revealed shared ancestry between wild dromedaries from the southeast coast of the Arabian Peninsula (Burger *et al.* 2019). After their domestication on the Arabian Peninsula, small numbers of dromedaries arrived in Mesopotamia and from there were probably introduced into northeastern Africa via the Sinai, possibly starting in the first millennium BCE. Another possible route for dromedary camel introduction into Africa might have involved a transfer from the south of the Arabian Peninsula by boat via the Gulf of Aden to Eastern Africa or further north across the Red Sea to

Egypt, which is supported by socio-ethological practices about the use of Eastern African dromedaries largely for dairying rather than for riding and transportation purposes (Burger *et al.* 2019).

Camels are remarkably strong, easy to feed and gifted with incredible endurance. They can withstand harsh climates prevailing in the arid zones. Camels can resist severe dehydration, high-temperature variations and a low energy and protein content diet and can regain up to 30% body water losses without suffering from intravascular haemolysis. The dromedaries are raised in a hot-desert area with temperatures ranging from 5°-45°C, the Bactrian camels inhabit areas where temperature varies from –20° to 40°C (Alhadrami and Fays 2022). Despite all the unique physiological traits and economic utility, camels did not spread worldwide and continue to be bred and utilized only in their native habitats or in the habitat with climatic extremes of Arabia and Inner Asia, possibly due to their comparatively late period of domestication, and the long maturation period. Also, many experiments to introduce the camel in other continents have been unsuccessful (Bulliet 2012). For example, dromedary camels were introduced into Australia in the 1800s as the most appropriate mode of transport for the challenging environment and served efficiently in the establishment of the modern infrastructure of the continent including the construction of the Transnational Railways. Today, the Australian dromedary exists in large numbers as feral and is looked upon as an animal that has served its economic purpose and is currently both out of place and time (Crowley 2014). However, Old World camels are typically multipurpose animals and continue to assume a special status in many Afro-Asian cultures.

No other domestic animal can provide such a variety of uses for human populations as imparted by the camel (Faye 2016). Over the centuries, domestic camels have contributed to human culture in several ways such as transport and carrying loads as pack or saddle animals, production of milk, meat, wool, hair, hide and manure, as a source of animal power in diverse agricultural activities like ploughing, weeding, harrowing, *noria*, water extraction, and as a source of leisure activities like racing, sports, tourism, and festivity (Burger *et al.* 2019, Fays 2016). Camels are also used in the army both in the form of cavalry and supply animals. The first recorded military use of the camel dates to the Battle of Qarqar in 853 BCE. Camel troops were employed for escort, desert policing and scouting duties during the late Roman empire (https://en.wikipedia.org/wiki/Camel_cavalry, accessed on 6-11-2023). Roman used both Bactrian and dromedary camels in the military, but named the camel-riding force *Dromedarii* (*droma*=running or runner in Greek). One of the roles of *Dromedarii* was to counter enemy cavalry (Jemmet *et al.* 2023).

Over time, camels have been bred and selected for different purposes. They are differentiated by their size, global conformation, and environment. According to their utility, camels are grouped as dairy and dual-purpose, draught power, meat-producing and wool-producing camels. Dairy camels are of large body size with a developed abdomen, large hump, prominent mammary vein, and an overall well-developed udder and > 3,000-litre annual milk yield. Dual-purpose (milk and meat or packing/ riding) camels have medium body and hump sizes with medium milk yield (1,500 and 3,000 litre). The wool-producing camels are mainly Bactrians, especially those found in Mongolia and China (Burger *et al.* 2019). Compared to dromedary camels Bactrian camels are low-yield dairy camels. However, the first-generation hybrids (F1) of the two types of camels showed improved milk and wool yield. In Kazakhstan, hybridization between dromedary and Bactrian camel is common to get higher milk yield (Alhadrami and Faye 2022).

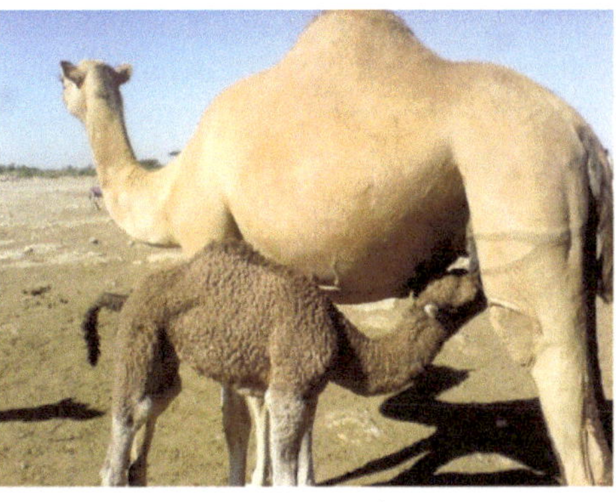

Fig. 1.6. *Apart from their traditional roles, camel dairy farming is a fast growing industry leading to rising trend in global camel population (Photo courtesy of Dr. A. Sahoo, ICAR-NRC on Camel).*

Box 1.3. Use of Camel Milk in Autism Spectrum Disorder (ASD)

Owing to its core value in pastoralists' life, culture and health benefits, camel milk is known as White Gold of Desert (Gebremichael et al. 2019, Oselu et al. 2022). It has been traditionally used for the treatment of some health conditions in humans such as jaundice, gastric ulcers, asthma, anaemia, and tuberculosis

Much of the scientific and public interest on therapeutic camel milk owe to its ameliorative potential in autism spectrum disorder (ASD), a neurodevelopmental disorder in children. Camel milk consumption reduces oxidative stress, which plays a vital role in pathophysiology of neurological disorders A double-blind clinical trial showed that 500 ml camel milk given daily for two weeks to autistic children reduced serum level of activation-regulated chemokines and improved childhood autism rating scale (Bashir and Al-Ayadhi 2014).

The use of camels as pack and draught animals has declined in the world of modern transport and fast connectivity. However, the growing demand for sustainable milk and meat production — especially in countries affected by climate change and increasing desertification — has renewed the focus of animal breeders and scientists on this valuable domestic species (Burger *et al.* 2019). The renewed interest in the camel and its products in the modern world is reflected by the global camel population trend, which showed a growth rate faster than the cattle, sheep, and horse populations, and like that of the buffalo population (Faye 2016, 2020). According to the FAO database, the estimated world population of camels in 2021 was 40.37 million which increased to 41.77 million in 2022. The camel raw milk and meat production was 4.1 million tonnes and 604,530 tonnes, respectively in

2022 (https://www.fao.org/faostat/en/#data/QCL, accessed on on 18-01-2024). Camels rank fifth globally in milk production, following cows, buffaloes, sheep, and goats. They excel as milk producers in arid and desert environments, surpassing other livestock in the same conditions. Moreover, they exhibit a longer duration of milk production, making them crucial for sustaining dairy production in drought-affected regions (Seifu 2022). Recent years have seen a significant increase in literature exploring various facets of dairy camel farming, including husbandry practices and the composition of camel milk, along with its nutritional, medicinal, and socioeconomic significance.

Traditionally considered a hospitality gift, and consumed raw or in naturally fermented form, camel milk plays a vital role in ensuring food security and bolstering the rural economy across arid regions in North and East Africa, Central Asia, and the Indian subcontinent (Seifu 2022). The urbanization and the modernization of the farming systems have facilitated development of a camel milk commodity channel leading to integration of camel milk in the market in many countries of the camel world (Faye *et al.* 2014). A notable transformation has occurred in the camel milk industry, marked by the adoption of pasteurization techniques and the diversification of product offerings. These include milk powder, cheese, yogurt, sweets, and ice cream, catering to varied consumer preferences. Furthermore, non-food products like soaps and cosmetic creams derived from camel milk have emerged, indicating a burgeoning market for camel-based goods. The current global interest in camel milk stems primarily from its perceived health benefits for consumers. Extensive research and development efforts are being pursued to transform technological advancements into widely available products (Konuspayeva and Faye 2021).

Scientific investigations, predominantly consisting of *in vitro* studies and experiments conducted on animal models, alongside a limited number of clinical trials, have revealed medicinal properties associated with camel milk. These include its antioxidative, antibacterial, antiviral, antihypertensive, antiulcerogenic, antiaging, antineoplastic, immune-boosting, hypoglycaemic, hepatoprotective, and neuroprotective effects. Furthermore, camel milk has emerged as a suitable alternative for infants allergic to bovine milk. The medicinal properties of camel milk can be attributed to its unique composition. It is rich in essential nutrients such as iron, zinc, magnesium, vitamin C, riboflavin (B_2), niacin (B_3), pyridoxine (B_6), folic acid (B_9), and cobalamin (B_{12}). Moreover, camel milk contains vital bioactive components like lysozymes, N-acetylglucosamine, lactoferrins, peptidoglycan, recognition proteins, A_2 beta-casein, α-hydroxyl acid, and tumour binding antibodies (Oselu *et al.* 2022, Seifu 2022).

Breeding camels for various purposes such as milk, meat, fibre, hides, skins, and energy is gaining global significance, particularly in regions where other livestock may not thrive. In Arabian countries, camel husbandry is undergoing industrialization, with large-scale camel dairy farms housing thousands of camels operating in these regions. New camel farms are also being established in Western Europe and the USA for both tourist attraction and dairy production purposes (Faye 2022). The utilization of racing camels and camels for beauty pageants represents additional facets of the regional camel industry (Köhler-Rollefson 2022). In many Arabian countries, dromedary camels are reared extensively for camel racing, an event of significant socio-economic importance. Bactrian camels are valued for their production of fine wool, which is utilized in the manufacturing of luxury coats. Camel hides find application in the production of shoes and sandals (Khomeiri and Yam 2015). Moreover, camel milk, urine, and meat are utilized in traditional remedies. A recent review highlighted the promising medicinal properties of camel urine, including its potential as an antidiabetic, anti-cancerous, antibacterial, antiviral, antifungal, and hepatoprotective agent, prompting further studies to validate these findings (Tharwat *et al.* 2023). In general, the role of camels is transitioning from multipurpose livestock to highly specialized animals, serving specific purposes such as dairy production, fattening, racing, or participation in beauty contests.

South American Camelids and Domestication of Llamas and Alpacas: South American camelids (SACs), also referred to as New World camelids are represented by four living species including two wild species — guanaco (*Lama guanicoe*) and vicuña (*Vicugna vicugna*) — and two domestic species, llama (*Lama glama*) and alpaca (*L pacos*). SACs have played a central role in the development of Andean societies, from ancient times and remain a core element in the rural communities all along the Andes (Goñalons 2008). These large herbivores are valued for their several material and non-material contributions to people and are a key component of Andean biocultural heritage. They constitute a nature component in the complex system of human interaction and Andean Mountain environment. In the indigenous and local knowledge, the wild species are considered as *Salaq* (natural, untamed), which are protected by the *Malkus* or mountain deity. The domestic species are *Uywa* or the one that belongs to people (Vilá and Arzamendia 2022).

The guanaco is the largest wild artiodactyl in South America having an adult body weight of 90-140 kg, and a height at withers 90-120 cm. Guanacos have the broadest distribution and occupy the most diverse habitat over an elevation range of sea level to 4,500 m. Their distribution range extends from northern Peru southward, to western Bolivia, Argentina, Chile, and Tierra del Fuego. There are two recognized subspecies of guanaco: the small-light colour *L. guanicoe cacsilensis* found in the northern part of the habitat between Northen Peru and Northen Chile, and the large- dark colour *L. guanicoe guanicoe* located in the southernmost guanaco distribution (Wheeler 1995, Hoffman 2014). Guanacos played an important role in prehistoric Patagonian life and were exploited for meat, fat, blood, bones, and skins for clothing and to build shelters (Vilá and

Arzamendia 2022). A mitochondrial genomic study confirmed that the now-extinct *Chilihueque* of Mocha Island in Southern Chile was a domestic form of guanacos. The *Chilihueque* played a major role in the island's society and was used for ritual sacrifice (Westbury 2016). Captive-borne guanacos may be tamed and handled similarly to llamas. They were used as pack animals by the Incas (Wheeler 1995). The guanaco has a skin of good quality and produces one of the finest wools, which is more valuable than the old-world camel. The pelt of guanaco is used for making bed covers, coats, and mantels (Khomeiri and Yam 2015). The population of guanacos was significantly impacted by indiscriminate hunting and commercial sheep rearing leading to a severe decline in their number from 30 to 40 million in the pre-Hispanic period to 7 million in the 19th century and around 0.6 million survived in the 20th century. In 1974, the International Union for the Conservation of Nature and Natural Resources (IUCN) declared the species as vulnerable (Wheeler 1995). Successful capture and shearing projects have been valuable for the sustainable use and conservation of guanacos (Vilá and Arzamendia 2022). They are presently classified as species of least concern on the IUCN Red List (Hoffman 2014).

Distribution of vicuña is limited to the areas of extreme elevation of the Andes. This wild species is the smallest of the SACs (adult body weight 40-55 kg and height at withers 70-90 cm). There are two subspecies of vicuña- the smaller Peruvian *V mensalis* with long growth of hair on the chest and the larger Argentinian, *Vicugna vicugna vicugna* (Wheeler 1995). The vicuña produces one of the finest fibres in the world. It was considered the property of the king in the Inca civilization, and only royalty was allowed to wear garments made of vicuña fibre garments (McLean and Niehaus 2022). Aymara and Quechua ethnic communities in Argentina hold this species in high respect and have cultural taboos against its killing. Other indigenous communities believe that the vicuña is owned by Pachamama, the mother-Earth deity (Vilá *et al.* 2020, Vilá and Arzamendia 2022). The vicuña holds a place of profound significance and revered status in Peru. It is the national animal of Peru and is represented across various national emblems and symbols of the country. Loss of habitat and excessive poaching and killing to meet the increasing demand of highly-priced vicuña fleece in the international luxury market caused a drastic decline in the vicuña population in the Andes, bringing it down to less than 10,000 individuals in the mid-half of the 20th century. From 1982 to 1994, the vicuña was placed under the critically endangered category by the IUCN. Subsequent conservation efforts including passing laws to protect vicuña by Argentina, Chile, Peru, and Bolivia helped in the recovery of the population and reclassification of the species as Least Concern in the IUCN Red List (Vilá *et al.*2020).

The two domestic species of SACs, the llama and alpaca, first appeared in the fossil record around 7,000 BP suggesting their status as domestic species. The Puna ecosystem in the tundra environment of the Peruvian Andes is suggested to be the probable site of SAC domestication. Approximately 12,000 years ago, both wild guanacos and vicuñas inhabited this ecosystem, and together with huemul deer were the primary prey of early hunters. The domestication of llama and alpaca is believed to have occurred from these two species after 7,500 BP (Wheeler 1995). However, the origin of domestic SACs is a scientifically debatable issue. There are four possible hypotheses: llamas and alpacas were domesticated from guanacos and vicuña, respectively; llamas were domesticated from guanacos, whereas, alpacas originated from hybridization between llamas and vicuña; llamas and alpacas were both domesticated from guanacos while vicuña was never domesticated; guanaco and vicuña were never domesticated and the two domestic species evolved from extinct wild precursors (Wheeler 1995).

Zooarchaeological indicators and contextual data point to the domestication of the alpaca in the Central Andes by 6,000 BP, and the llama in the Central and South-Central Andes sometime between 4,600 and 3,000 BP. Probably, the process of alpaca and llama domestication took place independently at different times and places within the Andes (Goñalons 2008). The hypothesis that the llama (*Lama glama*) is domesticated from guanaco (*Lama guanicoe*) and the alpaca (*Vicugna pacos*) from vicuña (*Vicugna vicugna*) has wide scientific acceptance (Wheeler 1995, Goñalons 2008, Marín *et al.* 2017, Vilá and Arzamendia 2022), and is supported by whole genome sequencing (Fan *et al.* 2020). The four SACs can interbreed and produce fertile offspring. They all have the same number (n=74) of chromosomes (Sánchez-Villagra 2022). Analysis of ancient mitochondrial genomes found guanaco ancestry within alpacas and vicuña ancestry within llamas pointing towards pre-contact bidirectional hybridization, and that interbreeding practices were widespread during the domestication process by the early camelid herders in the Atacama during the Early Formative period (Díaz-Maroto *et al.* 2021).

The llama is the largest (adult body weight 113-250 kg and height at withers 102-119 cm), whereas the alpaca is the second smallest (adult body weight 55-90 kg and height at withers 76-96 cm) of the four lamoid species. South American llamas are classified into heavy neck fibre (*chaku, lanuda,* and *tapada*), and short neck fibre (*ccara* and *pelada*) breeds (McLean, and Niehaus 2022). Woolly llamas are more common in Argentina, whereas non-woolly phenotype llamas are found in Peru, Bolivia, and Northern Chile (Wheeler 1995). Traditional herding communities of the Puna region hugely valued llamas and alpacas and regarded them as a kind of treasure, that was sent to mankind by the deities on loan. Their continuing presence was dependent primarily on the treatment these valuable animals received. Appropriate care of llamas and alpacas included providing adequate pasture and water, treating their maladies, protecting them from predators, and carrying out proper ceremonies annually. Elaborate rituals designed to protect the health and well-being of llamas and alpacas were held by the herder communities (Stephenson 2010).

Llamas have a long history of interaction with Andean people, supplying meat, leather, and fibre for garments, rope, burlap bags, etc., and serving as beasts of burden for transporting goods, as well as religious and sacrificial animals. Like old-world camels, llamas possess high thirst tolerance making them an important transport animal in the Andean region. An adult llama can carry up to 40 kg weight and can travel up and down in the mountainous region. Caravans of llamas played a critical role in the expansion of Pre-Incan Andean cultures. Apart from transporting loads, ancient Andeans raised llamas, alpacas, and pigs as sources of meat (Wakild 2021). Inca extended the use of llama. Armies on the move regularly used trains of thousands of llamas not only for carrying loads but also for food when their role as portage was no longer needed. The llamas and alpacas also served as the source of wool and leather for state personnel, especially for the soldiers of the empire (D'Altroy 2015). In the sixteenth century, the South American camelids, especially llamas found a unique yet less-recognized use as a source of bezoar stones, calcinated concretions somewhat like pearls, formed in the digestive tracts of ruminants. These stones were claimed to possess curative virtues against a range of diseases including an antidote for all kinds of poisons and were widely regarded as effective and excellent remedies for serious illnesses, including plague, typhus, and fevers by the physicians and apothecaries in Europe. The stones became a highly sought-after priceless commodity for both the European and traditional Andeans and played a dramatic role in shaping the social and economic history of early modern Europe and Spanish America. The medical interest in the claimed therapeutic value of bezoar stones declined and completely waned by the mid-nineteenth century (Stephenson 2010, Wakild 2021).

As per the latest data, the total number of other camelids (livestock category) was 8.66 million in South America in 2022, showing an increasing trend over the 2020 and 2021 populations (https://www.fao.org/faostat/en/#data/QCL, accessed on 18-01-2024). The population trend underlines the continuing socio-economic and cultural values of the domestic SACs in the Andean nations. Nowadays people tend to see llamas as working animals and the alpaca as source-animal for meal and wool (Sánchez-Villagra 2022). Till recently the Quechua-Spanish speaking people (*Llameros*) belonging to indigenous communities of Central Andes lead and travel in llama caravans to barter the pastoralist products such as fibre, dried meat, fat, and vegetables for industrial food products like flour, sugar, pasta, and other essential industrial products. These caravans are however becoming sparse or extinct (Vilá and Arzamendia 2022).

Alpacas are the premier fibre-producing animals. Their fibres are lightweight and strong, with high lustre and insulation properties, and are sold as luxury yarn. Alpaca fibres are used primarily for knitwear in addition to woven products such as shawls, rugs, and duvets. Haucaya (fibre with light crimps) and Suri (fibre without crimps) are the two breeds of alpaca (McLean, and Niehaus 2022). Peru owns the largest biological reserve of the alpaca in the world and is the main fibre-producing country (Bathrachalam *et al.* 2019, Galbraith 2019). The fibre of *crias* (young alpaca) has the smallest diameter and is considered lighter, warmer, and softer than cashmere fibre (Galbraith 2019). Their pelts are used to make fine rugs and wall hangings, and the leather to make ropes. Alpacas are also bred for meat in South America. In North America, alpacas serve as a source of fibre, and companion animals and are used for breeding and showing (McLean, and Niehaus 2022). To build up a wool business for European alpaca fibres, some owners in Europe import alpacas from different countries to breed special animals with fine and dense fibres and sell their fibres and offspring (Gunsser 2013). Alpacas were introduced into Australia and New Zealand in 1980-90s to establish a new animal fibre industry. In Australia, the alpaca industry is evolving from the initial breeding phase of industry development to a more commercial industry with a greater focus on financial returns from fibre production (McGregor 2006). In Australia, a common strategy to reduce predator attack on livestock is the deployment of guardian alpacas. Castrated male alpacas are usually used to guard lambing flocks at a stocking rate of one alpaca per 100 sheep. Some of the likely indicators of guardianship behaviour of the alpacas include travelling greater distance than the sheep, and sharing similar periods of activity and flock dynamics. The alpaca's apparent attraction towards lambs, the more vulnerable animals in the flock, is also concluded to be a behaviour that may be indicative of a protective attitude of alpacas towards lambs and add success as a guardian animal (Matthews 2020).

Utility of llamas and alpacas in their conventional roles might have declined to some extent in their home tract, but there is growing interest in these animals in other countries including the United States, Canada, Australia, New Zealand, and some European countries such as the United Kingdom, Germany, Italy, Austria, Switzerland, and France. In Northern America, llama predominates over alpacas. In contrast, alpacas are more popular in Europe, New Zealand, and Australia (Sharpe 2009, Kiesling 2019). Interestingly in Europe, the population of llamas was dominating over that of alpacas until 2008. The number of the alpaca increased steadily overtaking the llama. The estimated registered population of alpacas (14,203) was more than twice of the llama population (5,689) in 2017 (Kiesling 2019).

In Europe and North America, SACs are not only kept for breeding, wool, or hide reason, but also for numerous other purposes including pet, companion, and therapy animals, packing, promenade or trekking, landscape conservation, and educational purposes (Gunsser 2013, Neubert *et al.* 2021). In the UK, SACs were usually kept for breeding purposes and as pets (D'Alterio *et al.* 2006), whereas in Germany, these were mostly kept as a hobby rather than for breeding or wool purposes. Farmers did not use them for meat (Neubert *et al.* 2021). In North America, guarding sheep, and goat flocks from predation by coyotes is an important niche that the llama fills (McLean, and Niehaus 2022). Highly social SACs exhibit aggression towards their canid predators, such as coyotes, foxes, and dogs. Adult male guanacos are notably territorial, diligently guarding their turf and alerting their family group at the sight of predators. This instinct, inherited from their wild ancestors, persists in domestic SACs, leading to the utilization of llamas and alpacas as guard animals for protecting sheep and goat herds. Once introduced into a sheep flock, llamas quickly acclimate to their surroundings, forming strong bonds with the sheep. The pasture becomes the llama's territory, and the flock becomes its family, a behaviour observed even in gelded llamas. Guard llamas display proactive leadership, often taking the forefront to guide and shield their flocks (Franklin *et al.* 2006).

The modern llama and alpacas are also used in the medical context as registered therapy animals, and as a source of unique heavy chain-only antibodies, which possess exceptional physiochemical properties, and therapeutic potential against a range of human diseases. Llamas are particularly friendlier and good with people, especially those who are sick or in need. A well-trained, quiet llama can be ideal for taking to schools and convalescent hospitals and for interacting with emotionally and physically disadvantaged children and adults (McLean, and Niehaus 2022). Serum of camelids (dromedaries, Bactrian camel, llamas, alpacas, guanacos, and vicuña) contain both conventional antibodies consisting of two long pieces called heavy chains (HC) and two shorter pieces called light chains (LC) and a low molecular mass heavy-chain-only antibodies (HCAb) without LC. HCAb has a variable antigen-binding domain (VHH) that comprises full antigen-binding potential and strong affinity to cognate antigens. It is the smallest naturally occurring intact antigen-binding fragment. Owing to their low nanometre range size, VHHs were named nanobodies (Jovčevska and Muyldermans 2020). Small size of nanobodies allows them to bind cryptic binding sites on antigens, that are inaccessible to conventional antibodies. Also, nanobodies easily penetrate and are rapidly cleared from cells and tissues with low chances of toxicity, making them an ideal candidate for therapeutic diagnostics and drugs (Tai 2020). The nanobodies have three hypervariable antigen binding loops- complementarity degerming regions CDR1/2/3. CDR3 is the main contributor to assist in binding strength antigen recognition and specificity. An exceptionally shorter extended nanobody CDR3 loop is found in the llama nanobody that reduces the entropic penalty associated with the majority of nanobodies comprising a longer length of CDR3 (Jovčevska and Muyldermans 2020). The llama nanobodies are thus extremely suitable for nano therapy, developing diagnostic tests, and manipulating other proteins. Some of the examples of a wide range of applications of llama nanobodies with promising results included the treatment of cancer, neurodegenerative disorders, rotavirus diarrhoea, HIV 1 and SARS-CoV 2 virus, prevention of dandruff in shampoos, and development of more sensitive biosensor based diagnostic test for diagnosis of FMD. In general, the llama has become an important laboratory animal for modern biomedical research.

Reindeer, Rabbit, and other Domestic Farm Mammals: Besides above global farm animal species, several mammalian species were domesticated by humans in different parts of the world in due course of time to serve as source of food, draught power, hide and other animal product power. These farm animals such as reindeer, mithun, yak, and guinea pigs, though exist only in restricted regions of the world, play important roles in the human subsistence, lifeways, economy, and cultures in the specific geographical regions where they are kept. For example, reindeers are important multipurpose animals for all circumpolar peoples. The mithun (gayal) and yak are highly characteristic of the high Himalayan way of life, and the brief history of their domestication will be described in the next chapter. Guinea pigs are an important source of meat production in some South American countries where nearly 65 million are consumed yearly in Peru alone (Waibliger 2019).

Reindeer (Rangifer tarandus): Reindeer are a pan-Arctic ungulate species found in the northern parts of Eurasia and North America. The species, a biological resource of vital importance to the physical and cultural survival of arctic residents, has been exploited for food and subsistence for thousands of years (Røed *et al.* 2008). In the opinion of some scholars, the *Rangifer* was the most important game for millions of years, which could be hunted year-round in the extensive circumpolar region by the herd-followers. It was used by the people more intensively than any other animal. The *Rangifer* provided flesh for food, warmer fur for clothing, sinew, and antlers for making tools and other objects (Gordon 2003). Further, extraordinarily strong, and resilient antlers were one of the most important raw materials of pre-metal age and the reindeer is the only species in which females also regularly have antlers (Clutton- Brock 1999).

The morphology and ecology of the reindeer vary across the area and different subspecies or ecotype divisions divided into high arctic, tundra, and forest ecotypes (Salmi 2023). *Rangifer* species and subspecies are called reindeer in Eurasia and caribou in North America. The taxonomic conclusions, based on the review of available Latin and English names for distinct reindeer and caribou populations identified by molecular data, suggested following names for different ecotypes and phylogenetic clades of *Rangifer: R. tarandus* (Eurasian reindeer), *R. fennicus*, (forest reindeer) including junior synonyms *R. silvicola, R. transuralensis,* and *R. dichotomus, R. platyrhynchus* (Svalbard Reindeer), *R. caribou* (woodland caribou), *R. arcticus* (North American mainland barren-ground caribou) and *R. groenlandicus* (Greenland caribou) with 16 Rangifer type localities each in Eurasia and in North America (Harding 2022).

Reindeer is the only successfully domesticated cervid species, and perhaps the last species to follow a prey pathway to domestication. The species is considered in the early phase of domestication with wild and domestic herds still coexisting widely across Eurasia. In many ways, reindeer herding serves as a good model for the initial stages of domestication of other prey pathway domesticates like sheep and goats, and provides a unique opportunity to examine how domestication involves more than bodily changes in animals produced through selection (Røed *et al.* 2008, Zeder 2012, Losey *et al.* 2021). The process of reindeer domestication mainly included breeding for characteristics that make the animals easier to gather and handle, as well as enskilment where both people and reindeer learn new skills when engaging with each other (Skarin and Åhman 2014, Losey *et al.* 2021).

It is uncertain when and where reindeer domestication began. However, the long-term relationship between *Rangifer* and humans is documented across the Arctic region including Canadian Barren lands, Siberia, Northern Europe, and Ice-Age France. The transition to domestication is indicated by the Iron and Bronze Age petroglyphs and pictographs (Gordon 2003). There are two hypotheses about the origin of reindeer domestication. According to the monocentric diffusion theory, domestic reindeer first appeared a few thousand years ago east of the Urals in the southern part of the Siberian taiga from where they spread to other regions. On the other hand, proponents of the polycentric hypothesis argue that the domestication of reindeer occurred independently multiple times in different parts of Eurasia (Gordon 2003, Røed *et al.* 2008). The genetic analyses showed independent origins of domestic reindeer in Russia and Fennoscandia, and possibly also in Eastern Russia from the wild Eurasian tundra reindeer (*R tarandus tarandus*) most likely as the common ancestor (Røed *et al.* 2008, Weldenegodguad *et al.* 2020). Small-scale reindeer herding characterized by interspecies sociality, cooperation, and care developed during the Late Iron Age, with regional variations in the timing and details of the events (Salmi 2023). The earliest and most convincing artifact evidence for reindeer domestication comes from Ust'-Polui, an Iron Age archaeological site located within the modern city of Salekhard in Iamal (Arctic Siberia) dating from ca. 260 BCE to 140 CE. The artefactual evidence such as nine barbed L-shaped objects and several forms of swivel all made of antlers recovered from the site are considered by the present-day reindeer herders of Iamal and adjacent regions as the parts of headgear used for training young reindeer to pull sledges. It is argued that some of these objects were utilized for training young reindeer repeatedly for transport in the Yamal peninsula beginning at least 2,000 BP (Losey *et al.* 2021, Nomokonova *et al.* 2021). The North Eurasians domesticated reindeer for transport, meat, hide, milk, and medicine. In some cultures, reindeer were also saddled and ridden (Gordon 2003). Reindeer were crucial for the colonization of the northernmost parts of the region and have a central symbolic role in several indigenous cultures of Northern Eurasia (Weldenegodguad *et al.*2020). The spiritual influence of reindeer on people appears in taboos, legends, and art including wall and cave paintings. Also, *Rangifer* is reported to regulate human birth space through its seasonal availability and seasonal fat content (Gordon 2003).

Reindeer herding is still an essential way of life for people in much of northern Eurasia from Mongolia in the east through the Siberian tundra and taiga zones to the northern parts of Finland, Sweden, and Norway (Salmi 2023). Though many indigenous people have disappeared, nearly thirty reindeer herder groups exist across Eurasia with great variability in husbandry practices and purposes for the herding. For example, in the Sámi reindeer-herding area in northern Fennoscandia, the reindeer herding is generally extensive and animals move freely in the landscape for most of the year. Sámi herders used small domestic herds as decoys for hunting wild reindeer and for milking. Only some domestic reindeer were used for pulling sledges carrying freight. In Siberia, large herds composed of thousands of animals were common. The Tungusic people use reindeer only as pack or saddle animals, and occasionally both for riding and drawing sledges, particularly by the Northern group (Pelletier *et al.* 2020). Following the introduction of the snowmobile in the 1960s, reindeer are not used as frequently for transporting people and goods. However, reindeer have been rediscovered in new roles including as a valuable resource in the tourist industry, particularly by those companies that organize reindeer safaris. The reindeer is also used for racing in some parts of the world (Mazzullo 2020, Pelletier 2020). In many acratic pastoralist cultures like the Nentsy, reindeer continue to mean everything in all spheres of life. Nenets reindeer herders protect their animals from birth onwards, and reindeer, in turn, serve people as guides and teachers, as a means of transport, as sacrifice, as a vehicle for spiritual communication, and provide food, clothing, and housing. Even though fish enjoys broader popularity as a commodity than reindeer meat and can be economically more important than reindeer, the Nentsy still associate themselves mainly with reindeer, which they consider to be the highest prestige animal and the supreme property. Fishing is less prestigious than herding among the Nenets. These pastoralists value the reindeer as the supreme property (Stammler 2020).

Rabbit Domestication: Rabbit (*Oryctolagus cuniculus*), is amongst the most recently domesticated animals. It is the only *Lagomorph* species to have been domesticated (Clutton-Brock 1999). The European rabbit (*Oryctolagus cuniculus*), native to the Iberian Peninsula, is the single recognized progenitor of domestic rabbits. *Oryctolagus cuniculus* comprises two subspecies; *O. c. algirus,* which is found in the southwestern Iberian Peninsula, and *O. c. cuniculus* present in the northeastern Iberian Peninsula and France. The subspecies *O. c. cuniculus* is the possible direct source from which almost all the domesticated rabbit breeds including the English lop, the Angora rabbits, and the New Zealand white rabbit, have developed (Carneiro *et al.* 2011, Somerville and Sugiyama 2021).

Archaeological and biological research has provided evidence for thousands of years of interactions between humans and leporids (rabbits and hares) across the world (Somerville and Sugiyama 2021). The first written account of this interaction is provided by the Phoenicians (1100 BCE), who on reaching the shores of Spain, found wild rabbits (*Oryctolagus cuniculus*) in southern Europe. They may have named the place *I-Sephan-im* (land of rabbits), which was subsequently Latinized as *Hispania*, and began trading rabbits from Spain along the entire Mediterranean coastline (Sandford 1992, Dalle Zotte 2014)). Many ancient writings refer to both hare and rabbit and differentiate them. Polybius (ca. 204 – 122 BCE) called rabbit *kunikloi* and stated that the rabbit indeed at a distance looks like a small hare; but when taken in the hand, it is found to be widely different both in appearance and in the taste of its flesh; and it also lives generally underground. Roman author and satirist Marcus Terentius Varro (116 – 27 BCE) referred to the rabbit as the third variety of hare, found in Spain, which resembles in some measure our Italian hare, but it stands low. This is called cuniculus. Pliny the Elder (ca. 23-79 AD) mentions rabbit as a species of hare, in Spain, which is called cuniculus; it is extremely prolific, and produces famine in the Balearic Islands, by destroying the harvests. He also writes about the delicacy of rabbit meat as young ones, either when cut from out of the body of the mother, or taken from the breast, without having the entrails removed, are considered a most delicate food; they are then called laurices (Sandford 1992). Archaeological evidence demonstrates thousands of years of human–rabbit interactions in North America, particularly at the ancient city of Teotihuacan (ca.1–550 CE) in central Mexico where several studies suggest practices of rabbit management by humans. The rabbit was an important source of food for farming communities across Canada, the United States, and Mexico (Somerville and Sugiyama 2021).

While archaeological evidence indicates extensive exploitation of rabbits for meat during the Epipaleolithic, Mesolithic, and early Neolithic periods in the Iberian Peninsula and southwest France, there is no clear indication of their domestication. Rabbit bones, being fragile and small, are frequently destroyed and rearranged by predators, making it challenging to trace the origin and evolution of rabbits (Lukefahr *et al.* 2022). It is suggested that domestic rabbits likely originated from wild European rabbits, possibly through a directed pathway. The wild ancestors remained confined to the Iberian Peninsula, Southern France, and potentially North Africa from the end of the Pleistocene until the Roman period (Irving-Pease *et al.* 2018). Based on ancient records, Sandford (1992) concluded that rabbit domestication began around 2,000 years ago by the Romans. Even before domestication, humans transported rabbits from one location to another, where they established populations. However, some scholars argue that while the Romans facilitated the spread of rabbits out of Spain, they did not attempt to breed rabbits in captivity (Clutton-Brock 1999). Since no selective breeding was implemented, this may not be considered a genuine domestication. The most widely cited theory suggests that rabbit domestication was initiated by French monks around 600 CE, as a result of an edict by Pope Gregory the Great allowing Christians to consume newborn or foetal rabbits (laurices) during Lent, as they were not considered meat (Irving-Pease *et al.* 2019). The genetic structure of domestic rabbits further suggested a single origin of domestication in wild populations from France (Carneiro *et al.* 2011).

More recently, doubts have emerged regarding this widely cited opinion. According to *Encyclopedia Britannica*, a convergence of fossil and written records, along with DNA analysis, suggests that the domestication of rabbits likely originated between the retreat of the ice sheets and the 1st century BCE in southwestern Europe. Given that domestication is contingent upon multiple natural and human-driven factors working in tandem rather than a singular discrete event, the process of rabbit domestication likely unfolded over hundreds, if not thousands, of years. (Smith 2024). Rabbits were first intentionally transported across Europe in the northeast Atlantic in the Middle Ages when they were considered a high-status food. After the 18th century, European rabbits were introduced to other parts of the world including parts of Chile and Argentina, Australia, New Zealand, North America, and South Africa (Carneiro *et al.* 2011, Irving-Pease *et al.* 2018, Smith 2024). Although several varieties of different sizes and coat colours were recorded in rabbits in Europe by the 16th century, the development of most rabbit breeds has occurred during the last 200 years (Irving-Pease *et al.* 2018).

Today, rabbit farming is one of the most popular animal production systems in the world comprising 158.417 million rabbits and hares. There are more than 50 established strains of domestic rabbits, all selectively bred from one species for different purposes (Smith 2024). As a farm animal, rabbits are bred mainly to produce meat, fur, and wool. The rabbit and hare meat production reached 756,476 tonnes in 2022, which was 15.1% less than 861,739.35 tonnes produced in the previous year (https://www.fao.org/faostat/en/#data/QCL, accessed on 18-01-2024). However, rabbit farming for commercial meat production has considerable potential, particularly in developing countries facing population pressures and acute food shortages. The abundance of local vegetation that cannot be consumed directly by humans can be fed to rabbits in many of these countries. Also, rabbits have a staggering reproductive potential and can be bred throughout the year with significant feasibility of post-partum breeding. Another advantage of rabbits is their small size, rendering them suitable for small-scale and backyard farming by using weeds, tropical forages, vegetable tops, and table scraps as rabbit feed. Rabbits act as biological refrigerators because the meat from one animal can be consumed without the need for storage (Lukefarh *et al.* 2022). Rabbit meat offers excellent dietary nutritional properties. It contains high levels of essential amino acids and a significant proportion of long-chain PUFA. Rabbit meat is rich in lysine and sulphur-containing amino acids (Dalle Zotte 2014). Angora wool produced by rabbits is soft in touch and has good absorption of water. It is used to produce luxury knitted cloth items such as pullovers, scarves, socks, and gloves (Galbraith 2019). The best quality rabbit skin is used to make high-priced luxurious fur garments and is used in various apparel items like fur coats. Other skins are used to produce garments for children, toys, and felt hats. The glue made from shredded rabbit skins is especially strong, and is used mainly in furniture manufacturing (Lukefarh *et al.* 2022).

Rabbits are traditionally used as experimental animals for biomedical and fundamental research. Classical experimental use of rabbits includes antibody production, development of new surgical techniques, physiology, and toxicity studies for the testing of new drugs, nutritional studies, and study of human diseases (Bosze and Houdebine 2006, Lukefarh *et al.* 2022). Different transgenic rabbit models have been developed to study hypertrophic cardiomyopathy as small rodents like mice fail to accurately reflect some crucial features of human cardiovascular physiology. Also, the rabbit is the smallest animal that can be used to produce recombinant proteins in its milk or serum both on an experimental and a commercial scale (Bosze and Houdebine 2006). The attractive appearance, quiet manner, and easy management make the rabbit a fine pet for children and numerous breeds are raised specifically for this purpose. A special bond exists between children and rabbits. The rabbit is a very popular animal mainly through children›s literature and creative arts. It elicits positive feelings in children and enhances their imagination. The rabbit can also be used as an alternate animal species and complementary therapy for many diseases. It is an intelligent, friendly, and playful small animal, which is easily socialized and transported. It possesses very good communication through its body language (Loukaki 2010). In general, the domestic rabbit today is not only economically important as a farm animal, but also a valuable experimental animal model for biomedical research as well as a pet and therapy animal.

Avian Domestication: The chronology of avian domestication is divided roughly into three main epochs. The first epoch (Ancient) manifests the incipient stages of domestication. During this epoch, people of the ancient high cultures, who had domesticated mammals like sheep and goats a few millennia earlier, began domesticating the greylag goose (*Anser anser*), the rock dove (*Columba livia*) and the chicken (*Gallus gallus*) — the earliest bird species to be domesticated. Other avian species domesticated in this period comprised the swan goose (*Anser cygnoides*) in East Asia, the Muscovy duck (*Cairina moschata*), and the turkey (*Meleagris gallopaco*) in Central America, the helmeted guineafowl (*Numida meleagris*) in the Mediterranean area, the Indian peafowl (*Pavo cristatus*) in India; the ring-necked pheasant (*Phasianus colchicus*), the silver pheasant (*Lophura nycthemera*), and Bengalese finch (*Lonchura striata*) and the Java finch (*Padda oryzivora*), as pets in East Asia (Sossinka 1982).

Histological, geochemical, biochemical, and morphological analysis and conventional findings point out that the domestication of geese happened ca. 7,000 years ago in the lower Yangtze River in China, making gees the oldest domesticated poultry species (Eda *et al.* 2022). The domestication of chicken took place in at least two geographical regions involving several subspecies of Red Junglefowl (RJF) from South and South East and surrounding areas including India (Tixier-Boichard *et al.* 2011, Al-Qamashoui *et al.* 2014). Genetic evidence from Indian RJF populations also corroborated the multiple domestication of modern chicken occurring independently in different locations in Asia including India (Kanginakudru *et al.* 2008). Mitochondrial genome (mtDNA) analysis of local chickens from the Arabian Peninsula revealed that the most frequently observed haplotypes from the Arabian Peninsula (and Socotra) clustered in clade E originated on the Indian subcontinent (Al-Qamashoui *et al.* 2014). Some recent studies indicated that chickens were likely domesticated from the *G. g. spadiceus* subspecies of RJF in the Holocene in peninsular Southeast Asia and from there they dispersed south into Islands and west across Asia to Africa and Europe (Wang *et al.* 2020, Peters *et al.* 2022). Gallinaceous birds have an attraction for cereal grains. Most likely, the wild ancestors of these earliest domesticated birds were attracted to the human niche by kitchen scraps, animal dung, and the year-long availability of cultivated cereals like millet and rice, leading to their domestication via commensal pathway (Larson and Fuller 2014, Irving-Pease *et al.* 2018, Peters *et al.* 2022).

The second Epoch from middle age to the present, was marked by the global spread of ancient domesticated birds and the domestication of the Japanese quail (*Coturnix coturnix*) in Japan in the 17th Century and the successful breeding of Temminck's Cormorant in captivity in China. The Helmeted Guineafowl that probably became extinct in captivity at least in Europe was domesticated again. The turkey and Muscovy ducks which had been domesticated in Central America were introduced into Europe, and domesticated avian species that were bred in Europe were introduced to North America (Sossinku 1982). The Mexican turkey transported to Europe in the early 16th century by the Spanish spread quickly across the continent with an estimated rate of 40-50 km per year (Crawford 1992).

The third and the last Epoch of avian domestication began a century ago and is currently progressing with the unprecedented growth of the domestic avian farming system comprising an increase in the number of newly domesticated species and a significant increase in the number of different breeds within a species in some cases. Several new species that underwent successful domestication during the present epoch consist of the ostrich (*Struthio camelus*), the budgerigar (*Melopsittacus undulatus*), and the zebra finch (*Taeniopygia guttata castanotis*), cockatiel (*Nymphicus hollandicus*), red-rumped parrot (*Psephotus haematonotus*), Bourke's parrot (*Neophema bourkii*), peach-faced lovebird (*Agapornis roseicollis*), diamond dove (*Geopelia cuneata*), golden pheasant (*Chrysolophus pictus*), lady Amherst's pheasant (*Chrysolophus amherstiae*), California Quail (*Callipepla californica*), painted quail (*Coturnix chinensis*), Canada goose (*Branta canadensis*), wood duck (*Aix sponsa*), and several other species of avian families (Sossinku 1982).

Relationships between humans and birds go back several millennia. Humans exploited various species for many different purposes including as a source of meat and eggs for food, skins and feathers for clothing, egg shells, and feathers as well as whole taxidermized birds as decorative items, and feathers as quill, pens or as fletching for arrows and darts. Bones of birds have been used to make musical instruments, fish hooks, and other artifacts. Tamed birds assisted in hunting small mammals, and other wild birds and catching fish (Anderson 2010). Ancient Egyptians used ostrich egg shells as water carriers, and when broken for making jewellery (Wilkinson 2011). The precise aims of the ancient people for maintaining and breeding birds are not known. Probably, breeding birds provided a permanent supply of highly palatable flesh, eggs, grease, and other usable products and bred for aesthetic purposes. The chicks of waterfowl and junglefowl were kept as pets, releasing care-taking reactions in humans by their appearance. Birds are also thought to have been used for religious sacrifice; for that purpose, white varieties may have been selected at a very early phase of domestication (Sossinku 1982). Domestic pigeons (*Columba livia domestica*) were bred for the homing trait, inherited from the wild ancestor, to serve as a messenger for rapid communication. The messenger pigeons or mail pigeons were used in many places around the world to carry messages and have played a crucial role in post-services (pigeon-post), and in war (war pigeon) for thousands of years from ancient times till the current century. They have been critical to military intelligence during wartime and are credited with saving many human lives (Anderson 2010). The use of messenger pigeons declined after the advent of modern communication systems.

Birds have occupied a privileged place in the art, literature, tradition, religions, myths, and beliefs across cultures throughout the human history. Freedom and airy flight of birds made them often to symbolize the immortal human soul. Birds of many species appear in Christian art as soul symbols. The ancient Egyptians conceived the human being as comprising multiple components, most notably a visible human-headed bird, the *ba*, and the ineffable and, if free from sin, weightless *ka*. The soul bird, the *ba,* could fly to the heavens, leaving the body at death and returning at will. There are numerous myths in which birds speak to human beings, issuing warnings, carry messages, or conveying knowledge (Werness 2004). In several ancient cultures and tradition, birds are regarded as messengers of the god, purity, transformation, and wisdom. The ancient Egyptian god of wisdom and reason (truth, knowledge, learning and study, and writing and mathematics) has ibis's head. The sacred ibis was considered the living incarnation of *Thoth* on earth and the desperate search for wisdom led the Egyptians to mummify and bury up to two million birds at Saqqara alone. To keep pace with demand, ibises were bred on an industrial scale on the shores of nearby Lake *Abusir* and at other farms throughout Egypt. At *Khmun*, the principal cult centre of Thoth, a vast area was devoted to feeding the flocks of birds. When they died, even the tiniest parts of them — individual feathers, nest material, and fragments of eggshell were carefully gathered up for sale and burial (Wilkinson 2011). Muscovy ducks were significant in ancient Aztec culture. Aztec rulers wore cloaks made from the feathers of the Muscovy Duck, which was considered the totem animal of the Wind God, Ehecatl (https://thepeasantsdaughter.net/muscovy-ducks/). The dove has symbolized deliverance of God's forgiveness, and peace since ancient times. It remains one of the most recognizable icons as a symbol of peace in the modern world (Jerolmack 2007).

Birds are generally sensitive to their environment and have been frequently used as sentinel species to measure the levels and adverse effects of pollution. Till the last century, coal miners in the UK, USA, and Canada used canaries in coal mines as a sentinel for toxic gases, particularly carbon monoxide. Some of the classic examples of birds serving as sentinel to harmful effects of environmental pollution include the peregrine and other bird species that have acted as sentinel species for the harmful environmental effects of organochlorine (Furness 1993), discovery of the *Yushō* disease following alarming death rate in chicken due to polychlorinated biphenyl poisoning in Japan (Kuratsune *et al.* 1972), and potential residual toxicity due to diclofenac identified as cause of rapid decline in vulture populations across the South Asia. Captive and free-ranging birds such as chickens, house sparrows, and pigeons have also been used for decades as living sentinels in arbovirus surveillance programs (Komar 2001). Large numbers of birds, mostly domestic fowls, are used in biomedical research mainly to evaluate the pharmacokinetics and test the safety of drugs and vaccines designed to treat other birds. Smaller numbers of birds are also used as animal models for human diseases and disorders as well as for fundamental research or to evaluate the effects of substances on wild and domestic birds, for example in the safety testing of agricultural substances, industrial substances, toxicants, and additives for animal feeds. Genetically altered fowls are used for the expression of pharmacologically important substances in their eggs, and genetic studies to develop poultry resistant to diseases like avian influenza (Girling 2010).

Early people domesticated chicken for aesthetic, socio-cultural, and /or pure pleasure because of its beautiful plumage and fighting abilities, especially for the popular sport of cockfighting (Sossinku 1982, Keeling 2002, Lawal and Hanotte 2021). The domestic fowl is known for its fighting ability and was preferred for this trait in the early phase of domestication. The aims and methods of breeders changed substantially in the subsequent time and domestic chickens were used for meat and egg production. Ancient Romans though kept chickens for cockfighting, they had a well-developed poultry industry with breeds selected for high egg production (Keeling 2002). Except for a few countries, cockfighting is now prohibited globally and only small numbers of chickens are kept for sport and ornamental purposes. Most chickens are presently raised to produce meat (broiler chickens) or eggs (laying hens) worldwide (Millman *et al.* 2010).

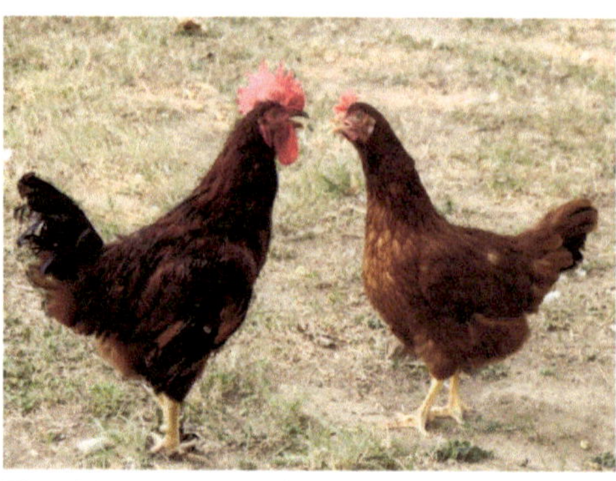

Fig. 1.7: *Domestic chicken is by far the most numerous and ubiquitous farmed species (Photo courtesy of Dr. A.K. Tiwari, ICAR-CARI).*

Domestic birds raised for eggs, meat, and feathers are referred to as poultry covering a wide range of avian species including indigenous and commercial breeds of chickens, geese, ducks, turkeys, guinea fowl, and pigeons (Eda *et al.* 2022). The rapidly growing, modern poultry sector is an important segment of the global animal production system with a crucial contribution to food security and the commercial livestock industry all over the world. The domestic chicken (Fig. 1.7), considered either a subspecies of Red Junglefowl (*G. g. domesticus*) or a separate species, *G. domesticus* (Kanakachari *et al.* 2023), accounted for ~ 92.9% of the world's poultry population followed by ducks (4.2%), turkeys (1.5%), and geese and other birds (1.3 %) (Eda *et al.* 2022). In 2022, the estimated number of chickens (26.561643 billion) was 17 times more than the cattle (1.5515156 billion), the most widely distributed mammalian livestock. The other poultry species included 1.126276 billion ducks, 255.76 million turkeys, and 366.478 million geese globally with an annual production of 123.63 million, 6.06 million, 5.08 million, 4.42 million, and 18,669.43 tonnes of fresh and chilled meat of chickens, ducks, turkeys, geese, and pigeons, respectively, and ~87 million tonnes and ~6 million tonnes eggs of hens and other domestic birds, respectively. (https://www.fao.org/faostat/en/#data/QCL, accessed on 01-02-2024). Large-scale breeding programmes have resulted in more than sixty chicken breeds representing four genealogical groups: egg, game, and meat-varieties along with bantamweight breeds (Moiseyeva *et al.* 2003). Ducks usually forage on aquatic weeds, algae, green legumes, fungi, earthworms, maggots, snails, and various types of insects (Padhi and Giri 2024). As such, rearing ducks is recommended as an effective biological control strategy for pest control and the snail-borne helminthic parasites such as *Fasciola, Paramphistomum,* and *Schistosomes*, thereby reducing the incidence of parasitic diseases in livestock.

Keeping birds as pets is an age-old practice. In the past, bird-keeping was predominantly a pastime for the wealthy, involving relatively low numbers of birds. Today, keeping birds as pets is one of the highly popular hobbies and is an expression of social status in many countries driving a growing and lucrative pet trade. An enormous trade and economy exist around keeping cage birds, particularly in developing countries such as Brazil, Mexico, and South Africa, and across China and Southeast Asia. It is reported that more than one million birds belonging to over a thousand species are legally traded annually around the world (Butchart 2008, Cassey *et al.* 2015, Dyer *et al.* 2017). Psychological studies focusing on the personality of bird owners or the therapeutic advantages of pet bird ownership showed that compared to horse owners, bird owners were better on the affiliation, nurturance, and nurturant parent scales. Avian companionship is qualitatively like that provided by cats and dogs. Social workers and other healthcare professionals believe that birds as pets help many people to lead healthier, happier lives (Anderson, 2003).

Outcomes and Sociocultural Significance of Human– Domestic Animal Relationships

Animal husbandry had a profound impact on the human lifestyle heralding an evolutionary change in the history of human civilization through changing the subsistence pattern of the hunter-gatherer culture of early men to a sedentary agricultural lifestyle ultimately giving rise to the formation of complex societies (Frantz *et al.* 2020). The animals, which were the sources of food, slowly assumed more diverse roles in agrarian societies to become the most crucial component for the onset and advancement of ancient civilizations across the world. The domestication of plants and animals stands as one of the most monumental changes in history, transforming the primary economic activity of early communities from food collection to food production, thereby enabling a steady food supply, introducing new sources of labour, and fostering companionship and protection. Animals also became integral to religious practices and symbolism. While closely linked with agriculture, many pastoral societies specialized in raising livestock without farming. Livestock further ensured food security in unstable environments and harsh climates, from Siberia and Mongolia to the deserts of Africa, and were highly valued in social customs such as bride price and gift exchanges (DeMello 2021). In general, the mutualistic relationship between man and domestic animals benefitted people in many ways leading to the growing importance of living animals to human society. At the same time, domestic animals helped shape human history and influenced socio-ecological, cultural, religious, political, economic, health, and almost all other aspects of human life. Humans in many ancient cultures were much dependent on their domestic animals for daily life activities.

Early Zoocentric Societies and Socio-Cultural Impacts of Domestic Animals

Domestic animals played a significant role in many ancient societies and assumed prominent place in art, tradition, symbolism, mythology, cosmology, kin relations, and social organizations. As the significance and value of livestock increased, the attitude of people towards animals changed. This was associated with the evolution of early human societies that were highly zoocentric. In these societies, a particular animal species influenced human life and attained a prominent place in spiritual beliefs and religious teachings, traditional practices, symbolism, and almost all other aspects of human life. The sheep was the first livestock and an early pastoralist zoocentric society of sheep-culture people likely evolved in the Fertile Crescent and from there spread to other ancient societies and civilizations (Schwabe 1978). Sheep was valued not only for economic reasons, but was involved in symbolism and worshipped as founders of wealth, order, and civilizations. Sirtur the Ewe is the goddess of flocks in Sumerian, Babylonian, and Akkadian mythology; and in the ancient Egyptian religion, the ram was the symbol of gods—Khnum and Heryshaf, while the great god of sun and air, Amun, was often depicted as a Ram-headed sphinx (Coulthard 2020).

Almost all great ancient civilizations were built by the bull-cow culture people. Cattle herding was an important occupation for the ancient Egyptians, Canaanites-Phoenicians, and Babylonians, who anthropomorphized and transformed the cattle as an object of worship (Zoolatry*[1]) giving rise to bull-cow god worshipping cattle-culture societies in which cattle signified wealth, power, and fertility (Schwabe 1994, Swabe 1999). Although both sheep herding and cattle herding people entered the fertile crescent, cattle herders discovered agriculture and built the towns (Schwabe 1978). The bull cults were popular in Ancient Egypt, from at least the First Dynasty. The people worshipped a great number of deities, who were either depicted entirely in cattle form or represented with bovine features like horns or ears. The bull god Apis was believed to be the incarnation of the creator god Ptah. The cow was sacred as the Mother of Apis and the incarnation of the goddess Isis and the cow goddess Hathor (Wilkinson 2011). The iconic Narmer Palette, a founding document of Ancient Egypt commissioned during the first dynasty (~3000 BCE), is decorated on both sides with a carving of a human face having bovine ears and highly curved horns. It is thought to represent the cow goddess Bat and Hathor (Wengrow 2001). The supreme Akkadian god Anu from *Uruk* was called the bull of heaven; the moon god shin was represented with bull horns and frequently referred to as the young bullock. The Babylonian main god of healing magicians, the Marduk was originally Amarutu (k), the young bull of the sun. An early interaction between the Ancient Egyptian and early Neolithic tribes promoted the Cattle culture in Northeast Africa (Schwabe 1978).

Domesticated cattle and their secondary products played a central economic role in supporting agricultural systems in Bronze Age Anatolia. The emerging elite class, situated at the apex of society used cattle as a material and symbolic source of power

*[1]Zoolatry: Sometimes spelled zooalotry: refers to the worship or veneration of animals, often regarding them as sacred beings

(Arbuckle 2014). For the Proto-Indo-European speakers, the cattle were symbols of the generosity of Gods and the productivity of the earth. They believed that humans were created from primordial cows. The cattle were held in high esteem comparable to sons. Cattle, sheep, and probably horses would have been used by these people as gifts to Gods and to pay bride-prices (Anthony 2007: p135, 139). Cattle was also of great significance in European culture. Cattle find a prominent place in Indus Valley seals and terracotta figurines, as well as in Vedic and post-Vedic writings. It is represented in almost 75% of Indus Valley terracotta figurines (Eraly 2002). Cows and bulls were not only economically important but had ritualistic, sacrificial, and cosmological contexts in ancient Indian societies, which were believed to be a part of cattle culture. India is the largest cattle culture that remains to date (Thrusfield 2018). It is commented that literally and figuratively human civilization rode into old world on the back of cows (Albright and Arave 1997).

While cattle remained the most prominent livestock in Egypt and many other ancient civilizations, the domestication of horses on the vast grassland Steppes of Eurasia resulted in the emergence of a new kind of culture in which everything in life centred on the horse (Guler 2016). The event transformed the future not only of equines but human history as well. The domestication of horses provided an impetus to cultural, technological, and military evolution, which otherwise would have been much slower had humans plodded on donkey backs and ox-driven carts. Endowed with the endurance and stamina of horses, the horse-culture people could travel faster and increasingly long distances to trade and conquest than ever before, ultimately converting the Eurasian steppes into a thriving intercontinental corridor of commercial, and cultural exchange including the dispersion of innovative advanced ancient technologies of copper mining, warfare, and patron-client political institution (Anthony 2007: p. 460).

The horse-culture spread swiftly across the most ancient civilizations in Europe, the Near East, Central and South Asia including China and India. The dependency on horses in these societies for numerous tasks became so profound that it no longer seemed possible to think of a society to perform without them (Willekes 2016). The popularity of the horse in the Bronze Age across the ancient civilizations is reflected in many ancient artworks, manuscripts, myths, beliefs, and symbolism. The horse is represented in Iranian, Greek, and Celtic pantheons (Thrusfield 2018), and is mentioned reverently in Vedic and post-Vedic Indian scriptures. The horse-driven chariot racing on a horseshoe-shaped course was a favourite pastime of Vedic people in India (Eraly 2002, p.148). Rig Veda uses the word *ashva* (horse) over 200 times, indicating that Vedic society must have been full of horses (Danino 2006). The horse was, though used in agricultural works to pull carts and ploughing the land, this species was more the vehicle of warriors than farmers, and ownership of horses was an indicator of wealth and social status (Swabe 1999).

There is a long list of horses by names, who have played vital roles in the life of many historical figures. One of the most notable examples in Indian tradition is found in the story of the Great Departure, one of the major episodes in the life of Lord Buddha. According to Buddhist legends, *Kanthaka* (Fig. 1.8) was the most skilful and able horse of Prince Siddhartha Gautam (6th century BCE), who carried the bodhisattva (the buddha-to-be) away in the middle of the night from the lavished and pampered life of the palace and kingdom into his true destiny as the Buddha (Chandra 2022). Once the Bodhisattva has renounced the world, *Kanthaka* returns to the kingdom and bears the brunt of the emotional reactions of the Bodhisattva's loved ones. The *Mahāvastu* recounts that *Kanthaka* overwhelmed by sorrow, eventually starved himself to death (Ohnuma 2017). Across cultures, many other famed horses have also become legendary: *Bucephalus*, the horse of Alexander the Great; *Babieca*, the warhorse of El Cid (Rodrigo Díaz de Vivar), the Castilian knight and ruler of medieval Spain; *Incitatus*, the favourite horse of the Roman emperor Caligula; *Llamrei*, the mare owned by the legendary King Arthur of Britain; *Chetak*, the loyal warhorse of Maharana Pratap; *Marengo*, the famed steed of Napoleon Bonaparte; and *Nelson* and *Blueskin*, the favoured mounts of George Washington during the American Revolutionary War (https://en.wikipedia.org/wiki/List_of_historical_horses, accessed on 19-02-2024).

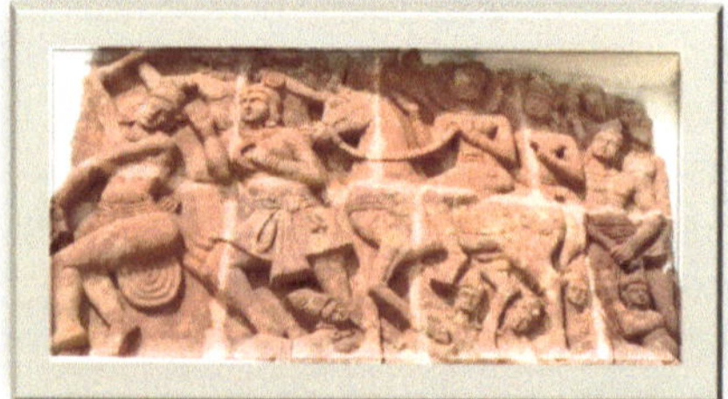
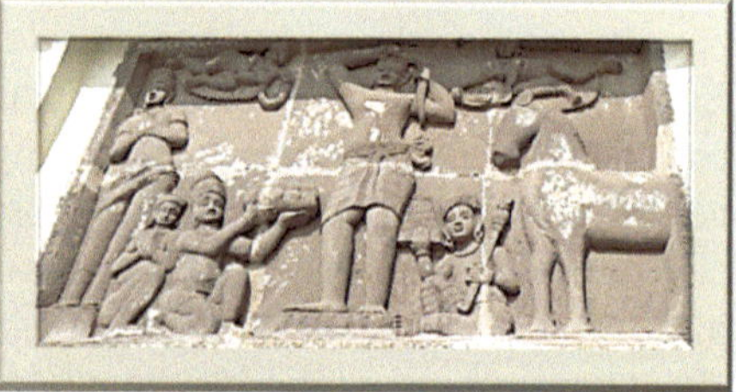

***Fig 1.8.** Carved stone panels on outer wall of Shanti Stupa (Dhauli, Odisha) featuring noble steed Kanthaka in 'the great departure' episode (Photo by the Author).*

Secondary Animal Product Revolution and Animal Draught Power

Almost all livestock species were domesticated initially for meat purposes. They were slaughtered young. The secondary animal products or products obtained from living animals (antemortem products named by some scholars) such as wool, dairy foods, traction power, and transport were discovered later. These instantly became the most sought-after animal products leading to the secondary animal products revolution (SPR). The SPR had profound effects on human economies across the Old World and increased both the economic value and the political importance of livestock (Anthony and Brown 2011).

Animal traction power, particularly, provided great impetus to the advancement of human civilizations. The bullock, horse, camel, donkey, buffalo, elephant, reindeer, and yak are the major draught animals used for agricultural operations, travel, trade, transport, and warfare. Sumerian pictograms and cylinder seals dating from the end of the fourth millennium BCE provide the first recorded use of cattle power in agriculture. Asses, donkeys, and later camels were harnessed and used as beasts of burden, although their meat and milk were also consumed long before they began to perform these roles in human society. Such pack animals could be used to transport agricultural produce over considerable distances and made trading with neighbouring or distant communities much easier (Swabe 1999). In *The History of Agriculture in India* (Vol.1 pp. 183-84), Randhawa (1980) observed that the working power of domestic animals was probably more important than their food value, and the degree of development of an ancient civilization is closely related to the relative efficiency of the domestic animals available in the country concerned. The Red Indians of North America, and Aboriginals of Australia, who had no draught animals remained in the primitive hunting stage for centuries when other civilizations with available domestic animal power progressed far ahead. The South American civilizations who domesticated llamas and alpacas were ahead of their kinsmen in North America, but lagged the Mesopotamian, Egyptian, and Indian Civilizations having working animals such as bullocks, asses, horses, camels, and elephants, which were more efficient than llamas and the alpacas. The draught animals relieved man of drudgery and provided him with surplus food, creating a leisure class of humans, who could think and imagine higher things. Thus, the domestication of animals provided a conducive milieu, in which ancient practices, and the quest for knowledge on different aspects such as art, literature, science, and philosophies flourished in human societies. As described in *The Horse, the Wheel, and Language,* the domestication of cattle and sheep changed life in the Neolithic Pontic-Caspian environment. The cattle and sheep were part of everyday work. Humans identified with their cattle and sheep, wrote poetry about them, and used them as currency for gifts, payment of debt, and calculation of social status. On the other side, because cattle and sheep could be easily stolen, unlike grain crops, cattle-raising people tend to have problems with thieves, leading to conflict and warfare (Anthony 2007: pp. 137-38).

Early Animal Husbandry Practices, Skills, Technologies, and Knowledge Base

Domestication of animals was associated with the invention and development of early animal husbandry practices, skills, and technologies, and the evolution of experience-based traditional knowledge on different aspects of domestic animals. Beginning from the innovative methods to capture and tame the wild ancestors of domestic animals, the next step in the process of domestication was to find the optimal ways to manage and breed the captured herds efficiently to exploit favourable traits of the domesticates. Early animal husbandry practices included selective breeding to reduce aggressiveness and for better production, housing to protect animals, management of herd size, effective grazing and feeding practices, raising newborns with low mortality, shearing, etc. Studies from northeastern Bulgaria on Neolithic cattle farming (ca. 6200-5500 ca. BCE) indicated that the initial rearing of cattle was intended for beef, which subsequently changed to the production of both beef and milk. The husbandry practices were accordingly shifted. Breeding strategies were developed to reduce adult body weight to maintain large herd size without stressing food resources, and to reduce the birth weight of calves to prevent birthing complications. Individual animals were slaughtered at their optimal weight when beef production was the goal. Strategic feeding, housing, and intensive post-lactation slaughter were performed for more milk production, and the calving season was manipulated to minimize calf mortality in winter (Kamjan *et al.* 2021).

Pastoralists were ought to be wise decision-makers with a detailed knowledge of the environment, close familiarity with the seasons and an acute sense of timing, which was essential for maintaining herds. It is believed that the purpose of the standing stones and the calendar circle found at Nabta, an early fifth millennium BCE ancient archaeological site in Egypt, was to predict the arrival of the all-important rains, which was essential for fresh supply of water for cattle and a matter of life and death for the whole community. The community would celebrate arrival of rains by slaughtering some of their precious cattle as a sacrifice of thanks, and burying the animals in graves marked on the surface with large, flat stones. Under one such mound, archaeologists found a huge sandstone monolith that had been carefully shaped and dressed to resemble a cow (Wilkinson 2011). By and large, cattle husbandry was more than the keeping of smaller livestock and required manpower for handling, housing, grazing, and feeding of herds of large animals, which may have contributed to uneven distribution of manpower, ultimately leading to the evolution of novel methods, technologies, and strategies for cattle husbandry and management. The most recent development, prompted by a more industrial approach to animal husbandry and the globalization of human society, has been an expansion of the most productive breeds at the expense of several traditional native germ-plasm (Ajmone-Marsan *et al.* 2010).

Farm implements, ox-driven sledges, and wheeled carts were invented to optimum utilization of bullock power in agriculture, travel, and transport. One of the most significant technological developments in the ancient world was the innovation of wheeled carts using cattle traction. The overall process of the innovation involved putting together various components of wheeled wagons, and training pairs of cattle to move together at the same pace to pull the vehicle. The construction of roads wide enough to drive carts on them was the aftermath of this innovation (Klimscha 2017). Attaching ploughs to the horns of cattle, particularly oxen, proved to be a significant technological advance. It allowed fields to be ploughed and kept fallow with far greater ease. Intensification of agricultural production in ancient Egypt took place to provide fodder for increasing livestock populations, particularly the cattle (Swabe 1999). The cattle culture people were also the first to use one or more of the earliest known surgical procedures namely bull-nose-ringing, castration, and dehorning. Early cattle-herders could have controlled cows easily, but restraining males, especially maturing bull calves, even in the initial stages of domestication would have been problematic, ultimately leading to the invention and use of the above surgical procedures. A bull with a ring in its nose is depicted in The Royal Standard of Ur, one of civilized man's oldest surviving relics (Schwabe 1978). The analysis of an almost complete cow cranium found in the Neolithic site of Champ-Durand in France (3400-3000 BCE) with trepanation in the right frontal bone reveals that Neolithic man honed the techniques of cranial surgery on domestic animals before treating and caring for humans. Possibly the mastery of techniques in cranial surgery shown in the Mesolithic and Neolithic periods was acquired through experimentation on animals. It is also possible that cranial surgery as a practice could have been performed to save the animal, presenting the earliest evidence of veterinary surgical practice (Ramirez Rozzi and Froment 2018).

The first domesticated sheep were not particularly useful for their wool and were raised primarily for meat. Milk soon became a useful secondary product. By 5000 BCE, when farming was the main system of food production for increasing human populations across the ancient societies, a new generation of improved sheep developed for wool, came out of the Fertile Crescent, and spread to Europe, Africa, and rest of Asia. Their breeding, interbreeding, and adaptation to new climates shaped most modern-day breeds. Interestingly, the flow of new generation sheep was not a one-way event, as the herders developed their own unique and successful breeds and returned the unique breeds to Western Asia and Europe for thousands of years via trade routes, war, and conquest. The evolution of wool-producing sheep might have taken place slowly through a series of experiments and accidental mutations. However, once the value of the wool became apparent, new methods and technologies were developed for improving wool production and to improve its efficient collection, including shearing. Five thousand years ago, sheep herders discovered the use of stone scrapers (called tabular scrapers) for shearing, which led to the invention of scissors. The first use of metal shears is recorded in the 5th BCE Babylonian text (Coulthard 2020).

The invention of spoked- two-wheeled light chariots around 4,000 BP and its use for horse-powered transportation is one of the technological landmarks of the ancient era. Horse-back riding was learnt by the beginning of the 4th millennium (Klecel and Martyniuk 2021). Horse-drawn chariots and horseback riding skills compounded with the fast speed of horses, and the evolution of effective training and tools such as saddle, metal bits, and the recurve bow converted horse into a versatile weapon of the war which altered the course of mankind's future (McMiken 1990, Willekes 2016). Noted the author of *The Horse, the Wheel, and Language*

– the horse-driven chariot, the first wheeled vehicle designed entirely for speed, was meant to intimidate the enemy. It required a specially trained team of fast, strong horses. When a squadron of javelin-burling chariot warriors wheeled onto the field of battle, assisted by the clients and soldiers on foot and horseback with axes, spears, and daggers, it was a new, lethal style of fighting that had never been seen before, something that even urban kings soon learned to admire (Anthony 2010). Besides, the use of the horse-driven chariots, light and heavy cavalry was also raised. Strong cavalry units and squadrons of chariots driven by well-trained horses guaranteed success in the war for several centuries during the history of mankind.

Riding also helped in the pastoral economy. A herder on horseback could care for and control larger herds of horses and other livestock more efficiently than he could do on foot with the help of his companion dog (Anthony and Brown 2011). The importance of horses and chariots and the substantial cost and expertise needed for their management led to the development of specialized horse-related professions (Klecel and Martyniuk 2021). Specialized horse trainers and chariot builders spread with the horse trade and riding. Innovative traditional knowledge and concepts also emerged on different aspects of management, breeding (including hybridization to produce mules), foal raising and weaning, feeding, and training of horses for specific purposes (Beawer 2019). Several important writings describing horse training systems, as well as various aspects of equine breeding, management, care, feeding, and cure were developed, many of which are still useful. *The Hittite Training Texts for Chariot Horses* (1350 BCE) written by *Kikkuli,* a master horse trainer (*assussanni*) of *Mittani* (= Hurrian state in northern Mesopotamia and Syria) and his colleagues, is the earliest known document of horse training and management. It contained the earliest written instructions on systematic conditioning, grain feeding, and on interval training of chariot horses. Some of these instructions are comparable to modern ideas and techniques in equine sports medicine and even superior to modern methods of horse training (McMiken 1990, Nyland 1992). Xenophon (ca. 430–354 BCE), an ancient Greek general, historian, philosopher, and equestrian penned *On Horsemanship*, one of the most detailed horse-training manuals of the ancient period. Most of the advice offered by Xenophon is sound and continues to influence horsemanship and training today (Willekes 2016).

Impacts on Human Health and Welfare

Interactions with animals have both favourable and unfavourable effects on human growth, health, and disease occurrence. It is beyond the scope of this chapter to describe all these effects in detail, and only a little scientific information related to the unwanted and beneficial effects of domestic animals on human health and welfare are summarized here.

Adverse Effects: Interaction with domestic animals may affect human health both directly and indirectly. Physical injuries, emergence and transmission of infectious diseases, antimicrobial resistance, and increased risk for non-infectious diseases including cardiovascular diseases (CVD) and allergies to animal products are some of the major negative health effects linked to animal domestication and close human–animal contact.. Animals are a major cause of work-related physical injuries to farmers. On dairy farms animals were involved in 24% to 38% of the accidental injuries to farmers and handlers in different regions of the world (Lindahl *et al.* 2016). Dog bites are one of the major causes of fatal and non-fatal injuries to humans, particularly among children throughout the world. In the United States, dog bites ranked as the 13th leading cause of nonfatal emergency department visits during 2018 (Tuckel and Milczarski 2020). In India, in response to rising dog bite incidents, the Union Government in 2024 proposed restrictions on certain dog breeds, but nationwide enforcement was withdrawn following judicial scrutiny.

Emergence of Infectious Diseases: The origin and evolution of novel infectious diseases in humans is one of the main health concerns associated with the Neolithic revolution involving the domestication of animals. It is not that pre-Neolithic hunter-gatherers were free from infectious diseases. They also suffered from diseases including those caused by pathogens contracted from non-human animals. Scientists argue that usually, human hunters had the greatest chances of killing or trapping old, crippled, or weak wild animals, many of whom might have been infected. Consumption of edible parts from these infected animals or even contact with them might have caused infection in people. For example, it is likely that during the Pleistocene era, cattle herds were affected by tuberculosis, and ingestion of meat from bovines having tuberculosis would have resulted in the possible transfer of infection to humans (Swabe 1999). However, Neolithization considerably increased the risks of infectious diseases. The Neolithic revolution transformed the human lifestyle, health, nutrition, population, and fertility. As compared to hunter-gatherers, the Neolithic man lived longer and the human population grew by 60 % post-Neolithization. The density of human populations also increased. The large dense human populations were necessary for the evolution and persistence of human crowd diseases, and large populations of domestic animals, with which farmers came into much closer and more frequent contact than hunter-gatherers had with wild animals, generated greater risks for transmission of zoonotic pathogens to man. Analysis of scientific information indicated that 60 % of the 202 emerging human infectious diseases (EID) events that occurred during 1940-2002 were zoonoses. Out of them, 74 (36.6 %) of the 202 were associated with livestock and 128 (63.4%) involved wildlife, pets/recreational animals, and environmental sources (Otte and Pica-Ciamarra 2021). Domestic animals serve as reservoirs and intermediate hosts for many pathogens and are efficient conduits for the transfer of several pathogens from wild animals to humans. For example, bats are the primary reservoir hosts for Nipah and SARS viruses, and humans acquire these viruses from intermediate hosts like domestic pigs and wild animals sold for food. Most probably, the pathogens of diseases like diphtheria, influenza A, measles, mumps, pertussis, rotavirus, smallpox, and tuberculosis likely reached humans from domestic animals (Wolfe *et al.* 2007). Further, humans can get rabies infection directly from bats, but more than 99% of rabies cases in humans occur from infection with dog rabies viruses (RABV) that circulates in dogs (Bourhy *et al.* 2008). Pet animals may also be a source of zoonotic infection and in the absence of proper care and preventive measures can pose a serious risk to public health with huge economic consequences. Dogs and cats are the reservoirs of a wide range of parasitic zoonoses such as toxocariasis, giardiasis, toxoplasmosis, cryptosporidiosis, leishmaniasis, echinococcosis, and dirofilariasis. In the absence of proper care and preventive measures, dog faeces harbouring infective parasitic forms (larvae, eggs, cysts of helminths, and oocysts of protozoan) are potential sources of environmental contamination, representing a high risk of infection for people (Pal *et al.* 2023). Other common pet-borne infections include ringworm, campylobacteriosis, salmonellosis, leptospirosis, yersiniosis and rotavirus (Kantere *et al.* 2014).

Antimicrobial Resistance: Antimicrobial resistance (AMR) represents one of the major global health challenges, posing a great risk to human health. Unscrupulous or exuberant antimicrobial usage is the major driver contributing to the unabated spread of AMR. Modern husbandry and veterinary practices are also associated with the emergence of AMR. In veterinary practice, antibiotics are amongst the most used veterinary pharmaceuticals. These are not only used to treat bacterial infections and prevent diseases in a herd but also at a subtherapeutic concentration as growth promoters, especially in farm animals and poultry. It is reported that 73% of global antimicrobial use (AMU) is in livestock, and the demand is likely to rise further, primarily in developing countries with large animal populations (Magnusson *et al.* 2021). This may ultimately magnify the already challenging situation of AMR.

Other Health Concerns: Industrialization of the modern livestock production system and heavy emphasis on meat consumption has resulted in new diseases of the circulatory system (DeMello 2012) as well as greater degrees of environmental degradation. Eggs and milk, the two most commonly dietary animal products, are also associated with human health risks. Though this remains debated, several authors state that dietary cholesterol from eggs could be an important risk factor for cardiometabolic diseases including CVD and diabetes. However, for healthy individuals, the nutritional benefits outweigh the concern surrounding the dietary cholesterol provided by one large egg (Miranda *et al.* 2015). Allergy to egg and cow milk is a serious health issue. According to a study, most allergic reactions to foods, particularly in children, occur primarily from eight foods, namely cow's milk, egg, wheat, soy, peanut, tree nuts, fish, and shellfish. Of these, milk and eggs were the most common cause of allergies in infants and children in Europe (Nwaru *et al.* 2014). Apart from nutrition-related risks, meat, egg, and milk consumption can also represent a risk for consumers derived by other factors, such as their microbiological status and the presence of chemical contaminants.

Beneficial Effects: A substantial body of scientific literature highlights the numerous benefits domestic animals provide to human health and well-being. These benefits span across their roles as livestock, companion and therapy animals, and experimental models. On balance, the positive effects of human–animal interactions far outweigh the negatives. Some key benefits include:

Nutritional Security: Domestic animals play a critical role in global nutrition. Beyond their traditional contributions—such as providing draught power for agriculture, transportation, hides, fur, and fibre—they are essential in enhancing food security. According to FAO (2023), animal-sourced foods contribute approximately 13.81% of global dietary energy (410 kcal per capita per day) and 28.34% of protein intake (an average of 32.8 grams per capita per day). These animals efficiently convert low-value, inedible, or unpalatable materials into high-quality milk, meat, and eggs. These animal products are among the best sources of complete proteins and micronutrients vital for optimal growth, development, and overall health (Smith et al. 2013). In fact, many critical nutrients are found exclusively—or in significantly higher concentrations—in animal products compared to plant-based foods. For example, dietary taurine, creatine, carnosine, anserine, and 4-hydroxyproline have important physiological roles in anti-oxidative and anti-inflammatory reactions, as well as in neurological, muscular, retinal, immunological, and cardiovascular function in healthy people. Adequate provision of these five nutrients is beneficial for preventing and treating obesity, cardiovascular dysfunction, and aging-related disorders, as well as inhibiting tumorigenesis, improving skin and bone health, ameliorating neurological abnormalities, and promoting well-being in infants, children, and adults. Taurine, carnosine, anserine, and creatine are absent from plants, and hydroxyproline is negligible in many plant-source foods. On the contrary, these are highly abundant in beef. An intake of 30 g dry beef can fully meet the daily physiological requirements for taurine and carnosine of a healthy 70-kg adult person. It can also provide large amounts of creatine, anserine, and 4-hydroxyproline necessary to improve human nutrition and health and prevent infections including coronavirus by enhancing the metabolism and functions of the immune cells (Wu 2020). Not only nutritional security, there are plenty of other direct and indirect benefits to human society that are derived from domestic animals. Animal products like milk of mare, Jenny, and she-camel are rich in bioactive ingredients with medicinal properties. These are used in traditional practices for the treatment of human diseases. Serum of llama possesses nanobodies, which are extremely useful in nano-therapy, developing diagnostic tests, and manipulating other proteins.

Animal Assisted Interventions (AAI): It is another important beneficial aspect of the human-domestic animal relationship, which is exploited to improve human health and welfare. AAI comprises animal-assisted therapy (AAT) and animal-assisted activities (AAA). AAT is a goal-directed intervention with animals as an integral part of the treatment process for a particular client; while AAA refers to a general category of interventions without a protocol. It provides opportunities for motivational, educational, recreational, and or therapeutic benefits to enhance the quality of life (Kruger and Serpell 2010). AAI are increasingly used in clinical practice for emotional support to improve the lives of elderly people and emotionally impaired children such as those affected by autism spectrum disorder (Cirulli *et al.* 2011). AAI can reduce aggression and depression; increased attention and strengthen social skills among youths (Flynn *et al.* 2020).

Dogs are particularly used for animal assisted therapy. In both Greece and Rome, there were special healing dogs known as cynotherapists. They were kept in temples and they licked the wounds of the sick and the dying, especially in the temple of Asklepios at Epidaurus. There were miraculous recoveries (Debroy 2008). Ownership of companion animals may stimulate positive social interaction and relationships, among people including those with disabilities pet ownership is found to have a positive economic impact in the form of reduced medical expenses. Studies from Australia and Germany have indicated that pet owners made fewer doctor visits annually than non-owners. Further, interaction with pets in childhood may have positive impacts on adult attitudes to animals (Serpel 2019). During the recent global COVID-19 pandemic, pets were reported to have provided substantial support to their owners to mitigate the emotional effects of confinement arising due to unprecedented lockdown (Bowen *et al.* 2020), and the AAT programmes effectively improved the social interaction and quality of life of patients with chronic schizophrenia during the pandemic (Shih and Yang 2023). In this regard, Green Care consisting of Care Farming, Social and Therapeutic Horticulture, Ecotherapy etc. is a fast-emerging new concept of AAI in many countries.

***Sentinels to Human Health Hazards due to Pollution*:** Domestic animals may act as potential sentinels to forewarn human health hazards due to environmental pollution. Farm animals are in the lower trophic of the food web, and they mostly live outdoors, consuming raw feed, and water from natural resources. They have shorter life spans than humans. Therefore, the impacts of pollution are usually greater in animals and biological effects may appear in animal species earlier than humans. In several instances, domestic animals have provided early warning for human health hazards due to pollution and have been used as environmental sentinels (Reif 2011). In a study, a population of sheep around a zinc smelter was established to serve as biological monitors and sentinel for community and public health hazards around the point source of pollution (Reif *et al.* 1989). While large animals are useful sentinels in outdoor environments, scientific studies have demonstrated the potential role of pets, particularly cats and dogs, as sentinels for human health effects resulting from exposure to several classes of indoor environmental contaminants such as metals, persistent organic pollutants, flame retardants, and polycyclic aromatic hydrocarbons (Poma *et al.* 2020).

Role of Domestic Animals in Biomedical Research and Developments: Although, rats and mice are the most used laboratory animals, domestic animal species like guinea pigs, rabbits, dogs, cats, birds, pig sheep, and other farm animals (horses, llamas, cows, goats, buffaloes) are also used in considerable number in research facilities and commercial organizations to produce immunobiological. These animals have played an indispensable role in the advancement of biomedical and pharmaceutical research and developments including the discovery, invention, and refinement of enumerable numbers of new drugs, vaccines, diagnostic methods, and technologies. Although many research studies now involve the use of computational, molecular, and cellular models, animal models are still a mainstay of biomedical research and have led to important discoveries (Ward and Osenkowski 2022). There are numerous examples where experiments on domestic animals have resulted in great biomedical breakthroughs. The discovery of insulin involving experimentation on dogs and knowledge of farm animal practices is worth mentioning. Sir Frederick Banting, a physician and scientist, was the co-discoverer of insulin along with his student Dr Charles Herbert Best. The discovery involved experiments in dogs. An extract of atrophied pancreas collected from dogs was injected into a sickly dog named Marjorie, whose pancreas had been removed several days earlier. The administration of the extract, named isletin resulted in a sharp decrease in the blood sugar level of the dog. However, the hypoglycaemic effect was temporary, and the discoverers realized the need for a larger source of pancreas extract. According to a scientific study, the pancreas of foetal and newborn animals contains a higher proportion of islet cells than an adult pancreas. Dr Benting, aware of farm animal activities from his childhood days, knew that farmers impregnated cows to increase their weight for the market, and would discard the embryos at the time of slaughter. The isletin from bovine sources worked just like the extract made from dogs, ultimately leading to the discovery of insulin (Tan 2017). The discovery of the function of the heart and the circulation of blood by William Harvey is one of the greatest medical discoveries of all time, in which domestic animals played an important role. William Harvey experimented on various animal species including sheep, pigs, and dogs. Harvey claimed that if the aorta of a dog or a sheep be tied at the base of the heart, and the carotid or any other artery be opened, the artery will be empty and the veins replete with blood. This is consistent with the notion that arteries receive blood from the veins in no other way than by transmission through the heart (Aird 2011). Harvey performed vivisections on dogs to demonstrate and prove his findings in the presence of the Fellows of the Royal College of Physicians of London for verification (Friedland 2009)

Domestic animals are also used as a suitable experimental model to study human diseases. The rabbit is an extremely valuable animal model for studying many human hereditary diseases such as aortic arteriosclerosis, cataracts, hypertension, hypertrophic cardiomyopathy, epilepsy, spina bifida, and osteoporosis. It is also commonly used in studies of *in-vitro* fertilization, embryology, organogenesis, and toxicology studies (Carneiro *et al.* 2011). There are similarities in aetiopathogenesis and other features of many human and canine diseases. As such, dogs have emerged as powerful and excellent large-animal models for the study of important human diseases notably including diabetes mellitus, cancer, hereditary diseases, aging, epilepsy, and urological diseases. For example, epilepsy is a common complex brain disease characterized by an enduring predisposition to generate spontaneous recurrent epileptic seizures in both humans and domestic dogs, making dogs an ideal translational model of epilepsy (Löscher 2022). The canine models have played important roles in identification of causative genes and/or in novel therapeutic approaches of interest to hereditary diseases. The dog is afflicted with approximately 450 hereditary diseases, about half of which have remarkable clinical similarities to corresponding diseases of humans, and there is a strong desire amongst pet owners to cure diseases of the dog (Tsai *et al.* 2007). Further, dogs are among a limited number of non-human species that require continence and socially appropriate urinary behaviours such as going to the bathroom outside, training to not have submissive urination, etc. These features make dogs unique in the animal kingdom and an ideal animal model for urologic research (Ruetten and Vezina 2022). Because of their anatomical and physiological similarities to humans and the availability of genomic, transcriptomic and, progressively more, proteomic tools for analysis, domestic pigs are used as a model for highly prevalent human metabolic diseases (diabetes, metabolic syndrome, obesity, and cardiovascular diseases), infections and inflammations, neurodegenerative and neuropsychiatric disorders, and transplantation and proteomics research (Bassols *et al.* 2014). The relative similarities of young pigs to young humans in terms of brain development, physiology, diet, and gastrointestinal function make pigs a potentially powerful animal model for human neonates to investigate the effects of early life events and later behavioural and neurological functions (Nordquist *et al.* 2017). There are many other human diseases, where different species of domestic animals have played important roles as animal models in the identification of causative agents, understanding of disease pathophysiology, and mechanisms of drug resistance, and in the development of novel drugs and therapeutic strategies, that have immensely benefited the overall human health and wellness.

Effects on Animal Welfare and Health

Several scholarly articles are available on welfare of domestic animals and effects of domestication on it. There are many definitions of animal welfare. According to the terrestrial code of World Organization for Animal Health (WOAH) animal welfare means the physical and mental state of an animal in relation to the conditions in which it lives and dies. It is a state where an animal is both healthy and gets what it wants. Good welfare is Five Freedoms: (i) freedom from thirst, hunger, and malnutrition, (ii) freedom from thermal and physical discomfort, (iii) freedom from pain, injury, and disease, (iv) freedom from fear and distress, and (v) freedom to express normal behaviour (Dawkins 2021). Standards for good animal welfare are defined based on five domain that include ready access to a diet to maintain full health and vigour, provision of a suitable environment including shelter and a comfortable resting area, prevention of diseases or rapid diagnosis and treatment, providing sufficient space, proper facilities and the company of the animal's own kind and ensuring conditions which avoid mental suffering.

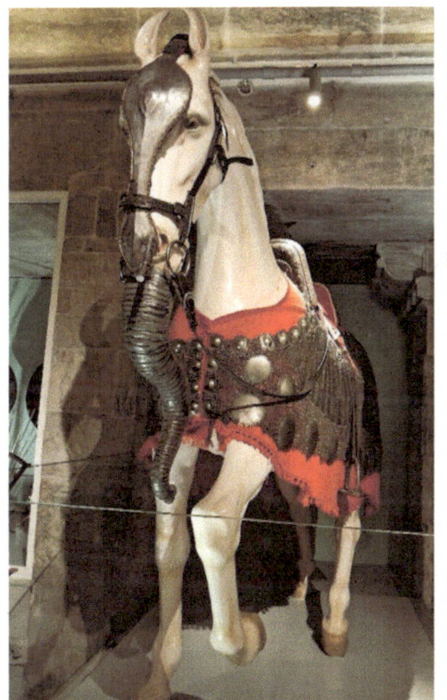

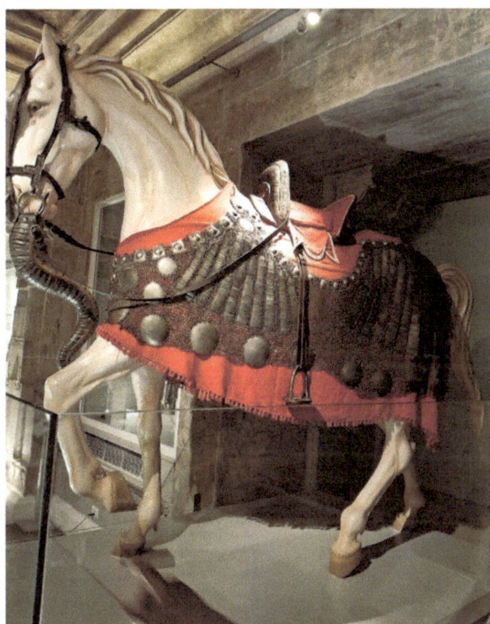

Fig. 1.9. *The chain mail and plate horse armour of the legendary Chetak (16th century) exemplifies the advanced protection provided to Indian warhorses. This intricate armour includes components such as the shaffron, crupper, pierced saddle, and carefully designed stirrups, all crafted to ensure the horse's safety and effectiveness on the battlefield. Notably, a false trunk near the horse's nose was added, creating the illusion of a baby elephant, likely to confuse enemy elephants. (Source: Armour of Chetak at City Palace, Udaipur. Photo by the Author).*

Quality of the welfare of animals largely depends on the attitude of people and the purposes for which animals are kept (Fig. 1.9). Pet and companion animals are usually treated by their owners like family members with lots of compassion and empathy. They are not utility animals and hence no production stress. However, they are deeply attached to their owners and may develop behavioural disorders due to bereavement and mistreatment. On the other hand, farm animals are mainly kept for production of animal products, and traction purposes, making them more prone to stress and metabolic diseases. Knowingly or unknowingly draught animals are subjected to excess workloads and mistreatment causing physical injuries. The existing health status is the foundation of good animal welfare. The freedom from disease and injury is listed as a key indicator of welfare. Most of the welfare schemes are therefore specifically aimed at maintaining animal health such as making sure that animals have adequate food and water, and are kept in safe comfortable environments to avoid injuries. A key feature of domestication is the increased occurrence of diverse metabolic diseases in cattle and other domestic animals. For example, increased milk outputs that have been achieved over the last 70 years have led to several health and pathophysiological conditions in high-yielding dairy animals, including metabolic diseases that were uncommon in the past. Cows genetically selected for high milk production are more likely to develop production-related diseases like mastitis, hypocalcaemia, rumen acidosis, ketosis, and laminitis, among others (Zachut *et al.* 2020). Selection for fast early growth rate, and feeding and management procedures to support growth have caused various welfare problems in modern broiler strains such as metabolic disorders associated with mortality due to sudden death and ascites. Fast growth rate is generally accompanied by decreased locomotor activity and extended time spent sitting or lying (Bessei 2006).

Rapid intensification of livestock production to feed the increasing populations during the present industrial era has resulted in advancement of many transboundary animal diseases notably including FMD, contagious bovine pleuropneumonia, classical swine fever, to cite a few (Otte *et al.* 2004). Introduction of susceptible animal populations like taurine cattle germplasm from abroad for crossbreeding to upgrade the local breeds in India and other countries of tropical region has led to re-emergence of ticks-borne parasitic infections like theileria, and babesia both in exotic and crossbred cattle. Since increased animal production is often required in peri-urban areas with large human populations, under suboptimal husbandry practices, the disease outbreaks affect a greater number of animals at a faster rate and speed, leading to heavy economic losses (Yadav *et al.* 2020).

Nutrition is vital for good welfare and optimum health of animals. Inadequate and erroneous feeding and management practices are not only associated with deficiency and metabolic diseases in animals, but have caused many devastating health problems, and occurrence of poisoning in domestic animals. The outbreak of bovine spongiform encephalopathy (BSE), or mad cow disease, is a glaring example. BSE was considered as the most economically important prion disease in veterinary medicine during the late 20th and early 21st centuries. The outbreak of diseases occurred in 1986 in the UK due to supplementation of cattle feed with rendered cattle meat and bone meal contaminated with BSE prions (PrPSc). Most cases of classic BSE reported so far are anthropogenic (Haley and Richt 2023). The disease had a devastating impact on the cattle industry. Scientists found that BSE prion was capable of crossing species and contaminated barriers, and authorities were forced to slaughter thousands of cattle. There are several other examples of adverse health impact in different species of animals due to substandard feed and feeding practices. Contaminated feed caused lead intoxication in more than 15,000 cattle on over 330 farms in north Netherlands during 1989-90 (Baars *et al.* 1990), and feeding of poor-quality feed supplement having high concentration of fluoride was responsible for fluorosis (Fig. 1.10) in large number of cattle in India (Singh and Swarup 1995).

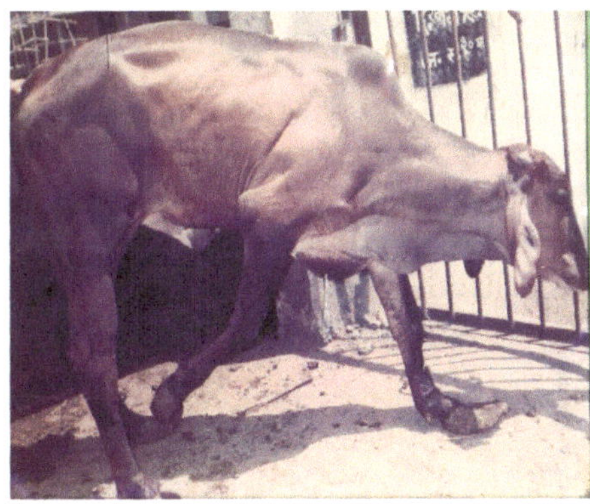

Fig. 1.10. *Fluorosis in cattle can occur due to feeding low grade feed supplement with high concentration of fluoride (Photo courtesy of Dr. J.L. Singh GBPUAT).*

Animal welfare is significantly influenced by locations, hygienic standards, and space of the animal houses, and overall quality of the environment and grazing areas in which animals are kept. The animals in urban, peri-urban, industrial, and mining areas are frequently allowed to graze on or fed with contaminated pastures or fodders and are continually exposed to toxic pollutants leading to various health hazards. Disease problems caused by environmental pollution have already been detected in veterinary diagnostic laboratories. The pollutants and the resulting health effects are in many forms. Many environmental contaminants accumulate preferentially in vital organs—particularly the liver and kidneys—resulting in a spectrum of adverse effects ranging from acute clinical toxicosis to subclinical toxicities. Globally, outbreaks of clinical poisoning in livestock have been attributed to anthropogenic contaminants, including heavy metals, fluoride (fluorosis), pesticides, nitrates and nitrites, and other agrochemicals. In addition to overt clinical and subclinical manifestations, pollutants may induce subtle yet biologically significant alterations, such as oxidative stress, immunotoxicity, cardiotoxicity, teratogenicity, enzyme inhibition, reproductive dysfunction, and endocrine disruption. For example, cows reared in industrial and mining areas have been reported to exhibit impaired liver function and altered endocrine profiles, characterized by elevated serum cortisol (stress hormone) levels and disturbances in triiodothyronine (T3) and thyroxine (T4) concentrations (Swarup *et al.* 2007).

The presence of non-decomposable wastes such as paper, rubber, plastic, leather, metal scrap, sharp objects like wires and nails, glass, ceramics, and stones in the animal surroundings can cause serious health problems such as foreign body syndrome in ruminants. A study reported that in the industrialized countries, majority of of normal cattle had metallic objects in the reticulum and residual traumatic lesions existed in as many as 70 % of the dairy cows (Leek 1968). Contamination of animal surrounding and pastures with non-indigestible non-metallic wastes like rubber, plastics, and leather ropes, cement bags, etc., may be ingested by cattle and buffaloes and accumulated in rumen leading to indigestion, bloat, intestinal obstruction, and death. A retrospective study from Ethiopia, revealed that out of 711 cattle subjected to rumenotomies, 350 had accumulated foreign bodies weighing above 9 kg, mainly comprising non-penetrating foreign bodies (Ramaswamy and Sharma 2011).

There are many issues concerning the welfare of pet and companion animals. Researchers believe that years of domestication and living in close contact with humans have led to dogs losing their natural wild instinct of problem solving. They have learned to rely more on human help instead of solving problems independently. Pet dogs failed the intelligence test, which was easily cleared by wild dogs and wolves. Wolves also outperformed dogs in their ability to follow causal cues, suggesting that domestication has altered these specific skills (DeMello 2012, Lampe *et al.* 2017). The pet and show industries have adopted selective breeding to produce pets with traits favourable to humans and have created several varieties of dogs, cats, and other companion animals. Pets, particularly dogs that have been created for aesthetic purposes by artificial selection today are at higher risk of several health problems. Changes in morphology and behaviour of many companion animal's breeds with odd proportions in body, head, and leg sizes are detrimental to their health (DeMello 2012). For example, extreme brachycephaly in many of the pug faced dog and cat breeds can result in severe respiratory problems. The other animal welfare issues related to pets include companion animal abuse and neglect leading to behavioural problems, provision of inadequate space, and exercise, over or under-feeding, use of aversive training and control methods, and the fate of unwanted or surplus pets (Serpell 2019).

Conclusion

For thousands of years, humans have coexisted and interacted with other animals in various ways. The relationship between animals and hunter-gatherers was typically one of mutual trust, where the environment and its resources were shared between animals and people. Animals hunted by humans were viewed as equals (Harari 2015). However, the advent of animal domestication marked a revolutionary shift in human-animal relationships. It represents the oldest and most profound evolutionary interaction between animals and humans. Although the association between humans and domesticated animals is often described as mutualistic, humans assumed the dominant role, controlling aspects such as breeding, feeding, housing, and reproduction. This transition transformed the relationship into one of dominance and control, with humans becoming masters and animals their property, to be owned and traded. On their part, animals have provided resources to human society, including protein for nutrition, fur and skin for clothing, draught animal power for farming and transportation, and manure for soil improvement. Companion animals have also offered physical and emotional support to people as trusted friends. However, the quality of life for domestic animals is often considered poorer and compromised compared to their free-living progenitors (Zeder 2012).

In modern society, advanced scientific tools and technologies have led to the mechanization of agriculture and transport, reducing the traditional roles of domestic animals, particularly draught and pack animals. However, domestic animals remain integral assets, as evidenced by the significant global livestock production. Livestock, led by cattle and poultry, comprises a vast portion of global mammal biomass (Waiblinger 2019, Ritchie *et al.* 2022). Pet keeping has also emerged as a popular hobby in urban dwellings. Today, companion animals are more abundant than ever before and global expenditure on commercial pet food and pet products has risen manifold in several countries (Serpell 2019). Today, domestic animals are ubiquitous, found in various human dwellings worldwide, from urban high-rises to remote rural areas. They contribute not only to farming communities but also to urban employment opportunities in the organized dairy, meat, egg, pork, wool, and fiber production sectors. Scientific institutions, pharmaceutical companies, and entrepreneurial ventures involved in animal-related products further demonstrate the socioeconomic significance of domestic animals. Moreover, domestic animals play essential roles in biomedical research and as therapy animals. Their historical and ongoing contributions to human society underscore the importance of compassionate treatment, care, and kindness towards them. As the ancient Greek fabulist Aesop famously said – *No act of kindness, no matter how small, is ever wasted* – and it is truly appropriate for domestic animals.

References

Agam A and Barkai R. 2018. Elephant and mammoth hunting during the Palaeolithic: a review of the relevant archaeological, ethnographic, and ethno-historical records. *Quaternary* **1** (1): 1-28 doi:10.3390/quat1010003.

Ajmone-Marsan P, Garcia JF and Lenstra JA. 2010. On the origin of cattle: how aurochs became cattle and colonized the world. *Evolutionary Anthropology: Issues, News, and Reviews* **19** (4): 148-57.

Albarella U, Dobney K and Rowley-Conwy P. 2006. The domestication of the pig (*Sus scrofa*): New challenges and approaches. In: *Documenting Domestication: New Genetic and Archaeological Paradigms.* pp. 209–27. (Eds) Zeder, M.A, Daniel G. Bradley D.G. Emshwiller B. and Smith RD. University of California Press, California, USA.

Albright JL and Arave CW. 1997. *The Behaviour of Cattle.* 306 p. CABI, Wallingford, , Oxfordshire, UK.

Alhadrami G and Faye B. 2022. Camel. In: *Encyclopaedia Dairy Science* 3rd edn, Vol 1. pp. 48-64. (Eds) Paul LH McSweeney PLH and McNamara JP. Elsevier, Academic Press: https://doi.org/10.1016/B978-0-12-818766-1.00364-0.

Al-Qamashoui B, Al-Ansari A, Simianer H, Weigend S, Mahgoub O, Costa V, Weigend A, Al-Araimi N and Beja-Pereira A. 2014. From India to Africa across Arabia: An mtDNA assessment of the origins and dispersal of chicken around the Indian Ocean Rim. In: *Towards Conservation of Omani Local Chicken: Management. Performance and Genetic Diversity.* PhD Dissertation. pp. 43- 60. Georg-August-Universität Göttingen, Germany.

Alves RRN. 2012. Relationships between fauna and people and the role of ethnozoology in animal conservation. *Ethnobiology and conservation* **1** (2): 1-69; doi: 10.15451/ec2012-8-1.2-1-69.

Amills M, Capote J, and Tosser-Klopp G. 2017. Goat domestication and breeding: a jigsaw of historical, biological, and molecular data with missing pieces. *Animal Genetics* **48** (6): 631-44.

Anderson DG, Harrault L, Milek KB, Forbes BC, Kuoppamaa M and Plekhanov AV. 2019. Animal domestication in the high Arctic: Hunting and holding reindeer on the I͡Amal peninsula, northwest Siberia. *Journal of Anthropological Archaeology* **55**: 101079; https://doi.org/10.1016/j.jaa.2019.101079.

Anderson P. 2003. A bird in the house: An anthropological perspective on companion parrots. *Society and Animals* **11** (4): 393-418.

Anderson PK. 2010. Human–bird interactions. In: *The Welfare of Domestic Fowl and Other Captive Birds*. pp 17-52. (Eds) Duncan IJ and Hawkins P. Dordrecht: Springer Netherlands.

Anthony DW and Brown DR. 2011. The secondary products revolution, horse-riding, and mounted warfare. *Journal of World Prehistory* **24** (2-3): 131-60.

Anthony DW. 2007. *The Horse, the Wheel, and Language*. pp. 134-222, 460-64. Princeton University Press, NJ, USA. Available at: https://archive.org/details/horsewheelandlanguage.

Arbuckle BS and Kassebaum TM. 2021.Management and domestication of cattle (*Bos taurus*) in Neolithic Southwest Asia. *Animal Frontiers* **11** (3):10-19.

Arbuckle BS, Öztan A and Gülçur S. 2009. The evolution of sheep and goat husbandry in central Anatolia. *Anthropozoologica* **44** (1):129-57.

Arbuckle BS. 2014.The rise of cattle cultures in Bronze Age Anatolia. *Journal of Eastern Mediterranean Archaeology and Heritage Studies* **2** (4):277-97.

Aspri M, Economou N and Papademas P. 2017. Donkey milk: An overview on functionality, technology, and prospects. *Food Reviews International* **33** (3): 316-33.

Atsenova N, Palova N, Mehandjyiski I, Neov B, Radoslavov G and Hristov P. 2022.The sequence analysis of mitochondrial DNA revealed some major centers of horse domestications: The Archaeologist's Cut. *Journal of Equine Veterinary Science* **109**: 103830: https://doi.org/10.1016/j.jevs.2021.103830.

Baars AJ, Beek HV, Visser IJ, Vos G, Delft WV, Fennema G, Lieben GW, Lautenbag K, Nieuwenhuijs JH, Coulander PD and Pluimers FH. 1990. Lead poisoning among cattle in North Netherlands between October 1989 and January 1990. *Tijdschrift voor Diergeneeskunde***115** (19): 882-90.

Bashir S and Al-Ayadhi L Y. 2014. Effect of camel milk on thymus and activation-regulated chemokine in autistic children: double-blind study. *Pediatric Research* **75** (4):559-63.

Bathrachalam C, Nocelli C, Pazzaglia I, Pallotti S, Pediconi D, La Terza A and Renier C. 2019. Interaction between ASIP and MC1R in black and brown alpaca. In: *Advances in Fibre Production Science in South American Camelids and other Fibre Animals*. pp. 163-70. (Eds) Gerken M, Renieri C, Allain D, Galbraith H, Gutiérrez JP, McKenna L Niznikowski R and Wurzinger M. Universitätsverlag Göttingen, Göttingen, Germany.

Beaver BV. 2019. The history of horses and their relationships to humans. In: *Equine Behavioral Medicine*. pp. 1-31. Academic Press, Elsevier, London, UK.

Beja-Pereira A, England PR, Ferrand N, Jordan S, Bakhiet AO, Abdalla MA, Mashkour M, Jordana J, Taberlet P and Luikart G. 2004. African origins of the domestic donkey. *Science* **304** (5678):1781.

Berg EL and Causey A. 2014. The life-changing power of the horse: Equine-assisted activities and therapies in the US. *Animal Frontiers* **4** (3): 72-75.

Bertino E, Agosti M, Peila C, Corridori M, Pintus R and Fanos V. 2022. The donkey milk in infant nutrition. *Nutrients* **14** (3): p.403. https://doi.org/10.3390/nu14030403.

Bertoni A, Álvarez-Macías A, Mota-Rojas D, Dávalos JL and Minervino AH. 2021. Dual-purpose water buffalo production systems in tropical Latin America: Bases for a sustainable model. *Animals* **11(**10): p.2910; https://doi.org/10.3390/ani11102910.

Bessei W. 2006. Welfare of broilers: A review. *World's Poultry Science Journal* **62** (3): 455-66.

Blumenschine RJ and Cavallo JA. 1992. Scavenging and human evolution. *Scientific American* **267** (4): 90-97.

Bollongino R, Burger J, Powell A, Mashkour M, Vigne JD, Thomas MG. 2012. Modern taurine cattle descended from small number of Near-Eastern founders. *Molecular Biology and Evolution* **29** (9): 2101–04.

Borghese A. 2005. Buffalo meat and meat industry. In: *Buffalo Production and Research* pp 197-217. (Ed) A Borghese. REU technical Series 67, Food and Agriculture Organization of the United Nations, Rome, Italy.

Bosse M. 2018. A genomics perspective on pig domestication. *Animal Domestication*. pp. 22-34. (Ed) Teletchea F. Intechopen: http://dx.doi.org/10.5772/intechopen.82646.

Bosze ZS and Houdebine LM. 2006. Application of rabbits in biomedical research: A review. *World Rabbit Science* **14:** 1-14.

Bourhy H, Reynes JM, Dunham EJ, Dacheux L, Larrous F, Huong VT, Xu G, Yan J, Miranda ME and Holmes EC. The origin and phylogeography of dog rabies virus. *The Journal of General Virology* **89** (Pt 11):2673. doi: 10.1099/vir.0.2008/003913-0.

Bowen J, García E, Darder P, Argüelles J, Fatjó J. 2020.The effects of the Spanish COVID-19 lockdown on people, their pets, and the human-animal bond. *Journal of Veterinary Behavior* **40**:75-91. https://doi.org/10.1016/j.jveb.2020.05.013.

Broushaki F, Thomas MG, Link V, López S, Van Dorp L, Kirsanow K, Hofmanová Z, Diekmann Y, Cassidy LM, Díez-del-Molino D and Kousathanas A. 2016. Early Neolithic genomes from the eastern Fertile Crescent. *Science* **353** (6298): 499-503.

Bulliet RW. 2012. Afterword: Camels and deserts. In: *Camels in Asia and North Africa. Interdisciplinary Perspectives on their Significance in Past and Present*. pp 231-36. (Eds) Eva- Knoll Maria and Burger P. Austrian Academy of Sciences Press, Vienna, Austria.

Burger PA, Ciani E and Faye B. 2019. Old World camels in a modern world–a balancing act between conservation and genetic improvement. *Animal Genetics* **50** (6): 598-612.

Butchart SH. 2008. Red List Indices to measure the sustainability of species use and impacts of invasive alien species. *Bird Conservation International* **18** (S1): S245-62. https://doi.org/10.1017/S095927090800035X P.

Camillo F, Rota A, Biagini L, Tesi M, Fanelli D and Panzani D. 2018. The current situation and trend of donkey industry in Europe. *Journal of Equine Veterinary Science* **65**: 44-49.

Carneiro M, Afonso S, Geraldes A, Garreau H, Bolet G, Boucher S, Tircazes A, Queney G, Nachman MW and Ferrand N .2011. The genetic structure of domestic rabbits. *Molecular Biology and Evolution* **28**(6): 1801-16.

Cassey P, Vall-Llosera M, Dyer E and Blackburn TM. 2015. The biogeography of avian invasions: History, accident, and market trade. In: *Biological Invasions in Changing Ecosystems: Vectors, Ecological Impacts, Management and Predictions*. pp. 37-54. (Ed). Canning-Clode J. de Gruyter Open, Poland:https://doi.org/10.1515/9783110438666-006.

Chandra Y. 2021. *The Tale of the Horse: A History of India on Horseback.* 384 p. Picador India, New Delhi, India.

Cirulli F, Borgi M, Berry A, Francia N and Alleva E. 2011. Animal-assisted interventions as innovative tools for mental health. *Annali dell'Istituto Superiore di Sanità*, **47** (4): 341-48.

Clutton-Brock J. 1999. *A Natural History of Domestic Mammals.* 2nd edn. pp.10-24, 177- 92. Cambridge University Press, UK.

Coulthard S. 2020. Why some sheep are so rooed: A mummy's tattoos, the invention of scissors and a ram on run. In: *A Short History of the World According to Sheep*. 320 p. Head of Zeus Ltd, London, UK.

Crawford RD. 1992. Introduction to Europe and the diffusion of domesticated turkeys from the Americas. *Archivos de Zootecnia* **41** (154):307-14.

Crowley SL. 2014. Camels out of place and time: the dromedary (*Camelus dromedarius*) in Australia. *Anthrozoös* **27** (2): 191-203.

D'Alterio GL, Knowles TG, Eknaes EI, Loevland IE and Foster AP. 2006. Postal survey of the population of South Ameri can camelids in the United Kingdom in 2000/01. *Veterinary Record* **158** (3): 86-90.

D'Altroy TN. 2015. Farmers, herders, and storehouse. In: *The Incas*. 2nd edn. pp. 392-417. Wiley-Blackwell, Chichester, Sussex, UK.

Dalle Zotte A. 2014. Rabbit farming for meat purposes. *Animal Frontiers* **4** (4): 62-67.

Danino M. 2006. The horse and the Aryan debate. *The Journal of Indian History and Culture* **13**: 33-59.

Dawkins MS. 2021. What is animal welfare? In: *The Science of Animal Welfare: Understanding What Animals Want*. pp. 3-14. Oxford University Press, USA.

Debroy B. 2008. *Sarama and Her Children*. 243p. Penguin Books, New Delhi, India.

Decker JE, McKay SD, Rolf MM, Kim J, Molina Alcalá A, Sonstegard TS, Hanotte O, Götherström A, Seabury CM, Praharani L and Babar ME. 2014. Worldwide patterns of ancestry, divergence, and admixture in domesticated cattle. *PLoS Genetics* **10** (3): e1004254.

DeMello M. 2012. *Animals and Society: An Introduction to Human-Animal Studies*. pp. 3-29, 84-96. Columbia University Press, New York, USA.

Díaz-Lameiro P, Rey-Iglesia A, Cartajena I, Núñez L, Westbury MV, Varas V, Moraga M, Campos PF, Orozco-terWengel P, Marin JC and Hansen AJ. 2021. Ancient DNA reveals the lost domestication history of South American camelids in Northern Chile and across the Andes. *Elife* **10**: p.e63390. DOI: https://doi.org/10.7554/eLife.63390.

Dolker Lamo S, Bharti VK and Chaurasia OP. 2023. Distribution and morphology of double-hump camel (*Camelus bactrianus*) in Ladakh region, India. *Indian Journal of Natural Sciences* **14** (77): 54743-52.

Dunne J, Evershed RP, Salque M, Cramp L, Bruni S, Ryan K, Biagetti S, and di Lernia S. 2012. First dairying in green Saharan Africa in the fifth millennium BC. *Nature* **486** (7403): 390-94.

Dyer EE, Cassey P, Redding DW, Collen B, Franks V, Gaston KJ, Jones KE, Kark S, Orme CD and Blackburn TM. 2017. The global distribution and drivers of alien bird species richness. *PLoS Biology* **15**(1): e2000942.

Eda M, Itahash Y, Kikuchi, H, Sun G, Hsu KH, Gakuhar T, Yoneda M, Jiang L, Yang G and Nakamura S. 2022. Multiple lines of evidence of early goose domestication in a 7,000-y-old rice cultivation village in the lower Yangtze River, China. *Proceedings of the National Academy of Sciences* **119** (12): p.e2117064119. https://doi.org/10.1073/pnas.2117064119.

Eraly A. 2002. *Gem in the Lotus*. pp 37-55, 514-16. Penguin Books, New Delhi, India.

Fagan B.M. 2017. Bountiful waters. In: *Fishing: How the Sea Fed Civilization*. pp.1-14. Yale University Press, USA.

Fan R, Gu Z, Guang X, Marín JC, Varas V, González BA, Wheeler JC, Hu Y, Li E, Sun X and Yang X. 2020. Genomic analysis of the domestication and post-Spanish conquest evolution of the llama and alpaca. *Genome Biology* **21**: 1-26.

FAO. 2023. *World Food and Agriculture – Statistical Yearbook* 2023. Rome, Italy: https://doi.org/10.4060/cc8166en, downloaded on 8-12-2023.

Faye B. 2016. The camel, new challenges for a sustainable development. *Tropical Animal Health and Production* **48** (4): 689-92.

Faye B. 2020. How many large camelids in the world? A synthetic analysis of the world camel demographic changes. *Pastoralism* **10**(1):1-20.

Faye B, Madani H and El-Rouili SA. 2014. Camel milk value chain in Northern Saudi Arabia. *Emirates Journal of Food and Agriculture* **26** (4):359-65.

Felius M. 2007. *Cattle Breeds: An Encyclopedia.* 799 p. Trafalgar Square Books, New York, USA.

Flynn E, Gandenberger J, Mueller MK and Morris KN. 2020. Animal-assisted interventions as an adjunct to therapy for youth: Clinician perspectives. *Child and Adolescent Social Work Journal* **37**(6): 631-42.

Franklin S. 2002. Dolly the world-famous sheep. In: *Identity and Difference in the Global Era.* pp. 221-32. (Ed.) Larreta ER. Unesco, ISSC, Educam, Rio de Janeiro, Brazil.

Franklin WL, Powell KJ and Youngs CR. 2006. Guard llamas. A part of integrated sheep protection. *The Camelid Quarterly* **March 2006**: 1-7.

Frantz LA, Bradley DG, Larson G and Orlando L. 2020. Animal domestication in the era of ancient genomics. *Nature Reviews Genetics* **21**(8): 449-60.

Friedland G. 2010. Discovery of the function of the heart and circulation of blood. *Cardiovascular Journal of Africa* **20** (3):160.

Frisch JE, O'neill CJ, and Kelly MJ. 2000. Using genetics to control cattle parasites—the Rockhampton experience. *International Journal for Parasitology* **30** (3): 253-64.

Fuks D and Marom N. 2021. Sheep and wheat domestication in southwest Asia: a meta-trajectory of intensification and loss. *Animal Frontiers* **11**(3): 20-29.

Furness RW. 1993. Birds as monitors of pollutants. In: *Birds as Monitors of Environmental Change*. pp. 86-143. (Eds) Furness RW and Greenwood JJ. Dordrecht: Springer, Netherlands.

Galbraith H. 2019. Animal fibre production in Europe: biology, species, breeds, and contemporary utilisation. In: *Advances in Fibre Production Science in South American Camelids and other Fibre Animals*. pp. 23-41. (Eds) Gerken M, Renieri C, Allain D, Galbraith H, Gutiérrez JP, McKenna L Niznikowski R and Wurzinger M. Universitätsverlag Göttingen, Germany.

García-Sancho M. 2015. Animal breeding in the age of biotechnology: the investigative pathway behind the cloning of Dolly the sheep. *History and Philosophy of the Life Sciences* **37** (3): 282-304.

Gebremichael B, Girmay S and Gebru MU. 2019. Camel milk production and marketing: Pastoral areas of Afar, Ethiopia. *Pastoralism* **9** (1):1-11.

Germonpré M, Lázničková-Galetová M, Sablin MV and Bocherens H. 2018. Self-domestication or human control? The Upper Palaeolithic domestication of the wolf. In: *Hybrid Communities*. 1st edn. pp. 39-64. (Eds) Stépanoff C and Vigne J-D. Routledge: https://doi.org/10.4324/9781315179988.

Germonpré M, Van den Broeck M, Lázničková-Galetová M, Sablin MV and Bocherens H. 2021. Mothering the orphaned pup: The beginning of a domestication process in the Upper Palaeolithic. *Human Ecology* **49** (6): 677-89.

Girling SJ. 2010. The welfare of captive birds in the future. In: *The Welfare of Domestic Fowl and Other Captive Birds*. pp 115-33. (Eds) Duncan IJ, Hawkins P. Drodrecht: Springer, Netherland.

Goñalons GLM. 2008. Camelids in ancient Andean societies: A review of the zooarchaeological evidence. *Quaternary International* **185** (1): 59-68.

Greenfield HJ, Shai I, Greenfield TL, Arnold ER, Brown A, Eliyahu A and Maeir AM. 2018. Earliest evidence for equid bit wear in the ancient Near East: The "ass" from Early Bronze Age Tell eṣ-Ṣâfi/Gath, Israel. *PLoS One* **13** (5): p.e0196335.

Griffin JA, McCune S, Maholmes V and Hurley K. 2011.Human-animal interaction research: An introduction to issues and topics. In: *How Animals Affect us: Examining the Influence of Human-animal Interaction on Child Development and Human Health*. pp. 3–9. (Eds) McCardle P, McCune S, Griffin JA and Maholmes V. American Psychological Association, Washington, DC, USA.

Groenen MA .2016. A decade of pig genome sequencing: a window on pig domestication and evolution. *Genetics Selection Evolution* **48** (1): 1-9.

Groeneveld LF, Lenstra JA, Eding H, Toro MA, Scherf B, Pilling D, Negrini R, Finlay EK Jianlin H, Groeneveld EJ and Weigend S. 2010. Genetic diversity in farm animals–a review. Animal Genetics **41** (Suppl. 1): 6-31.

Guil-Guerrero JL, Tikhonov A, Ramos-Bueno RP, Grigoriev S, Protopopov A, Savvinov G and González-Fernández MJ. 2018. Mammoth resources for hominins: From omega-3 fatty acids to cultural objects. *Journal of Quaternary Science* **33** (4): 455-63.

Guler K. 2016. Ancient Horse-Cultures of the Eurasian pes Steppes. *The Saber and Scroll Journal* **5** (2): 69-85.

Gunsser I .2013. Animal welfare problems in alpacas and llamas in Europe. In: *Symposium on South American Camelids and other Fibre Animals, .* pp. 25-30. 64th EAAP Annual meeting. 25-30 August 2013, Nantes, France.

Haley NJ and Richt JA. 2023. Classical bovine spongiform encephalopathy and chronic wasting disease: two sides of the prion coin. *Animal Diseases* **3**(1):24: https://doi.org/10.1186/s44149-023-00087-7.

Hanotte O, Bradley DG, Ochieng JW, Verjee Y, Hill EW and Rege JE. 2002. African pastoralism: genetic imprints of origins and migrations. *Science* **296** (5566): 336-39.

Harari YN. 2015. *Sapiens–A Brief History of Humankind.* 498 p.Vintage, Penguin Random House, London, UK.

Harding LE. 2022. Available names for *Rangifer (*Mammalia, Artiodactyla, Cervidae) species and subspecies. *ZooKeys* **1119**: 117–51. https://doi.org/10.3897/zookeys.1119.80233.

Helmer D, Gourichon L and Vila E. 2007. The development of the exploitation of products from Capra and Ovis (meat, milk, and fleece) from the PPNB to the Early Bronze in the northern Near East (8700 to 2000 BC cal.). *Anthropozoologica* **42** (2): 41-69.

Hendricks BL. 2007. *International Encyclopedia of Horse Breeds*. University of Oklahoma Press, USA.

Herbeck YE, Eliava M, Grinevich V and MacLean EL. 2022. Fear, love, and the origins of canid domestication: An oxytocin hypothesis. *Comprehensive Psychoneuroendocrinology* **9:** https://doi.org/10.1016/j.cpnec.2021.100100.

Hill E. 2013. Archaeology and animal persons: toward a prehistory of human-animal relations. *Environment and Society* **4** (1): 117-36.

Hoffman E. 2014. *Lama guanicoe:* Animal Diversity Web: https://animaldiversity.org/accounts/Lama_guanicoe/, accessed on 07-12-2023.

Hosey G, Birke L, Shaw WS and Melfi V. 2018. Measuring the strength of human–animal bonds in zoos. *Anthrozoös* **31** (3): 273-81.

Hosey G and Melfi V. 2014. Human-animal interactions, relationships, and bonds: A review and analysis of the literature. *International Journal of Comparative Psychology* **27** (1): 117-42.

Hosey G and Melfi V. 2019. *Anthrozoology: Human-animal Interactions in Domesticated and Wild Animals*. pp.1-17. Oxford University Press, New Delhi, India.

Irving-Pease EK, Frantz LA, Sykes N, Callou C and Larson G. 2018. Rabbits and the specious origins of domestication. *Trends in Ecology and Evolution* **33** (3): 149-52.

Irving-Pease EK, Ryan H, Jamieson A, Dimopoulos EA, Larson G and Frantz LA. 2019. Paleogenomics of animal domestication. In: *Paleogenomics: Genome-Scale Analysis of Ancient DNA*, pp. 225-72. (Eds) Lindqvist C and Rajora OP. eBook Springer Nature, Switzerland.

Jacques G, Guedes JDA and Shuya Z .2021. Yak domestication. *Ethnobiology Letters* **12** (1): 103-14.

Jeannin S. 2018. Cognition and emotions in dog domestication. In: *Hybrid Communities: Biosocial Approaches to Domestication and Other Trans-species Relationships*. pp. 235-47. (Eds) Stépanoff, C and Vigne JD. Routledge, London, UK.

Jemmett AM, Groombridge JJ, Hare J, Yadamsuren A, Burger PA and Ewen JG. 2023. What's in a name? Common name misuse potentially confounds the conservation of the wild camel *Camelus ferus*. *Oryx* **57** (2): 175-79.

Jerolmack C. 2007. Animal archeology: Domestic pigeons and the nature-culture dialectic. *Qualitative Sociology Review* **3** (1):74-95: http://www.qualitativesociologyreview.org / ENG/archive_eng.php, retrieved 16- 01-2024.

Jovčevska I and Muyldermans S. 2020. The therapeutic potential of nanobodies. *BioDrugs* **34** (1): 11-26.

Kamjan S, de Groene D, van den Hurk Y, Zidarov P, Elenski N, Patterson WP and Çakırlar C. 2021. The emergence and evolution of Neolithic cattle farming in southeastern Europe: New zooarchaeological and stable isotope data from Džuljunica-Smărdeš, in northeastern Bulgaria (ca. 6200–5500 cal. BCE). *Journal of Archaeological Science: Reports* **36** (April 2021): 102789. https://doi.org/10.1016/j.jasrep.2021.102789.

Kanakachari M, Chatterjee RN, Reddy MR, Dange M and Bhattacharya TK. 2023. Indian Red Jungle fowl reveals a genetic relationship with South East Asian Red Jungle fowl and Indian native chicken breeds as evidenced through whole mitochondrial genome sequences. *Frontiers in Genetics* **14**: doi: 10.3389/fgene.2023.1083976.

Kanginakudru S, Metta M, Jakati RD and Nagaraju J. 2008. Genetic evidence from Indian red jungle fowl corroborates multiple domestication of modern-day chicken. *BMC Evolutionary Biology* **8**: 174. https://doi.org/10.1186/1471-2148-8-174.

Kantere M, Athanasiou L, Chatzopoulos D, Spyrou V, Valiakos G, Kontos V and Billinis C. 2014. Enteric pathogens of dogs and cats with public health implications. *American Journal of Animal and Veterinary Sciences* **9** (2): 84-94.

Keeling L. 2002. Behaviour of fowl and other domesticated birds. In: *The Ethology of Domestic Animals. An Introductory Text.* pp.101-17. (Ed) Jensen P. CABI Wallingford, UK: https://cabidigitallibrary.org by 2402: e280:210b:57:7c37:df01:339e:af4b, downloaded on 01-02-2024.

Khandai V and Shrivastava P. 2023. Evolution of research on human–animal interaction: A review. *Journal of Entomology and Zoology Studies* **11**(2): 115-18.

Khomeiri M and Yam BAZ. 2015. Introduction to camel origin, history, raising, characteristics, and wool, hair, and skin: A review. *Research Journal of Agricultural and Environmental Management* **4** (11): 496-508.

Kiesling C. 2017. The camelid registry LAREU: What are we breeding in Europe? In: *Advances in Fibre Production Science in South American Camelids and other Fibre Animals*. pp. 97- 110. (Eds) Gerken M, Renieri C, Allain D, Galbraith H, Gutiérrez JP, McKenna L Niznikowski R and Wurzinger M. Universitätsverlag Göttingen, Göttingen, Germany.

Kimura B, Marshall F, Beja-Pereira A, Mulligan C. 2013. Donkey domestication. *African Archaeological Review* **30**: 83-95.

Klecel W, Martyniuk E. 2021. From the Eurasian steppes to the Roman circuses: A review of early development of horse breeding and management. *Animals* **11** (7): 1859. https://doi.org/10.3390/ani11071859.

Klimscha F. 2017. Transforming technical know-how in time and space. Using the digital atlas of innovations to understand the innovation process of animal traction and the wheel. *eTopoi Journal of Ancient Studies* **6** (2017): 16-63.

Köhler-Rollefson I, Rathore S, Rollefson A and Hardy K. 2013. *The Camels of Kumbhalgarh. A Biodiversity Treasure*. Lokhit Pashu-Palak Sansthan, Sadri: http://www. lpps. org/wp-content/uploads/2013/10/Camels Of_ Kumbhalgarh_web. pdf.pdf, accessed on 17-11-2023.

Köhler-Rollefson I. 2018. *Camel Cultures of India*: https://www.sahapedia.org/camel-cultures-of-india, accessed on 17-11-2023.

Komar N. 2001. West Nile virus surveillance using sentinel birds. *Annals of the New York Academy of Sciences* **951** (1): 58-73.

Kondybayev A, Loiseau G, Achir N, Mestres C and Konuspayeva G. 2021. Fermented mare milk product (Qymyz, Koumiss). *International Dairy Journal* **119:** p.105065. https://doi.org/10.1016/j.idairyj.2021.105065.

Konuspayeva G and Faye B. 2021. Recent advances in camel milk processing. *Animals* **11**(4): 1045-66:https://doi.org/10.3390/ani11041045.

Koufariotis L, Hayes BJ, Kelly M, Burns BM, Lyons R, Stothard P, Chamberlain AJ and Moore S. 2018. Sequencing the mosaic genome of Brahman cattle identifies historic and recent introgression including polled. *Scientific Reports* **8** (1): 17761.

Kruger KA and Serpell JA. 2010. Animal-assisted interventions in mental health: Definitions and theoretical foundations. *Handbook on Animal-Assisted Therapy*. 3rd edn. pp. 33-48. (Ed) Fine AH. Academic Press: San Diego, CA, USA.

Kumar S, Nagarajan M, Sandhu JS, Kumar N, Behl V and Nishanth G. 2007. Mitochondrial DNA analyses of Indian water buffalo support a distinct genetic origin of river and swamp buffalo. *Animal Genetics* **38** (3): 227-32.

Kuratsune M, Yoshimura T, Matsuzaka J and Yamaguchi A. 1972. Epidemiologic study on Yusho, a poisoning caused by ingestion of rice oil contaminated with a commercial brand of polychlorinated biphenyls. *Environmental Health Perspectives* **1**: 119-28.

Larson G and Fuller DQ. 2014. The evolution of animal domestication. *Annual Review of Ecology, Evolution, and Systematics* **45** (1): 115-36: https://doi.org/10.1146/annurev-ecolsys-110512-135813.

Larson G, Liu R, Zhao X, Yuan J, Fuller D, Barton L, Dobney K, Fan Q, Gu Z, Liu XH and Lu Y. 2010. Patterns of East Asian pig domestication, migration, and turnover revealed by modern and ancient DNA. *Proceedings of the National Academy of Sciences* **107** (17): 7686-91.

Lassaletta L, Estellés F, Beusen AH, Bouwman L, Calvet S, Van Grinsven HJ, Doelman JC, Stehfest E, Uwizeye A and Westhoek H. 2019. Future global pig production systems according to the shared socioeconomic pathways. *Science of the Total Environment* **665**:739-51: https://doi.org/10.1016/j.scitotenv.2019.02.079.

Lawal RA and Hanotte O. 2021. Domestic chicken diversity: Origin, distribution, and adaptation. *Animal Genetics* **52**(4): 385-94.

Lee RB and Daly R. 1999. Introduction: Foragers and others. In: *The Cambridge Encyclopedia of Hulnters and Gatherers*. pp 1-19. (Eds) Lee RB, Daly RH and Daly R. Cambridge University Press, Cambridge, UK.

Levine MA .2005. Domestication and early history of the horse. In: *The Domestic Horse: The Origins, Development, and Management of its Behaviour.* pp.5-22. (Eds) Mills DS and McDonnell SM. Cambridge University Press, UK.

Librado P, Fages A, Gaunitz C, Leonardi M, Wagner S, Khan N, Hanghøj K, Alquraishi SA, Alfarhan AH, Al-Rasheid K A and Der Sarkissian C. 2016. The evolutionary origin and genetic makeup of domestic horses. *Genetics* **204** (2): 423-34.

Librado P, Khan N, Fages A, Kusliy MA, Suchan T, Tonasso-Calvière L, Schiavinato S, Alioglu D, Fromentier A, Perdereau A and Aury JM. 2021. The origins and spread of domestic horses from the Western Eurasian steppes. *Nature* **598** (7882): 634-40.

Lindahl C, Pinzke S, Herlin A and Keeling LJ. 2016. Human-animal interactions and safety during dairy cattle handling—Comparing moving cows to milking and hoof trimming. *Journal of Dairy Science* **99** (3):2131-41.

Löscher W. 2022. Dogs as a natural animal model of epilepsy. *Frontiers in Veterinary Science* **9**: https://doi.org/10.3389/fvets.2022.928009.

Losey RJ, Nomokonova T, Arzyutov DV, Gusev AV, Plekhanov AV, Fedorova NV, and Anderson DG. 2021. Domestication as enskilment: harnessing reindeer in Arctic Siberia. *Journal of Archaeological Method and Theory* **28** (1): 197-231.

Loukaki K, Koukoutsakis P and Kostomitsopoulos N. 2010. Animal welfare issues on the use of rabbits in an animal assisted therapy program for children. *Journal of the Hellenic Veterinary Medical Society* **61**(3): 220-25.

Lukefahr S D McNitt JI, Cheeke PR and Patton NM .2022. *Rabbit Production.* 10th edn. pp. 1-11. CABI, Oxfordshire, UK: https://www.cabidigitallibrary.org/doi/pdf/10.5555/20220190938., downloaded on 24-02-2024.

Magnusson U, Moodley A and Osbjer K. 2021. Antimicrobial resistance at the livestock-human interface: implications for Veterinary Services. *Revue Scientifique et Technique International Office of Epizootics* **40** (2): 511-21.

Manteca Vilanova X, Beaver B, Uldahl M and Turner PV. 2021. Recommendations for ensuring good welfare of horses used for industrial blood, serum, or urine production. *Animals* **11**(5):1466 https://doi.org/10.3390/ani11051466.

Marín JC, Romero K, Rivera R, Johnson WE and González BA. 2017. Y-chromosome and mtDNA variation confirms independent domestications and directional hybridization in South American camelids. *Animal Genetics* **48** (5): 591-95.

Marshall FB, Dob*ney* K, Denham T and Capriles JM. 2014. Evaluating the roles of directed breeding and gene flow in animal domestication. *Proceedings of the National Academy of Sciences* 111(17): 6153-58.

Mateescu RG. 2020. Genetics and breeding of beef cattle. *Animal Agriculture*. pp.21-35. (Eds) Fuller W. Bazer, G. Cliff Lamb and Guoyao Wu. Academic Press: https://do*i.org/1*0.**1**016/B978-0-12-817052-6.00002-1.

Matthews PT, Barwick J, Doughty AK, Doyle EK, Morton CL, *and Brown WY. 2020.* Alpaca field behaviour when cohabitating with lambing ewes. *Animals 10* (9): 1605. doi:10.3390/ani10091605.

Mazzullo N. 2020. More than meat on the hoof? Social significance of reindeer among Finnish Saami in a rationalized pastoralist economy. In: *Good to Eat, Good to Live With: Nomads and the Animals in Northern Eurasia and Africa.* 2nd edn. pp. 101-19. (Eds) Florian Stammler F and Takakura H. University of Lapland, Finland.

McGregor BA. 2006. Production, attributes, and relative value of alpaca fleeces in southern Australia and implications for industry development. *Small Ruminant Research* **61** (2-3): 93-111.

McLean K and Niehaus AJ. 2022. General biology and evolution. In: *Medicine and Surgery of Camelids.* 4th edn. pp 1-18. (Ed) Niehaus AJ. Wiley-Blackwell Hoboken NJ, USA.

McMiken DF. 1990. Ancient origins of horsemanship. Equine Veterinary Journal 22 (2):73-78.

Millman ST, Mench JA and Malleau AE. 2010. The future of poultry welfare. *The Welfare of Domestic Fowl and Other Captive Birds*. pp. 279-302. (Eds) Duncan IJ, Hawkins P. Dordrecht, Springer, Netherland.

Minervino AH, Zava M, Vecchio D, Borghese A. 2020. *Bubalus bubalis*: A short story. *Frontiers in Veterinary Science* **7***:* 570413: https://doi.org/10.3389/fvets.2020.570413.

Miraglia N, Salimei E and Fantuz F. 2020. Equine milk production and valorization of marginal areas—A review. Animals 10 (2): p.353. https://doi.org/10.3390/ani10020353.

Miranda JM, Anton X, *Redondo-V*albuena C, Roca-Saavedra P, Rodriguez JA, Lamas A, Franco CM and Cepeda A. 2015. Egg and egg-derived foods: effects on human health and use as functional foods. *Nutrients* **7**(1): 706-29.

Mitchell P. 2018. *The Donkey in Human History: An Archaeological Perspective.* pp. 1-13, 72-107. Oxford University Press, UK.

Mithen S. 1999. The hunter—gatherer prehistory of human—animal interactions. *Anthrozoös* **12** (4): 195-204.

Moiseyeva IG, Romanov MN, Nikiforov AA, Sevastyanova AA and Semyenova SK. 2003. Evolutionary relationships of Red Jungle Fowl and chicken breeds. *Genetics Selection Evolution,* **35** (4): 403-23.

Naderi S, Rezaei HR, Pompanon F, Blum MG, Negrini R, Naghash HR, Balkız Ö, Mashkour M, Gaggiotti OE, Ajmone-Marsan P and Kence A. 2008. The goat domestication process inferred from large-scale mitochondrial DNA analysis of wild and domestic individuals. *Proceedings of the National Academy of Sciences* **105** (46): 17659-64.

Nagarajan M, Nimisha K and Kumar S. 2015. Mitochondrial DNA variability of domestic river buffalo (Bubalus bubalis) populations: genetic evidence for domestication of river buffalo in Indian subcontinent. *Genome Biology and Evolution* **7** (5): 1252-59.

Neubert S, von Altrock A, Wendt M and Wagener MG. 2021. Llama and aalpaca management in Germany—Results of an online survey among owners on farm structure, health problems and self-reflection. *Animals* **11** (1):102: https://doi.org/10.3390/ani11010102.

Ní Leathlobhair M, Perri AR, Irving-Pease EK, Witt KE, Linderholm A, Haile J, Lebrasseur O, Ameen C, Blick J, Boyko AR and Brace S. 2018. The evolutionary history of dogs in the Americas. *Science* **361**(6397): 81-85.

Nomokonova T, Losey RJ, Fedorova NV, Gusev AV and Arzyutov DV. 2021. Reindeer imagery in the making at Ust'-Polui in Arctic Siberia. *Cambridge Archaeological Journal* **31(**1): 161-68.

Nordquist RE, Meijer E, van der Staay FJ and Arndt SS. 2017. Pigs as model species to investigate effects of early life events on later behavioral and neurological functions. In:

Animal Models for the Study of Human Disease. pp. 1003-30. (Ed). Michael CP. Academic Press: https://doi.org/10.1016/B978-0-12-809468-6.00039-5.

Norman HD, Hubbard SM and VanRaden PM. 2010. Dairy cattle: Breeding and genetics. *Encyclopedia of Animal Science.* 2nd edn. pp. 262-65. (Eds) Ullrey DE, Baer CK and Pond WG. Taylor & Francis Boca Raton, Florida, USA.

Nwaru BI, Hickstein L, Panesar SS, Roberts G, Muraro A and Sheikh A. 2014. Prevalence of common food allergies in Europe: a systematic review and meta-analysis. *Allergy* **69 (1)**: 992–1007:https://doi.org/10.1111/all.12423.

Nyland A. 1992. Penna-and parh-in the Hittite horse training texts. *Journal of Near Eastern Studies* **51**(4):293-96.

Ohnuma R. 2017. Scapegoat for the Buddha: The horse Kanthaka. *Unfortunate Destiny: Animals in the Indian Buddhist Imagination. Online edn.* pp. 101–28. Oxford Academic, New York: https://doi.org/10.1093/acprof:oso/9780190637545.003.0005, accessed on 19-02-2024, USA.

Olsen SL. 2006. Early horse domestication on the Eurasian steppe. *Documenting Domestication: New Genetic and Archaeological Paradigms*. pp. 245-269. (Eds) Zeder, M.A, Daniel G. Bradley D.G. Emshwiller B. and Smith RD. University of California Press, Berkeley and Los Angeles, California.

Oselu S, Ebere R and Arimi J M. 2022. Camels, camel milk, and camel milk product situation in Kenya in relation to the world. *International Journal of Food Science* **2022:** https://doi.org/10.1155/2022/1237423.

Otte J and Pica-Ciamarra U. 2021. Emerging infectious zoonotic diseases: The neglected role of food animals. *One Health* **13**:100323: https://doi.org/10.1016/j.onehlt.2021.100323.

Otte MJ, Nugent R and McLeod A. 2004. Transboundary animal diseases: assessment of socio-economic impacts and institutional responses. *FAO Livestock Policy Discussion Paper No 9*. 46 p. Food and Agriculture Organization, Livestock Information and Policy Branch, Rome, Italy.

Ottoni C, Girdland Flink L, Evin A, Geörg C, De Cupere B, Van Neer W, Bartosiewicz L, Linderholm A, Barnett R, Peters J and Decorte R. 2013. Pig domestication and human-mediated dispersal in western Eurasia revealed through ancient DNA and geometric morphometrics. *Molecular Biology and Evolution* **30** (4): 824-32.

Padhi M and Giri S. 2024. Status of duck breeding in India. *The Indian Journal of Animal Sciences* **94**(1):3-10.

Pal M, Tolawak D and Garedaghi Y. 2023. A comprehensive review on major zoonotic parasites from dogs and cats. *International Journal of Medical Parasitology and Epidemiology Sciences* **4**(1): 3-11.

Pelletier M, Kotiaho A, Niinimäki S and Salmi AK.2020. Identifying early stages of reindeer domestication in the archaeological record: a 3D morphological investigation on forelimb bones of modern populations from Fennoscandia. *Archaeological and Anthropological Sciences* **12**(8): 1-25: https://doi.org/10.1007/s12520-020-01123-0.

Perri AR, Feuerborn TR, Frantz LA, Larson G, Malhi RS, Meltzer DJ and Witt KE. 2021. Dog domestication and the dual dispersal of people and dogs into the Americas. *Proceedings of the National Academy of Sciences* **118** (6): 1-8: https://doi.org/10.1073/pnas.2010083118.

Peters J, Lebrasseur O, Irving-Pease EK, Paxinos PD, Best J, Smallman R, Callou C, Gardeisen A, Trixl S, Frantz L and Sykes N. 2022. The biocultural origins and dispersal of domestic chickens. *Proceedings of the National Academy of Sciences* **119** (24): 1-9, p.e2121978119: https://doi.org/10.1073/pnas.2121978119.

Pierotti R and Fogg B R. 2017. The beginnings. In: *First Domestication: How Wolves and Humans Coevolved.* pp.1-23. Yale University Press, New Haven, and London, UK.

Pitt D, Sevane N, Nicolazzi EL, MacHugh DE, Park SD, Colli L, Martinez R, Bruford MW and Orozco-terWengel P. 2019. Domestication of cattle: Two or three events? *Evolutionary Applications* **12** (1): 123-36.

Poma G, Malarvannan G and Covaci A. 2020. Pets as sentinels of indoor contamination. In: *Pets as Sentinels, Forecasters and Promoters of Human Health.* pp. 3-20. (Eds) Pastorinho Mand Sousa A. Springer, Cham: https://doi.org/10.1007/978-3-030-30734-9_1.

Porter V. 2020. *Mason's World Dictionary of Livestock Breeds, Types and Varieties.* CABI, Wellington, Oxfordshire, UK.

Prabhu VR, Arjun MS, Bhavana K, Kamalakkannan R and Nagarajan M. 2019. Complete mitochondrial genome of Indian mithun, *Bos frontalis* and its phylogenetic implications. *Molecular Biology Reports* **46** (2): 2561-66.

Prakash V, Jyotsana B, Sawal R K and Sahoo A. 2021. Promising Camel breed of India-Exploring Dairy Traits. pp 15-26 In: (Eds) Sahoo A and Sawal RK. *Opportunities and Constraints in Camel Production System and its Sustainability. Souvenir-Cum Proceeding, Interactive Meet.* August 3, 2021. ICAR-National Research Centre on Camel, Bikaner, Rajasthan, India.

Price M and Hongo H. 2020. The archaeology of pig domestication in Eurasia. *Journal of Archaeological Research* **28**: 557-615: https://doi.org/10.1007/s10814-019-09142-9.

Prieto A, Martins Almeida, Ayupe K, Nemetala Gomes L, Saúde AC and Gutierres Filho P. 2022. Effects of equine-assisted therapy on the functionality of individuals with disabilities: systematic review and meta-analysis. *Physiotherapy Theory and Practice* **38** (9): 1091-1106.

Pringle H. 1997. Ice Age communities may be earliest known net hunters. *Science* **277** (5330): 1203-05.

Purugganan MD. 2022. What is domestication? *Trends in Ecology & Evolution* **37**(8): 663-70: https://doi.org/10.1016/j.tree.2022.04.006.

Ramaswamy V and Sharma HR. 2011. Plastic bags–Threat to environment and cattle health: A retrospective study from Gondar City of Ethiopia. *The IIOAB Journal* **2** (1): 6-11.

Ramirez Rozzi F and Froment A. 2018. Earliest animal cranial surgery: From cow to man in the Neolithic. *Scientific Reports* **8** (1):5536. DOI:10.1038/s41598-018-23914-1.

Ramos-Onsins SE, Burgos-Paz, W, Manunza, A and Amills M. 2014. Mining the pig genome to investigate the domestication process. *Heredity* **113** (6): 471-84.

Randhawa MS. 1980. *A History of Agriculture in India.* Vol I, II, II, IV. Indian Council of Agricultural Research, New Delhi, India.

Reed SA. 2022. Horses as athletes: the road to success. *Animal Frontiers* **12**(3): 3-4.

Reif JS. 2011. Animal sentinels for environmental and public health. *Public Health Reports* **126** (Suppl.1) : 50–57.

Reif JS, Ameghino E and Aaronson MJ. 1989. Chronic exposure of sheep to a zinc smelter in Peru. *Environmental Research* **49** (1): 40-49.

Ritchie H, Rosado P and Roser M. 2022. *Environmental Impacts of Food Production.* OurWorldInData.org. Retrieved from: https://ourworldindata.org/environmental-impacts-of-food' [Online Resource].

Røed KH, Flagstad Ø, Nieminen M, Holand Ø, Dwyer M.J, Røv N and Vilà C. 2008. Genetic analyses reveal independent domestication origins of Eurasian reindeer. *Proceedings of the Royal Society B: Biological Sciences* **275** (1645): 1849-55.

Ruetten H and Vezina CM. 2022. Relevance of dog as an animal model for urologic diseases. *Progress in Molecular Biology and Translational Science* **189** (1): 35-65.

Sahrhage D and Lundbeck J. 2012. *A History of Fishing*. 1st edn. 348 p. Springer Verlag, Berlin Heidelberg, Germany.

Salmi AK. 2023. The archaeology of reindeer domestication and herding practices in Northern Fennoscandia. *Journal of Archaeological Research* **31**(4): 617-60.

Sánchez-Villagra M. 2022. Domesticated mammals and birds; Species account. In: *The Process of Animal Domestication*. pp. 36-66. Princeton University Press, New Jersey, USA.

Sanders JO. History and development of Zebu cattle in the United States. 1980. *Journal of Animal Science* **50** (6): 1188-200.

Santana Jr ML, Pereira RJ, Bignardi AB, Ayres DR, Menezes GD, Silva LO, Leroy G, Machado CH, Josahkian LA and Albuquerque LG. 2016. Structure and genetic diversity of Brazilian Zebu cattle breeds assessed by pedigree analysis. *Livestock Science* **187**: 6-15.

Savalia K B, Ahlawat A R, Gamit VV, Parikh SS and Verma AD. 2019. Recently recognized indigenous cattle breeds of India: A review. *International Journal of Current Microbiology and Applied Sciences* **8** (12): 161-68.

Scanes CG. 2018. The neolithic revolution, animal domestication, and early forms of animal agriculture. *Animals and Human Society*. pp. 103-31. (Eds) Scanes C.G. and Toukhsati S. Academic Press, London, United Kingdom. doi.org/10.1016/B978-0-12805247-1.00006-X.

Schatz T, Thomas S, Reed S and Hearnden, M. 2020. Crossbreeding with a tropically adapted *Bos taurus* breed (Senepol) to improve meat quality and production from Brahman herds in Northern Australia. 1. Steer performance. *Animal Production Science* **60** (4): 487-91.

Schwabe C W. 1978. How men first learned to heal. In: *Cattle, Priests and Progress in Medicine, The Wesley W. Spink Lectures on Comparative Medicine Vol 4*. pp 8-48. University of Minnesota Press, Minneapolis, USA.

Schwabe C W. 1994. Animals in the ancient world. In: *Animals and Human Society: Changing Perspectives*. 1st edn. pp. 36-58. (Eds) Manning, A and Serpell J. Routledge, London, UK https://doi.org/10.4324/9780203421444

Seifu E. 2022. Recent advances on camel milk: Nutritional and health benefits and processing implications—A review. *AIMS Agriculture and Food* **7**(4): 777-804.

Serpell JA. 2019. Companion animals. In: *Anthrozoology: Human- Animal Interactions in Domesticated and Wild Animals*. (South Asia edn.). pp. 17-31. (Eds.) Hosey G and Melfi V. Oxford University Press, New Delhi, India

Sewell A. 1877. *Black Beauty: The Autobiography of a Horse: https://en.m.wikisource.org/wiki/Black_Beauty.*

Seyiti S and Kelimu A. 2021. Donkey industry in China: current aspects, suggestions, and future challenges. *Journal of Equine Veterinary Science* **102**: p.103642:https://doi.org/10.1016/j.jevs.2021.103642.

Sharpe MS, Lord LK, Wittum TE and Anderson DE. 2009. Pre-weaning morbidity and mortality of llamas and alpacas. *Australian Veterinary Journal* **87** (1-2): 56-60.

Shih CA and Yang MH. 2023. Effect of animal-assisted therapy (AAT) on social interaction and quality of life in patients with schizophrenia during the COVID-19 pandemic: An experimental study. *Asian Nursing Research* **17** (1): 37-43.

Singh JL and Swarup D. 1995. Clinical observations and diagnosis of fluorosis in dairy cows and buffaloes. *Agri-Practice (USA)* **16** (5): 25-30.

Singh MK, Shakyawar DB, Bajpai P and Gangwar AK. 2023. Pashmina fiber blended woven fabrics for high functional performances. *Journal of Natural Fibers* **20** (1): 1-12: https://doi.org/10.1080/15440478.2022.2139324.

Skarin A and Åhman B. 2014. Do human activity and infrastructure disturb domesticated reindeer? The need for the reindeer's perspective. *Polar Biology* **37** (7): 1041-54.

Smith AT. 2024. Rabbit. In: *Encyclopedia Britannica:* https://www.britannica.com/animal/rabbit, retrieved on 08-01-2024.

Smith J, Sones K, Grace D, MacMillan S, Tarawali S and Herrero M. 2013. Beyond milk, meat, and eggs: Role of livestock in food and nutrition security. *Animal Frontiers* **3** (1): 6-13.

Sofi AH, Wani SA, Shakyawar DB, Malhotra VK, Ahmad SR, Pal MA, Beig S and Khan AA. 2018. Subjective evaluation of Pashmina and Pashmina blended knitted fabrics. *Journal of Pharmacognosy and Phytochemistry* **7** (2): 2686-89.

Somerville AD and Sugiyama N .2021. Why were New World rabbits not domesticated? *Animal Frontiers* **11**(3): 62-68.

Sossinka R. 1982. Domestication in birds. In: *Avian Biology Vol 6*. pp.373-403. (Eds) Donald S. Farner DS, King J R and Parkes KC. Academic Press, Inc. New York, USA.

Stammler F. 2020. Animal-diversity and its social significance among Arctic pastoralists. In: *Good to Eat, Good to Live With: Nomads and the Animals in Northern Eurasia and Africa.* 2nd edn. pp. 215-43. (Eds) Stammler F and Takakura H. University of Lapland, Finland.

Stephenson M. 2010. From marvelous antidote to the poison of idolatry: the transatlantic role of Andean bezoar stones during the late sixteenth and early seventeenth centuries. *Hispanic American Historical Review* **90** (1): 3-39.

Stock F and Gifford-Gonzalez D. 2013. Genetics and African cattle domestication. *African Archaeological Review* **30**: 51-72: DOI: 10.1007/s10437-013-9131-6.

Stokstad E. 2015. Bringing back the aurochs. *Science* **350** (6265): 1144-47 DOI: 10.1126/science.350.6265.1144.

Swabe J. 1999. *Animals, Disease, and Human Society: Human-Animal Relations and the Rise of Veterinary Medicine.* Taylor & Francis e-Library. http:// www.ir.juit.ac.in:8080/jspui/bitstream/123456789/6114/1/Animals.Disease. 1998.pdf downloaded on 8-2-2023.

Swarup D, Naresh R, Varshney VP, Balagangatharathilagar M, Kumar P, Nandi D and Patra RC. 2007. Changes in plasma hormones profile and liver function in cows naturally exposed to lead and cadmium around different industrial areas. *Research in Veterinary Science* **82** (1): 16-21.

Tai LL. 2020. Small antibodies from no so small organisms: harnessing the unique immune system of llamas, camels, sharks, and lampreys: https://www.immpressmagazine.com/small-antibodies-from-not-so-small-organisms-harnessing-the-unique-immune-system-of-llamas-camels-sharks-and-lampreys/, accessed on 24-12-2023.

Tan SY, Merchant J and Frederick Banting (1891–1941). 2017. Discoverer of insulin. *Singapore Medical Journal* **58(**1):2-3.

Teletchea F. 2019. Animal domestication: A brief overview. *Animal Domestication*. pp. 1-19. (Ed) Teletchea F. IntechOpen; DOI: 10.5772/intechopen.86783.

Thayer ER and Stevens JR. 2019. Human-Animal Interaction In: *Encyclopedia of Animal Cognition and Behavior*. pp. 1-5. (Eds) Vonk J and Shackelford, T. Springer, Cham: https://doi.org/10.1007/978-3-319-47829-6_2058-1.

Thrusfield M. 2018. Development of veterinary medicine. In: *Veterinary Epidemiology.* 4th edn. pp. 1-27. (Eds) Thrusfied M and Christley R. John Wiley & Sons Ltd. Oxford, UK.

Tixier-Boichard M, Bed'hom B and Rognon X. 2011. Chicken domestication: from archeology to genomics. *Comptes Rendus Biologies* **334** (3): 197-204.

Todd ET, Tonasso-Calvière L, Chauvey L, Schiavinato S, Fages A, Seguin-Orlando A, Clavel P, Khan N, Pérez Pardal L, Patterson Rosa L and Librado P. 2022. The genomic history and global expansion of domestic donkeys. *Science* **377(**6611): 1172-80.

Treves A and Bonacic C. 2016. Humanity's dual response to dogs and wolves. *Trends in Ecology and Evolution* **31**(7): 489-91.

Tsai KL, Clark LA and Murphy KE. 2007. Understanding hereditary diseases using the dog and human as companion model systems. *Mammalian Genome* **18**: 444-51: https://doi.org/10.1007/s00335-007-9037-1.

Tuckel PS and Milczarski W. 2020. The changing epidemiology of dog bite injuries in the United States, 2005-2018. *Injury Epidemiology* **7**(1): 57: https://doi.org/10.1186/s40621-020-00281-y.

Uerpmann HP and Uerpmann M. 2017. The "commodification" of animals. In: *Ancient West Asian Civilization: Geoenvironment and Society in the Pre-Islamic Middle East*, pp.99-113. (Eds) Tsunek A Yamada S and Hisada, Ki. Springer, Singapore: https://doi.org/10.1007/978-981-10-0554-1_7.

Utsunomiya YT, Milanesi M, Fortes MR, Porto-Neto LR, Utsunomiya AT, Silva MV, Garcia JF, Ajmone-Marsan P. 2019. Genomic clues of the evolutionary history of *Bos indicus* cattle. *Animal Genetics* **50** (6) : 557-68.

van der Geer A. 2008. *Animals in Stone*: *Indian Mammals Sculptured through Time*, pp. 140-49, 171-74. Brill NV, Leiden, The Netherland.

Verdugo MP, Mullin VE, Scheu A, Mattiangeli V, Daly KG, Maisano Delser P, Hare AJ, Burger J, Collins MJ, Kehati R and Hesse P. 2019. Ancient cattle genomics, origins, and rapid turnover in the Fertile Crescent. *Science* **365** (6449): 173-76.

Vigne JD. 2011. The origins of animal domestication and husbandry: Amajor change in the history of humanity and the biosphere. *Comptes Rendus Biologies* **334** (3):171-81.

Vigne J D. 2015. Early domestication and farming: what should we know or do for a better understanding? *Anthropozoologica* **50** (2): 123-50: http://dx.doi.org/10.5252/az2015n2a5.

Vilá B and Arzamendia Y. 2022. South American Camelids: their values and contributions to people. *Sustainability Science* **17**(3): 707-24.

Vorobiev DV. 2018. Ethnozoology or the interaction of humans with the world of fauna? (An Introduction). *Etnograficheskoe Obozrenie* **4**: 5-12: https://ras.jes.su/ethnorev/s086954150000195-4-1-en.

Vozzi PA, Marcondes CR, Magnabosco CD, Bezerra LA, Lôbo RB. 2006. Structure and genetic variability in Nellore (*Bos indicus*) cattle by pedigree analysis. *Genetics and Molecular Biology* **29**: 482-85.

Waiblinger S. 2019. Agricultural animals. In *Anthrozoology: Human-Animal Interactions in Domesticated and Wild Animals*, 1st edn. pp.32-58. (Eds) Hosey G and Melfi V. Oxford University Press, New Delhi, India.

Wakild E. 2022. Learning from the llama: on the broad contours of cultural contributions and geographic expansion. *História, Ciências, Saúde-Manguinhos* **28** (Suppl.): 141-159: https://doi.org/10.1590/S0104-59702021000500006.

Wang GD, Zhai W, Yang HC, Wang LU, Zhong LI, Liu YH, Fan RX, Yin TT, Zhu CL, Poyarkov AD and Irwin DM. 2016. Out of southern East Asia: the natural history of domestic dogs across the world. *Cell Research* **26** (1): 21-33.

Wang MS, Thakur M, Peng MS, Jiang YU, Frantz LA, Li M, Zhang JJ, Wang S, Peters J, Otecko NO and Suwannapoom C. 2020. 863 genomes reveal the origin and domestication of chicken. *Cell Research* **30** (8): 693-701.

Wang S, Chen N, Capodiferro MR, Zhang T, Lancioni H, Zhang H, Miao Y, Chanthakhoun V, Wanapat M, Yindee M and Zhang Y. 2017. Whole mitogenomes reveal the history of swamp buffalo: initially shaped by glacial periods and eventually modelled by domestication. *Scientific Reports* **7**(1): p.4708: https://doi.org/10.1038/s41598-017-04830-2.

Wang Y, Hua X, Shi X and Wang C. 2022. Origin, evolution, and research development of Donkeys. *Genes* **13** (11): p.1945. https://doi.org/10.3390/genes13111945.

Ward SL and Osenkowski P. 2022. Dog as the experimental model: Laboratory uses of dogs in the United States. *ALTEX-Alternatives to Animal Experimentation* **39** (4): 605-20.

Weldenegodguad M, Pokharel K, Ming Y, Honkatukia M, Peippo J, Reilas T, Røed KH, and Kantanen J. 2020. Genome sequence and comparative analysis of reindeer (*Rangifer tarandus*) in northern Eurasia. *Scientific Reports* **10** (1): 8980. doi: 10.1038/s41598-020-65487-y.

Wengrow D. 2001. Rethinking 'cattle cults' in early Egypt: Towards a prehistoric perspective on the Narmer Palette. *Cambridge Archaeological Journal* **11**(1): 91-104.

Werness HB. 2004. *The Continuum Encyclopedia of Animal Symbolism in Art*. Continuum International Publishing Group, New York, USA.

Westbury M, Prost S, Seelenfreund A, Ramírez JM, Matisoo-Smith EA and Knapp M. 2016. First complete mitochondrial genome data from ancient South American camelids-The mystery of the chilihueques from Isla Mocha (Chile). *Scientific Reports* **6** (1): 38708 https://doi.org/10.1038/srep38708.

Wheeler JC. 1995. Evolution and present situation of the South American Camelidae. *Biological Journal of the Linnean Society* **54** (3): 271-95.

Wilkinson T. 2011. *The Rise and Fall of Ancient Egypt*. 672 p. Bloomsbury Publishing, London, UK.

Willekes C. 2016. Introduction horses and humans. In: *The Horse in the Ancient World: from Bucephalus to the Hippodrome*. pp 1-5. IB Tauris, London, UK.

Wolfe N, Dunavan C and Diamond J. 2007. Origins of major human infectious diseases. *Nature* **447**: 279–83:https://doi.org/10.1038/nature0577.

Wu G. 2020. Important roles of dietary taurine, creatine, carnosine, anserine and 4-hydroxyproline in human nutrition and health. *Amino acids* **52**(3): 329-60.

Yadav MP, Singh RK and Malik YS. 2020. Emerging and transboundary animal viral diseases: Perspectives and preparedness. Emerging and transboundary animal viruses. In: *Emerging and Transboundary Animal Viruses*. pp.1-25. (Eds) Malik YS, Singh RK and Yadav MP. Springer Nature, Singapore: https://doi.org/10.1007/978-981-15-0402-0.

Zachut M, Šperanda M, de Almeida AM, Gabai G, Mobasheri A and Hernández-Castellano LE. 2020. Biomarkers of fitness and welfare in dairy cattle: healthy productivity. *Journal of Dairy Research* **87** (1): 4-13.

Zava MA. 2012. Present situation and future perspective of buffalo production in America. *The Journal of Animal and Plant Sci*ences **22** (3 Suppl.): 262-69.

Zeder MA. 2012. The domestication of animals. *Journal of Anthropological Research* **68** (2): 161-90.

Zeder MA. 2008. Domestication and early agriculture in the Mediterranean Basin: Origins, diffusion, and impact. *Proceedings of the National Academy of Sciences* **105** (33): 11597-604.

Zhang M, Yang Q, Ai H and Huang L. 2022. Revisiting the evolutionary history of pigs via de novo mutation rate estimation in a three-generation pedigree. *Genomics, Proteomics and Bioinformatics* **20**(6): 1040-52.

Zhang Y, Colli L and Barker JSF. 2020. Asian water buffalo: domestication, history, and genetics. *Animal Genetics* **51**(2): 177-91.

Zhang Z, Khederzadeh S and Li Y. 2020b. Deciphering the puzzles of dog domestication. *Zoological Research* **41** (2): 97-104.

2

Brief History, Socio-Economic Roles, and Current Status of Domestic Animals in India

D. Swarup

A gāvo agmannuta bhadramakrantsīdantu gosthe ranayantvasme. Prajāvatiḥ pururūpā iha syuri-ndrāya pūrvīrusaso duhānāḥ.
Let the cows come as rays of the sun. Let them sit and rest in the stalls, be happy and comfortable. They bring happiness and good fortune. May they be fertile, rich with progeny, abundant rich and various by growing, yielding plenty of milk for the health and prosperity of the nation, and thereby let them be harbingers of light as morning dawns.

(Atharva Veda 4.21.1; translation by Sharma 2013)

Introduction

India stands among the world's ten most ancient civilizations, with a rich evolutionary history spanning over 50,000 years. One of the earliest migrations out of Africa—the cradle of modern humans (*Homo sapiens*)—led to the settlement of India around 50,000 years ago. Since then, successive waves of migration from various regions have shaped India into a remarkable genetic melting pot of the ancient world (Majumder and Basu 2015). Today, home to about 1.46 billion people, India is one of the world's 17 richest regions in terms of biodiversity. It has a huge variety of plants and animals, both wild and domesticated. Despite covering only 2.4% of Earth's land area, the megadiversity country accounts for 7-8% of all recorded species, including over 45,000 species of plants and 91,000 species of animals globally (India | IUCN, accessed on 21-07-2025). Domestic animals, comprising a plethora of breeds and species including bovine, canine, equines, camelid, swine, avian, and semi-domestic species like elephant and pet birds, constitute a significant portion of Indian faunal biodiversity. They hold immense economic, cultural, and practical value in human life. This chapter serves as a synthesis and summation of existing knowledge regarding the history of domestic animals in India, their socio-cultural and economic influences, and their current status in modern society.

Pre-Agricultural Hunter- Gatherers in India

Approximate timeline of major archaeological periods in India (South Asia) is suggested as Paleolithic-ca. 53000 – 10000 BCE; Mesolithic- ca.10000 – 6500 BCE; Neolithic- ca. 6500 – 4000 BCE (up to ca. 2000 BC in some areas); Chalcolithic- ca. 4000 – 2000 BCE; Bronze Age (Indus Valley Civilization)- ca. 3100 – 1100 BCE; Iron Age- 1100 – 500 BCE; Proto- history (known as Vedic period) ca. 1500 – 500 BCE; and Historical Period- after 500 BCE (https://en.wikipedia.org/wiki/List_of_archaeological_periods, accessed on 28-03-2024). During the Palaeolithic and early Mesolithic periods, India teemed with hunter-gatherer societies whose sustenance relied upon the hunting of wild animals, fishing, and the gathering of various wild plants. It was not until the late Mesolithic period that the initial transition towards agricultural practices commenced.

As many as 2,740 Paleolithic sites, along with several pieces of microlithic evidence from the Mesolithic period, dot the Indian subcontinent. These findings suggest that the subcontinent played a significant role in the evolution of fauna and hominins in Asia (Chauhan 2020). Paleolithic sites are scattered in the Indian landscape from the periglacial sub-Himalayan regions such as Kashmir and the Kangra valley, to coastal zones like Konkan, Saurashtra, and Tamil Nadu. They also extend into arid or semi-arid tracts of Rajasthan and Kutch, the heavy-rainfall areas of Assam, and the densely forested regions of Bihar. These sites are present across various river basins in peninsular India and within rock shelters like Gudiyam in Tamil Nadu. The extensive distribution of Paleolithic artifacts underscores the early dispersal of humans across India, navigating diverse terrains, climates, vegetation, and to some extent, animal habitats (Ghosh 1990). Archaeological evidence, including depictions of hunting scenes in ancient rock art, indicates that the lifestyle of early humans in India closely resembled that of their counterparts in other ancient civilizations. They coexisted with various animal species, relying on hunting, foraging, and gathering a diverse array of foods, both plant and animal in origin. However, what set them apart was their ingenuity and capacity to adapt creatively to challenges (Eraly 2002). Humans made various stone tools such as hand axes, cleavers, and scrapers, primarily for activities like hunting, digging, and fishing. They also used bones and wood to fashion tools and honed hunting strategies, often operating in groups to target small herds of larger game. During the Mesolithic period, people advanced to crafting smaller and more refined tools called microliths, which facilitated more effective hunting and gathering (Fig. 2.1). Despite these advancements, Mesolithic societies did not adopt agriculture or domesticate animals, aside from dogs, which potentially were domesticated by specialized hunter-gatherers of the period and served as hunting companions.

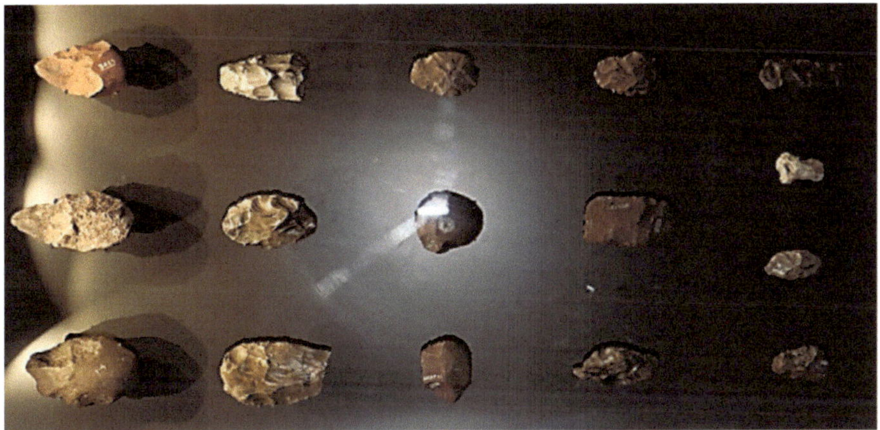

Fig. 2.1. *Stone tools, including microliths, which were utilized by early humans for hunting, digging, and fishing, have been unearthed at Paleolithic and Mesolithic sites scattered across India, as showcased at the Bihar Museum (Photo by the Author).*

Domestic Dog

The origin of domesticated dogs in India is not well documented. The earliest indisputable evidence of domestic dogs in India comes from Mesolithic level of Adamgarh in Madhya Pradesh (Gosh 1990) Comparison of available mt DNA sequences of dogs with those obtained from wolves from across lowland peninsular India, the Himalayas and Tibetan Plateau has indicated that Bhutia, Twang, Tibetan Mastiff and local Pariah dog breeds were brought into the Himalayas and peninsular India by humans, and were not domesticated independently from Indian wolves (Shannon *et al.* 2004). Probably, Indian dogs evolved from wolves elsewhere (Europe?) and migrated to India with humans. Kashmir is cited as the laboratory for canine domestication and the possible place for the domestication of dogs during the Neolithic period and maybe a place for the evolution of Indian dog breeds (Rissman 1989). A study based on genomic data from 5,392 dogs, including a global set of 549 village dogs suggested that domestication of dogs occurred in Central Asia perhaps near present-day Nepal and Mongolia and early dogs carrying nearly the full complement of Mt and Y haplotypes spread to nearby Asian regions, including Afghanistan, India, and Vietnam (Shannon *et al.* 2015).

The dog finds frequent representation in Bhimbetka rock shelters paintings and 5 of the 14 images are from Mesolithic period (8000 BCE), but there is near absence of wild or Dhole dog (Tiwari 2000). The discovery of bones of dogs, the copper-dog of Lothal, terracotta dog figurines, and soapstone figures of dogs, some of them with collars, from archaeological sites indicate the existence of domestic dogs during the Indus Valley Civilization (IVC). A brick found at Chanhudaro shows characteristic foot-prints of dog and cat providing evidence for their domestication (Eraly 2002). Archaeologists believe that IVC people had at least three kinds of domesticated dogs, a mastiff-like breed with a tightly twisted tail, a pariah dog, and a hunting dog resembling greyhound or Afghan dogs. The mastiff-like dogs were kept as pets, sometimes for hunting as well as a watch-dog (Bollée 2020). Ancient Greek historian Diódōros Siculus (active First Century BCE) noted that Alexander was fascinated by ferocious hunting dogs of Punjab, which were remarkable for their size and strength (Eraly 2002). Dog also finds reference in Vedic and post-Vedic classic texts including Rig Veda, Ramayana, Mahabharata, and other ancient Indian texts. Mentioned for the first time in the Rig Veda, the eponymous Sarama, the dog of Indra was regarded as the ancestor of all dogs. The dog was used for hunting, guarding and tracking cattle as well as for keeping watch at night (Macdonell 1899). According to Panini (4th century BCE), the grammarian, and revered scholar of ancient India, the dogs bred in royal kennels were called *Kauleyaka* (Agrawala 1953). Kautilya's Arthaśāstra (4th–3rd century BCE), seminal ancient treatise on statecraft, economic policy, and military strategy, refers to dog-keepers and prescribe rations for domestic dogs. The *Jataka* fables (2nd century BCE), which are ancient Buddhist stories, often include moral lessons and depict various aspects of life, including the treatment of animals. The mention of thoroughbred dogs maintained by kings reflects the social status and significance of dogs in ancient times. The Bhimbetka Rock Art, dating back thousands of years, provides a glimpse into prehistoric life, including the animals that were present in ancient Indian society. The depiction of dog figuring 21 times in the rock art (Dubey-Pathak 2014) suggests that dogs held some significance in the lives of the people who created these artworks, whether as companions, hunters, or symbols with cultural or religious importance. Together, these references offer valuable insights into the historical relationship between humans and dogs in ancient India, showcasing the multifaceted roles that dogs played in various aspects of life. There were herd dogs, watchdogs, and hunting dogs, as well as those used as beasts of burden (Debroy 2008). According to a 19th-century account detailing the role of animals in Indian society, it was noted that the Banjara community maintained the finest breeds of hound dogs. These canines were described as robust and sizable, highly esteemed for their dual capabilities as vigilant watchdogs and skilled hunters. Sheep dogs kept by the

Himalayan shepherded garnered glowing praise from their keepers, who would say that amidst the obscuring mists shrouding mountain pathways, these faithful dogs were invaluable guides (Kipling 1904).

Currently, five indigenous dog breeds are officially registered in India: Rajapalayam and Chippiparai, both native to Tamil Nadu; Mudhol Hound from Karnataka; Gaddi from Himachal Pradesh; and Changkhi from Ladakh (https://nbagr.res.in/geese-dog, accessed on 30-08-2025). The overall population of pet dogs in India was over 27 million in 2021, which is likely to reach more than 43 million by 2026. The growth in dog population has led to an increase in sales of pet food. The retail sales value of dog food in India amounted to approximately 393 million U.S. dollars in 2021 and projected to reach 879 million dollars by 2026. The compound annual growth rate (CAGR) for retail sales of dog food was estimated to be 17.2 % between 2021 and 2026. Market of veterinary drugs and other pet-need products also increased substantially across the country (https://www.statista.com/statistics/1061130/india-population-of-pet-dogs/, accessed on on 25-03-2024), indirectly contributing to the national economy. Apart from being the most common pet animal, the dog serves many other roles in modern society. Indian Army, Border security Force, Central Reserve police, Central Industrial Force, and the Special Protection groups employ dogs for guarding, patrolling, sniffing explosives and contraband drugs, detection of mines, and in search operations to locate fugitives and terrorists. The dog is also an important experimental animal for biomedical research. Though the population of stray dogs has declined by 10.61 % between 2012-2019, a huge population estimated at 15.309 million, still roams as the stray animal in India (Anonymous 2019). Contrary to pet-dogs, the stray dogs pose serious public health, welfare and environmental issues. A study reported human to stray dog ratio of 28-38.1 in urban and 32-42.1 in rural areas of Punjab with a density of 256-577 dogs per km^2 of built-up area (Gill *et al.* 2022). The faecal shedding of pathogens by stray dogs contaminates the environment and is a potential risk to human health. Over 90% cases of rabies in India are due to dog bites, involving stray dogs. Mauling by dogs causing injury and even death has emerged as a serious public health issue. The stray dogs may also act as invasive species causing large-scale edge effects on wildlife within and around protected areas as predators or competitors (Home *et al.* 2018).

Transition to Agricultural Production and Domestication of Farm Animals

During the Paleolithic and early Mesolithic periods, India teemed with hunter-gatherer societies whose sustenance relied upon the hunting of wild animals, fishing, and gathering of various wild plants. During the late Mesolithic period only the initial transition towards agricultural practices commenced. The images, discovered in the rock shelters of Bhimbetka in Madhya Pradesh, India, depict various scenes of humans interacting with animals. They provide valuable insights into the ancient relationship between humans and animals, showcasing hunting, domestication, and possibly even ritualistic practices spanning from Paleolithic and Mesolithic period to the historic and modern period (Fig. 2.2). Evidence from archaeological sites scattered across the Indian subcontinent suggests the nascent stages of farming, animal husbandry, and pastoralism, dating back to at least the late Mesolithic era. Skeletal and dental remains of domesticated animals were unearthed from Mesolithic strata at Adamgarh in Madhya Pradesh. Furthermore, historical records document instances of full-fledged plant and animal domestication in Northern Rajasthan. It is theorized that Mesolithic communities inhabiting the savannahs of Rajasthan used periodic fires, likely to stimulate the growth of fresh grasses for their domesticated animals as early as 8000 BCE. Moreover, they gradually incorporated pastoralism into their hunting and foraging strategies by capturing certain wild animal species around 5000 BCE. By 3000 BCE, pastoralists residing along the Ghaggar river had begun cultivating fodder crops to support their domesticated animals (Mehra 2007). The presence of plant remains, agricultural tools, and evidence of dental pathology all point to a smooth, gradual transition from a hunting and gathering lifestyle in the late Mesolithic period towards farming and herding in regions spanning the Ganga – Vindhya and the Northwestern subcontinent (Misra 2008). This pastoral adaptation continued to spread, encompassing an expanding savanna stretching from the Thar desert to Karnataka and Andhra Pradesh (Murphy and Fuller 2016).

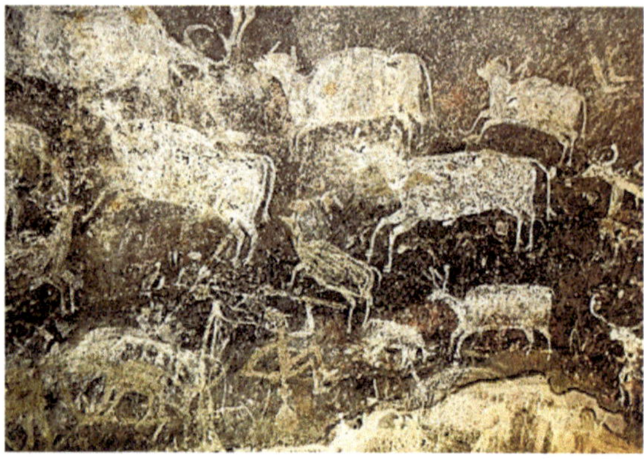

Fig. 2.2. *Neolithic-Chalcolithic panel from rock shelters of Bhimbetka depicting numerous animal figures and a 'shaman' sitting at lower right (Photo courtesy of Dr. Meenakshi Dubey-Pathak, description based on Dubey Pathak 2014).*

Neolithization in India

The Neolithic period was indeed a transformative era marked by the shift from a nomadic lifestyle to settled communities based on agriculture and animal domestication. This transition occurred at different times and in various regions across the subcontinent, resulting in a diverse array of Neolithic cultures. Evidence of sedentary settlements, cultivation of crops, and domestication of animals has been unearthed in different parts of India, viz., northwestern India, Kashmir, the Vindhyan region, the middle Ganga valley, the Southeastern India, the Northeastern India and the Southern India (Singh 2008). The characteristic features of the emerging Neolithic culture were domestication and diffusion of different crops and farm animal species and occurrence of polished celts; and introduction of handmade pottery (Misra 2008). Skeletal remains, encompassing limb bones, maxillae, teeth, pelvic and pectoral girdles, vertebrae, scapulae, and metapodials, have been unearthed in excavations across India. These remains belong to as many as 10 species of domesticated animals. Among these animals were both crop-robbers as well as those primarily utilized for food, such as cattle, pigs, buffalo, sheep, and goats. Additionally, horses, camels, donkeys, and elephants were domesticated primarily for traction purposes (Ghosh 1990). During the late Neolithic period, livestock emerged as a significant component of the economy owing to their versatile utility. For instance, the animal husbandry techniques embraced by the Harappans constituted a vital aspect of the thriving cultural and economic advancement witnessed in the urban-industrial Bronze Age Indus Valley Civilization (Deshpande-Mukherjee and Goyal 2022). Cattle, in particular, held a pivotal position in the transportation of goods. The inhabitants of the Indus Valley also kept domestic buffaloes, sheep, goats, domestic fowl, and possibly pigs, asses, and even elephants (Eraly 2002). These animals were domesticated either as a primary (domesticates derived from local populations of wild progenitors) or secondary centre (introduced as cultigens from other geographical areas) during the period spanning over several millennia post-Neolithization. This section provides an overview of the historical and contemporary sociocultural roles of major livestock species. Additionally, the elephant, which has had a profound socio-political and cultural influence throughout Indian history, is also included in the list.

Sheep and Goat Domestication: The Zagros region is widely regarded as the probable source of an eastern expansion of domestic plants and animals in southwestern Asia (Broushaki *et al.* 2016). It is suggested that sheep and goats may have reached the Indian subcontinent as part of this Neolithic package. Alternatively, some researchers propose that certain populations of domestic sheep and goats could have been independently domesticated within the Indian subcontinent. Zooarchaeological evidence, such as faunal remains identified as sheep and goats dating back to 12000–8000 BCE, has been discovered from the Indo-Gangetic Plain and the Belan River valley region of Central India. This discovery is noteworthy as it places these remains hundreds of miles away from their natural habitats in the foothills of Baluchistan and the Himalayas. These findings are often cited as indicative of the possible domestication of sheep and goats during the Upper Palaeolithic period in India (Alur 1980). Significantly, after cattle, the goat and sheep were the most prevalent animals bred and slaughtered at prehistoric sites in India (Ghosh 1990).

Domestic Sheep: The world populations of sheep belong to five maternal haplogroups (A, B, C, D and E), with most modern sheep breeds, including those in India belonging to haplogroups A, B and C (Meadows *et al.* 2011,

Kamalakkannan *et al.* 2021). Lineage A is the most predominant in sheep breeds of India. A study based on the high levels of genetic diversity in sheep breeds of north China and Mongolian Plateau, suggested that lineage A was brought into the Indian subcontinent from the Middle East via Arabia, whereas the lineage B and C entered the subcontinent from Middle East via Mongolian Plateau (Lv *et al.* 2015). Archaeological evidences and recent mtDNA analyses of Indian sheep breeds countered this view, and it is concluded that the domestication of lineage A type sheep occurred in Indian subcontinent much earlier than previously reported; whereas the lineage B type sheep possibly migrated to India from Middle East via Arabian sea route (Kamalakkannan *et al.* 2021).

There are references of existence of an ancient trade linking Arabia, East Africa and Asia via sea route in Indian ocean provided opportunity for the diffusion of crops and livestock and that the ancient Indians used the sea routes to export elephants and buffaloes from India to other countries. The present-day breeding tract of the Sonadi breed of sheep lies in a region considered peripheral to the broader Harappan cultural sphere of the Indus Civilization, with the major ancient port of Lothal located further south in Gujarat. This port played a pivotal role in trading connections with distant regions of West Asia and Africa during the Indus civilization era. The notable prevalence of lineage B in this Indian region can be construed as circumstantial evidence supporting the hypothesis that this port served as a major entry point for this lineage into the Indian subcontinent (Singh *et al.* 2013). Remains of the Asiatic Urial have been identified at archaeological sites such as Harappa and Mohenjo-Daro, as well as at ancient locales in Hastinapur and Maski. Additionally, breeds like Hunia, Barwal, and Dumba, found in the Himalayan and Tibetan Mountain ranges, exhibit traits suggestive of Urial descent (Sheshadri 2014). These discoveries further substantiate the notion of sheep domestication and the presence of sheep-rearing societies in ancient India (Fig. 2.4). It is plausible that local domestication events in India occurred concurrently with agricultural dispersals from other regions worldwide, forming an intricate tapestry of cultivation, pastoralism, and sedentism (Fuller and Murphy 2014).

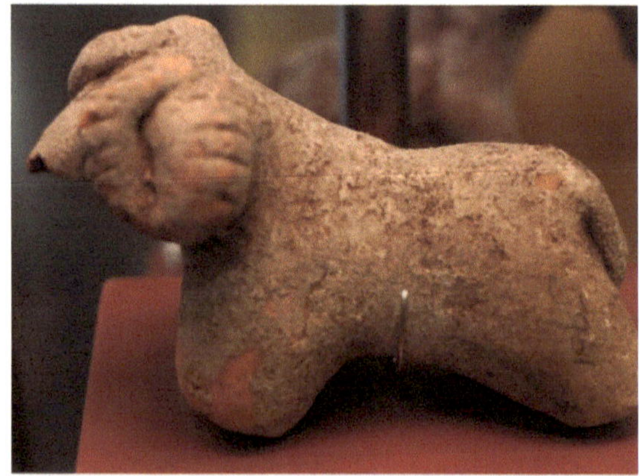

***Fig. 2.3.** Terracotta ram excavated from the Prehistoric Bhir mound in Taxila, displayed at Bihar Museum (Photo courtesy of Dr Pallav Shakhar, BVC, BASU).*

The domesticated sheep exhibits a notable presence across numerous excavated sites in India, with ample evidence indicating extensive slaughtering during the

Mesolithic period. Initially, sheep were primarily domesticated for meat, but like other contemporary cultures, they were later utilized also for wool and milk. Archaeological evidence from Neolithic sites in the Deccan region suggests a pattern of raising small flocks of sheep, with the selective slaughter of animals aged between two and three years for meat production. It is likely that lambs were reserved for meat consumption while ewes were primarily utilized for milk and wool production (Ghosh 1990). The Rigvedic people utilized sheep wool to weave cloths, often variegated and occasionally adorned them with gold. The Rig Veda also makes reference to numerous tribes within the Aryan community. Among these, the most north-westerly are the *Gandhāris,* who, based on the context in which they are mentioned, evidently engaged in sheep breeding. They were later well known as *Gandhāras* or *Gāndhāras.* The sheep was also used for gift (Macdonell 1899). The *Aṣṭādhyāyī* (Ashtadhyayi) of Pānini refers flock of rams to as *aurabbraka* and sheep as *avi* and *avika* (Agrawala 1953).

Arthaśāstra (Arthashastra) places sheep under the head-herds, and specifies that a flock of 100 sheep should contain 10 males. Sheep were sheared every six months for wool, which was utilized to make garments and blankets of various hues, including white, pure red, or as vibrant as a lotus flower. Blankets were made of worsted threads by sewing (*khachita*); or by weaving woollen threads of various colour (*vānachitra*); or from different pieces (*khandasanghātya*); or from uniform woollen threads (*tantuvichchhinna*). Sheep were also utilized for dairy production, with their milk yielding approximately 1.5 times more butter than cow milk, as noted in the Arthashastra (Shamasastry 1951). Domestic sheep were also valued for bones, sinews, fat, and even their bladders found utility in crafting musical instruments or bags. Additionally, trained rams served purposes beyond mere sustenance. They were used as sport animal for fighting and were occasionally ridden, predominantly by children (van der Geer 2008). Moreover, rams functioned as draught animals for pulling small carts and beast of burden, especially in mountainous region. It is reported that bags full of asafoetida, borax and other commodities were brought to India from Tibet on backs of large flocks of sheep (Kipling 1904). In Indian societies, domestic sheep are favoured sacrificial animals. Rams carry religious significance as they are associated with Vedic God Agni, serving as his divine mount or *Vahana* (van der Geer 2008).

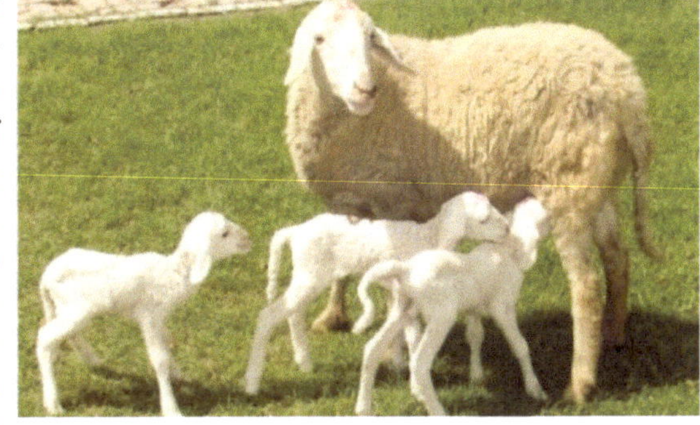

Fig. 2.4. *A Muzaffarnagari sheep with her triplets at the ICAR-CIRG farm, a rare occurrence in this breed known for its exceptional body weight (Photo source: ICAR-CIRG).*

The sheep, a versatile livestock, plays vital role in the contemporary rural economy of India. Presently, the country ranks second globally in terms of sheep population, with approximately 74.26 million sheep, constituting around 13.8 % of the nation's total livestock population (Anonymous 2019). These encompass 46 well-described breeds (https://nbagr.res.in/sheep-breed, accessed on 30-08-2025) alongside numerous non-descript populations. Some of the most renowned sheep breeds in India include Chokala, Magra, and Nali, known for their carpet wool; Garole and Kendrapada, for their prolificacy; Patwaardhani, for milk yield; and Muzaffarnagari for superior body weight. Additionally, new strains for specific purposes have been developed through breeding and selection strategies by the ICAR-Central Sheep and Wool Research Institute, e.g., Avimaans for mutton, Bharat Merino and Avivastra for fine wool, Avikalin for superior carpet wool, and Avishaan for enhanced prolificacy. Terminal crosses of Dumba rams with Malpura breed can produce lambs with higher weight (Kumar *et al.* 2021).

Ewe's milk is a rich source of proteins, minerals, and lipids, primarily utilized by industries for cheese manufacturing globally. Bioactive peptides found in sheep milk exhibit specific biological activities, including antihypertensive, antimicrobial, opioid, antioxidant, immunomodulatory, and mineral binding properties. Dairy sheep farming has been found more profitable, providing 2.2 times more net income per flock and per ewe compared to non-dairy sheep farming (Shinde and Naqvi 2015). While Asia is a major contributor to global sheep milk production, India's share in this production remains minimal. Most sheep breeds in India produce less than 500 g of milk on average, which is mainly utilized for the requirements of young lambs. Surplus milk is generally used for in-house consumption or for the preparation of ghee or curd (Kumar *et al.* 2021). Dairy sheep farming has tremendous potential in India, necessitating selective breeding to develop dual-purpose (milk and meat) breeds and the creation of markets for value-added sheep milk products, including their therapeutic applications. Overall, sheep, as well as goats, offer several advantages over other large ruminants — their grazing preferences enable them to feed on weeds and shrubs, their smaller size requires less space and reduces soil damage and compaction, and they are generally easier and more affordable to manage. Sheep production can thus serve as a significant source of income for farmers and rural economy, particularly in arid and semi-arid regions of India.

Domestic Goats: Evidence from pre-Harappan settlements indicates that goats were a widely represented domestic species across various cultural strata at archaeological sites in India. They are reportedly found at all Neolithic sites prior to the appearance of sheep. At several sites, goat bones predominate over those of sheep in the earlier levels, although this trend reverses later, possibly due to changing ecological conditions and preference for sheep meat and wool. Like sheep, goats were typically slaughtered between the ages of 2 and 3 years. Notably, the goat population exhibited a marked increase during the Iron Age (Ghosh 1990).

The initial dispersal of goats into Indian subcontinent is believed to have taken place from Fertile Crescent through two primary corridors: firstly, by traversing the Khyber Pass to reach India, and secondly, via the Eurasian Steppe belt which connects the Middle East with Mongolia and northern China. Subsequently, from the Indian subcontinent, goats spread to southeastern Asia through both overland and maritime routes. The possibility of independent goat domestication within the Indian subcontinent is suggested based on archaeological findings. However, the status of Indian subcontinent as an additional primary centres of goat domestication lacks support from modern phylogeographic studies (Amills *et al.* 2017).

Domestic goat populations in the world are classified into six maternal haplogroups (A, B, C, D, F, and G), comprising a total of 22 haplotypes. Notably, the majority of domestic goats fall under haplogroup A (Naderi *et al.* 2007). In India, goat populations are distributed across four haplogroups (A, B, C, and D), with haplogroup A being the most prevalent, constituting 93.5 % of the haplotypes nationwide, followed by haplogroup B, making up 4.1 %. Interestingly, haplotype A is rarely found (6 %) in Bezoar goats, while haplogroup C, uncommon in domestic goat populations (0.2 %), emerges as the predominant haplogroup in wild goat populations (39%). The identification of four haplogroups among Indian goat populations, out of the six recognized globally, underscores the intricate maternal genetic history of Indian goats. Molecular marker-based phylogeographic studies suggest that goat domestication likely occurred not only in Eastern Anatolia, as indicated by haplogroup A and supported by zooarchaeological data, but also possibly in Central Iran (the Zagros Mountains and Iranian Plateau). However, there is no evidence supporting the domestication of goats in the Indus Valley region. The limited geographical structuring of goat mitochondrial variability in Indian goats could be attributed to the frequent transportation of goats along terrestrial and maritime migration and commerce routes, particularly during the early phases of domestication (Diwedi *et al.* 2020, Darji *et al.* 2022).

The domestic goat held significant economic importance as a livestock species during the Harappan civilization, providing essential resources such as meat, milk, and skin for the inhabitants. Goats served pivotal roles in agricultural, economic, and cultural aspects, and possibly even in certain rituals of the society. Their presence greatly contributed to the subsistence of Harappan culture. Evidence of the goat's significance are evident from artifacts crafted by the Harappan people, including paintings on pottery, terracotta and metal figurines, as well as depictions on seals (Kumar 2023). Following the transition from early to late Harappan cultures, the widespread utilization of goats as a resource became more pronounced, paralleling the utilization of cattle during the same period. Both goat and sheep held significant place within Vedic societies as well, and were regarded as valuable assets requiring careful protection. In the Atharva Veda, sages express the sentiment of welcoming and ensuring the happiness of cows, sheep, and goats within their homes - 'Let cows be happy and welcome here. Let sheep and goats be welcome and happy (in our homes)' (Atharva Veda 7.60.5, Sharma 2013) and proclaim that 'Whatever mischief they have done to the cock and the peacock or to the goat and the ram or the sheep, that I counter, defuse and return to the doer (by way of punishment)' (Atharva Veda 5.31.2, Sharma 2013). The Aṣṭādhyāyī refers to a flock of goats to as *ajāka*. The sheep and goat together were called *ajaida* (Agrawala 1953).

By the Mauryan era, goats gained prominence, categorized under the broader classification of herd alongside cows, buffaloes, sheep, asses, camels, horses, and mules. Beyond their significance for meat and hide, goats were also valued for their milk production. Notably, the milk from goats and sheep was recognized for its superior butter yield, producing half a *prastha* more butter compared to an equivalent quantity of cow's milk. According to the share in inheritance rule, goats were designated to the eldest sons, born of the same mother, as a distinct share (Shamasastry 1951). The goat is also used for ritual purposes and immense numbers of males are sacrificed as offerings to the god and during festivities. In the 19th century, it was commonplace to witness the daily procession of milch goats being herded into urban centres both in the mornings and evenings. Local inhabitants exhibited a marked preference for goat meat over mutton due to the widely held belief that goats were notably cleaner feeders compared to sheep, resulting in a more appealing taste. Additionally, the utility of goat skin did not go unnoticed, as it was commonly repurposed for crafting water-bags known as mashk. These water-bags were essential tools utilized by water-carriers, known as Bhistis, for transporting water intended for drinking purposes as well as for irrigating gardens and maintaining roads (Kipling 1904).

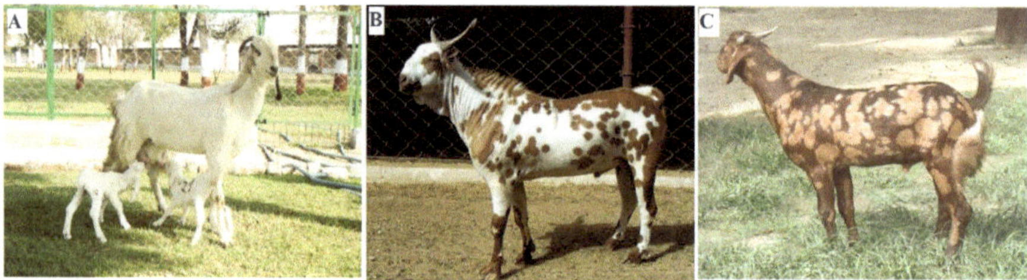

Fig 2.5. *Jamunapari (A), an outstanding dairy breed, and Barbari (B) and Sirohi (C) dual purpose goat breeds of India at ICAR-CIRG farms (Photo source: ICAR-CIRG).*

The goat, traditionally regarded as the poor man's cow, is emerging as a pivotal component of India's rural economy in the modern era. Presently, India's goat production system comprises 148.88 million goats as per 20th Livestock Census (Anonymous 2019). Along with 41 recognized breeds (https://nbagr.res.in/goat-breed on 30-08-2025), numerous non-descript populations are widely distributed across the country's four major agro-ecological regions: Northwestern arid and semi-arid, Southern peninsular, Northern temperate, and Eastern regions (temperature ranging from – 20° C to 50° C). This extensive genetic diversity significantly contributes to the national economy. Globally, Indian goat breeds are renowned for their distinct attributes, including excellent milk production (Jamunapari or Jamnapari and Jakhrana breeds), high prolificacy (Black Bengal and Beetal breeds), and rapid growth rate (Beetal and Sirohi breeds). Furthermore, some breeds are valued for their luxurious natural fibre, such as the Pashmina, which is sourced from breeds like Changthangi and Chegu. India boasts a substantial output in goat-related products, producing 1.09 million tonnes of meat (13.53 % of global production) and 6.17 million tonnes of milk, representing 33 % of global goat milk production. Typically, goats in India are raised for multifaceted purposes. Scientific endeavours are underway to enhance genetic potential focusing on specific breeds for dual purposes, such as Malabari, Osmanabadi, Sangamneri, and Sirohi for meat and milk; Surti, Beetal, Barbari, Jamunapari, and Sirohi breeds (Fig. 2.5) for milk and meat, and Changthangi breed for fibre and meat.

The consistent increase in the goat population over the past few decades in India is reflective of massive contribution of goats in ensuring livelihood, nutritional, and financial security of millions of marginal farmers and landless people (Fig. 2.6). Goat production systems are very efficient due to the animal's short gestation and early maturity. Goats have a better potential for rearing even under constraints of limited land and forage area, higher environmental stress, and disease prevalence. They can be raised with minimal resources such as locally available feed and fodder, and can perform better under intensive and/or semi-intensive grazing systems. Further, goat husbandry is viewed as economically more viable and profitable with low investment and high consistent returns. It offers flexibility for farmers in capital investment (space and feed, management). Goats are saleable at any point in time, thereby, constituting a ready and steady source of income, signifying – sell one bunch get another ready. Goat milk and milk products are increasingly being recognized for their nutraceutical properties and may be used as a functional food. Goat butter is rich in short and medium-chain fatty acids and goat milk powder has the potential to be promoted as a good substitute for conventional baby milk powder available in the market. These properties of goat milk have given the impetus to commercial dairy goat production in India. Owing to these favourable features, the goat once referred to as the poor man's cow, is now fast emerging

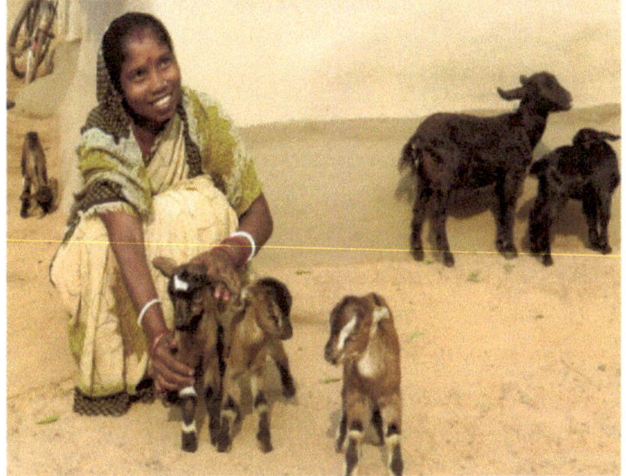

Fig. 2.6. *The goat, often referred to as the poor man's cow, serves as a vital source of livelihood, nutritional security, and empowerment for women in rural areas (Photo source: ICAR-CIRG).*

as a popular choice for commercial livestock entrepreneurship and is projected as the Future Animal in India. The ICAR-Central Institute of Research on Goats is organizing regular training programmes on scientific methods in goat farming, which is one of the most sought-after programmes of the institute drawing participants from different regions, economic classes, and communities. The institute has also developed scientific technologies including many value-added milk and meat products for better income return.

Box 2.1. Goat Milk for Cosmetics and Skin Health

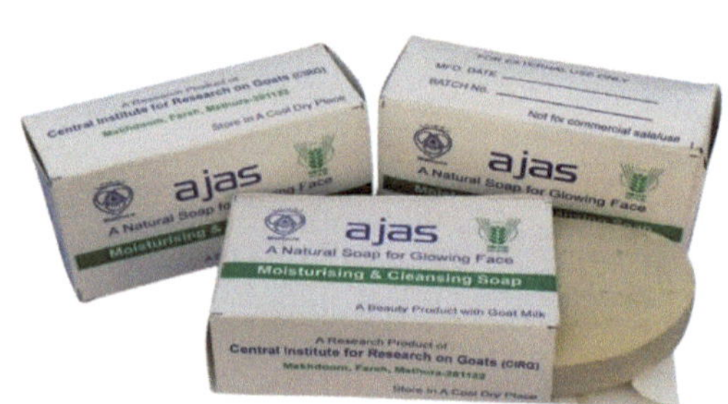

(Ajas a goat milk-based soap developed and patented by ICAR-CIRG)

Goat milk is recognized not only for its nutritional value but also for its potential medicinal properties. Several studies have demonstrated that goat milk is rich in calcium, phosphorus, potassium, vitamin A, vitamin B_2 *(riboflavin), and vitamin D and contains bioactive components such as oligosaccharides and fatty acids, and proteins and peptides like casein, lactoferrin, lysozyme and immunoglobulins. Goat milk exhibits inherent anti-inflammatory, barrier-enhancing, antimicrobial, antioxidant, and immunomodulatory activities, which hold significant therapeutic potential in the management of chronic skin conditions such as eczema and psoriasis. Additionally, certain oligosaccharides and fatty acids present in goat milk exert anti-inflammatory effects by modulating immune responses and reducing inflammatory cytokine production and may help to mitigate underlying inflammation associated with eczema and psoriasis, thus contributing to symptom relief and improved skin health. Lipid profile of goat milk, characterized by high content of medium chain fatty acids and triglyceride contributes to excellent moisturizing and emollient properties The caprylic acid found in goat milk helps to remove dead skin cells results in a mild, non-irritating, and highly natural moisturizing effect. From its anti-inflammatory and antimicrobial activities to its moisturizing and antioxidant effects, goat milk offers a holistic approach to managing these chronic skin conditions. The goat milk skincare products such as soaps, lotions, creams, and cleaners made of goat milk are increasingly finding their ways into mainstream beauty markets around the world. The Goat milk cosmetics market was valued at $3 billion in 2021, and is projected to reach $5 billion by 2027. (Ref. Ncube et al. 2024, Input and photo courtesy of Dr. Ashok. Kumar, ICAR-CIRG)*

Domestic Cattle: Since their domestication in the Indus Valley, indicine cattle have played a significant role in the socio-economic and cultural evolution of India, occupying a prominent place within Neolithic -Chalcolithic Indian societies. Among the various sites of the Indus civilization in India, Bhirrana, situated on the banks of the river Ghaggar in Haryana, is deemed as the oldest Archaeozoological sites. The identification of domestic cattle remains in pre-Harappan layers (9,500–8,000 BP) at this settlement, suggests that the predecessors of the Harappan people were already engaged in cattle management before the onset of the Harappan cultural phases. Cattle are the most frequently represented domestic animal in the Mesolithic rock paintings in Bhimbetka and other rock shelters in the country (Tiwari 2000). Cattle husbandry persisted from the Early Harappan to the Mature Harappan period, establishing a robust cattle-based faunal economy despite a decline in climatic conditions (Deshpande-Mukherjee and Goyal 2022, Atkulwar *et al.* 2024).

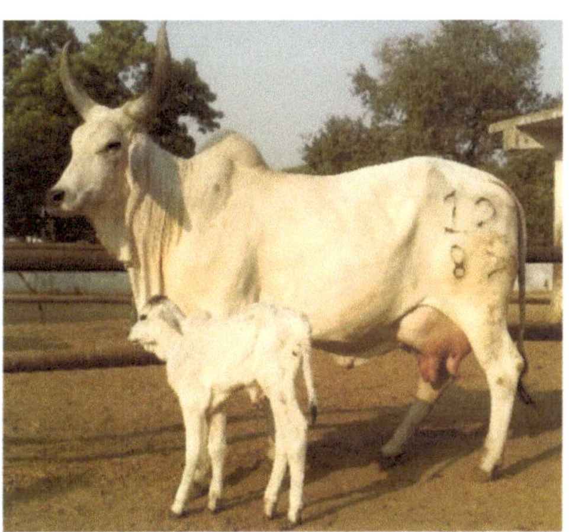

Fig. 2.7. Kankrej cow at LRS-JAU Junagarh. The breed is renowned as one of India's premier modern dual-purpose breeds. The bull figurine depicted on the Indus seals bears a striking resemblance to the males of this breed (Photo courtesy of Dr. A.K. Mohanty, ICAR-CIRC).

Cattle breeding was one of the main occupations for the Indus and Saraswati Valley people in India. Seals and clay toys recovered from Indus Valley sites depict verities of cattle, mainly the bull. The depiction on these seals resembles bulls of modern Kankrej (Fig. 2.7) and Red Sindhi breeds (Randhawa 1980). The wheeled bullock cart, a significant invention, revolutionized trade in the Indus Valley Civilization by facilitating the transportation of goods. The presence of a cart as a toy (Fig. 2.8) indicates its prevalence in the society and that animal husbandry was at an advanced stage. Its introduction not only aided in the expansion of their culture but also fostered enhanced opportunities for cultural exchange and trade with neighbouring civilizations. A comprehensive analysis of lipid residues extracted from vessels unearthed at both rural and urban sites across the Indus Valley in Northwest India reveals the presence of milk, meat, various plants, or combinations thereof, suggesting a prevalent cultural inclination towards beef consumption among the Indus populations. Moreover, the evidence points towards the practice of cow rearing specifically for dairy purposes (Suryanarayan *et al.* 2020). Cattle in the Harappan Civilization served not only as a primary source of meat but also played a crucial role due to their multipurpose applications.

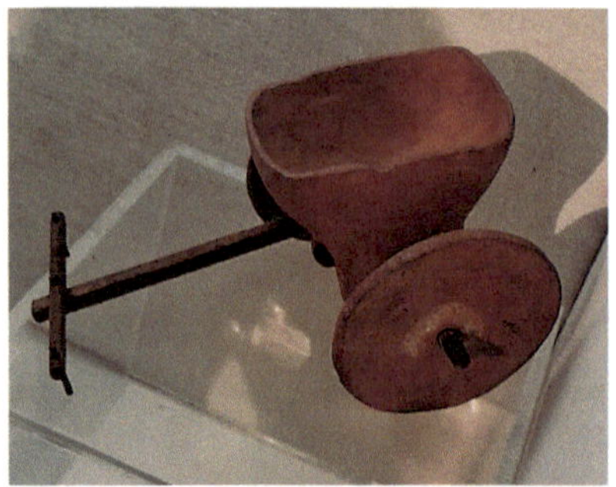

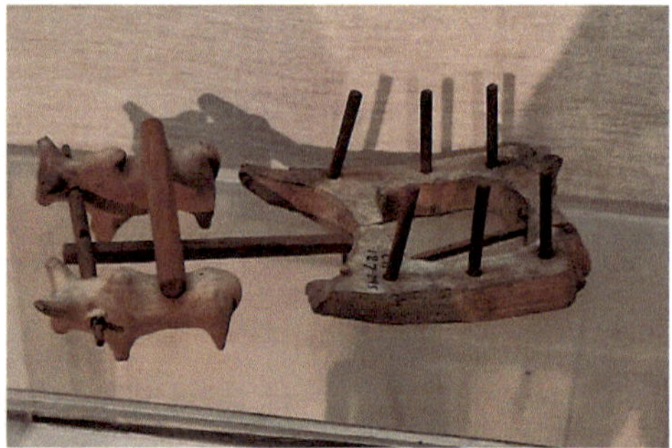

Fig. 2.8. The people of Indus Valley invented the wheeled cart and used bullocks for various traction and draught tasks such as pulling carts. A toy wheeled cart and a bullock cart from this civilization are displayed at Harappan Gallery in National Museum, New Delhi (Photo by the Author)

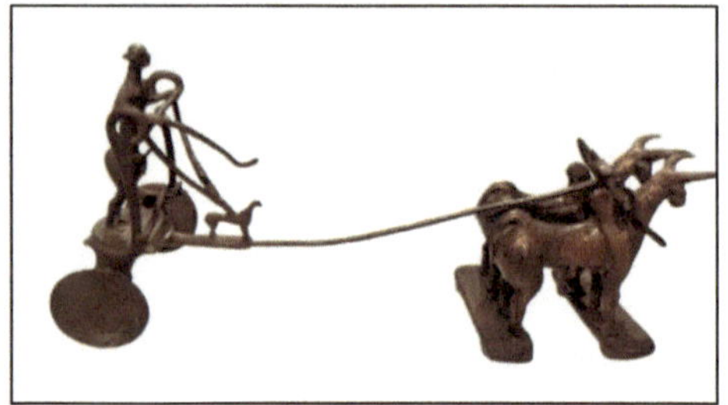

Fig. 2.9. A bronze sculpture (c-2000 BCE) of bullock driven chariot unearthed from Diamabad displayed at Harappan Gallery in National Museum New Delhi (Photo by the Author).

Beyond providing meat, their secondary products such as milk and their ability to provide traction, held significant importance in the Harappan economy. It is conceivable that all the three exploitations of cattle in Harappan culture resulted in production of milk, meat, and labour (Goyal 2013). Cows were bred primarily for their milk, while male cattle were utilized for various traction and draught tasks such as pulling carts, ploughing fields, threshing grains, lifting water, and operating the *Ghani* — a wooden contraption akin to a mortar and pestle — devised by the Harappans for extracting oil from oilseeds. It is speculated that the Harappans also used cattle in sporting activities. Evidence from the Chalcolithic period, notably a bronze sculpture of a chariot unearthed in Diamabad (Maharashtra), depicts a man standing in a chariot yoked to two oxen (Fig. 2.9), suggesting their role in transportation. Further, a seal discovered at an Indus site indicates that bullfighting was a significant aspect of Harappan culture (Kumar 2009). The sport of taming the bull—*Eru Thazhuvuthal* (meaning "embracing the bull")—is prominently mentioned in Sangam literature (100 BCE–250 CE). This enduring tradition, known today as *Jallikattu* in Tamil Nadu, stands as a living example of the ancient practice of bull-taming. It continues to inspire communities to preserve their bulls and conserve indigenous breeds such as the Pulikulam and Kangayam, native to Tamil Nadu. Overall, cattle were not only a prominent form of wealth, but must have been a source of great prestige and social status for the Indus people.

The Neolithic period in the Deccan Plateau of South India is believed to have commenced around the onset of the third millennium BCE. One notable cultural aspect of this period is the emergence of ashmounds, which made their first appearance circa 3000 BCE. Ashmounds, formed over a relatively brief period — potentially spanning just a few human generations—resulted from repetitive and symbolic dung-burning practices. These events led to the creation of prominent mounds on the landscape, likely serving as focal points for various activities such as goods exchange, cattle trading, communal feasts, social and ritual gatherings, and possibly the exchange of marriage partners (Boivin *et al.* 2008). The process of ashmound formation involved burning agricultural waste, including crop residues and dung, alongside other organic materials. Cattle dung played a significant role due to its rich nutrient content. Interestingly, similar burnt and sometimes vitrified cattle dung deposits have been observed in regions of Southern Africa associated with societies centred around cattle husbandry and millet cultivation. This suggests that cattle held central importance in the social and agricultural dynamics of Neolithic Southern India. Over time, they acquired symbolic significance, as evidenced by rituals associated with ashmounds (Murphy and Fuller 2016). Morphological changes such as anchylosis of the hock joint and bony growth (exostosis) on the third phalanx observed in cattle bones excavated from Neolithic sites in Southern India indicate joint compression resulting from heavy labour (Ghosh 1990). These findings suggest that akin to the Indus Valley civilization, cattle were utilized as draught animals in this region as well.

Cattle migrated eastward from the Indus Valley to the Ganges plains, where they likely interbred with the native wild aurochs, already a part of the hunting menu (Murphy and Fuller 2016). Their presence became widespread in the region, and cattle breeding rapidly emerged as the predominant activity during the initial centuries of the Ganges civilization (Fig. 2.10), with cattle serving as the primary form of wealth. Much like their significance in the Indus culture, cattle held a crucial role in Vedic society as well. While the bull was prominent in Harappan culture, the cow assumed a unique and revered status in Vedic India. The cow is the most largely referred animal in Rig Veda. Family communities relied on each other as clans, often engaging in conflicts over cattle

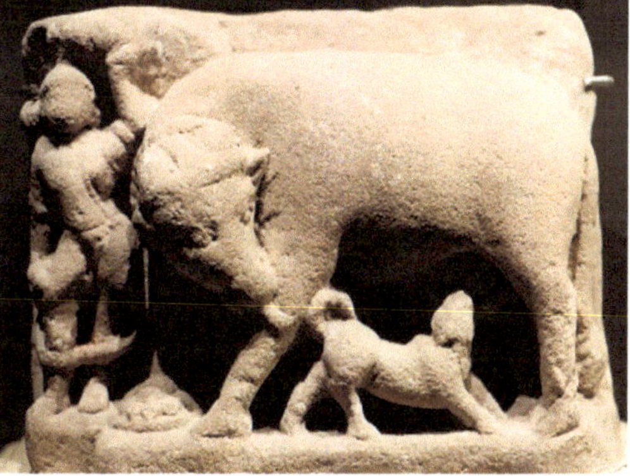

Fig. 2.10. *A stone panel from the Gupta period (4th-6th Century AD) displayed at the Bihar Museum portrays a woman holding the cord of a cow with a suckling calf, highlighting the cow's pivotal role as the primary dairy animal in ancient India (Photo by the Author).*

ownership. The Sanskrit term for war, *gavisti*, literally translates to 'searching for cows' (Macdonell 1899). The Atharva Veda (4.21.7) reflects this reverence, expressing a wish for the well-being of cows: 'O fertile and abundant cows blest with progeny, feeding on fine green grass and drinking pure water from clear pools, may no thief, no sinner, ever rule over you, may no strike of the cruel butcher ever slaughter you' (Sharma 2013). Though Vedic people consumed the meat of other domestic animals, the cow was considered *aghnyā*, inviolable and not to be harmed. In various Vedic texts, cows are depicted as bestowers of fortune and metaphors of the universe. The Atharva Veda (Sharma 2013) dedicates two *Suktas* namely, *Gavah* and *Goshala Devata* (3.14), and *Gavah Devata* (4.21) entirely to the welfare and development of cows. The sage in the Atharva Veda articulates care and concern for cows: 'O cows, we provide you with comfortable stalls, a nurturing environment, and proper nourishment. We strive to care for you diligently each day'. Another verse (Atharva Veda 3.14.1) emphasizes the desire for mutual growth and prosperity: 'Let the cows thrive under my guardianship and may our goshala be a place of abundance and auspiciousness. Through the wealth of milk, health, and breed, may they flourish joyfully, and may we, as caretakers, improve their breed and quality' (Atharva Veda 3.14.6). Professor Macdonell, the renowned Sanskrit scholar of the 19th century, eloquently expressed the sentiment that 'nothing gladdened the eye of Vedic Indian more than the cow returning from the pasture and licking her calf fastened by a cord; no sound was more musical to his ears than the lowing of milch kine'. For added security, cows were confined to stalls upon returning from nightly pastures, only to be released once more in the morning (Macdonell 1899). The paramount significance of the cow in Vedic societies stemmed primarily from its invaluable secondary product: milk, often described as nectar in Vedic texts. Milk served not only as sustenance but also as a medicinal elixir and a vital ingredient, known as *grtha*, essential for *yajna* rituals (Atharva Veda 2.26.4). The cow's dung was utilized as fertilizer for crops, as expressed in the invocation of the Sage of Atharva Veda: 'Let the cows come and move around in this stall and on the meadows, free from disease, free from fear, bearing honey sweet of milk, most delicious, eating well and giving plenty of natural manure for crops' (Atharva Veda 3.14.3, Sharma 2013). Furthermore, while cows were esteemed for their milk, bulls and oxen played pivotal roles in agricultural endeavours, being regularly used for ploughing and cart-pulling (Macdonell 1899). Although horses were preferred for pulling war chariots, oxen-driven chariots found their place in auspicious processions. According to the Mahabharata, after the war Yudhisthira entered the city of Hastinapur in a new chariot adorned with blankets and deer skins, and drawn by sixteen white oxen, the symbols of good fortune (*Shanti Parva* 37: 31-33).

Cattle as draught animal for pulling carts and ploughing also find mention in *Jātak* tales, one of the oldest classes of Buddhist literature dating back to the 4th century BCE. The Ashtadhyayi of Panini provides valuable insight into prevailing cattle husbandry practices, encompassing breeding, feeding, and housing during pre-Mauryan Period. Draught bulls were categorized based on their tasks and age. For instance, *Rathya* bulls were designated for drawing chariots, *Yugya* for yokes, *Dhurya* and *Daureya* for carts, *Sakata* for loaded carts, and *Balika* or *Sairika* for ploughing (Figs. 2.11-2.12). A young draught bull was referred to as *Vatsa*, then as *Damya* upon being broken in, and finally as *Balivarda* when matured into a bullock. Yoked bullocks were also used for pulling large leather buckets tied with ropes (known as *varatrā*) to lift well-water (*udañchana*) for crop irrigation. This method, along with the term *varat* from *varatrā,* persisted in many regions of the country till date. Panini also mentions the renowned *Salvaka* breed of draught bulls, which appears to be akin to the modern celebrated Nagori breed of draught cattle (Agrawala 1953).

During the Mauryan period, bullocks were used for draught, while bulls were primarily utilized for breeding. Cows held significant value for their milk production, which served as a staple food and was also utilized in the preparation of ghee and cheese (*kalita*). According to the Arthashastra, herds of cattle were referred to as *vraja*, with cattle categorized into various types such as calves, steers, trainable ones, draught oxen, bulls to be trained for yoking, bulls reserved for breeding, female calves, female steers, heifers, pregnant cows, milch cattle, and calves at different stages of growth. The slaughter of cattle, including calves, bulls, or milch cows, was strictly prohibited. Officials known as the Superintendent of Cows and the Superintendent of the Slaughter-House were appointed to oversee animal husbandry practices, ensure the welfare of cattle, and regulate the proper slaughter of cattle and other animals. Cattle dung was utilized for preparing manure and fuel, while various cattle by-products such as milk, ghee, urine, horns, bones, and bile were utilized for medicinal purposes (Shamasastry 1951).

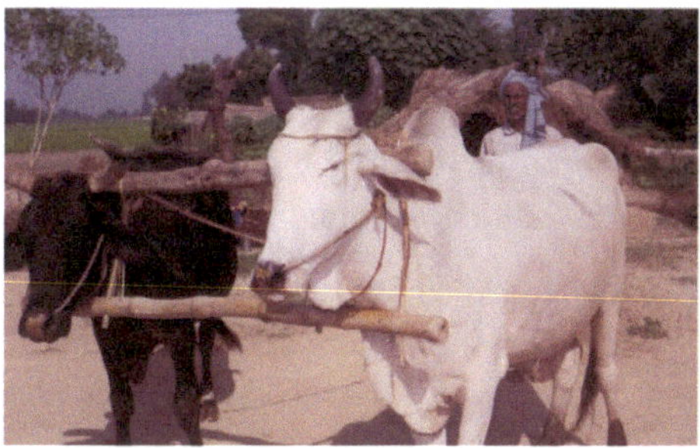

Fig. 2.11. *Bullocks continue to play a crucial role in conventional farming operations. A pair of bullocks is valued for a range of agricultural tasks and rural transport (Photo by the Author).*

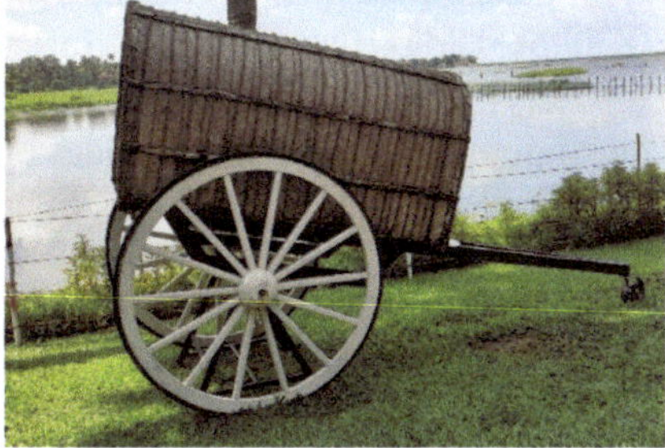

Fig. 2.12. *Ox- and horse-drawn light carts remain a readily accessible mode of travel and transport in numerous parts of the country (Photo by the Author).*

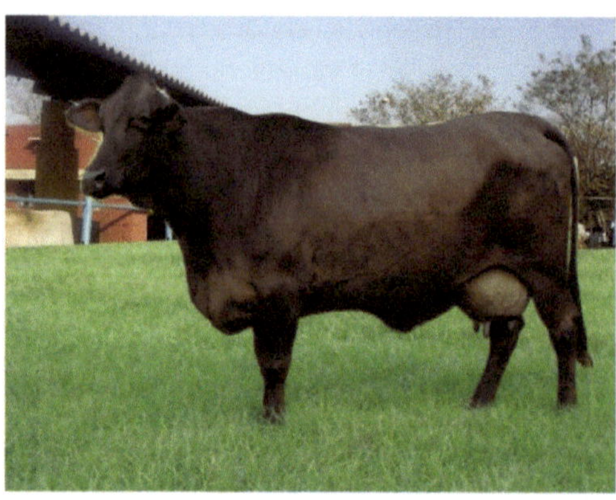

Fig. 2.13. Vrindavani cattle represent a synthetic crossbred strain developed in India, incorporating genetic inheritance from exotic breeds such as Holstein-Friesian, Brown Swiss, and Jersey, alongside indigenous genetics from the Hariana breed (Photo courtesy of Dr. S. Dey, ICAR-IVRI).

Throughout history, cattle have consistently played multifaceted roles in Indian societies, serving as a cornerstone of animal husbandry and rural economies. Cows have primarily functioned as dairy animals, while oxen have been indispensable for transportation and a variety of agricultural tasks (Fig. 2.11), including ploughing, sowing, and threshing crops. They were also used for lifting ground and surface water for irrigation, pulling traditional oilseed presses (*Ghani*), as well as transporting agricultural goods and other commodities. Before the introduction and wider accessibility of motorized vehicles, ox-driven vehicles were the primary mode of public transport in India. Scores of bullock carts carrying commercial goods, construction materials, and agricultural products such as grains, sugarcane, paddy, straw, and other domestic items were a common sight on Indian roads until a few decades ago. These carts were utilized for both intercity and intra-city transportation. According to a 19th-century account, farmers relied on oxen for working the land, while the bullock cart, in its diverse forms, was the primary vehicle in Indian traffic. A small hack carriage known as the *Rekla* filled the streets of Bombay. This neat vehicle, equipped with a sensible canopy to protect cattle from the sun, was preferred for travel in the city due to its affordability and speed (Kipling 1904). Ox-driven chariots, frequently used by affluent individuals and for ferrying brides and grooms during wedding ceremonies, were esteemed as prestigious and comfortable modes of transportation. In rural India, the number of bullocks owned by a farmer was indicative of their social standing and prosperity.

According to the 20th Livestock Census, India's total cattle population is estimated at 192.49 million, comprising 50.42 million exotic and crossbred and 142.11 million indigenous and non-descript cattle. While the overall cattle population has increased by 0.8% since the previous census, there has been a notable 6% decline in the population of indigenous and non-descript breeds compared to the previous census (Anonymous 2019). The decline in the population of indigenous/nondescript cattle is mainly due to decrease in their utility in agricultural work and farmers' preference for exotic/crossbred cows as milch animal. India boasts 54 registered breeds of cattle including a synthetic breed–Frieswal ((https://nbagr.res.in/cattle-breed, 30-08-2025). These breeds are broadly categorized based on their utility into milch, draught, and dual-purpose. Among the notable indigenous breeds, the dairy breeds include Gir, Sahiwal, Red Sindhi, Tharparkar, and Rathi; draught breeds include Nagori, Poda Thurpu, Kenkatha, Malvi, Kherigarh, Hallikar, Amritmahal, Khillari, Nimari (Khargoni), Bargur, Bachaur, and Gaolao; and dual-purpose breeds consist of Hariana (Hariyana), Gangatiri, Mewati, Kankrej, Deoni, Ongole, Kangayam, Red Kandhari, Siri, Krishna Valley, and Mewati. Certain breeds like Badri, Belahi (Morni, Desi), Kherigarh, Ponwar, Siri, and Malnad Gidda (Gidda, Uradana, Varshagandhi) are found in various hilly regions across the country. They are often utilized, with males employed for mild work on small fields amidst hilly terrains, while cows are reared for their milk production. Pulikulam, a well-known breed in Tamil Nadu, serves as a popular choice for the traditional sport of Jallikattu. Furthermore, Kangayam, Hallikar, and Ongole bulls are also used in traditional bull races.

Cow dung and urine have been utilized for various purposes across India, with recent applications extending to the creation of commercial products (Box 2.2). Indigenous cow urine, in particular, is purported to possess numerous medicinal properties (Talokar *et al.* 2013). Notably, cow-urine distillate has been patented for its efficacy as an activity enhancer and anti-infective agent (US Patent No. 6410059), as well as its role as a bioavailability facilitator and pharmaceutically acceptable additive for anti-cancer therapy (Patent No. 6896907 and 7235262). Among the 12 mutations of bovine -Casein gene (CSN2), A1 and A2 variants are the most common. They differ only at the 67th amino acid position. A1 contains histidine, whereas A2 has proline. The researchers reported that due to this amino acid change, the A1 allele breaks down into casomorphin-7, posing potential risks to humans consuming raw or processed milk rich in the A1 allele. In contrast, the A2 allele is less harmful. Studies demonstrated that the milk of indigenous zebu cattle breeds Kosali, Tharparkar, Gangatiri, Sahiwal, Gir, Khariar, Motu, and Pulikulam has a higher frequency of the A2 allele. This milk may provide various health benefits, including protection against type-1 diabetes, coronary heart disease, autism, and schizophrenia (Khan *et al.* 2023, Selvaramesh and Narmatha 2024). Ongoing research, development, and extension programs are being conducted under the auspices of the Department of Animal Husbandry and Dairying (Ministry of Fisheries, Animal Husbandry, and Dairying), the Indian Council of Agricultural Research, the National Dairy Development Board, Animal Husbandry Departments of different States, and Veterinary and Agricultural Sciences Universities. These efforts aim to enhance farmers' income through economically sustainable cattle production systems in India. The development of the Vrindavani cattle breed (Fig. 2.13) stands as a notable outcome of these collective endeavours. Additionally, there is a concerted effort underway to enhance the Kankrej breed, renowned for its dual-purpose utility, encompassing superior milk production, draught capacity, and adaptability to subtropical dry climates. This initiative is being actively pursued at Junagadh Agricultural University, as part of the All India Coordinated Research Project on Cattle, which is coordinated by the ICAR-Central Institute for Research on Cattle, located in Meerut Uttar Pradesh.

Box 2.2. Commercial Cow-dung Cakes and Home Paints

In addition to its traditional use as manure, cow dung has been utilized in Indian households for centuries, employed for daubing homes and the production of cow-dung cakes for cooking fuel and religious rituals. More recently, a multitude of commercial products derived from cow dung and cow urine have emerged in the Indian market, including mosquito repellents, incense, and even paint.

One notable example is the cow dung-based paint named Khadi-Prakriti Paint, developed by the Khadi and Village Industries Commission (KVIC) under the Ministry of Micro, Small, and Medium Enterprises (MSME). This paint is available in two variants: distemper paint and plastic emulsion paint. These cost-effective products are purportedly devoid of toxic heavy metals such as lead, mercury, arsenic, and chromium. Similarly, numerous commercial entities are now marketing cow dung cakes for various applications.

Mithun *(Bos frontalis)*: The mithun or gayal (*Bos frontalis*) is an endangered semi-domestic bovine species native to the hilly areas of India, Bhutan, Bangladesh, Myanmar, and China. Although there are conflicting hypotheses about the origin of the mithun, the widely held view is that *B. frontalis* evolved around 8,000 years ago (BP) at Indo-Myanmar border through the direct domestication of the wild gaur or Indian bison (Rajkhowa *et al.* 2004, Prabhu *et al.* 2019, Khan and Mitra 2020). The shift in climate and the onset of aridity are recognized as significant factors contributing to the domestication of wild animals. As food and water resources decline, the hungry and thirsty wild animals congregated around the scattered oasis, where human settlements already existed, presenting an opportunity for their potential domestication (Randhawa 1980). The gaur, the largest extant wild bovid, is found as a rare animal in India and Southeast Asia (Fig. 2.14). These animals rely on water sources for grazing and browsing, displaying a preference for green grass and other vegetation found in forest clearings. The creation of clearings by human activity, primarily for agriculture, offered abundant food

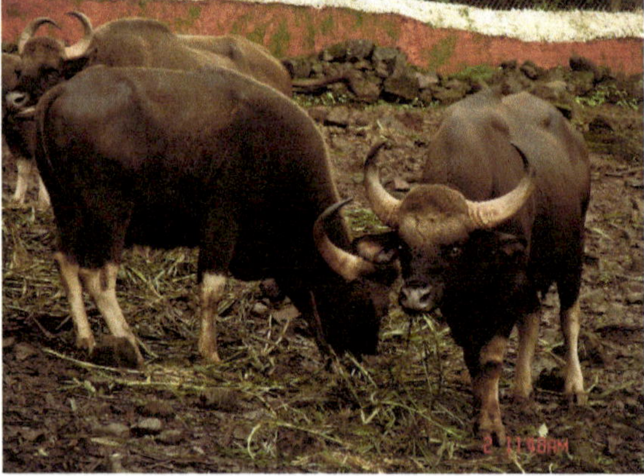

Fig. 2.14. *The Gaur (Indian Bison): Ancestral to the Mithun, is listed as vulnerable on the IUCN Red List of Threatened Species and is protected under Schedule I of the Wildlife Protection Act (WPA) in India. This species holds the distinction of being the state animal of Bihar and Goa (Photo courtesy of Dr. Asit Das, ICAR-IVRI).*

sources for gaurs. Combined with the proximity of settlements to water sources and the protection from predators provided by human habitation, this environment facilitated the self-domestication of gaurs. The culmination of self-domestication process occurs when animals lose their innate fear of humans to the extent that they can be utilized for sustenance and trade (Estes 2009). A few studies, however, propose alternative theories suggesting that the mithun may be either an independent species or a hybrid descendant of the gaur and domestic cattle. While mithuns and gaurs share notable similarities in appearance and geographic distribution, mitochondrial DNA diversity analyses have indicated that *B. frontalis* constitutes a distinct species (Baig *et al.* 2013). Karyotype analysis conducted on Indian mithun and gaur demonstrated the same number of chromosomes (2n = 58) possessed by both species, which differs from the number (n=56) possessed by Malaysian and Chinese gaur. Phylogenetic assessments of Indian mithun, alongside other *Bos* species, have shown a very close genetic relationship between Indian mithun and the gaur, supporting the notion that Indian mithuns might have evolved from the gaur (Prabhu *et al.* 2018). A recent study utilizing SSR markers for genetic characterization of the Indian mithuns (*Bos frontalis*), the Indian bison or wild gaur (*Bos gaurus*), and Tho-tho cattle (*Bos indicus*), has proposed that both mithun and gaur share a common lineage, tracing back to a now-extinct wild bovine ancestor (Mukherjee *et al.* 2022).

Smaller than the gaur and possessing shorter legs, the mithun is a large size animal, standing 140–160 cm tall at the shoulder and weighing an average of 400-650 kg. Bulls typically outweigh cows by 20–25 %. Unlike the gaur, the mithun lacks a massive shoulder hump, and its skull is shorter, wider, and flatter. Both males and females have horns that protrude from the sides of their heads; these horns are thicker but shorter compared to those of the gaur (Estes 2009). A distinctive feature of the mithun lies in its head, which exhibits a well-developed, broad frontal bone and a flat-shaped face. From a frontal view, it resembles an inverted triangle, with two horns emerging laterally. Horn coloration ranges from whitish yellow to a salty black in most individuals. Another prominent feature of the mithun is its dorsal ridge, which is flat and tapers on the shoulder, extending up to the middle of the back. Mithuns primarily browse on a variety of natural tree leaves, shrubs, and bushes found in their native vegetation. Traditionally, they are reared in a free-range forest ecosystem as a community herd, released into designated forest areas specifically by the mithun society (Kamni *et al.* 2020).

India has the highest population of mithun in the world, distributed exclusively in four Northeastern states: Arunachal Pradesh, Nagaland, Mizoram, and Manipur, each hosting distinct strains — Arunachali, Nagami, Mizorami, and Manipuri (Prabhu *et al.* 2018). As per the 20th Livestock Census, the total mithun population in the country was 3.9 lakh in 2019, reflecting a 29.5 % increase since the 19th Livestock Census in 2012. Arunachal Pradesh (40.62 %) and Mizoram (20.38 %)

observed population growth, while Nagaland (-33.69 %) and Manipur (-10.58 %) experienced decline (Anonymous 2019). Despite population fluctuations, mithun holds significant cultural, social, and religious importance for more than 20 tribal communities in these states (Dorji *et al.* 2021). The mithun is not only playing a crucial role in sustaining mountain agriculture, which forms the foundation of food and nutrition security for tribal communities, but is also involved in socio-cultural roles (Fig. 2.15 A,B). It is revered as a symbol of peace and communal harmony, and holds a revered position as a sacrificial animal during festivals and religious ceremonies. Among the Adi tribes of Arunachal Pradesh, it symbolizes peace and communal harmony, notably celebrated during the annual *Soulung* festival, which marks the birth and arrival of the mithun on earth (Kamni *et al.* 2020). Additionally, in various ceremonies such as the *Mopin* festival, the Adi people offer mithun sacrifices to invoke good fortune, a bountiful harvest, and a prosperous new year. Similarly, during the *Etor* festival, mithun is sacrificed as an expression of gratitude to God for domestic animals, while the *Reh* festival, observed by the Idu Mishmis, emphasizes the maintenance of brotherhood and social cohesion through mithun sacrifices (Dorji *et al.* 2021). Ownership of a mithun carries significant social status, with possession of these bovids conferring prestige, and generally the village leader or clan or wealthier people who own the mithun. Indeed, an individual's wealth is often gauged by the number of mithuns they own. Furthermore, mithuns are utilized to settle social and legal fines and serve as valuable commodities in trade and exchange. A customary tradition involves offering a live mithun as a bride price in marriage ceremonies. Among the Adi tribe of Arunachal Pradesh, a marriage is considered incomplete until the bride's family receives the mithun offered by the groom's family (Dorji *et al.* 2021).

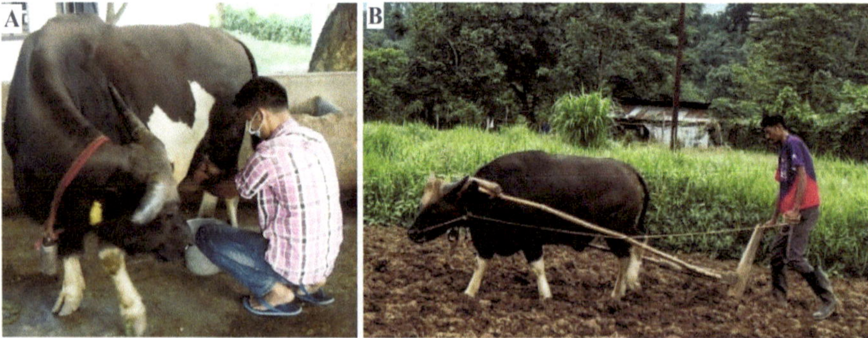

***Fig. 2.15.** The Mithun (Bos frontalis), has significant potential as both a dairy **(A)** and draught animal **(B)**. Its utilization holds promise for bolstering the rural economy within the Northeastern region of India through the establishment of sustainable animal production systems (Photo courtesy of Dr. Girish Patil, ICAR-NRC on Mithun).*

The mithun is primarily bred for its meat, known as *meef*, which among native tribes is highly esteemed due to its distinctive texture, taste, and flavour (Mukherjee *et al.* 2022). Renowned for its tenderness, this meat holds a revered position as a traditional delicacy within tribal communities, often favoured over other types of meat. Moreover, their rapid growth rate (450-600 g/day) and substantial adult body weight (400-600 kg), combined with a high dressing percentage of 58-62% compared to cattle and buffalo, establish mithuns as superior meat-producing animals in North East region (Khan and Mitra 2020). Mithuns exhibit remarkable potential for milk production, yielding approximately 1-2.5 litre of milk daily. Notably, mithun milk is distinguished by its high nutritional value, being rich in fat, protein, and non-fat solids (SNF). It contains significant quantities of polyunsaturated fatty acids, with linoleic and linolenic acids being particularly abundant. Additionally, it is rich in essential amino acids such as glutamic acid, lysine, proline, and isoleucine. Key vitamins such as A, D, and E, along with calcium, are also present in notable amounts (Devi *et al.* 2023). Furthermore, the calorific value of 1 litre milk of mithun is approximately equivalent to that of 2 litres of cow milk and yields around 400-450 g of high-quality paneer. Mithun milk is also highly suitable for the production of various traditional dairy products, including lassi, curd, ghee, barfi, etc. (Khan and Mitra 2020). The combination of these attributes underscores the potential of the mithun as a highly nutritious food source, with significant implications for improving human nutrition and health. The milk of this minor bovine dairy species holds a commercial potential for the preparation of value-added milk products, which can fetch better prices in the market.

In the traditional rearing system, *B. frontalis* is seldom milked and rarely utilized as a draught or plough animal. Calves typically suckle their dam without constraints. However, in recent times, farmers have embraced a semi-intensive mithun production system characterized by controlled grazing, improved animal housing, supplementary feeding, appropriate healthcare measures, and suitable milking facilities. Consequently, farmers are effectively collecting milk from mithun. Mithun and its hybrids with cattle are being milked in the West Kameng and Tawang districts of Arunachal Pradesh, as well as certain parts of Mizoram. In Bhutan, Jatsham (a crossbreed of mithun cow and male cattle) are utilized as dairy animals (Dorji *et al.* 2021). Beyond milk and meat production, mithun can serve as a draught animal, and its dung can be utilized as input for fish ponds and biogas plants as part of an integrated farming system (Khan and Mitra 2020). High-quality leather can also be processed from the hide of the mithun. Essentially, this distinctive species, commonly referred to as mountain cattle, holds a crucial position within the socio-economic and cultural framework of numerous local communities in the Northeastern states of India. The conservation and preservation of the mithun are of utmost importance as it faces threats such as inbreeding, inter-species breeding with cattle, and the indiscriminate destruction of its habitat. The ICAR-National Research Centre on Mithun is at the forefront of these efforts. They are actively engaged in conducting systematic studies on the scientific husbandry and breeding of mithun, as well as exploring its diversified uses (Kamni *et al.* 2020).

Domestic Yak (*Bos grunniens*): The yak is a large, sturdy bovid species native to the Himalayan region and parts of Central Asia. Yaks possess unique traits suited to high-altitude environments. With their thick coat, they stay warm in freezing winters. They also have enlarged heart and lung capacities, along with an adapted tongue that enables them to efficiently graze on the low-lying forage grasses abundant in plateau regions. Yaks are primarily domesticated for their milk, meat, and fibre, which is used for textiles (Jacques *et al.* 2021). Yaks are sure-footed and can traverse rugged terrain, making them valuable pack animals in mountainous areas where other livestock struggle to survive. In addition to their practical uses, yaks also hold cultural significance in the regions where they are found, often featuring prominently in local traditions and folklore. Often termed as 'Ship of Snow' (Fig. 2.16), yak plays a crucial role in maintenance of agro-biodiversity in the fragile ecosystem of their habitat by utilizing low growing grasses and its refurbishing by seed dispersal (Ahlawat 2013).

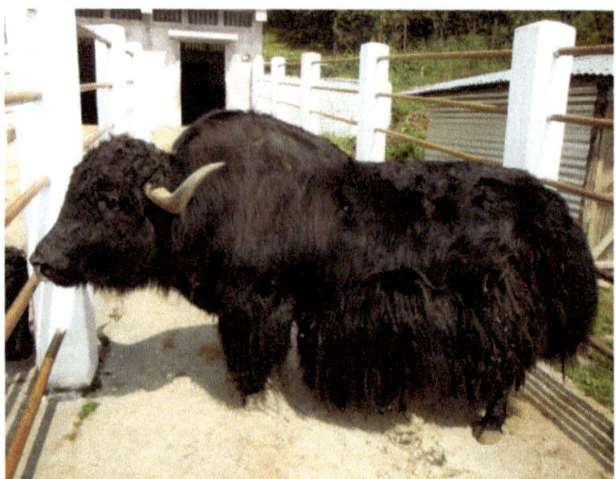

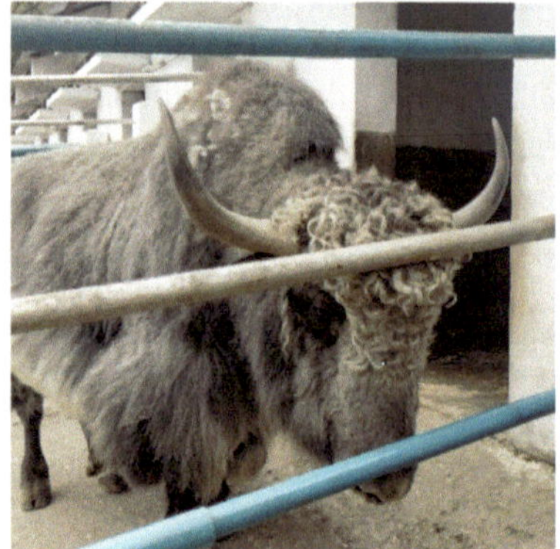

Fig. 2.16. *Known as ship of snow, several communities in Northeastern states and Ladakh rely on yaks and other livestock for their livelihoods (Photo courtesy of Dr. S. Bandhyopadyay, ICAR-IVRI and Dr. R.B. Sharma, ICAR).*

Limited information is available about the timing and processes of yak domestication, with currently very little concrete evidence in the archaeological record. The extant wild yak (*Bos mutus*) is believed to be the direct ancestor of the yak. Some genetic studies suggested that domestication process may have commenced as early as approximately 10,000 BP by the nomadic Qiang people (Han 2014). However, arguments based on modern genetic data regarding yak population expansion and information on pollen and linguistic shifts propose that yak domestication occurred following hybridization with taurine cattle from the end of the fourth millennium BCE. It is suggested that the original domesticators of yaks included not only the ancestors of the Tibetans but also Rgyalrongic-speaking people from Eastern Tibet (Jacques *et al.* 2021). The process involved selection on wild yaks by mid-Holocene hunter-gatherers and/or late yak domestication at approximately 4000 to 3000 calibrated radiocarbon years before the present, somewhat after the introduction of cattle, sheep, goats, wheat, and barley around 3,900 BP in the region. Archaeological and genetic findings have substantiated that people managed yaks and cattle together at approximately 3,700 to 4000 meter above sea level (MSL), providing opportunities for interbreeding and experimentation (Chen *et al.* 2023). Hybridization of female yaks with male taurine or indicine cattle has been suggested to have been practiced since 1100 BCE, intensifying in the 19th century in order to achieve heterosis in milk and meat production (Han 2014).

The domestic yak is distributed across a vast area spanning ten countries: Afghanistan, Bhutan, China, India, Kyrgyzstan, Mongolia, Nepal, Pakistan, Russia, and Tajikistan, forming both southern and northern zones connected in the west by the Pamir Mountains (Joshi *et al.* 2020, Jacques *et al.* 2021). In India, yak populations are found in the Union territory of Ladakh and states of Sikkim, Himachal Pradesh, Arunachal Pradesh, and West Bengal. In these regions, several communities rely on yaks and other livestock for their livelihoods. Some of the yak-herding ethnic groups of India are the Bhutia, Bhotia, Changpas (also called Champa, Fangpa, or Phalpa), Dokpas, and Pangwals. They inhabit altitudes ranging from 3,000 to 4,500 MSL and follow a semi-migratory free-range system of livestock management. These communities have a long history of yak rearing, which serves various purposes and is deeply embedded in their culture. For them, the yak is a source of milk, meat, hair, wool, and draught power (Joshi *et al.* 2020).

Yak-rearing communities utilize a variety of yak milk and meat products, including curd, whey, butter, buttermilk, wet cheese, yak fat and cream, creamy cheese, and traditionally processed meat products (smoked, sun-dried, air-dried, or fermented). Similarly, yak wool, hair, and tendons are used to craft various value-added products such as clothes, ropes, tents, caps, blankets, handbags, doormats, slings, and handwoven carpets. The fat and dung of yaks are used as fuel, while their meat is consumed as food. Yak hides and stomachs are utilized in the creation of storage bags. Yaks are also utilized as pack animal for carrying load during migration (Lachungpa 2009, Ghatani and Tamang 2016). Yak tails hold significant religious value and are utilized in the creation of holy *Chamar* (yak tail fans), which find application in temples, gurudwaras, and by the business community for religious purposes. The preference lies towards white tails for these holy *Chamar*, resulting in a substantial demand (Ramesha *et al.* 2009). An intriguing detail from the transport of the relics of Buddha depicted on the Upper Drum slabs of the Great Stupa at Kanaganahalli (1st Century BCE–3rd century

CW) is the ceremonial use of the flywhisk in reverence of the relics (Menon and Sinha 2023). This strongly suggests the historical use of the yak tail flywhisk in India since ancient times (Fig. 2.17).

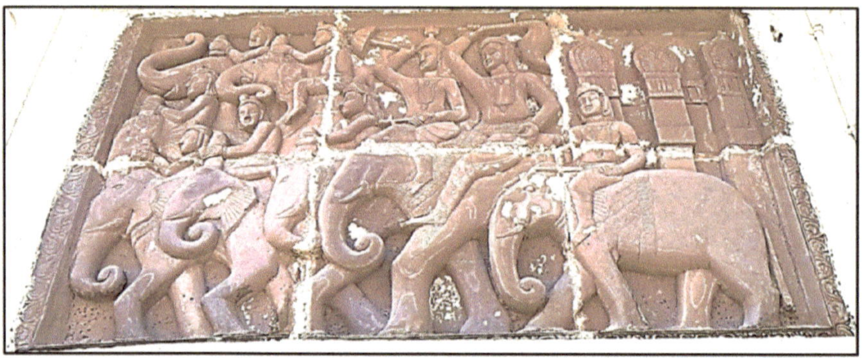

Fig. 2.17. *A slab from outer wall of Shanti Stupa in Dhauli depicting the transport of the relics of the Buddha. A man can be seen holding a flywhisk (Photo by the Author).*

According to the 20th Livestock Census, the total yak population in the country was 57,570, with the highest number in Ladakh (26,221), followed by Arunachal Pradesh (24,075) and Sikkim (5,219). The total population of yaks in the country declined by nearly 25 % during 2012-2019, principally due to a steep decline in the Northern states and West Bengal. However, the population of yaks showed over a 71 % and 29 % increase in Arunachal Pradesh and Sikkim, respectively, during the two census periods (Anononymous 2019). These populations have been geographically isolated from each other since ancient times, leading to considerable phenotypic variations in yaks found in different geographical locations (Ahlawat 2013). Based on their geographical distribution, Indian yaks are classified into four types: Arunachali, Ladakhi, Sikkimi (Sikkimese), and Himachali (Behl *et al.* 2020). Among these, the Arunachali and Ladakhi types are officially recognized as registered breeds in the country (https://nbagr.res.in/camel-donkey-yak, accessed on 30-08-2025).

Ladakhi yaks are of medium size and possess a moderate temperament. Their coat colour ranges from dark brown to black with glossy sheen. Their skin, muzzle, eyelids, and tail switch are black, while their horns vary in shades of grey to black (Behl *et al.* 2020). These animals, along with their hybrids such as the *Dzo* (the sterile first-generation male resulting from the crossbreeding of a male yak and a local female cattle), *Dzomo* (the fertile female offspring of a male yak and a local female cattle), *Gar* (the sterile male offspring of a male yak and a dzomo), and *Garmos* (the fertile female offspring of a male yak and a dzomo), constitute indispensable resources for the livelihoods of the people of Ladakh. This importance stems primarily due to their resilience in the extremely harsh climatic conditions of the region, which are unsuitable for crop cultivation (Wani *et al.* 2022). The Changpa community residing in the Changthang region raises substantial herds of sheep, goats, and yak hybrids. These animals serve multiple purposes, including providing milk, meat, and labour for their own use, as well as for bartering for grains and other necessities. Historically, Changpas were self-sustaining, with livestock providing them food and shelter, and they maintained a significant population of yaks (Bashin 2012). However, in recent decades, there has been a decline in the region's dependence on yaks, leading to a notable decrease in the yak population in Ladakh. Several factors contribute to this decline, including a lack of high-quality breeds for breeding, low productivity of yaks, insufficient pastureland, and increased competition for grazing areas from high-yielding cattle hybrids. Additionally, the region has seen significant changes such as substantial defence investments, improved communication infrastructure, proliferation of government departments, introduction of development initiatives, provision of basic amenities, shifts in traditional subsistence economies towards commercialization, and dissemination of knowledge through governmental and non-governmental organizations. Furthermore, the growth of tourism has heightened aspirations for improved living standards among locals, prompting them to transition away from traditional livestock-based livelihoods (Bhasin 2012, Wani *et al.* 2022).

The north-eastern state of Arunachal Pradesh in India is home to Arunachali yak. The majority of Arunachali yaks exhibit a black coloration. Some animals feature distinctive white markings, such as a white forehead, face, or a dorsal stripe extending from the hump to the tail. Yaks in Arunachal Pradesh are reared mainly by Brokpa pastoralists, belonging to Monpa tribe in Tawang district in the northwestern part of the state, and are treated as an asset by the rural community (Behl *et al.* 2020). Yaks play an essential role not only as a source of food but also as material for cloth or religious tools and bride-price. The yak dance, indicating the legend of introducing yaks into the region a long time ago, is performed at the *Lossar* festival, celebrated to mark the Monpa's New Year in February, reflecting the socio-cultural significance of yaks and their crossbreeding (Pandey *et al* 2020). The Arunachali yak is also known for its pack performance. Male yaks have a working life of 10-12 years, and the bulls not intended for breeding purposes are castrated at an early age for use as pack animals. *Dzos* are generally used to carry loads during migration (Das *et al.* 2022). *Dzomo*, the F1 female hybrid of yak and cattle is economically important livestock for Brokpa community. The hybrid has a better milk yield than yak (Pandey *et al.* 2020).

The native Sikkimese yak is a pastoral treasure that has been raised through centuries-old transhumance practices and has evolved in response to natural and man-made selection. These yaks are medium-size animals with a usually docile temperament. Their coat, along with the skin, muzzle, eyelids, and tail switch, is black in majority of animals. They have a broad and straight forehead with horizontal or diagonal ears. Horns are usually black and curved upwards and outwards. The hump is small to medium-size, whereas the dewlap and naval ap are small. In females, the udder is mainly bowl-shaped, although a round shape is also prevalent, whereas teats are mostly cylindrical in shape (Aggarwal *et al.* 2023). Sikkimese yaks are found in Lachen, Gurudongmar Lake, Chopta valley, Lachung valley, and Yumthang in the North district, Tsomgu Lake, Kupup, Thegu, Nathang in the East district, and Yuksom-Dzongri in Western Sikkim region (Ghatani and Tamang 2016). The yaks are arbitrarily divided into *Bho* and *Aho* types, depending on the communities that rear them. *Bho* is found in the western part of Sikkim. *Aho*, which is compact and smaller than *Bho,* is distributed in the eastern part (Bhel *et al.* 2020). Bhutias are Buddhist by religion, and the yak, called *gyag* in the Bhutia language, is the only livestock adapted to high-altitude conditions. They take their yaks to higher pastures during summer and descend to lower pastures for winter. The Bhutia community considers yak horns holy and also uses them for decorative purposes. The tails are also used as a fly whisker in some areas of India. Yak skins are used for decorative purposes and hides for making *mura* (stools) and tents to resist the cold (Ghatani and Tamang 2016). Besides the production of utility commodities, yak is also used in tourism. Tourists from far-off places come to Sikkim to enjoy a tranquil ride on a yak. Department of Tourism and Civil Aviation, Government of Sikkim organizes yak safari across the state (www.sikkimtourism.gov.in/Public/ThingsToDo/adventuretourismtype/Yak_Safari).

The Himachali yaks are hardy animals with elongated yet compact bodies. They possess wide foreheads and small eyes, with black being the predominant coat colour. Many of these animals feature a line of white hair along their dorsal line, extending to the forehead and tail. They are primarily found in the Lahul Spiti, Kinnaur, and Chamba districts of Himachal Pradesh (Behl *et al.* 2020). Similar to Ladakh, yak rearing and its associated traditions have been losing appeal in recent years, leading to a significant decline in the yak population in this state as well. This decline may be attributed to modernization and various environmental issues (Joshi *et al.* 2020).

Domestic Buffaloes: India is the birthplace of the domestic buffalo, an animal of multifaceted utility since ancient times. Compared to cattle, historical records provide scant information on the socioeconomic and cultural significance of buffaloes. However abundant archaeological evidence underscores their pivotal role in Indian society since antiquity. Buffalo figures frequently feature in the Bhimbetka rock art, which dates back to the Mesolithic period (ca. 8000 – 2500 BCE), as well as the Neolithic-Chalcolithic periods and the Early Iron Age (2500 –300 BCE). Mesolithic images depict buffaloes and bison of significant size (Dubey-Pathak 2014). The wild buffaloes, in particular, are prominently depicted, with as many as 88 drawings identified in Bhimbetka. They are usually shown alone in most of the rock paintings of central India (Tiwari 2000). The earliest evidence of domestic buffalo dates back to around 5500 BCE, originating from Adamgarh. Archaeological excavations at Nāgārjunikoṇḍa in Andhra Pradesh have unearthed both wild and domestic buffalo remains, indicating a probable local domestication process. The number of buffalo bones discovered at various archaeological sites suggests the existence of small herds that were selectively bred. Zooarchaeological findings also provide compelling evidence of buffalo being used for meat consumption. Excavations at Navdatoli, a Chalcolithic site in Madhya Pradesh, reveal crossbreeding between larger and smaller buffalo varieties, likely aimed to enhance milk production. The bulls were used for traction purpose (Ghosh 1990).

The renowned Harappan Pashupati seal (DK 5175/143), featuring an anthropomorphic depiction of Shiva, highlights the significance of the buffalo within the Indus Valley civilization. This seal (Fig. 2.18) portrays yogic figure (Pashupati) adorned with buffalo horns and surrounded by a diverse array of wild animals, including buffaloes and elephant (https://nationalmuseumindia.gov.in/en/collections/index/6). Another seal depicts a buffalo at a feeding trough, affirming its domesticated status. Further evidence of the buffalo's importance emerges from archaeological findings, such as a bronze sculpture discovered in Daimabad. This sculpture, depicting a buffalo standing upon a four-legged platform supported by four solid wheels, dates back to the late Harappan period (Fig. 2.19). Analysis of lipid residues from Indus pottery has revealed traces of both cattle and buffalo meat and milk, underscoring the integral role of these animals in the civilization's diet and economy (Suryanarayan *et al.* 2020). These findings provide evidence that, akin to cattle, buffaloes were utilized by the Harappans for both meat and milk production. They also used buffaloes in diverse agricultural activities. Limited information is available regarding the role of buffalo in Vedic India. Later Vedic traditions associated the buffalo with Yama, and it was likely used in ritual sacrifice. The Arthashastra classifies buffalo under the category of herd and describes it as a valuable dairy animal. According to the text, buffalo milk yields approximately 1/7th *prastha* more butter than cow milk. It is evident that during the Mauryan period, buffaloes were used as draught animals, and their horns were utilized in crafting sword handles (Shamasastry 1951).

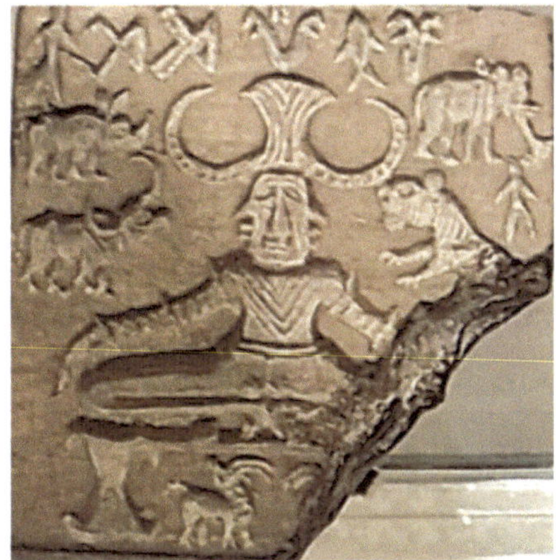

Fig. 2.18. *The famous Pashupati seal displayed at the Harappan Gallery in the National Museum, New Delhi (Photo by the Author).*

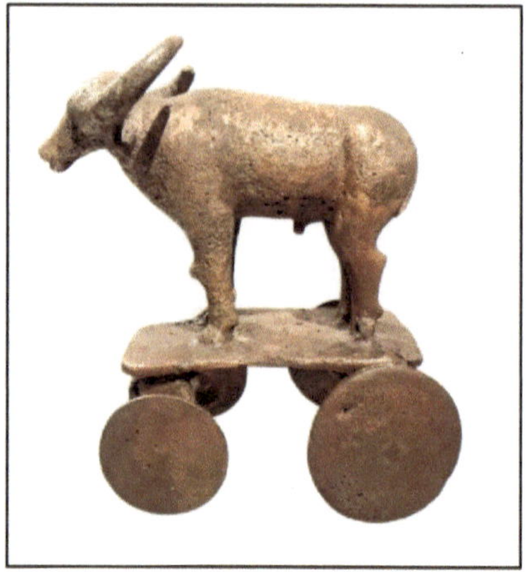

Fig. 2.19. A bronze sculpture of buffalo (c-2000 BCE) from Diamabad displayed at the Harappan Gallery in the National Museum, New Delhi (Photo by the Author).

The buffalo has long served as a significant resource in India, providing meat, milk, skin, and animal power for agricultural activities, traction, and transportation since its domestication. As of 2019, India had a buffalo population of 109.85 million, comprising over half of the world's estimated buffalo population for 2021. This population has shown a steady increase, with a growth rate of approximately 1.0% since the previous census in 2012 (Anonymous 2019). There are 21 registered breeds of buffaloes, spread across the country (https://nbagr.res.in/node/114, accessed on 30-08-2025). In terms of productivity, buffaloes are formidable, contributing over 99.15 million tonnes of raw milk, 4.35 million tonnes of meat and 0.95 million tonnes of raw hide and skins in 2022 (FAOSTAT, accessed on 14-04-2024). Buffaloes are well-suited to the country's hot and humid climate with superior adaptability to less digestible feeds compared to cattle. They can thrive on poor-quality pastures for extended periods, making them indispensable in areas where cattle farming might become impractical due to the projected impacts of climate change, leading to hotter and more humid conditions (Zhang *et al.* 2020). Buffalo milk, in particular, is valued for its nutritional composition, appealing to health-conscious consumers. It contains lower cholesterol, sodium, and potassium levels while being richer in calcium, phosphorus, and vitamins E and A— the latter derived from beta-carotene pigment conversion. Higher fat and solid contents make buffalo milk more valuable than cattle milk, serving as an economical raw material for various dairy products. These products provide technological advancements and also contribute to social benefits such as employment opportunities, income generation, and dietary improvements. Buffalo milk is favoured for the production of most traditional Indian dairy products, except for *Chhena*, for which cow milk is preferred (Pandya *et al.,* 2006). For example, in the 19th century Indian society, despite historical superstitions associating buffalo rearing with ill-fortune, buffaloes were valued for their gentleness and as a prime source of milk, particularly for ghee production. Interestingly, a significant portion of the ghee consumed in urban areas was meticulously crafted on a large scale from buffalo butter in remote districts and efficiently transported to cities via railways (Kipling 1904). Today, India leads the world in the population of buffaloes, comprising approximately 54 %, and also in milk production, boasting a share of approximately 68.51 %. This underscores the pivotal role of buffaloes as primary dairy animals in the country. Today, India is home to some of the finest milk breeds of dairy buffaloes, including Murrah, Nili-Ravi, Surti, and Jafarabadi. Renowned for their high potential in milk and fat production, these breeds also serve as valuable work animals and supplementary livestock for meat production (Borghese and Mazzi 2005).

The Murrah buffalo is widely distributed not only across India but also globally, spanning from Bulgaria to South America and throughout Asia. This breed is renowned for its exceptional milk performance, boasting up to 2,086 kg in a 305-day lactation period, with daily peak milk yields reaching 13 kg, and a remarkable lactation length of up to 321 days (Kumar *et al.* 2019). Originating from Haryana state, its name stems from the Hindi word *Muranā* denoting the characteristic spiral shape of its horns. Murrah buffaloes have found their way to numerous countries worldwide, including China, Brazil, Egypt, Bulgaria, and Bangladesh, where they were utilized to improve native buffalo breeds. China and Indonesia introduced Murrah germplasm to augment milk production, as the indigenous swamp-type buffaloes exhibit limited milk-producing capabilities; the same applies to many Asian countries, in which the original buffalo population is of the swamp type. Bulgarian Murrah is the only breed of buffalo, which was developed by crossbreeding the Indian Murrah and the local Mediterranean breed. Many animals were exported from Bulgaria to neighbouring Romania and Germany (Minervino *et al.* 2020). Recognized for its superior milk production potential, adaptability to various environmental conditions, and efficient feed conversion, the Murrah buffalo is aptly dubbed the 'Black Gold' or the 'Holstein-Friesian of the Buffalo World' (Kumar *et al.* 2019). Additionally, powerful Murrah bullocks are excellent draught animals, increasingly used in agricultural operations. Their robustness, resilience, and greater carrying capacity compared to cattle have made them a preferred choice among farmers, particularly in Northern Indian states, for transporting heavy cart-loads. The Nili Ravi buffalo is the second most widely distributed breed globally, hailing from the Murrah group. While bearing similarities to the Murrah breed, Nili Ravi buffaloes (Fig. 2.20) are distinguished by white markings on their extremities, walled eyes, and less curved horns. Originating from the Punjab regions of India and Pakistan, this breed is primarily chosen for dairy purposes and ranks among the top milk-producing buffalo breeds, with lactation milk yields reaching as high as 3,000 kg. Another significant dairy buffalo-breed in India is the Jafarabadi, known

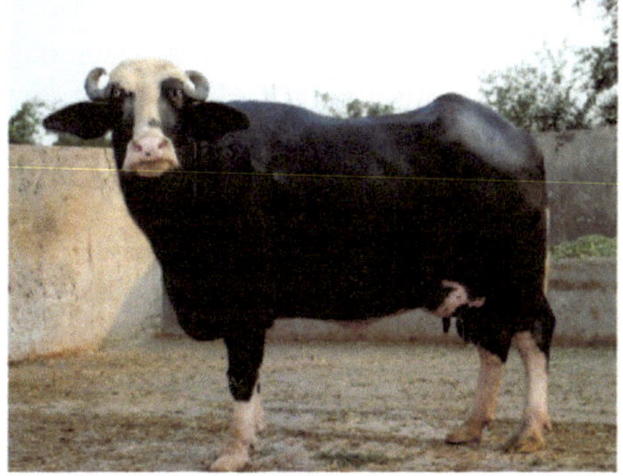

Fig. 2.20. *Nili Ravi breed ranks among the top dairy breeds of buffaloes (Photo source: ICAR-CIRB; courtesy of Dr. Naveen Kumar).*

for its lactation milk yield ranging from 1,800 to 2,700 kg and a lactation duration of 35 days. Indigenous to the North-Western parts of India, particularly Gujarat, Jafarabadi buffaloes are classified among the large-size buffalo breeds alongside Murrah, Banni, and Nili Ravi. Their substantial size and muscular build have garnered attention globally, with some countries, including America, selecting them for breeding purposes. Jafarabadi buffaloes have been exported from India to Brazil, where they are represented by two varieties: the medium-size, widely spread Gir and the larger Plitana breed, used for crossbreeding. Further, Jafarabadi buffaloes were instrumental in the creation of the Buffalypso breed in Trinidad, Tobago, and Cuba through crossbreeding with Bhadawari bulls (Minervino *et al.* 2020). India is also home to other notable buffalo breeds, such as the Bhadawari, originating from the former Bhadawar state covering parts of Uttar Pradesh and Madya Pradesh. Renowned for its high milk fat content ranging from 8 to 13 % and total solid percentage of 17 %, the Bhadawari breed is an exceptional dairy animal. Similarly, the Surti buffalo, a smaller-size breed native to Southern Gujarat, produces milk with a high-fat content averaging 7.9 %, alongside an average lactation milk yield of 1,289 kg (Borghese and Mazzi 2005).

Male buffaloes are increasingly recognized as an important draught animal. They have large hooves and flexible foot joints, and are referred to as the living tractor of the east. Their draught power is often utilized in traction of traditional oilseed milling (*Ghani*), and sugarcane crushing, as well as in transporting agricultural products and other domestic good. Buffaloes are also integral to certain renowned traditional sports, most notably the celebrated *Kambala*, an annual event in Tulunadu (coastal Karnataka). During *Kambala*, adorned with colourful *jhūls* and metal headpieces, buffaloes race through slushy paddy fields. This rural sport made its debut in Bengaluru city in 2023, marking a significant expansion of its cultural reach.

Domesticated Pigs: India is regarded as one of the potential centres for pig domestication. However, the historical documentation of domestic pigs in India remains incomplete. Indian wild boars, considered potential ancestors of domestic pigs, have interacted with humans on the Indian Subcontinent since the Upper Paleolithic period. The oldest depiction of wild boar is found in the Bhimbetka rock-shelter paintings, dating back to the early Mesolithic period. There are also five images of mythical boars, suggesting the sacrificial significance of wild boars in prehistoric societies. In many rock-shelters, including one in Mirzapur, the agony of the depicted animals can be observed, which might indicate they belonged to domestic pigs (Tiwari 2000). Bones of pigs (*Sus scrofa cristatus*), an Indian subspecies of wild boar (*S. scrofa*), were also discovered in the Mesolithic layers at Adamgarh and Bagor archaeological sites. At Bagor, wild boar bones dominate in the earlier layers, while those of domestic pigs become more prevalent in later layers. The teeth found at these sites resemble those of wild boars, suggesting that initially, boars were hunted rather than kept in captivity. The pig bones recovered from Ahar, Ropar, and Hastinapur archaeological sites predominantly belong to 1–2-year-old pigs, indicating that pigs were bred and slaughtered for pork during the Chalcolithic period. However, pig bones are found infrequently at Neolithic sites in South India (Ghosh 1990).

It is speculated that the Indus Valley people may have domesticated and bred pigs. Although pigs constitute 2-3 % of the total faunal assemblages across Indus sites, their domestic status remains uncertain (Suryanarayan *et al.* 2020). Archaeological discoveries in Iraq provide evidence that small pigs were commonly domesticated animals during the early third millennium BCE. Concurrently, settlements within the Indus Valley, either contemporary or emerging later, share a similar timeframe. It has been speculated that remains of *Sus scrofa* found in sites like Lothal were those of domestic pigs. However, these remains predominantly belong to large animals, and a noteworthy terracotta swine figurine unearthed in Mohenjo-Daro depicts distinct manes, indicative of a wild boar rather than a domesticated pig (van der Geer 2008). An initial increase followed by a rapid decrease in pig remains during successive periods at the Mehrgarh site of the Harappan civilization raises the possibility that efforts were made to domesticate pigs during the late fourth millennium BCE but were later abandoned (Larson *et al.* 2010).

Information on the status of domestic pigs and swine husbandry in the Vedic period is scanty. Ethnoarchaeological and historical records, however, highlight interactions between humans and wild boars, which were significant game animals often hunted with dogs (Macdonell 1899). *Dharmashastra,* the ancient Indian body of jurisprudence rooted in the literary tradition of the Vedas, categorizes pigs living in the wild (*mriga*) as edible animals, whereas village pigs were deemed inedible due to their close association with humans (van der Geer 2008, pp. 395-414). However, the significance of pigs as a food source increased once the cow was declared sacred (Ghosh 1990). Probably later Vedic people began keeping domestic pigs for pork. It is mentioned that the last meal of Buddha was pork (*sukaramaddava*) hosted by a metalworker named Cunda (Vajira and Story 1998). According to a study, he succumbed to the disease pig-bel, a necrotizing enteritis caused by toxins from *Clostridium perfringens* infection in tainted pork (Chen and Chen 2005). Pigs are not classified under herds in Arthashastra but the regulations defined for grazing herds of cattle, horses, asses, camels, and hogs were consistent. Provision for rations for boars was same as that of goats and rams. Furthermore, according to the Arthashastra persons rearing cocks and pigs were required to surrender half of their stock to the government; stealing or destroying pigs was a punishable offense (Shamasastry 1951). It appears that pig rearing was practiced in India during the Mauryan period.

The genetic evidence suggests that modern Indian domestic pigs have descended from local wild boars (Larson *et al.* 2010). Approximately five decades ago, indigenous or *desi* pigs predominated in pig production across the country.

Indigenous pigs, raised on garbage and other human wastes, represented the most economical meat source among all livestock. However, they were perceived as inferior compared to other livestock species. Consequently, pig farming remained largely disorganized and confined to specific communities, structured along caste lines. The commencement of the All-India Research Project on Pig Improvement during the IV Five-Year Plan in the 1970s marked the advent of a new era in the scientific management and enhancement of pig performance throughout the country. The study investigated the performance of indigenous pig breeds across various agro-climatic conditions, comparing their economic traits with those of exotic breeds and their crossbreeds under scientific management. Research efforts were directed towards developing region-specific packages of practices and improving the quality of germplasm. Currently, India has 15 registered pig breeds (https://nbagr.res.in/pig, accessed on 30-08-2025). Notable indigenous breeds include Ghoongroo (West Bengal), Niang Megha (Meghalaya) (Fig. 2.21), Doom (Assam), Nicobari (Andaman and Nicobar Islands), Agonda Goan (Goa), Banda (Jharkhand), Purnea (Bihar), and Gurrah (Uttar Pradesh). More recently, two additional breeds—Punhri from Assam and Ankamali from Kerala—have been characterized and recognized (Refer to Chapter 3, Fig. 3.5 for the distribution map). In 2019, the country had 9.06 million pigs, marking an overall decline of 1.7% compared to the 2012 population (Anonymous 2019), possibly due to socio-economic factors leading to a decrease in pork consumption. According to an estimate, over 0.29 million metric tonnes of pork were consumed across India in 2023, slightly lower than the previous years (https://www.statista.com/statistics/826720/india-pig-meat-consumption/). The pig farming, however, remains an important livelihood in many states, particularly in the North Eastern region of the country, where the pig population has shown a rising trend. Assam has the highest pig population, increasing by 28.30 % during 2012-2019. Meghalaya (29.99 %), Jharkhand (32.69 %), Chhattisgarh (20.01 %), and Karnataka (6.25 %) have also shown increase in pig population (Anonymous 2019).

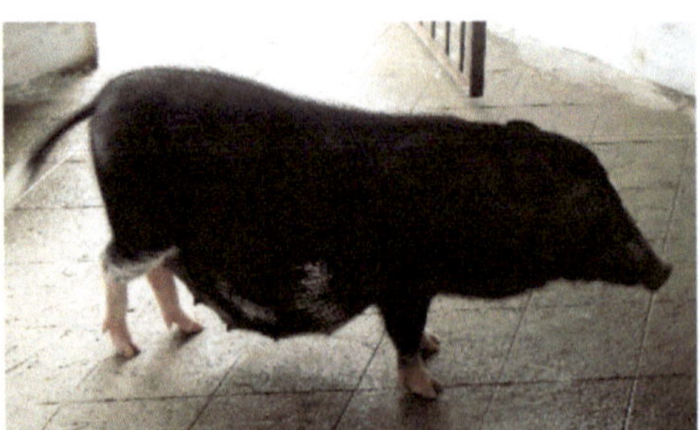
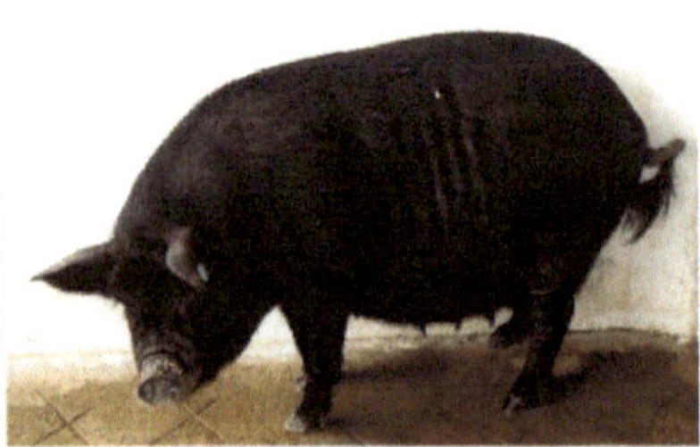

Fig..2.21. *Niang Megha and Ghoongroo sows. Indigenous breeds are known for their unique features such as better heat tolerance, meat quality, early sexual maturity and good quality bristles (Photo courtesy of Dr. V. K. Gupta, ICAR-National Research Centre on Pig).*

Domestic Horse: The horse holds a significant place among the most cherished animals in India, exerting profound influence across various facets of human life throughout history. Alongside the cow and elephant, it is regarded as one of the fourteen gems said to have emerged from the mythical ocean churning. However, the origins of the domestic horse remain one of the most contentious subjects in Indian archaeology. The earliest evidence of domesticated horses in India dates back to around 4500 BCE, discovered at Mesolithic sites like Bagor in Rajasthan. Subsequent findings of horse remain, dating to the Neolithic period, have been reported at sites such as Kodekal in Gulbarga and Hallur in Raichur, Karnataka. Additionally, late Harappan levels at Mohenjo-Daro have yielded evidence of true horse presence (Ghosh 1990, Danino 2006). Bones of horses (*Equus caballus*) and asses (*E. asinus)* have been unearthed at mature Harappan (ca. 2300-1900 BCE) and late Harappan (ca. 1900-1700 BCE) cultural sites in Gujarat (Thomas *et al.* 1997). Important Iron Age sites like Ujjain and Hastinapur have also yielded domestic horse remains, with cut marks on the bones suggesting the slaughter of horses as food (Ghosh 1990). Based on archaeological, anthropological (Fig. 2.22), genetic, literary, and cultural evidence, some scholars propose that various *Equus* species, including the true horse (*E. caballus*), likely existed during the Indus-Sarasvati civilization, albeit in limited numbers. It is plausible that horses may have entered India over a longer timeframe than traditionally believed, owing to interactions between people of the Indus-Sarasvati civilization and neighbouring regions (Danino 2006).

In Vedic India, horses and cows held a prominent status among domesticated animals. In the Rig Veda the term *ashva* is frequently used not only to denote horses but also to symbolize power and vitality. Throughout Vedic texts, the horse consistently emerges as a prized possession and a symbol of precious wealth. It was valued next to cattle, as wealth in steeds is constantly prayed for along with an abundance of cows (Macdonell 1899). The Atharva Veda (11.3:5) delineates the horse, stating, *Aśvāh kanā gāvastandulā maśakāstụsāh,* translating to 'Horses are grains, cows are the clean rice, flies and mosquitoes, the chaff' and placing it as one of the five forms of living beings, affirming, *Taveme pañcha paśhvao vibhaktā gāvo aśvāh purusā ajāvayah* (Atharva Veda 11.2:9) which means 'all these five forms of living beings – cows, horses, humans, goats, and sheep – are yours each distinct in its own way' (Sharma 2013). For the Vedic people, the horse was an important war tool, and the horse-driven chariot race was a favourite amusement. Though the horse was not used for riding during the Rigvedic period, there are indications that riding on horseback was at least known to the Rig Veda, with distinct references occurring in the Atharva Veda and the Yajur Veda (Macdonell 1899). Beyond its role as a linchpin in warfare, horses were used in land transport and agricultural activities, including ploughing, even during the Vedic era. An excerpt from the Atharva Veda (3.17.6) echoes this sentiment, urging 'Let the oxen and horses draw the plough and carry the burdens happily for growth and prosperity' (Sharma 2013).

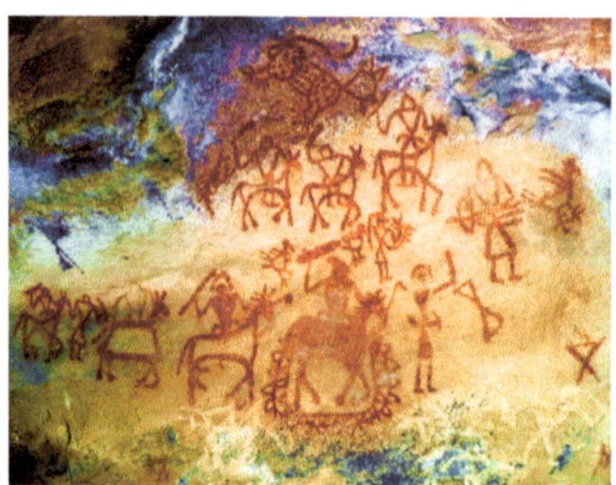 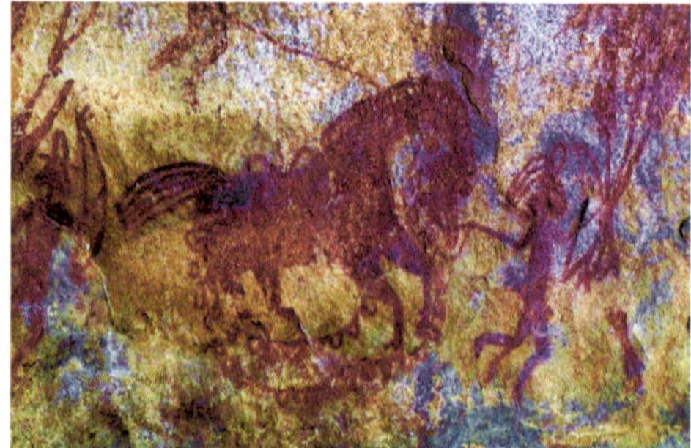

Fig. 2.22. The images of animals in Bhimbetka rock art are significant as they provide insights into the lives and beliefs of prehistoric peoples. Famous historic period panels from Bhimbetka rock shelter depicting soldiers on horseback, dancers and various animals and a man leading horse (Photo courtesy of Dr. Meenakshi Dubey-Pathak).

Horses and elephants were the two main war animals in the Mauryan army and were provided with the utmost care and security. Hurting or killing of any of these species invited the death penalty. According to the Arthashastra, the superintendent of horses was responsible to register the breed, age, colour, classes, and native place of the horse, and report the king of such animals as are inauspicious, crippled, or diseased. He was to be attended by the king daily during the 7th part of the day. The Arthashastra also holds that 'a prince shall spend the forenoon in receiving lessons in military arts concerning elephants, horses, chariots and weapons' (Shamasastry 1951). Horse-driven chariots constituted one of the four divisions of Indian armies from the time of Mahabharata to the late Mauryan period. Two horse-driven two-wheeled chariots used in early Vedic times were lethal in battle. But over the centuries, chariots grew into huge and ponderous vehicles and lost their swiftness and use in battle. The enervating influence of the climate, coupled with the scarcity of horses that needed to be imported from the region of the Indus, might have also contributed to the gradual decline in the use of the chariot, both for warfare and racing (Macdonell 1899). By the Gupta age (300-550 CE), horse chariots virtually lost their relevance in actual wars, but the cavalry division remained the main fighting division. The horses were given more importance than elephants in Samudragupta's army because of their speed and easy manoeuvrability. The emperor also performed *Ashvamedha yagna* to proclaim his imperial power and issued a gold coin depicting a horse. Use of saddled horses in warfare and spending of a huge amount of money on purchase of good horses from Persia and Afghanistan by emperor Harshavardhan of Kannauj empire (606–647 CE) is also mentioned in history. The importance of cavalry in warfare is reflected by a statement in *Kathāsaritsāgara,* the famous 11th -century collection of Indian legends, histories and folk tales, which suggest that for a king having strong cavalry force, war becomes almost a sport, and that the cavalry is the key to fame. A king in possession of cavalry need entertain no apprehension regarding his territory said Chalukya king Somesvara III (Eraly 2014). During the reign of Krishnadevaraya the Vijayanagar kingdom possessed the finest cavalry, which played a pivotal role in numerous triumphant conquests against the traditional rivals of the renowned king (Fig. 2.23). However, a large number of war horses were imported, both via sea route and land routes from the Middle East (Chandra 2021).

Parts of Punjab and Sindh are mentioned in historical records as centres of breeding horses, perhaps as an extension of the breeding complex that sprawled Afghanistan and Central Asia. Panini mentions *Pārevadavā*, a special breed of mares from across the Indus. The best class of horses were imported from Kamboja, Sindhu, Bahlika and Sauvira (Agrawala 1953). The European merchant Marco Polo, who visited Southern India from 1292-94 CE during the reign of Rudramma Devi of the Kakatiya Dynasty, noted that 'here are no horses bred; and a great part of the wealth of the country is wasted in purchasing the horses' (Eraly 2014). The imported horses deteriorated rapidly due to unsuitable climates and poor maintenance. The breeding of Indigenous horses started in the 16th century in many parts of India, with the Western Punjab, Haryana, Western Uttar-Pradesh, different Himalayan regions and foothills of Rajasthan and Gujarat being the most prolific horse breeding belt and 'in a short time Hindustan ranked higher in this (breeding) respect than Arabia, whilst many Indian horses cannot be distinguished from Arab and [Iraqi] breed' recorded Abul Fazl, the official historian of Akbar's reign (Chandra 2021). The importance of horses in warfare in India continued till late 19th century.

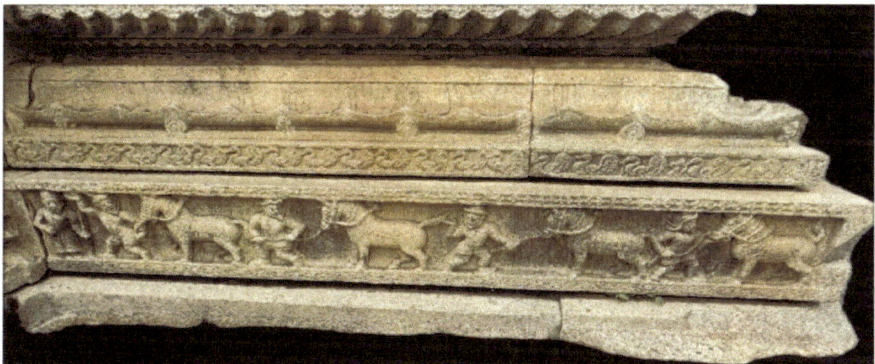

Fig. 2.23. *Vijayanagar empire possessed finest cavalry in 16th century. A frieze on outer wall of Ramachandra temple Humpi depicting fasten-up horses being led by their handlers or riders (Photo by the Author).*

Until the late 20th century, horse-drawn vehicles such as two-wheeled ekkas, tongas, as well as four-wheeled carriages like Victoria and coaches, were prevalent means of both private and public transport in India. Ekkas and tongas served as the equivalent of modern-day cabs, taxis, or private hire vehicles. Ekka, pulled by one horse, hence its name from the Hindi word *Ek*, is an indigenous technology. This small, springless horse-carriage featuring a tea-tray top was predominantly used in Northern India and parts of Bengal in the 19th century. In contrast, the Tonga (Fig. 2.24), a low, hooded two-wheeled dog-cart mounted on strong springs, was widely used in the Deccan region and also as post-cart (*dāk gāri*) on routes to Shimla, Murree, and the new Kashmir-road (Kipling 1904). Tonga stands, designated parking areas for these vehicles, were common in most towns and cities. The two-wheeled horse carts were extensively utilized for local public transport in rural areas, often serving as the livelihood of the less affluent. Before their prohibition in 2015, Victoria horse carriages were a significant tourist draw in Mumbai.

Presently, horses in India are bred mainly for draught work, production of biologicals, equestrian activities such as horse racing, sports, leisure riding and training, and for the police work. Horses and horse-driven carriages remain in demand for various ceremonies, including weddings, often providing livelihood for the less affluent. The Remount Veterinary Corps and the Army Service Corps also play a significant role in maintaining equine populations for military and ceremonial purposes. The foremost horse-drawn carriage in post-independent India is the open, six-horse-drawn Presidential buggy, an iconic black carriage with gold-plated rims, a red velvet interior, and an embossed Ashoka Chakra, used exclusively by the President for ceremonial occasions. After a 40-year hiatus, the buggy made a grand return during the Republic Day celebrations of 2024, accompanied by the President's Bodyguard mounted on majestic Bay and Dark Bay horses. The President's Bodyguard, an elite household cavalry regiment, holds the highest position in the order of precedence among all Indian Army units. India has a well-established horse racing and breeding industry, with major turf clubs in Delhi, Bengaluru, Mysuru, Hyderabad, Pune, Mumbai, Chennai, and Kolkata. However, the country lacks dedicated racecourses or clubs for its 0.34 million indigenous horses (Mehta and Bhattacharya 2023). A study in Rajasthan and Punjab found that most horses are used for ceremonial functions (36%), followed by tourism and leisure riding (28.6%), breeding (25.8%), and equestrian sports (9.6%). These findings highlight the need to promote traditional equestrian activities—such as endurance races like *Rewal Chaal*—and develop structured frameworks for equestrian sports to ensure the economic sustainability and conservation of indigenous breeds (Mehta and Bhattacharya 2023). Notably, in 2024, the Government of India included the promotion of entrepreneurship for horses, donkeys, mules, and camels under the National Livestock Mission.

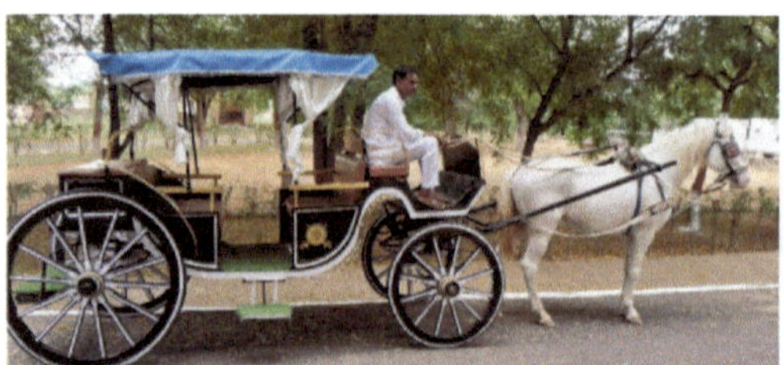

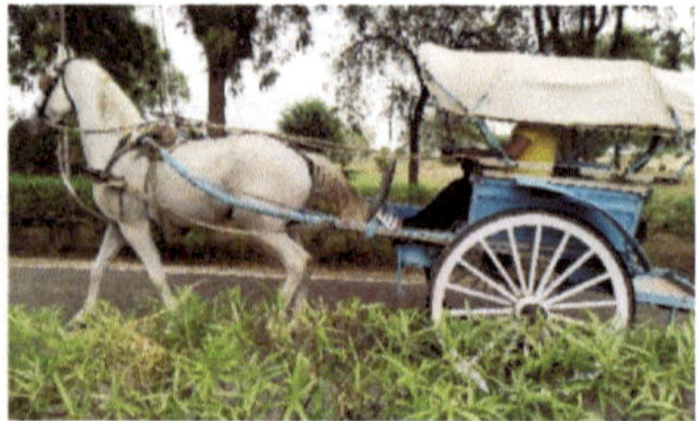

Fig. 2.24. *Horse-driven carriages (Buggy and Tonga) are used to promote equine ecotourism (Photo by the Author and Courtesy of Dr. Remash Dedar, ICAR-NRCE).*

According to the 20th Livestock Census, there were only 3.4 lakh horses and ponies in the country in 2019, showing a decline of 45.6% (Anonymous 2019). There are eight registered indigenous breeds of horses and ponies in India (https://nbagr.res.in/brc, accessed on 01-07-2025). These include Marwari, Kathiawari, Bhutia, Spiti, Manipuri, Kachchhi-Sindhi, Zanskari and recently registered Bhimthadi (Deccani) breeds, each recognized for its distinct characteristics and traditional roles (Mehta *et al.* 2024). For example, Manipuri ponies are famous for polo, and Kachchhi-Sindhi horses for their great speed and stamina to covering the long distance as well as for their excellent heat and draught tolerance. Marwari and Kathiawari horses are also known for their unique style of running (Rewal Chaal). Admired for their beauty, animated gait, and intelligence, Marwari horses (Fig.2.25) are particularly well-suited for dressage. They also possess exceptional hearing ability, which alerts riders to danger as well as amazing homecoming instinct and can always find their way home (Singh and Yadav 2004, Swinny 2019). Today, Marwari horses are used in safari in many parts of Rajasthan and they are preferred by foreign tourists (Pal *et al.* 2020).

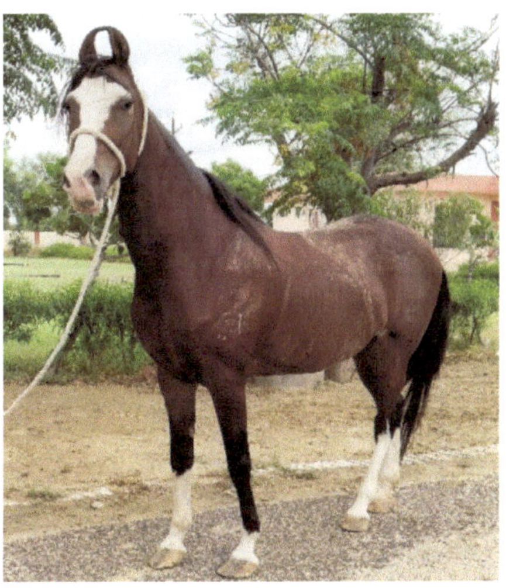

Fig. 2.25. *Known as the Pride of India, the Marwari breed is celebrated for its remarkable endurance and homing instinct (Photo courtesy of Dr. Naveen Kumar, ICAR-NRCE).*

Notwithstanding the glorious past and socio-cultural influence, the equine population in India has declined considerably over the years, mainly due to the replacement of horse driven carriages by motorized vehicles, high maintenance cost of horses and recent outbreaks of diseases. Considering the declining population of indigenous equines, the ICAR-National Research Centre on Equines initiated efforts to conserve and promote these animals for alternative roles, such as ecotourism and equine safaris at its Bikaner campus. Initiatives by the institute have also played a vital role in bringing indigeneous equestrain sports, including horse race and Rewal Chaal into the national spotlight. There is also potential for developing other agri-entrepreneurial ventures based on equine husbandry, such as equine harness making, equine farriery, shoeing and nailing, establishing equine riding academies, and utilizing equine by-products like milk, meat, hair, and leather for manufacturing various goods (Singh *et al.* 2022). The horse is used in animal assisted therapy and can serve as a significant part of animal care-farm or a therapeutic farm, where animals are kept and cared for as part of therapeutic or rehabilitative programmes for people with various physical, mental, or emotional challenges.

Donkeys and Mules: The origin of the donkey in India is not well defined. Although donkeys were not domesticated in the Indian subcontinent, their presence and use in the Indus Valley civilization and South Asia are substantiated by zooarchaeological data. A recent genetic study suggested that donkeys were introduced to the Indus Valley by traders from Africa, the Middle East, and the Near East, and subsequently to the Indian subcontinent (Earnist *et al.* 2022). There is strong evidence of flourishing trade between Mesopotamia and the Indus Valley cultures in the mid-third millennium BCE. Traders from the ancient Sumerian city of Ur travelled by donkey caravan, river barges, and seagoing ships to all parts of the Fertile Crescent, Persia, Telmun, Magan, and Melukka in the Indus Valley. They imported copper, precious stones and woods, and ivory, and exported woollen clothing, cloth, barley, and locally grown foodstuffs (Alexander and Violet 2012). Thus, the donkey reached South Asia before the end of the third millennium BCE and became an important part of transportation (Mitchell 2018). There were considerable building activities in Harappan towns, and perhaps the Harappan people used donkeys to transport bricks and other building materials (Randhawa 1980).

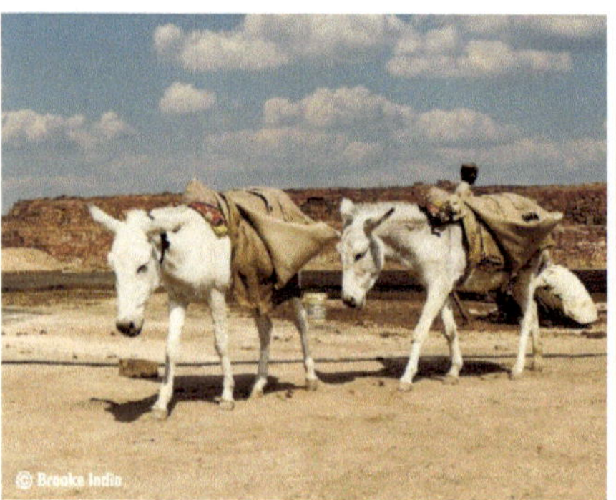

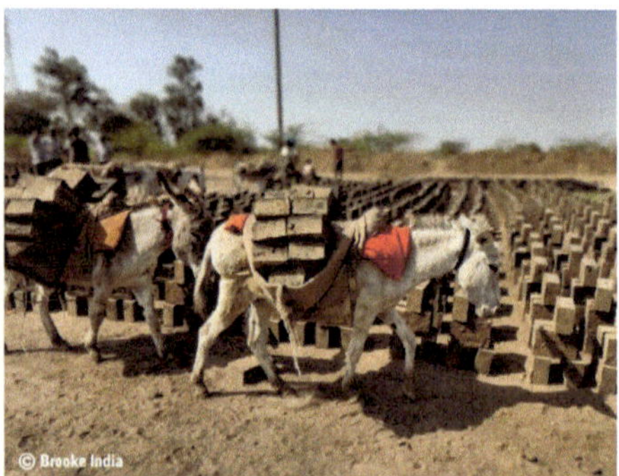

Fig. 2.26. *Over the centuries, donkeys have remained crucial pack animals in India, particularly for transporting loads of laundry, agricultural goods, and construction materials (Photo courtesy of Brooke India).*

The presence of domestic donkeys during the Vedic and post-Vedic periods is attested by Vedic and post-Vedic scriptures. The Arthashastra classifies asses and mules under the category of herd. The stables for asses were situated in the same direction as those of camels and working horses within the city. The recommended diet for donkeys and mules was similar to that for cows. It also specifies that a herd of 100 heads of asses and mules should have 5 males. The Arthashastra states that trade routes traversable by asses or camels, regardless of countries and seasons, were favourable, indicating that donkeys were utilized for transportation by traders. The use of donkeys and mules for transport is also recommended. Kautilya suggests, 'Against a country with characteristics like little rain and muddy water, one should march with an army mostly comprising asses, camels, and horses' (Shamasastry 1951). 'Donkeys ridden by throngs of boys accompanied the march of the army of Harshvardhan' (606–647 CE) noted Bana (Randhawa 1980). Describing the status and usefulness of donkeys (asses) in 19th century India, the author of *Beast and Man in India* writes, 'While the ass is among the most despised of creatures, it is also one of the most useful. There are regions where the donkey is yoked to the plough, but its primary occupation is carrying clothes for the washerman, and earth, burnt and unburnt lime, and stone for the potter, the builder, and the railway contractor. The grand works in the west are constructed by strong-armed men, but in India, railway banks, waterworks dams, and Queen's highways are built by the slender, unskilled woman labourers and the humble donkey. Its step is the first in the peaceful halls that mark the new civilization, but its loads are often too heavy for its weak limbs' (Kipling 1904).

According to the 20th Livestock Census, India had 1.2 lakh donkeys and 84 thousand mules (Anonymous, 2019). These animals are traditionally reared by washerman and potter communities, and they are primarily engaged in various activities such as transporting bricks and clay soil in brick kilns, carrying sand from river beds, and transporting other construction materials (Fig. 2.26). Additionally, they carry agricultural commodities such as grains, hay, straw, and wooden logs. Donkeys and mules are particularly suitable for transporting goods in swampy and waterlogged areas during the rainy season and through narrow lanes and roads that are inaccessible to motorized vehicles (Jadhav *et al.* 2023). In many parts of the country, donkeys and mules serve as carting animals and breeding stock. There is a growing interest in donkey milk and milk-based products in the Indian market, prompting many entrepreneurs to consider opening donkey farms to meet the demand. Donkey milk can fetch a high price in the market, sometimes reaching as high as Rs. 5,000 per litre.

The sight of caravans consisting of donkeys and mules, laden with bricks, clay soil, sand, and various other construction materials or agricultural products, was a common site in India, particularly in rural and hilly regions. However, the utility of donkeys as pack animals has considerably diminished over the last two decades, resulting in a 61.23% decline in their population from 2012 to 2019 (Anonymous 2019). Despite this decline, a significant number of impoverished individuals still rely on donkeys for their livelihoods, as they provide both direct and indirect sources of income. The higher population of donkeys in rural areas compared to urban ones, along with the dense concentration of mules in hilly states, underscores their importance in rural regions and challenging mountainous terrains.

Indian donkeys have white, grey, or black coats, and four registered breeds: Spiti, Halari, Ladakhi and Kacchhi (https://nbagr.res.in/camel-donkey-yak, accessed on 30-08-2025). Spiti donkeys primarily inhabit the Lahaul-Spiti and Kinnaur districts of Himachal Pradesh. They are small-size, body colour ranging from brown to dark brown or black, and are known for their sure-footedness, with an average height at the withers ranging from 80 to 90 cm. Spiti donkeys serve as pack animals, capable of carrying loads of up to 100 kg in the low-oxygen, high-altitude mountainous regions. Hailing from the Saurashtra (Kathiawar) region in the southwestern part of Gujarat state, Halari donkeys are predominantly white. They are relatively larger, with an average height at the withers of about 110 cm. Halari donkeys are characterized by their long ears (Fig. 2.27) and gentle nature. They are utilized as pack animals during pastoralist migrations and for carting, able to pull loads twice their body weight. Milk of Halari donkey is known for its sweetness. Kacchhi donkeys are native to the Kachchh District of Gujarat. They are primarily grey, followed by white, brown, and black variations. The average height at the withers for Kacchhi donkeys ranges from 77 to 110 cm. These donkeys exhibit a docile temperament and are employed in agriculture for inter-cultivation, weed removal, and transportation during pastoralist migrations. As pack animals, Kacchhi donkeys can carry nearly 80-100 kg on their backs and pull loads of 200-300 kg on carts (Pal *et al.* 2020, Jadhav *et al.* 2023). The Ladakhi donkey, a newly registered breed, is known for its adaaptability to the harsh climatic conditions of Ladakh. These small-sized animals weigh about 82 kg (males) and 78 kg (females) with coat colours ranging from light brown to black, though brown and black are most common (Niranjan *et al.* 2024).

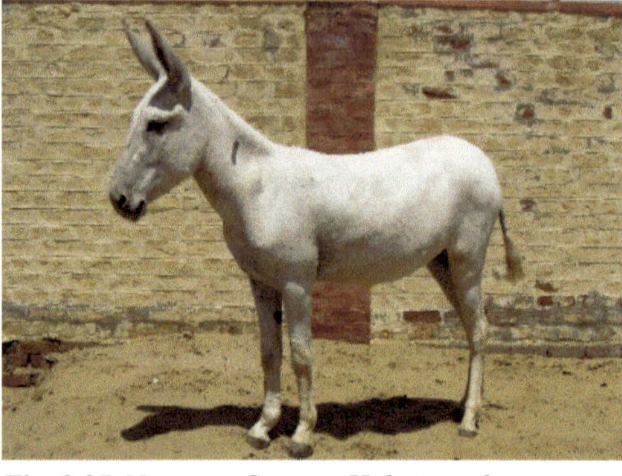

Fig. 2.27. *Native to Gujarat, Halari is a large size yet docile donkey. These donkeys can pull a load twice their body weight (Photo courtesy of Dr. Ramesh Dedar, ICAR-NRCE, Bikaner).*

Apart from registered indigenous breeds, India also possesses several lesser-known donkey populations distributed in different parts of the country. These include light or dark grey-coated, sure-footed sturdy donkeys in Rajasthan, the brown type donkeys of Kurnool and Anantapur districts in Andhra Pradesh, small (75 cm to 90 cm) to medium (91 to 105 cm) size dark grey to light grey colour donkeys in Bihar, the grey type donkeys of the Braj region of Uttar Pradesh, and the Kaikadi donkey from the Vidarbha region of Maharashtra (Jadhav *et al.* 2023). Additionally, India has imported Poitou donkeys for breed improvement, which are being maintained by ICAR-National Research Centre on Equines, and State Animal Husbandry Departments of Uttar Pradesh and Haryana. Furthermore, two types of wild asses - Kiang (*Equus homionus kiang*) and Indian wild ass (*E. hominous khur*) are also found in India (Ghosh 1990).

A study conducted by the International Livestock Research Institute (ILRI) provides insights into the issues facing the Indian donkey and mule population and their dependents (families that own and/or work with these animals). The main reasons for the decline in the donkey population flagged in the report include a decrease in demand for donkeys at brick kilns due to mechanization and a shift in the design of brick kilns from traditional continuous to advanced energy-efficient models for large-scale production, the use of earthmovers and tractors for excavation and transport of riverbed sand, the death of donkeys due to poor health and diseases including glanders outbreak, the preference of horses and mules over donkeys as pack animals, and the lack of interest among youth in donkey-owning communities (Ravichandran *et al.* 2023). The report also highlights the implications of declining donkey populations and recommends measures to improve the situation. Some of the recommendations include enhancing the livelihoods of donkey owners through integrated farming systems and capacity building, implementing effective disease surveillance and improving the health delivery system, developing guidelines for the donkey milk value chain and cooperatives for donkey milk producers and entrepreneurs, and designing carts that reduce the load on working donkeys. Organizations like Brooks India are endeavouring to improve the livelihoods of donkey owners by maintaining donkey health, organizing them through equine welfare groups—a kind of self-help group—and linking them with government schemes and banks for credit linkage. The rising demand for highly digestible donkey milk products in the country is also anticipated to support the growth of donkey farming and check the rapid decline in the donkey population.

Domestic Camels: The history of domestic camels in India can be traced to the Indus Valley Civilization. The remains of the camel bones, including a complete skeleton of a juvenile, have been recovered from Mohenjo-Daro and Harappa. These were initially thought to belong to dromedary but later attributed to Bactrian camels. Depiction of an animal with one large hump on the copper plate recovered from Mohenjo-Daro, indicates the existence of dromedary camels in the Indus Valley (van der Geer 2008). The ancient Greek historian Herodotus (c. 484 – c. 425 BCE) recorded that camels used by Indians were as swift as a horse suggesting that dromedaries were in use in India in the fifth century BCE (Randhawa 1980). It can be assumed that both types of camel existed in ancient India. References to camel are also found in Vedic scriptures. *tā me aśvinā sanīnāṃ vidyātaṃ navānām; yathā cic caidyaḥ kaśuḥ śatam uṣṭrānāṃ dadat sahasrā daśa gonām* 'become appraised, Aśvins, of my recent gifts, how that Kaśu, the son of Chedi, has presented me with a hundred camels and ten thousand cows,' and *ud ānaṭ kakuho divam uṣṭrāñ caturyujo dadat śravasā yādvaṃ janam.* Translated as the 'exalted [prince] has been raised by fame to heaven, for he has given camels laden with four [loads of gold], and Yādva people [as slaves]' (Rig Veda 8.5.37, 8.6.48. vedicheritage.gov.in, and https://www.wisdomlib.org/hinduism/book/rig-veda-english-translation/d/doc835679.html, accessed on 16-11-2023). These hymns clearly underline the importance of the camel as a domestic animal and its use as a pack animal in the Vedic society. Panini refers camel (*Ushtra*) as a multipurpose animal. Camel units (*ushtra sādi*) in the army were used for quick transport. Several articles (*aushtraka*) were made from the parts of dead camels such as large and small sacks (*goni* and *gonitari*) from hair, and large and small leather jars (*kutu* and *kutupa*) made from the camel hide and intestinal teguments (Agrawala 1953). Arthashastra includes the camel among the ranks of herd animals, highlighting its significant role in various spheres, including military endeavours. Repeated mentions within the text underscore its versatility and importance in the socio-political landscape of the Mauryan period. Arthashastra further states that, the king who has a small number of horses may use bulls with horses; likewise, when he is deficient of elephants, he may fill up the centre of his army with mules, camels, and carts (Shamasastry 1951). Apparently, camel was utilized for milk, meat, and transportation and also found its place in military strategies, including chariot pulling and serving as a substitute for elephants.

Pack camels emerged as indispensable assets for long-distance trade routes, where the establishment of wagon roads would have incurred exorbitant costs. Consequently, they became integral components of trade caravans, royal retinues, and wartime logistics, facilitating the movement of supplies and personnel across vast distances. Hundreds of camels were used to carry water to cross desert. The strategic significance of camel in military operations, is evidenced by historical accounts, such as Emperor Jahangir's entourage, which boasted 50 camels solely dedicated to transporting essential provisions. Similarly, during the era of British India, Governor-General Lord Auckland's retinue comprised a formidable force of 850 camels, in addition to elephants and horses, highlighting their pivotal role in logistical support (Akbar 2022). Noteworthy developments in camel utilization include the establishment of camel corps during the Mughal period by Emperor Akbar, and the formation of the renowned Ganga Risala in 1889 under the patronage of Maharaja Ganga Singh of Bikaner. This specialized unit, comprising both men and camels, exemplifies the enduring legacy of camel-mounted warfare, blending traditional methods with evolving military strategies. After independence, the cavalry and camelry of the Rajasthan regions were merged with that of the Indian Army and camelry became part of the Artillery Regiment. the camel-breeding herd was dissolved and animals were taken over by Raikas, the traditional camel herders (Köhler-Rollefson 2018). Camels, formerly belonging to the Indian Army, were transferred to the Border Security Force (BSF), which was established in 1965. This force utilizes camels for both operational duties and ceremonial purposes. Camels played a significant role in the 1971 war. The camel squad of the BSF is a notable feature in the Republic Day Parade. During the 74th Republic Day parade, the nation witnessed women riders in the camel contingent of the Rajasthan Frontier of the BSF for the first time. Camels also participate in thrilling sports events such as camel races and camel polo. In essence, the multifaceted contributions of camels as dependable carriers, logistical assets, and even combatants underscore their enduring significance throughout Indian history. They transcend mere utility to symbolize resilience, adaptability, and strategic innovation.

India was once renowned for its substantial camel population, ranking as the third largest country globally in camel population with over 1 million camel heads until the 1990s. The Raika community, also known as Rebari, hailing from Rajasthan, holds a profound connection with these majestic creatures. Their distinct pastoral lifestyle is marked by traditional customs prohibiting the slaughter of camels or consumption of their meat, alongside restrictions on selling camel milk, wool, or female camels (Köhler-Rollefson *et al.* 2013, Köhler-Rollefson 2018). Beyond the Raika community, various castes and communities across Rajasthan, Uttar Pradesh, Haryana, Madhya Pradesh, and Gujarat have long been involved in camel husbandry. Camels serve as indispensable assets in agricultural operations, functioning as draught and pack animals, facilitating rural transportation, and carting goods. Apart from their role in transportation and labour, camels significantly contribute to the rural economy by providing materials such as hair, wool, bones, leather, and dung. The versatile utility of camels extends to industries such as textile production, where camel wool is utilized to craft durries (carpets), fine wool shawls, and even fashionable mobile phone covers. Notably, innovative ventures have emerged, including the production of environmentally friendly paper from camel dung and the creation of artisanal soap using camel milk, particularly pioneered in Sadri, Rajasthan. These endeavours have not only provided additional sources of income for Raikas but have also showcased the resourcefulness and adaptability of camel-based economies The two-wheeled camel carts, equipped with used aeroplane tyres, were highly popular in the mid-20th century and made the camel an indispensable draught animal in the 1960s, leading to a rise in demand for the camel and an increased population that peaked at about 1.1 million in 1960s (Köhler-Rollefson 2018). These carts facilitated the transportation of diverse goods, including farm produce, construction materials, and daily necessities, along with providing a mode of short-distance travel. However, the proliferation of modern road infrastructure has led to a decline in the use of camel carts, as contemporary transport systems become more accessible. Many camel owners have repurposed their carts for recreational activities, offering joy rides at tourist destinations and during local fairs and festivals. Despite these shifts, the enduring legacy of camels in Indian culture persists, symbolizing resilience, tradition, and adaptability in the face of evolving socio-economic landscapes.

Until 1995-97, the population of camels in India remained higher than the baseline population figure in 1961; but a continuous decline occurred in their population after the 1990s with a negative annual growth trend of -1.5% (Faye 2020). As per the 20th livestock census, India is now left with only 2.5 lakh camels comprising 80 thousand males and 1.7 lakh females. The number is less than half of the camel population in 2007 and 37 % that in 2012 (Anonymous 2019). There are 9 registered breeds of camel (Fig. 2.28, 2.29) in India namely Bikaneri, Jaisalmeri, Jalori, Kutchi (Kachchhi), Malvi, Marwari, Mewari, Mewati, and Kharai (https://

nbagr.res.in/camal-donkey-yak, accessed on 30.08.2025). The majority of the Indian camel breeds are developed in Rajasthan, not by different tribal groups, but instead by the occupation of a specialized caste, the Raikas who looked after the royal camel breeding herds owned by local Maharajahs to meet the requirement of camels for desert warfare. As a consequence, the distinct breeds, such as Bikaneri, Jaisalmeri, Marwari, and Mewari are known after the former kingdoms of their origin (Köhler-Rollefson 1993).

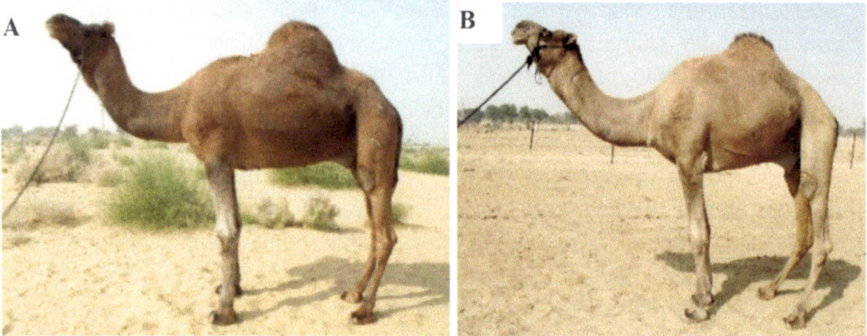

Fig. 2.28. A. *Heavy-built Bikaneri camels are renowned for their milk and draught capabilities, whereas lightly-built* ***B.*** *Jaisalmeri camels excel in riding and racing (Photo courtesy of Dr. A. Sahoo, ICAR-NRCC).*

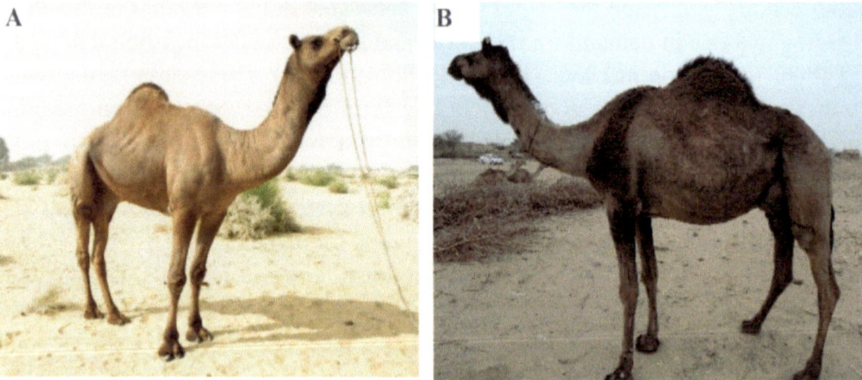

Fig.2.29. A. *Kachchhi camels are multipurpose animals, whereas brown or sand brown colour,* ***B.*** *Sindhi camels are primarily used as baggage animal (Photo courtesy of Dr. A. Sahoo, ICAR-NRCC).*

The camel breeds in India are mainly draught or dual-purpose animals. Heavy-built Bikaneri camels are known for better draught potentials, and also for milk and hair production with an average milk yield of 7.25 litre/ day and that of hair 800 g annually. The lightly built gracious Jaisalmeri camels are better suited for riding and racing. Malvi camels are found in the Mandsore district in Madhya Pradesh; males are used mostly for carrying loads and females for milk production.

Kachchhi and Mewari are good milk producers breeds with lactation yield of 1908±165.0 kg and 1410± 122.2 kg of milk respectively (Prakash *et al.* 2021). A small population of Bactrian camels also exists in India. According to a recent study, these camels numbering 304 (150 males and 154 females) are distributed in the Nubra Valley's Hunder, Diskit, and Sumur villages in Ladakh UT (Fig. 2.30). They were used as pack animals for the supply and transportation of logistics. This role is now replaced by motorized vehicles. However, due to recent increase in the tourism industry in Ladakh, the camel safari is emerging as the primary recreational activity in the Valley creating a new role for the camel and improving the socioeconomic status of camel farmer. A single camel earned approximately INR. 40,000 to 1 lakh per season from camel safari. Interestingly the study also revealed that the number as well as the price of these economically important animals is increasing in their home tract. The cost of an adult camel in 2022 was INR.1.5 to 4 lakh (Dolker Lamo *et al.* 2023).

Several factors are accounted for decline in the camel population in India, main being the significant reduction in traditional use of camels for draught purposes due to mechanization of agriculture and transport system, increasing role of synthetic fertilizers in local agriculture rather than camel manure, depleting camel grazing areas due to the closure of forests, intensification of agriculture and irrigation schemes, and also the Camel Act enacted by Rajasthan Government declaring camel as the State Animal. The Act prohibited slaughtering, selling and transporting camel outside the State of Rajasthan thus blocking disposal of unproductive animals (Köhler-Rollefson 2018, Faye 2020, Prakash *et al.* 2021). The absence of system for processing and marketing camel milk, absence of buyers for male camels, closure of traditional markets, and spread of diseases, especially mange and trypanosomiasis have also contributed to decline of camel population (Köhler-Rollefson *et al.* 2018).

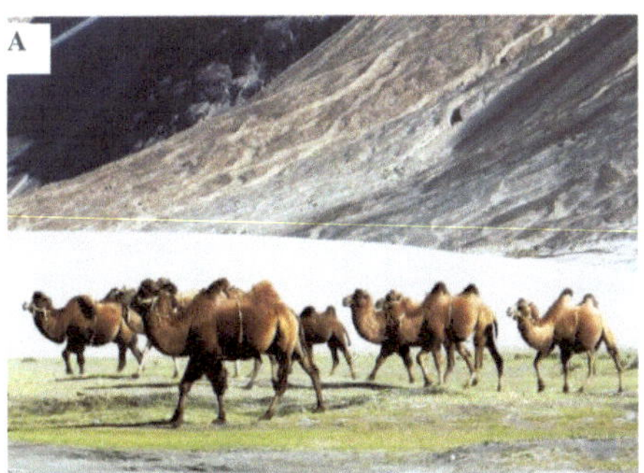

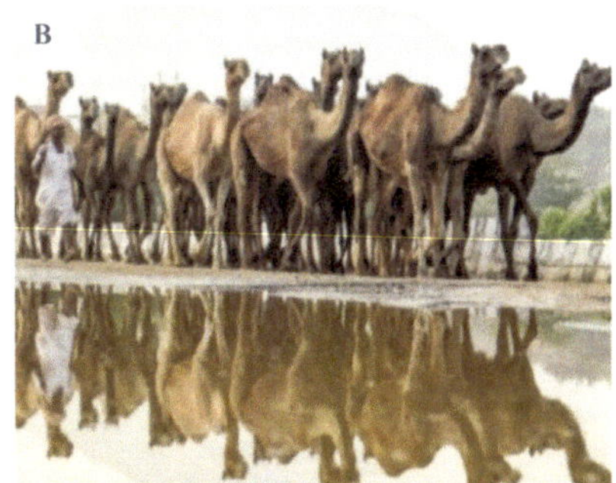

Fig. 2.30. A. *Bactrian camels found in Ladakh are now utilized for camel safaris and have become an important source of income for herders in their newfound role.* ***B.*** *Kharai camels, popularly known as swimming camels, are a rare breed found in the salt marshes of Kutch in Gujarat. (Photo courtesy of Dr. A. Sahoo, ICAR-NRCC).*

The nutritional value and health benefits of camel milk have been known in India since ancient times as well as to the present-day camel pastoralists. Ayurveda mentions the health benefits of camel milk (*Ushtra Ksheera*) in the treatment of a range of diseases including gastric ulcers, bloat, piles, haemorrhoids, parasitic (*Krimi*) infections, inflammatory conditions, ascites, and other ailments due to vitiation of *Vata* and *Kapha.* Raikas and traditional camel herders of Ladakh also know about the health benefits of camel milk (Köhler-Rollefson *et al.* 2013, Dolker lamo *et al.* 2023). The Raikas, who are traditionally reluctant to sell camel milk, carry *Aak* leaves in their turban which they use as vessels to drink fresh camel milk. They possess extensive knowledge of the effects of various trees and herbs on the health of camel as well as on the quality and taste of the milk (Köhler-Rollefson *et al.* 2013). Raikas, who regularly consume camel milk have zero prevalence of diabetes (Agrawal *et al.* 2007). Studies on the benefits of camel milk on human health undertaken by ICAR-National Research Camel (ICAR-NRCC) in collaboration with different agencies showed encouraging effects of raw camel milk in the management of type-1 diabetes and tuberculosis in human patients, recommending the use of camel milk as an adjunct therapy for faster recovery and effective management of these diseases. The institute has also conducted a clinical assessment of camel milk in autistic children with promising findings. Inclusion of a daily intake of 600 ml of camel milk for 3 months in the conventional therapeutic protocol enhanced the rate of recovery in 31 of the 42 autistic and mentally retarded (Anonymous 2015). Overall camel milk, can be an adjunct and nutritional supplement with conventional therapy in a range of human diseases for better recovery.

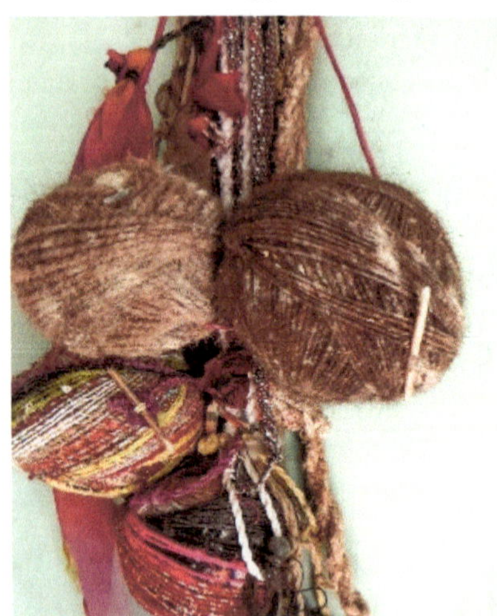

Fig. 2.31. *Camel hair threads are used for making range of products (Photo courtesy of Dr. Rakesh Ranjan ICAR-NRCC).*

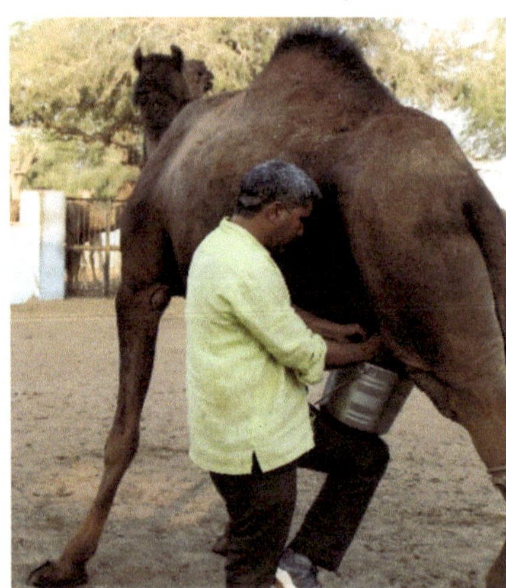

Fig. 2.32. *Raising camel for milk is the most promising new role and economically viable options for promoting camel husbandry (Photos courtesy of Dr. A. Sahoo, ICAR-NRCC).*

It is important to relook and explore camels beyond their traditional role as a source of economically viable livestock farming in modern India, where the traditional role of the camel is rapidly declining. Camels have immense potential as dairy animals. Despite its economic importance, the potential of milk has remained underestimated and underutilized in India due to limited awareness, lack of value-added products, and the absence of an organized marketing system for camel milk (Köhler-Rollefson *et al.* 2013, Dolker Lamo *et al.* 2023). Although, most camel breeds in India are primarily draught or dual-purpose type, some individuals within these breeds, possess good milk-yielding potential. The estimated peak milk yield of Mewari, Kachchhi, Bikaneri, and Jaisalmeri ranges between 6.7 and 8.6 kg. Genetic resources from these breeds can be explored for camel dairy establishment (Prakash *et al.* 2021). FSSAI has recognized camel milk in the food category and an operational standard for camel milk was developed by combined efforts of ICAR-NRCC and FSSAI. It is expected to promote the production and marketing of camel milk in the Indian market ultimately opening avenues for farmers/camel keepers to sell their produce in the National and International markets (Sahoo A 2023, Personal communication). Setting up camel milk collection and processing points in the camel herding areas, developing a cool chain to transport milk to the consumers and training youths in processing camel milk hygienically are also important for the success of camel dairy farming (Köhler-Rollefson *et al.* 2013, Köhler-Rollefson 2018). Value-added camel milk products (pasteurized milk, flavoured milk, fermented drinks, ghee, ice cream, and soaps) developed with technical interventions are gaining considerable consumer interest. Raising camel for milk is the most promising new role and economically viable option for promoting camel husbandry and arresting population decline in India. There is a need to create market opportunities and support the manufacturing and marketing of camel milk and value-added milk products, carpets and shawls manufactured from camel hair/wool (Fig. 2.31), and manure and bio-diverse papers. The camel safaris are gaining popularity in many tourist places and traditional fairs. Nubra Valley in Ladakh, the home tract of Bactrian camels, and Bikaner, Jaisalmer, Mandawa, and Pushkar in Rajasthan are some of the camel safari hotspots in India. In Gujarat, camel safaris (Fig. 2.33) are an essential part of the 100-day annual Rann Utsav, organized every year in Dhordo village near Rann of Kutch, by the State Tourism Department. Camel polo, first introduced in India by the British military, is gaining popularity in recent years, especially in Rajasthan (Fig. 2.34). The state government is planning to organize a camel polo competition in the famous Pushkar cattle fair in 2023 to make it as a tourist attraction.

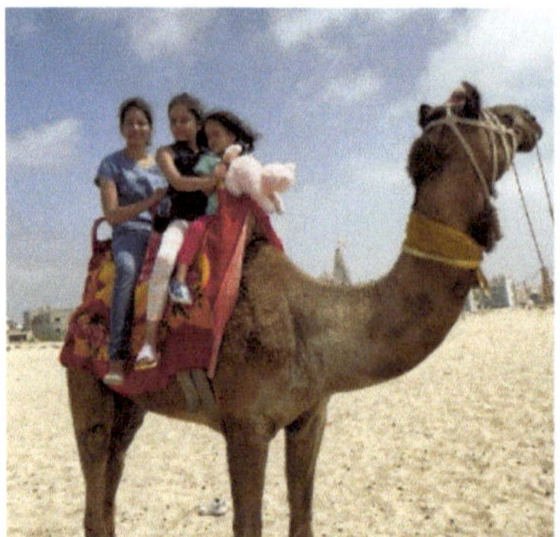
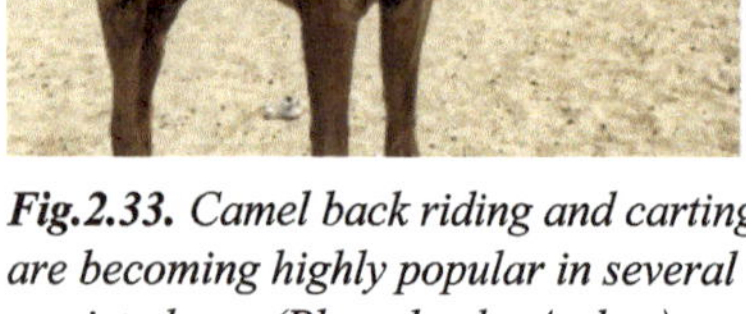

Fig.2.33. *Camel back riding and carting are becoming highly popular in several tourist places (Photo by the Author).*

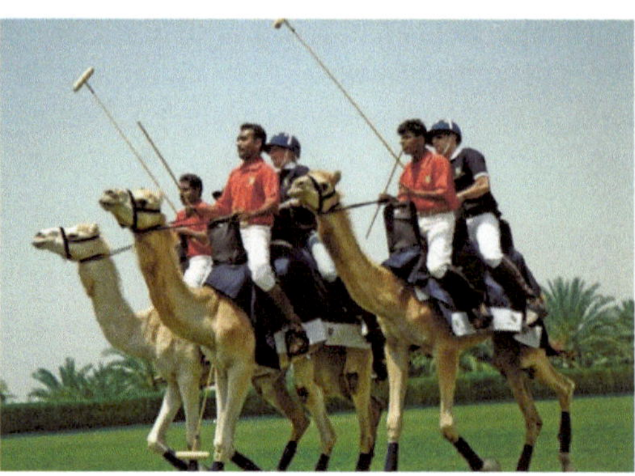

Fig. 2.34. *Camel polo, thrilling sport event has gained much popularity in the recent years (Photo courtesy of Dr. A. Sahoo, ICAR-NRCC).*

Asian Elephant (*Elehas maximus*): The extant species of elephants are Asian elephants (*Elephas maximus*), African savannah/bush elephants (*Loxodonta africana*), and African forest elephants (*Loxodonta cyclotis*). They are the largest land animals and the only living members of the order Proboscidea, which also included mastodons and mammoths. Although there are some physiological differences across species such as in their ear shape, tusk presence, and overall size, the three species are often grouped together when it comes to their behavioural, social, and cognitive traits (Raviv *et al.* 2023). Comparatively smaller in size than African elephants, Asian elephants are classified as endangered on the IUCN Red List. They are distributed throughout the Indian subcontinent and Southeast Asia, with three recognized subspecies: the Indian elephant (*Elephas maximus indicus*), the Sri Lankan elephant (*Elephas maximus maximus*), and the Sumatran elephant (*Elephas maximus sumatranus*). However, phylogeographic studies based on mitochondrial DNA data do not support the distinct subspecies or evolutionarily significant units (ESUs) and place Sri Lankan and Indian elephants within the same phylogenetic group (Fleischer *et al.* 2001).

Elephants are found both in free ranging (wild) and captive states. The captive elephants belong to the category of tame captive domestic animals. Tame captive animals are subjected to human control for specific purposes. While they are not typically bred in captivity, they qualify in some ways, as domesticates since their movement, feeding, and protection being primarily controlled by humans within a sustained, multigenerational relationship (Zeder 2012). It is suggested that all elephant species have undergone a form of self-domestication, as elephants exhibit as many of the traits associated with self-domestication such as reduced aggression, increased prosocial behaviour, an extended juvenile period, heightened playfulness, socially regulated cortisol levels, and intricate vocal behaviour (Raviv *et al.* 2023). It is also noted that there is no evidence indicating that Asian elephants, which were likely tamed as beasts of burden, were subjected to the pressure of artificial selection by humans.

The boundary between wild and captive or domestic elephants, however, remains permeable, as elephants incorporated into human societies for labour, warfare, tourism, religious purposes or display have not been irrevocably separated from their wild counterparts. They may continue to intermingle. In India, wild elephants served as the source of war elephants, and kings endeavoured to protect their habitats to ensure a supply of domestic elephants for warfare. The Arthashastra mentions the establishment of elephant forests at the country's extreme limits, separated from wild tracts, emphasizing the king's responsibility not only to care for existing elephant forests but also to establish new ones. These forests supplied war elephants for the king and were supervised and maintained by a superintendent of elephant forests and their retinue of forest guards. The penalty for killing an elephant in the elephant forest was a death sentence. Capturing of elephant calves, tuskless bulls, cow with calves and diseased pachyderm was prohibited (Shamasastry 1951). To address the perplexing terminological issues surrounding captive elephants, anthropologists propose to adopt the perspective of ethnoelephantology — an integral approach to study human-elephant relationships that recognizes the complex histories of interconnection by which human and elephant mutually affect each other (Locke 2013, 2014).

India inherits a captivating history featuring both domesticated and wild elephants. In Indian mythology, alongside the cow and the horse, the elephant is revered as one of the fourteen gems said to have emerged from the mythical ocean churn known as *Sāgara Manthana*. Elephants find a wide spectrum of representations across almost all spheres of human life in India. Indeed, it is difficult to imagine India without the elephant. A rock painting at Bhimbetka, dating back to the Mesolithic period or even earlier, portrays a strikingly large single elephant image, alongside depictions of hunters chasing elephants, bison, and antelopes (Dubey-Pathak 2014). Zooarchaeological findings from various sites across India further suggest that early humans engaged in hunting or scavenging of megafauna, including elephants, to procure meat for sustenance. Besides yielding substantial amounts of meat, elephants likely served as sources of skin, bones, and tusks for purposes such as shelter, clothing, and tool-making (Bose 2020) The domestication of elephants traces back to India, with the earliest definitive evidence of their domestic status found in seals recovered from the Indus Valley site of Mohenjo-daro. Several of these seals depict rugs placed over the backs of elephants, indicating their domestication during that era (Clutton-Brock 2012). It is probable that elephants were initially captured from the wild and then utilized in captivity primarily for draught purposes, but soon they became a crucial part of ancient war technologies.

References to trained elephants can be found in Vedic literature. The elephant, as an animal, is explicitly mentioned in two passages of the Rig Veda. One passage relates to the name *mriga,* meaning beast, with the addition of *hastin,* suggesting a hand applied to it. Another passage relates to attempts made to catch wild elephants (Macdonell 1899). The sages of the Atharva Veda (3.22.6) mention elephants several times, particularly emphasizing their strength, grace, splendour, and energy. They regard elephants as steady, sure, and comfortable among animals, without disturbance. Domestic elephants were also considered precious gifts (Atharva Veda 20.131.5) in the Vedic time (Sharma 2013). It is likely that Vedic people did not use elephants in warfare. However, literary evidence from both the Ramayana and Mahabharata indicates the use of elephants in warfare during the epic period. By the 6th century BCE, the art of catching and taming elephants had become refined, and the elephant emerged as a crucial component of military power in India (Bist *et al.* 2002).

The Arthashastra provides valuable guidelines for capturing, training, managing, and ensuring the welfare of elephants. Guards of elephant forests, assisted by elephant caretakers, forest dwellers, and elephant catchers, were tasked with tethering wild elephants with the help of five or seven female elephants. The whereabouts of elephant herds were traced by following the course of urine and dung left by elephants, along with forest tracts covered with branches of the *Bhallātakī* (marking nut tree, *Semicarpus anacardium*). Observations were made at spots where elephants slept or sat, where they left dung, or where they had destroyed the banks of rivers or lakes. Experts in catching elephants had to follow the instructions given to them by the elephant doctor (*anīkastha*). Elephants bred in Kalinga, Anga, Karūsa, and the east were considered the best, while those from western countries were of moderate quality. Elephants from Saurashtra and Panchajana were rated as of lower quality. However, the might and energy of all elephants could be improved through suitable training (Shamasastry 1951). Many of these guidelines retain their value today. Over time, various methods of capturing and training elephants have evolved across different geographical regions in the country. For instance, the pit method was popular in the southern region until recently. In the northeast, *Mela shikar*, involving noosing from the back of trained elephants, was commonly practiced. The *khedda* (Stockade method) was introduced in the Mysore region in the 19th century. Indian experts also travelled to other Asian countries to impart the art of catching and training elephants (Bist 2002).

There is no evidence, in either literature or sculpture from early times, of the provision of a *howdah* on elephants during warfare. Depictions of elephants at ancient Kanaganahalli stupa show riders, whether mahouts or royalty, riding bareback. The elephants are usually encircled with a girth chain or rope. One image clearly shows the girth rope, as well as a unique harness attached to it, presumably to prevent the rear rider from tipping off. The sculptor accurately depicts the manner in which the rider at the rear of the elephant, where its back begins to slope downwards, tucks up his legs to prevent toppling over backward. The goad (*Ankush*) has been used to control elephants since ancient times (Menon and Sinha 2023).

According to the Arthashastra, the victory of kings in battles mainly depends on elephants. Elephants, being of large bodily frame, are capable not only of destroying the enemy's arrayed army, fortifications, and encampments, but also of undertaking dangerous tasks (Shamasastry 1951). In the historic battle between Porus and Alexander in 326 BCE, the army of Porus had 50,000 infantry, 4,000 cavalry, 300 chariots, and 200 elephants. While Alexander also had elephants in his army, he primarily used them for transportation. The deployment of elephants was a significant advantage for Porus and at one point the elephants proved formidable, even demolishing the phalanx formation of the Macedonians, as documented by Arrian. In the Seleucid–Mauryan War (305–303 BCE), the forces of Chandragupta backed by considerable contingent of war elephants (Eraly 2002). By the 1st century CE, the elephant began to play an increasingly important role in armies, as well as in myths and religious rites. The king was entitled as Gajapati, or the master of elephants, and the cult of Ganesha, the elephant-headed deity, was introduced, with various myths created around elephants. The significance of elephants in warfare persisted into medieval India. Under the Mughal emperor Akbar, the imperial stables reportedly housed 32,000 elephants, and during the reign of his son, Emperor Jehangir, the number rose to 113,000. With the advent of more efficient weapons, such as mobile cannons, the role of elephants in war gradually declined. Elephants were relegated from the front lines to logistical support during the British colonial period (Lahiri-Choudhary 1995). However, the British used elephants to mobilize their resources in Northeast India against Japanese forces during the Second World War. An insight into the domestication of elephants during the 19th and 20th centuries can be visualized from historical records of captured elephants in the Indian subcontinent. Estimates suggest that between 1868 and 1980, approximately 30,000 to 50,000 elephants were captured. A census conducted in the year 2000 reported a total of 3,400 to 3,600 captive elephants in India. Among these, the northeast region possessed the highest numbers, with 1,903 to 1,907 elephants, followed by southern India with 860 to 920 elephants (Bist 2002).

Aside from its pivotal role in battles, the elephant has been a source of precious ivory since ancient times. According to Panini, the tusks of elephants, known as *danta*, were utilized for ivory, and a tusker was referred to as *dantāvala* (Agrawala 1953). The Arthaśāstra stipulates rewards for individuals who bring tusks from elephants that have died of natural causes. Elephants were also used in royal and religious processions, entourages, travel, load-pulling, traction, and even for amusement. The Ancient Greeks who journeyed to India perceived elephants as mild, gentle, and the most intelligent of all beasts. Some elephants were known to assist their fallen drivers in battle, carrying them off the field. Strabo, the ancient Greek geographer, philosopher, and historian, witnessed elephants playing cymbals (Eraly 2002). Another interesting ancient use of elephant was to fixing the boundaries of land granted for religious purposes by kings. The elephant was set free, and the course taken by the wise creature was acknowledged as the boundary of the grant. Additionally, the elephant was often made to serve as public executer by Mughals emperors and local kings (Kipling 1904). Elephants have been used to hunt game since the 4th century BCE. Mughal miniatures depict emperors hunting from elephant back, and there was a large-scale deployment of elephants in big-game hunting (*shikar*) during the 2nd quarter of the 19th century (Lahiri-Choudhary 1995).

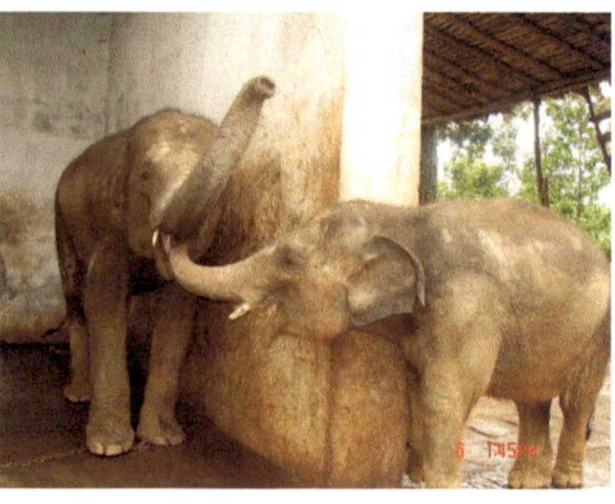

Fig. 2.35. *Elephants are a major attraction in Indian zoos drawing crowds, particularly children, who flock to see them (Photo courtesy of Dr. Asit Das, ICAR-IVRI).*

Placed under Schedule I and Part I of the Indian Wildlife (Protection) Act (1972), thereby bestowed with the highest level of protection, the elephant is the India's national heritage animal. India harbours 60% of the global Asian elephant population, estimated at 29,964 individuals across 23 states in 2017. Karnataka is the home of the highest elephant population, with 6,049 individuals, closely trailed by Assam (5,719) and Kerala (5,706). As of December 2022, there were 33 Notified Elephant Reserves covering an area of 80,777.778 square kilometres (https://moef.gov.in/moef/division/forest-divisions-2/project-elephant-pe/introduction/ index. html, accessed on 26.04.2024). While the majority of the elephant population roams freely in the wild, approximately 2,800 captive elephants are maintained in select zoos, state forest department camps, rescue facilities, and private ownership (Lakshminarayanan 2022). The forest departments primarily utilize elephants for a range of forestry and wildlife activities, including patrolling and mitigating human-elephant conflicts. India bears the highest death toll from human-animal conflicts, with an annual average of 200-250 human fatalities and 100 elephant casualties (Koehl 2024). *Kumki* (from Persian *aid*) elephants, are specially trained for capturing wild elephants. A good *kumki* can perform many roles. *Kumkis* are strategically deployed to assist in managing and guiding wild elephants, thus minimizing damage to crops, human settlements, and the potential loss of both human and elephant lives. Much of the exploitative use of captive elephants has been discontinued due to welfare concerns. However, they are still revered for their various traditional roles. In southern states, elephants are traditionally maintained in temples for religious purposes and processions. In northeastern states, a significant number of captive elephants belong to private owners who utilize them in the timber industry (Sarma 2022). Kerala, which accounts for the highest number of captive elephants (402), maintains the largest herd (44) at the *Guruvayur Devaswom* elephant camp for religious rituals (Koehl 2024). Elephants also serve as a major attraction in Indian zoos (Fig.2.35) and ceremonial processions drawing crowds, particularly children, who flock to see them. The Vijayadashami traditional procession, known as *jumbo savari,* featuring decorated elephants, stands as one of the main highlights of the renowned Mysore Dasara festival in Karnataka. Post-independence, India sent numerous elephants – as symbols of the nation and emissaries of its goodwill and friendship – to zoos in Japan, China, the Soviet Union, the United States, Germany, Turkey, Iran Canada and Netherlands (Menon 2019).

The elephant is a keystone species and playing a vital functional role in tropical forest ecosystems by dispersing seeds, cycling nutrients, removing biomass, and facilitating vegetation growth through trampling and other effects that ultimately influence forest communities. Biologically, elephants play a crucial role in supporting large assemblages of invertebrates, such as dung beetles, and lower plants, including algae and fungi, in semiarid tropical forests (Krishna 2010). These plants are preferred nutrient sources for some reptiles, such as monitor lizards and star tortoises. The presence of dung beetles attracts many insectivorous birds. Moreover, dung deposition into water holes benefits fish and amphibians. Strong sense of elephants enables them to identify subsoil water and natural salt licks, which is utilized by other animals, especially herbivores. Intake of minerals from natural soil is vital for many physiological activities of herbivores (Ramakrishnan *et al.* 2018). Consequently, tropical forests inhabited by elephants are usually rich in biodiversity. Elephants also act as water source for any perennial Indian rivers in India. Elephant-inhabited forests sequester tons of carbon emitted into the atmosphere, thereby mitigating the adverse impacts of climate change. Because of their pivotal role in shaping and preserving forest environments, elephants are frequently referred to as ecosystem engineers (https://moef.gov.in/moef/division/forest-divisions-2/project-elephant-pe/introduction/index.html, accessed on 26. 04. 2024). While human-elephant conflicts can pose challenges, many tribal communities have co-existed with elephants and benefitted in numerous ways. By encountering wild elephants frequently in their natural habitat, they have developed much knowledge on elephant ethology and have become expert elephant handlers carrying out a variety of forestry and wildlife activities. It is reported that most of the elephant handlers in Tamil Nadu Forest camps are from tribal communities. In Annamalai Tiger Reserve, the tribal communities of Malasars are engaged as Mahouts, and Betta Kurumba, Jenu Kurumba and Kattunaickers are the elephant handlers in Mudumalai Tiger Reserve. Tribals belonging to Gond, Oraons and others are engaged in elephant management (Manoharan 2022).

Mahouts believe that elephants are generally resilient animals with few health problems, and that in most cases they can heal themselves by utilizing the resources available in their environment. This unique relationship between mahouts and their elephants holds significant potential for enhancing our understanding of the origins of both human and veterinary medicine (Dubost *et al.* 2019). A study conducted in Thailand revealed that elephants consume 84 % of ethnoveterinary plants as part of their natural diet. Moreover, 8% of plant uses in ethnoveterinary and ethnomedicine practices likely stem from observed elephant self-medicating behaviours (Greene *et al.* 2020).

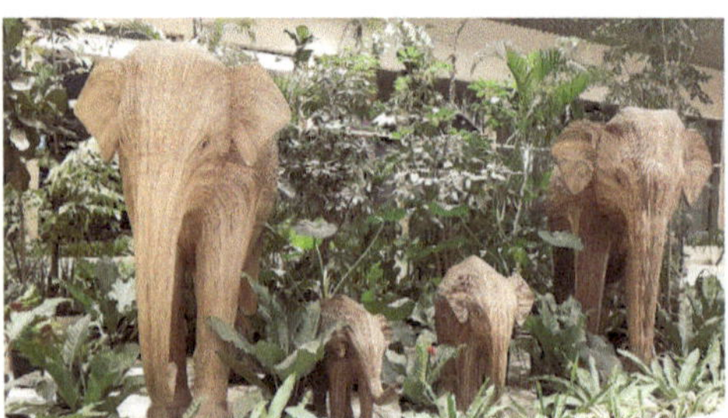
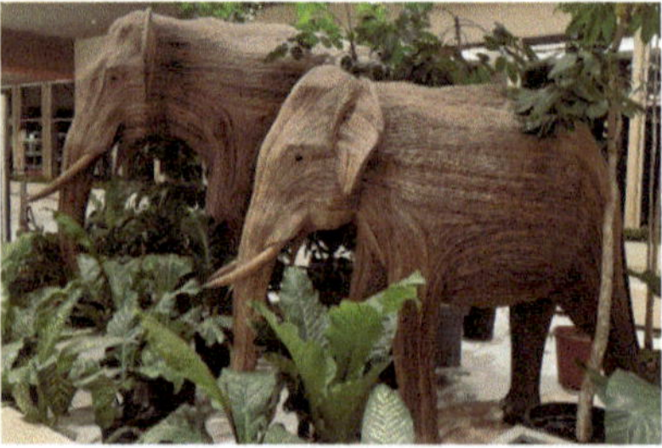

Fig.2.36. *Magnificent elephant sculptures replicate individual elephants from the wildlife reserves of Bandipur and Masinagudi. Crafted by indigenous artisans and tribal communities residing in the forests of Karnataka, Tamil Nadu, and Kerala, these sculptures are made from Lantana camara, a prevalent exotic invasive weed in India. This weed profoundly affects wildlife movements, disrupts feeding and hunting grounds, thus endangering various species, notably elephants. Truly novel idea for transforming an invasive weed into majestic elephants (Description and Source: KIA, Bengaluru; Photo by the Author).*

Despite the extensive literature on elephant management and healthcare, ensuring proper management and welfare of domestic elephants remains a significant challenge. According to the Prevention of Cruelty to Animals Act, 1960, domestic animals are defined as any animals that are tamed or being sufficiently tamed to serve some purpose for the use of humans or have become wholly or partly tamed. Consequently, captive elephants fall under the provisions of this act. Cruelty to domestic elephants may manifest in various forms, such as beating, over-riding, over-loading, torturing, subjecting elephants to unnecessary pain, confining them in cages, and failing to provide sufficient food, water, or shelter, as well as wilfully or unnecessarily administering injurious substances to them (Bist 2002). The use of captive elephants for commercial activities is a contentious issue. While captive elephants generate income for their owners, their welfare is often compromised, and they are knowingly or unknowingly subjected to cruelty. Moreover, not all elephants receive proper veterinary care due to a lack of expert veterinary professionals. Most zoos in the country have one or two veterinarians, often on deputation from the state animal husbandry department, who may leave once their deputation ends. However, some veterinary doctors are permanently employed at zoos and state forest departments, and have possessed extensive experience with captive elephants and made significant contributions to elephant management and healthcare. Wild elephants also face threats from habitat loss and various anthropogenic activities. The fragmentation, loss, and degradation of their habitats, combined with increasing elephant populations in certain areas (and the cessation of elephant captures), have exacerbated human-elephant conflicts in the country. These conflicts result in manslaughter, damage to cultivated crops, and property destruction (Baskaran *et al.* 2011).

Over the past four decades, significant strides have been made in addressing the challenges of managing healthcare, welfare, and conservation of elephants in India (Fig. 2.36). The Government of India launched Project Elephant in 1991-92 as a Centrally Sponsored Scheme under the Ministry of Environment, Forests & Climate Change. Its primary aim was to offer financial and technical assistance to the elephant range states of India to safeguard elephants, their habitats, and corridors, while also tackling human-animal conflicts and promoting the welfare of captive elephants. In 1984, the ICAR-Indian Veterinary Research Institute established the Centre for Wildlife Conservation, Management, Disease Surveillance, and introduced a diploma program on Wildlife Health and Conservation. Additionally, the Wildlife Institute of India (WII), in collaboration with the US Wildlife and Fish Service, initiated the Indian Wildlife Health Cooperative (IWHC) program, involving five veterinary colleges, one in each of the country's North, East, West, South, and Central zones. Most veterinary colleges now have dedicated wildlife departments or sections actively involved in advancing the knowledge and skills of veterinary graduates in wildlife-related areas. Presently, the Wildlife Institute of India, along with many veterinary colleges and other academic institutions, offers Masters, PG Diploma, short courses, short-term certificates, and training programs on various aspects of wildlife management and health for veterinarians and biologists. Workshops and training programs are also conducted for elephant handlers and mahouts. Wildlife SOS recently established an elephant conservation and care centre at their facility in Uttar Pradesh to provide treatment and care for captive and rescued elephants. The trade of captive elephants is now banned, including that at the famous Sonepur Cattle Fair in Bihar, the largest livestock fair in Asia, where a large number of elephants were sold until 2004. In an effort to ensure that no commercial transactions involving elephants take place at the fair, the forest department has introduced DNA profiling for elephants participating in the event. In southern India, state governments have effectively used a significant portion of the tribal population to combat ivory poaching in Protected Areas and beyond. A network of camps was established at strategic locations, staffed by local tribals under the supervision of departmental personnel. These camps are interconnected through a wireless network and provided with food supplies and arms for protection (Baskaran *et al.* 2011). In managing domesticated elephants, multiple contributions from various scientific and technical disciplines such as biology, forestry, veterinary medicine, animal husbandry, and law are evidently essential. However, the caretaking function performed by mahouts and owners, though less apparent, necessitates the integration of humanities such as social anthropology, alongside more specialized fields including comparative religion, social history, and linguistics (Locke 2013).

Rabbit Farming in India: Renowned for producing quality meat, fur, and exceptionally fine animal fibre, domestic rabbits are becoming increasingly important livestock. India does not have any indigenous breeds of domestic rabbit (*Oryctolagus cuniculus*). The endangered Hispid hare (*Caprolagus hispidus*), also known as the bristly hare or Assamese rabbit, is the closest related species to the domestic rabbit. Hares differ from rabbits in both behaviour and habitat. They prefer to live more solitarily, do not burrow like rabbits, and live above ground. The Indian hare, a large leporid widely distributed across the subcontinent, is mainly found in open grassy areas, cultivated plains, semi-arid and arid plains, and hills. It is divided into three subspecies: the black-napped hare (*Lepus nigricollis nigricollis*) found mainly in southern India, the rufous-tailed hare (*Lepus nigricollis ruficaudatus*) distributed roughly from the north of Madhya Pradesh to the Himalayas and down to the Godavari River, and the desert hare (*Lepus nigricollis dayanus*) found in the arid zones of northwestern India (ven der Geer 2008). Many Indian hares live near villages and cultivated areas. Hares are hunted mainly for meat and, to some extent, for their pelts. Historically, they are mentioned in ancient Indian art and literature. The earliest depiction of a hare (*Lepus nigricollis*) in India can be traced to the Bhimbetka rock shelter paintings. As many as 11 figures of hares have been identified in these rock paintings, some of which belong to the Mesolithic period. Interestingly some scholars used term rabbit synonymously with hare to describe these figures (Tiwari 2000). Steatite seals from Harappa (2300–1750 BCE) also depict hare. The rabbits found in the wild are feral domestic rabbits originating from the rabbits that were brought by British (van der Geer 2008).

Rabbit farming was introduced in India by isolated private owners, with New Zealand White rabbits being brought to southern India by the British in the 1940s. After independence, the first rabbit farm, involving the rearing of British Angora rabbits, was established in Dharamshala in 1962. Subsequently, Angora rabbit farms were set up in Kullu-Manali and Kangra districts of Himachal Pradesh, and in the Nilgiris hills of Tamil Nadu by various individuals and agencies (Mahajan 1987, Risam *et al.* 2005). Rabbit farming gained momentum as the country aimed to enhance meat production to address food security and nutrition challenges. Rabbits were considered suitable for small-scale farming and backyard rearing, making them an accessible source of income and nutrition for rural households. This initiative was part of broader agricultural and livestock development efforts. In the 1970s and 1980s, several agricultural universities and research institutes in India began promoting rabbit farming due to its potential to provide high-quality protein at a low cost. The Central Sheep and Wool Research Institute of the Indian Council of Agricultural Research (ICAR-CSWRI) pioneered research and development in rabbit farming by importing New Zealand White and White

Giant rabbits (meat breeds) from the UK, and Russian Angora rabbits (wool breed) from Russia (formerly the USSR) in 1978 and 1979. A full-fledged division on Fur Animal Breeding (FAB) was established at the North Temperate Regional Station (NTRS) in Garsa, Kullu Valley, Himachal Pradesh (Acharya 1982). Studies found that Angora, New Zealand White, and Soviet Chinchilla rabbits had better adaptability and survival rates, with the fur quality of Soviet Chinchilla and New Zealand White being the best. The New Zealand White rabbit project also exhibited the highest combining ability and maximum growth rate. In 1988, the ICAR Research Complex for the NEH Region introduced rabbit farming in the region, popularizing it in all seven states of the Northeast and neighbouring states. Kerala Agricultural University initiated a rabbit breeding project in 1984, leading to the start of commercial rabbit farming in both the private and government sectors. In Kerala, rabbit development schemes were implemented in Trivandrum, Idukki, Kollam, and Pathanamthitta districts (Das *et al.* 2014).

According to the 20th Livestock Census, the total rabbit population in India is approximately 5.50 lakh. The highest number of rabbits are reared in Kerala (92,693), followed by West Bengal (76,151) and Nagaland (57,729). There are more female (307,779) than male rabbits (242,162) in the country (Anonymous 2019). Various rabbit breeds available in India include the New Zealand White, Soviet Chinchilla, Grey Giant, and White Giant for meat and fur, and the Russian, British, and German Angora for wool (Das *et al.* 2014, Bharathy *et al.* 2022). Rabbit production is viewed as an alternative means of alleviating food shortages in several countries, including India. Rabbits have a small body size, rapid growth rate, high prolificacy, early maturity, and a shorter generation interval. They efficiently utilize low grain and high roughage diets and fibrous agricultural by-products. Rabbit farming is growing in many states of the country, primarily for meat and fur production. Rabbits are also kept as pets, and are used by numerous organizations as experimental animals for biomedical and pharmaceutical research and development. Low investment costs and the breeding and feeding traits of rabbits, coupled with the rising demand for quality food, have made rabbit rearing an attractive livestock farming opportunity. This has created significant demand among unemployed educated youth, who see rabbit farming as an alternate means of employment and entrepreneurship.

Human-Avian Interaction and Domestication of Poultry and Other Birds: India is home to a diverse range of resident and migratory birds, including the Red Junglefowl (RJF), the progenitor of the domestic chicken. These varied avian species, endowed with the ability to fly, have fascinated people since time immemorial and hold a prominent place in human history. Mediated by culture, religion, diverse beliefs, affections, and care, the relationship between humans and birds in India is rich and complex. This connection blends reverence, coexistence, and conservation, reflecting the country's rich biodiversity and cultural heritage. Birds hold an important place in Indian mythology and religion, prominently featured in symbolism, art, literature, and traditional practices. Vedic literature often describes the Sun as a celestial bird or eagle (falcon) traversing space (Macdonell 1899).

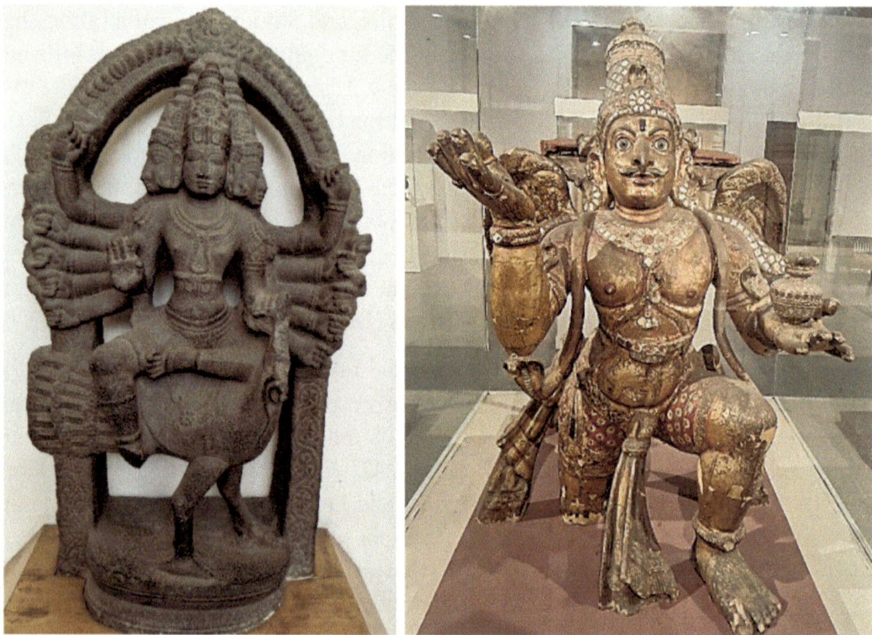

Fig. 2.37. *A 12th-century stone sculpture of Kartikeya on peacock and a 19th-century anthropomorphic wooden sculpture of Garuda displayed at the National Museum in New Delhi (Photo by the Author).*

In Hindu mythology, many birds are associated with various deities as their vehicles (*vahanas*), assisting them in their divine duties (Fig.2.37). They embody philosophical and moral qualities, reinforcing the virtues and powers of the deities they accompany. For example, Kartikeya, the god of war, rides a peacock, symbolizing beauty, splendour, and the ability to destroy harmful influences; and Saraswati, the goddess of wisdom and knowledge, rides a swan or sometimes a peacock, symbolizing discernment and beauty. Garuda, mighty eagle-like bird and the lord of birds, serves as the mount of Lord Vishnu and appears on his banner. Garuda symbolizes speed, martial prowess, Vedic wisdom and preservation of cosmic order–atributes associated with Lord Vishnu himself. He is believed to have recited the Garuda Purana, an ancient Hindu scripture from the first millennium. The text covers diverse topics such as cosmology, mythology, the theory of yoga, heaven and hell, karma and rebirth, soteriology, geography, and the listing of plants, herbs, and various diseases along with their treatments.

Birds find a prominent place in the ancient rock-shelter paintings in India. The bird species identified in the rock paintings of central India include peacock and peahen, junglefowl, chicks, cattle egret, sarus crane, blue magpie, pochard, spoonbill, heron, duck, owl, and vulture (Tiwari 2000). Ducks and swans are depicted in the mural paintings of the Sittanavasal Cave Temples, which date back to the 2nd century BCE (Mariyapillai *et al.* 2021). Anthropomorphic images with bird heads, and human figures wearing beaked and feathered head masks with claws, are found in several rock paintings across the country, including Kilvalai, Alambadi, Kiradipatti, Sirumalai, and Velleri Kombai rock art sites in Tamil Nadu. At Kilvalai, four human figures are shown standing in a row on a boat, all facing left, with noses resembling a bird's beak (Balaji 2018). Many scholars suggest that these masked figured humans had significant roles in their communities (Tiwari 2000). Fowl, peacock, pigeon, eagle, owl, and duck are depicted in various forms in Indus Valley art. The eagle (*Suparna, Śyena,* Garuda), peahen (*Mayūrī*), wild goose or swan (*Hamsa*), ruddy goose (*Chakravāka*), parrots (*Suka*), and common myna (*Sarika*) are some of the historical and literary important birds mentioned in Vedic scriptures. Peahens are spoken of in the Rig Veda as removing poison. By the time of the Yajur Veda, the parrot had already been tamed and is described as mimicking human speech (Macdonell 1899).

While hunting birds was once a popular pastime in India, religious attitudes and traditional practices such as feeding birds and maintaining water feeders during the summer remain auspicious acts, aiding in the conservation of diverse bird species. A remarkable example of community-driven bird conservation efforts is seen in Khichan village, Rajasthan, where thousands of Demoiselle Cranes (*Kurja* or *Koonj*, *Anthropoides virgo*) migrate every year. The practice began in the 1970s when local resident Ratanlal Mallo started feeding pigeons, gradually attracting a few cranes and other birds. Over time, this modest effort grew into a large-scale feeding program for migratory cranes, supported by residents, organizations, and visitors. Today, donations for crane conservation are managed by the *Kuraj Samrakshan Vikas Sansthan* and *Pakshi Chugha Ghar*. Recognizing these efforts, the Rajasthan government has promoted Khichan as a tourist destination, attracting birdwatchers, ornithologists, and wildlife photographers from around the world (Aiyadurai *et al.* 2023). In April 2023, the State Forest Department officially declared the *Kurja Conservation Reserve* at Khichan — India's first conservation reserve dedicated to the Demoiselle Crane. There are several more examples of traditions and provisions of caring birds in India. Bird watching is a popular activity in India, attracting both domestic and international tourists. The annual congregations of flamingos at the Rann of Kutch and the Siberian Cranes at Bharatpur are major attractions. Birds contribute to the ecological balance by acting as pollinators, seed dispersers, and pest controllers.

On the flip side, despite their importance, birds sometimes come into conflict with humans, especially in agricultural areas where they may damage crops. They also face numerous threats, the most significant being habitat loss due to deforestation, industrial pollution, overuse of agro-chemicals and fertilizers in modern agricultural practices, and illegal trade and hunting. In urban areas, birds like pigeons, crows, and sparrows are a common sight and have adapted well to human environments. They often rely on human activities for food and nesting sites. However, urban infrastructural developments, loss of trees, and pollution from urban waste, traffic, and industry have negatively impacted the richness of bird species in these areas. In general, anthropogenic factors have caused widespread declines in populations of numerous bird species, including those once abundant in the region. For example, the house sparrow (*Passer domesticus indicus),* commonly found around human dwellings rather than in forests, has experienced a decline in both urban and rural areas in India, mainly due to pollution and loss of nesting sites. Interestingly, a survey in the Coimbatore district of Tamil Nadu revealed that compared to the 2007-2008 period, the sparrow population in urban and agricultural areas increased by 128-369 % during 2020-2021. The study suggested that the lockdown during the COVID-19 pandemic, which reduced outdoor human activities and travel, was a potential cause of this population increase (Sundarapandian and Raman 2023). Similarly, the veterinary use of the nonsteroidal anti-inflammatory drug (NSAID) diclofenac in South Asia has led to the collapse of populations of three vulture species of the genus *Gyps*. These species, which numbered in the millions until the 1990s, have dwindled to merely a few thousand today. However, efforts are underway to address this crisis through sustainable practices, awareness programs, and conservation measures including a ban on the veterinary use of diclofenac and other toxic NSAIDs.

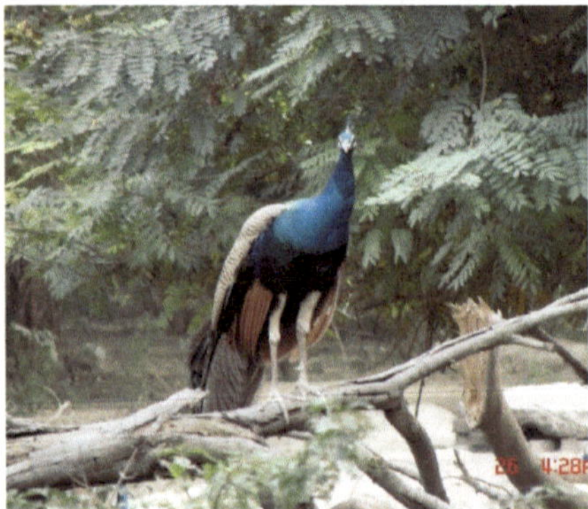

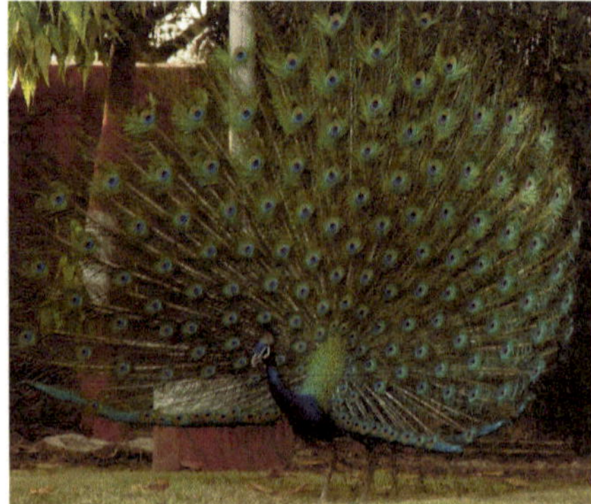

Fig. 2.38. *Largest amongst pheasants, the Indian peafowl or blue peacock (Pavo cristatus) is one of the most beautiful birds in the world. Declared as the national bird of India in 1963, the peacock is listed under Schedule I of Wildlife (Protection) Act, 1972. Like other indigenous wild birds, trapping wild peacock and trading or keeping them, pet is illegal in the country (Photo courtesy of Dr. Asit Das, ICAR-IVRI).*

Historically, people in India have domesticated birds for various purposes. Poultry species such as chickens, ducks, turkeys, and Japanese quails are primarily raised for their meat, eggs, and feathers. Birds like Indian peafowl, parakeets, bulbuls, doves, cuckoos, and common mynas (*Acridotheres tristis*) have been kept as pets both indoors and outdoors for companionship, amusement, and hobbies due to their unique personalities (Fig. 2.38). According to the Arthashastra, peacocks, partridges (*chakora*), parrots, and myna birds (*sarika*) were kept along with red-spotted deer (*prshata*), mongoose, and monkeys in the projected front entrance of the horse stable (Shamasastry 1951, p. 146). Some of these birds might have been used for meat, as evident from the First Rock Edict of King Asoka- 'Formerly, in the kitchen of Beloved-of-the-Gods, King Piyadasi, hundreds of thousands of animals were killed every day to make curry. But now with the writing of this Dhamma edict only three creatures, two peacocks and a deer are killed, and the deer not always. And in time, not even these three creatures will be killed' (Dhammika 1993). Moreover, apart from being used for entertainment by enthusiasts, domestic pigeons (*Columba livia domestica*) were effectively employed to carry messages from the Mauryan period until recently (Fig. 2.39). It is noteworthy that the last of the pigeon-post service in the world was the one instituted in 1946 by the Odisha police force in Cuttack, which existed till 2008. After discontinuation of this service, approximately 150 pigeons are still kept for ceremonial purposes in Cuttack and at the Police Training College in Angul (https://en.wikipedia.org/wiki/Pigeon_post, pdf downloaded on 25-01-2024).

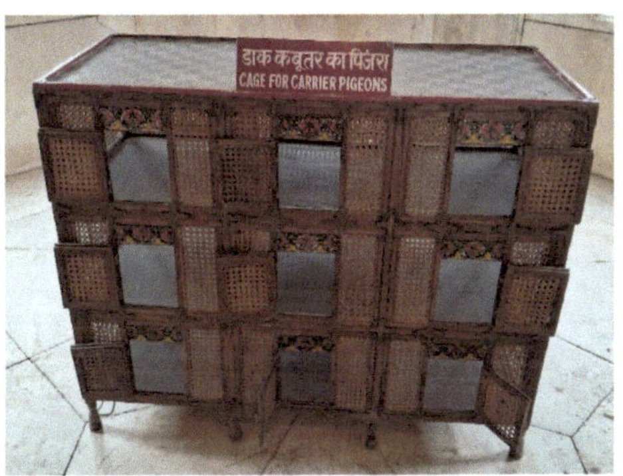

Fig. 2.39. *Cage for messenger pigeons displayed at City Palace Udaipur (Photo by the Author).*

Domestic Chicken: The domestic fowl or chicken (*Gallus gallus domesticus*) is the most numerous and economically important poultry species in India. It is believed to have originated from multiple domestication centres around 7,000-10,000 years ago from the Red Junglefowl (*Gallus gallus*), native to the tropical forests of Southeast Asia, including parts of India (Scanes 2018). Archaeological evidence indicates that Indus Valley populations domesticated poultry and engaged in poultry farming during the Mature Harappan period. Chickens from the Harappan culture of the Indus Valley (2500-2100 BCE) may have been a primary source for the spread of domesticated chickens worldwide (Al-Nasser *et al.* 2007). It is argued that Indus hunters were familiar with the Red Junglefowl found in the foothills of the Himalayas at the northern end of their civilization, as well as the Grey Junglefowl living on the southeastern border around the Gujarat state, facilitating domestication. From the Indus Valley, domestic chickens travelled westward on reaching the Middle East. Possibly the bird could have been carried across to the Arabian Peninsula via as cargo or provision. A 2000 BCE Mesopotamian Cuneiform tablet refers to the bird of Meluhha–the likely place name of Indus Vally. The chicken reached ancient Egypt around 1300-1100 BCE attaining special status as royal bird. Besides raising chickens for meat, the Harappan people kept them for cockfighting, and tandoori-style ovens found at Indus sites were used to cook chickens (Adler and Lawler 2012, Lawler 2016). However, Peters *et al.* (2022) reviewing all available evidence of ancient chicken remains in the subcontinent, suggested that poultry farming in the Indian subcontinent was a post-Harappan development, dating to around 1200 BCE.

Although the exact timing of chicken domestication remains debatable, it is widely accepted that the Red Junglefowl (*Gallus gallus*) is the primary wild ancestor of the domestic chicken. The domestic traits evolved in an insular population of South Asian Junglefowl (*G. gallus* ssp. *spadiceus*) involving hybrids of subspecies, across its expansive range from Thailand to India (Peters *et al.* 2024). The Red Junglefowl subspecies (*Gallus gallus murghi*) and the Grey Junglefowl (*Gallus sonneratii*) are endemic to the Indian subcontinent (Peters *et al.* 2022). The *G. gallus murghi* is a magnificent bird with beautiful plumage and curved wings that enable swift flight. It once had a wide natural range, but is now restricted to wildlife reserves. *G. sonneratii* is found in the evergreen hill forests of Western and Southern India (Ahlawat 2013). Archaeologists have identified nine images of fowl in the Bhimbetka rock-shelter paintings, some of which belong to the early historic period (before the 6th century BCE). However, it is uncertain whether these paintings depict wild or domestic chickens (Tiwari 2000). Genetic studies indicated that the Indian subspecies (*G. gallus murghi*) has made a substantial genetic contribution to domestic chickens. For instance, the genetic makeup of White Leghorn shows a significant influence from *G. g. murghi* (Wang *et al.* 2020).

Chickens in India were most likely first domesticated for cultural and entertainment purposes. It was only later that they began to be used as a food source. The spread of domesticated chickens throughout India was facilitated by trade and cultural exchanges, making chickens an integral part of Indian cuisine and agriculture. Selective breeding has led to the development of various breeds suited for different purposes such as egg production, meat, and ornamental use, resulting in a wide range of variations in body weight, plumage and skin colour, feathering, and comb type among different breeds. Presently, chickens are primarily raised for meat (broilers) or egg (layers) production, and occasionally for cockfighting associated with religious rituals in some regions. There are two distinct poultry rearing practices in the country: backyard farming and commercial farming. Until the second half of the 20th century, backyard poultry farming was a small-scale venture traditionally patronized by the landless poor and weaker sections of society in rural areas of the country. These resource-poor people reared small flocks of chickens of locally available breeds under free range system, which required almost zero investment.

The native birds typically scavenge and thrive on kitchen and agricultural waste, as well as leftover feed. They are hardy, excellent brooders, and have strong mothering abilities. Additionally, they are highly adaptable to hot and humid tropical climates. They also show resilience to certain deadly infections, such as Newcastle disease and infectious bursal disease. Generally, native breeds possess unique traits, including superior meat quality, quick running and flying abilities, defensive behaviours to protect against predators, and efficient performance with low inputs in hot and humid conditions (Kumar *et al.* 2021b, Kanakachari *et al.* 2022). Although the importance of native breeds has declined due to modernization and the rapid growth of commercial poultry sector, they still play a significant role in the rural economy. Currently, native chickens make up 37.2 % of the total poultry population in India and contribute approximately 17.8 % of total egg production, providing subsidiary income and nutritional security to people in the country (Kanakachari *et al.* 2022). There are 20 registered indigenous breeds (https://nbagr.res.in/chicken-breeds accessed on 30.08.2025) found in different parts of the country. Theses include Ankaleshwar (Gujarat), Aseel (Andra Pradesh, Chhattisgarh and Odisha), Busra (Gujarat), Kadaknath (Madhya Pradesh), Chittagong (Meghalaya and Tripura) Daothigir and Miri (Assam), Danki and Kalahasthi (Andhra Pradesh), Ghagus (Andhra Pradesh and Karnataka), Harringhata black (West Bengal), Mewari (Rajasthan), Nicobari (Andaman and Nicobar Islands), Kaunayen (Manipur), Hansali (Odisha), Kashmir Faverolla (Jammu and Kashmir), Punjab Brown (Punjab and Haryana), Tellichery (Kerala) and Uttara (Uttarakhand). Apart from these indigenous breeds, various organizations, including the ICAR-Central Avian Research Institute, ICAR- Directorate of Poultry Research (formerly Project Directorate on Poultry), and Agriculture, Animal Science, and Veterinary Universities, have developed several improved layer and broiler chicken breeds. These include CARI-Sonali, CARI-Priya, CARI-Debendra, CARI-Vishal, CARI-Bro- Dhanraja, CARI-Bro-Mrityunjay, CARI-Nirbheek, CARI-Shyama, CARI-Upcari, CARI-Hitcari, Vanaraja, Gramapriya, Srinidhi, Krisi-Bro, Krishi-J Gramalaxmi, and Girirani. Compared to the native breeds, these improved breeds demonstrate better production performance and feed conversion efficiency. They can thrive well in tropical climates and exhibit greater disease resistance than exotic breeds. Backyard poultry plays a vital role in rural India by providing supplementary income, nutrition through eggs and meat, and livelihood security, particularly for small and marginal farmers and women. Improved breeds developed for backyard farming not only have more attractive plumage than native hens but are also resilient, capable of withstanding adverse environmental conditions such as poor housing, limited feeding, and minimal healthcare (Kumar *et al.* 2021b).

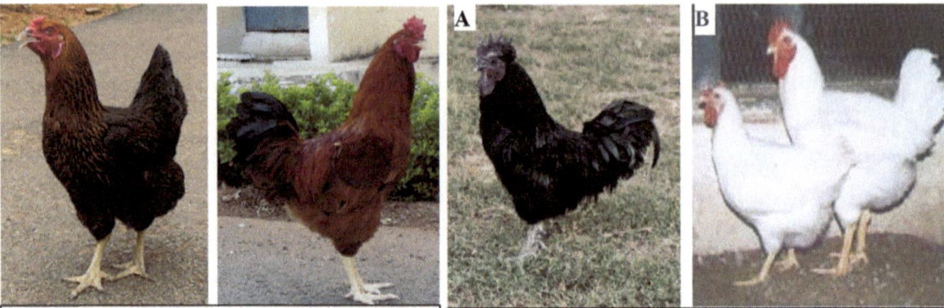

Fig 2.40. Vanaraja is a hardy, dual-purpose breed, well-suited for free-range poultry farming in rural and tribal areas even under harsh climatic conditions (Photo courtesy of Dr. Vijay Kumar Tiwari, ICAR-DPR).

Fig. 2.41. A. Kadaknath, a dual-purpose breed found in Madhya Pradesh, is known for its black flesh; ***B.*** CARI- Vishal, a broiler breed with superior growth and high disease resistance (Photo courtesy of Dr. A.K. Tiwari ICAR-CARI).

Over the past five decades, the poultry sector, particularly chicken farming, has undergone a significant transformation. What was once a simple backyard activity has now become a major commercial agri-entrepreneurship, with phenomenal growth in the number of birds and poultry farmers. In 2019, the total chicken population in India reached 807.894 million with 16.8 % increase over 2012 population, which constituted approximately 95 % of the overall poultry population (851.81million). Compared to 2012 population, the backyard poultry population grew by over 45.79 % in 2019 (Anonymous 2019). According to reports, 28 % of the total layer chicken population comprises indigenous fowl, while the remaining 72 % improved varieties. Backyard poultry contributes to 21% of egg production (Kumar *et al.* 2021b). Native chicken breeds (Fig. 2.40, 2.41) continue to play a crucial role in backyard poultry farming, while modern hybrids and exotic breeds are exclusively used in intensive production systems (Ahlawat 2013).

The success of the poultry industry can be attributed to high-yielding layer varieties, which produce 310-340 eggs annually, and broiler varieties that reach 2.4-2.6 kg within six weeks. Standardized practices in nutrition, housing, management, and disease control have driven significant growth rates in egg production (4-6 % per annum) and broiler production (8-10 % per annum) in India. Consequently, the annual per capita availability of eggs and meat has also risen steedily due to increased production (Chatterjee and Rajkumar 2015). Chicken meat production in the country rose from around 3.76 million tonnes in 2017 to 4.90 million tonnes in 2022, demonstrating a 30 % increase over five years. India produced a staggering 119.47 billion hen eggs (FAOSTAT, accessed on 14-04-2024). While nearly 79 % of total egg production comes from commercial farms, the share of backyard poultry was nearly 21 %. However, backyard chickens efficiently convert waste materials such as home kitchen waste, vegetable scraps, and green grass into high-quality eggs and meat for human consumption and their significance extends beyond mere production—it contributes to nutritional security, income generation, women's empowerment, and youth employment (Kumar *et al.* 2021b).

Domestic Ducks: Ducks have a rich history of domestication in India, spanning centuries. These versatile birds have been raised for various purposes, including their eggs, meat, and feathers. Ducks are also kept as show animals and pets. The majority of domestic duck varieties in India (*Anas platyrhynchos domesticus*) trace their lineage back to the Mallard or wild duck (*Anas platyrhynchos*). Male (drake) and female (hen) ducks can be distinguished based on their external appearance, vocalizations, behaviour, and internal anatomy. Drakes typically exhibit more colourful plumage and bills, possess a prominent curled feather near the tail, and emit a softer yet harsher quack (Naik *et al.* 2022).

Ducks are the second most numerous poultry species in India, following chickens. They offer a viable livelihood option for small and marginal farmers due to their resilience against diseases, extended production cycles, ease of training, large-sized eggs, and early morning egg-laying behaviour. Ducks require less attention and adapt well to scavenging conditions. They primarily forage on aquatic weeds, algae, green legumes, fungi, earthworms, maggots, snails, and various insects. The natural foraging behaviour of ducks reduces feed costs and is an effective tool for biological control of rice pests and snail vectors. Moreover, hardiness of ducks makes them suitable for diverse environments and they can thrive in marshy and wetland areas where other poultry birds struggle (Padhi and Giri 2024). Ducks are also suitable for integrated farming systems, such as duck-cum-fish farming and duck farming with rice cultivation. They are effective exterminators of potato beetles, grasshoppers, snails, and slugs. In areas plagued with liver flukes and snail-borne parasitic infections, ducks (2 to 6 ducks per 0.405 hectares of land) can serve as biological control agents (Akbar *et al.* 2014).

Duck farming has gained significant popularity in India, especially in coastal states and regions blessed with abundant water bodies. According to the 20th livestock census, the country hosts a substantial duck population of 33. 511 million with 42.4% growth over 2012, which was more than the chicken (16.6%). Notable concentrations of ducks exist in West Bengal (12.44 million), Assam (11.74 million), Jharkhand (1.65 million), Manipur (1.23 million), Kerala (875545) and Odisha (3377150). Remarkably, approximately 96% (31.19 million) of these ducks thrive in rural areas as backyard poultry (Anonymous 2019). The duck breeds in India comprise both exotic and indigenous genotypes. The exotic duck breeds available in India include White Pekin, Khaki Campbell, and Indian Runner. In contrast, the indigenous duck genetic diversity consists of both descriptive and non-descriptive breeds. Four registered indigenous duck breeds are – Pati from Assam, Maithili from Bihar, Andamani from the Andaman and Nicobar Islands, and Tripureshwari from Tripura (https://nbagr.res.in/geese-dog, accessed on 30-08-2025). In addition to these registered breeds, several non-descriptive indigenous varieties are also recognized, including Nageshwari or White-breasted Naga, Kuttanad, Sylhet Meta, Chara, Chambali, Desi (Kuzi) ducks of Odisha, as well as Kollam, Arni, Sanyasi, and Keeri ducks from Tamil Nadu (Ahalawat 2013, Naik *et al.* 2022, Padhi and Giri 2024). Indigenous duck breeds are known for their adaptability to the environment and their resistance to diseases. Typically, poultry farmers prefer indigenous breeds for rearing under a scavenging system, with flock sizes ranging from 2 to 9 ducks (Kamal *et al.* 2023). Other poultry birds raised in India include turkeys, geese, and quails.

Other Poultry Birds: The population of other poultry birds, such as turkeys, geese, and quails, in India has declined from 13,025 in 2012 to 10,405 in 2019 (Anonymous 2019). However, domestic geese, with interesting biological characteristics such as high juvenile growth, good adaptation to free-range rearing systems, and foraging behaviour, have immense potential as quality meat producers. Nutrient-rich geese meat is an excellent source of several nutrients and quality protein. Consumption of goose meat is suggested as a natural source of manganese for people struggling with mental disorders (depression, anxiety disorders), lipid disorders (hypercholesterolemia), and carbohydrate metabolism (reduced glucose tolerance), in whom reduced concentration of this element has been confirmed in blood (Goluch and Haraf 2023). Kashmir Anz, found in Jammu and Kashmir, is the only registered breed of domestic geese in India (https://nbagr.icar.gov.in/en/registered-geese/, accessed on 26-05-2024). It grows fast and has higher hatchability than domestic ducks reared in Kashmir (Hamadani 2014). Indigenous geese of Assam, locally called Rajhanh (king of ducks), are heavy birds and pristine germplasm of geese. They are usually reared for meat purposes in rural areas as backyard poultry under a traditional extensive system with low input. These birds are grass foragers and also scavenge kitchen waste, grains, and rice bran. They are let loose early in the morning for foraging and are housed in small pens made of locally available materials. They also act as guards for households and biological weeders and can be easily maintained by womenfolk (Hoque *et al.* 2023).

Pet and Game Birds: In India, several avian species have been kept as pets and game birds for recreational purposes. Birds such as Junglefowl, partridges, quails, bulbul have been used as game birds since the ancient time. Archaeological findings, including a clay figure of a man holding a fowl-like bird calmly against his chest, a rooster spur found at Harappa, and a clay seal depicting two roosters facing each other, provide circumstantial evidence that the Indus people raised chickens for cockfighting as well (Lawler 2016). In fact, the males of the *Gallus gallus* species can be quite fierce when trained for fighting. They are naturally armed with a bony spur on their legs. Humans have taken advantage of this feature by strapping metal spurs and knives onto the legs of fighting roosters, making them even more dangerous (Adler and Lawler 2012). The ancient practice of cockfighting still remains prevalent in some parts of India, particularly in Andhra Pradesh, Tamil Nadu, Kerala, Karnataka, Odisha, and West Bengal. Additionally, several tribal communities continue this tradition. In these regions, cockfighting often intertwines with religious rituals, and events are frequently organized during festivals and local gatherings. However, it is essential to note that cockfighting is illegal in India under the Prevention of Cruelty to Animals Act, 1960 and was banned in 2015 by the Supreme Court (https://en.wikipedia.org/wiki/Cockfighting_in_India, accessed on 28-05-2024) It is allowed only as a sport to be held in a traditional way, with the stipulation that there should not be any injury caused to the birds, the birds should not be intoxicated with any alcoholic substance, and no knives should be tied around the legs of the birds with the tip of the knives dipped in poisonous substances. A veterinary doctor is required to ensure compliance with these regulations before the event begins (https://indiankanoon.org/search/? formInput=cock%20fighting, accessed on 28-05-2024).

Keeping birds as pets is popular in India since ancient time. Pet birds provide companionship and a touch of nature to many households. They primarily belong to the Passeriformes (canaries, finches, sparrows) and Psittaciformes (parrots, parakeets, budgerigars, love birds) and Columbiformes (pigeons and doves) groups (Durge *et al.* 2022). These birds are appreciated for their vibrant colours, playful behaviour, and in some cases, their ability to mimic human speech. According to a report, the population of pet birds in India was over 171 thousand in 2021, which is projected to reach over 212 thousand by the end of 2026. The growth in the number of pets in India has led to an increase in pet food sales, rising from approximately 172 million U.S. dollars in 2016 to around 403 million dollars in 2021 (https://www.statista.com/statistics/1061203/india-population-of-pet-birds/, accessed on 20-05-2024). Importantly, certain native bird species in India are protected under the Wildlife Protection Act of 1972 making it illegal to capture and keep them as pets.

Conclusion

India, with its rich and mega-diverse culture and abundant natural resources, has a long history of human-animal interaction and a legacy of biodiversity conservation. The profound association and importance of animals in ancient India are evident through zooarchaeological remains, representations of various animals in ancient rock and cave art, Indus Valley seals, figurines, and other artifacts. There are also frequent mentions of different wild and domestic animals in Vedic and Post-Vedic scripts, edicts, and inscriptions of Emperor Ashoka, as well as in other historical records spanning several centuries. The UNESCO World Heritage-listed rock shelters in Bhimbetka, known to be the earliest rock art in India, feature 1,377 images of wild and domestic animals from more than 29 species. These images depict bulls, cows, bison, wild buffalo, gaur, wild boar, horses, elephants (with or without riders), lions, tigers, leopards, cheetahs, small mammals, various bird species and insects (Mathpal 1984, Tiwari 2000, Dubey-Pathak 2014). By analysing the changing styles and patterns of human and animal images during different periods, these paintings provide insights into the lives, beliefs, and human-animal relationships of prehistoric peoples. They also shed light on the evolution of animal husbandry practices in India. The representation of almost all kinds of domestic and wild animals, including bulls, buffaloes, donkeys, bison, sheep, goats, elephants, tigers, rhinoceroses, and various birds (such as cocks, peacocks, pigeons, owls, eagles, and ducks) in Indus Valley art further underscores the close association between humans and animals in the first urban civilization of the country (Kadgaonkar 2008).

The domestication of animals and birds has profoundly influenced socio-cultural, political, and economic aspects ingrained in India's social fabric. This process was not instantaneous; rather, it unfolded gradually over time. It began with the companionship of dogs during the Mesolithic period and extended to the domestication of livestock species. Simultaneously, humans successfully exploited various species of wild plants, fostering cultural and economic development from approximately 10,000 to 6,000 years ago. Paleofaunal evidence from numerous Neolithic sites across India reveals the presence of domesticated animals such as cattle, buffalo, sheep, goats, and pigs. Among these, cattle played a pivotal role in sustaining Neolithic communities (Sarkar 2021). Notably, cattle had great socio-economic significance during the Indus Valley-Saraswati civilization. However, as India transitioned into the Vedic and post-Vedic periods, the introduction of horses and the taming of elephants shifted great focus toward these two important animal species, which were highly valued for their utility in warfare and transportation. Furthermore, the cow declared inviolable, while bull was identified as *Nandi* (Fig. 2.42) the Shiva's vehicle since the Kushan

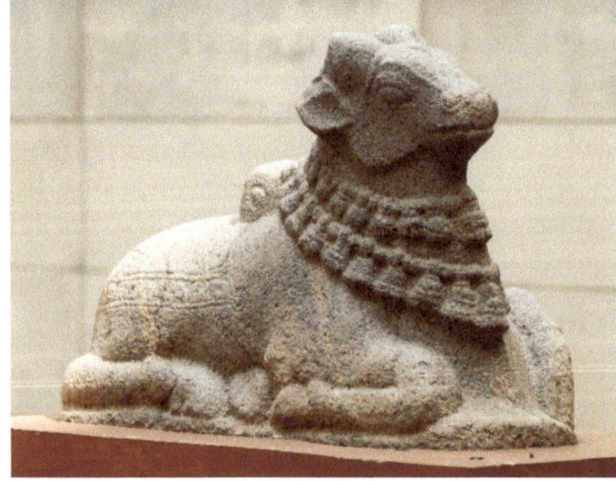

Fig. 2.42. *A finely carved sandstone sculpture of Nandi, displayed in the courtyard of the Śuṅga Gallery, Bihar Museum, Patna. Typically depicted in a seated posture on a pedestal, with three legs folded beneath him, Nandi—the divine mount of Shiva—symbolizes reverence toward bulls, a sentiment that has indirectly contributed to the conservation of indigenous bovine germplasm over generations (Photo by the Author).*

dynasty (ca. 1st century CE). Consequently, the significance of pigs, sheep, and goats as food sources increased, reflecting the intricate interplay between human-animal relationships and cultural dynamics in ancient India.

Despite modern scientific advancement, rapid urbanization, and industrial growth, domestic animal continue to play a vital a socioeconomic role in modern India. The country is home to over 535.78 million farm animals, including sheep, goats, cattle, buffaloes, mithuns, yaks, horses, mules, donkeys, camels, and pigs. Additionally, there are 0.55 million rabbits and 851.81 million poultry birds (Anonymous, 2019). Among these, a total of 230 indigenous breeds of domestic animals have been officially registered, comprising 54 cattle, 21 buffaloes, 41 goats, 46 sheep, 8 horses and ponies, 9 camels, 15 pigs, 4 donkeys, 2 yaks, 20 chickens, 4 ducks, 1 goose, and 5 dogs. Notably, 78 of these breeds have been registered in the past decade (https://nbagr.res.in/brc, accessed on 01-07-2025) States like Rajasthan, Gujarat, and the North Eastern regions exhibit rich breed diversity due to unique production systems. However, there has been a significant decline in the indigenous population, primarily driven by intensive production systems that replace traditional methods. Additionally, there is a preference for highly specialized exotic breeds in commercial animal farming. The indigenous breeds including Belahi, Pulikulum, and Punganur (cattle), Chilika (buffalo), Sumi-Ne, Chegu, Karnath and Teressa (goat), Kachaikatty black, Tibetean and Nilgiri (sheep), Agonda, Goan and Tenyi Vo (pig), Kharai, Marwari, Mewari, Mewati, Malvi and Jalori (camel), and Zanskari, Kachchi- Sindhi, Bhutia, Spiti and Mewari (horse) are currently at risk (Mishra and Niranjan 2022). Challenges related to animal health, welfare, and production systems in India also include prevailing and emerging economically important diseases, transboundary infections, antimicrobial resistance associated with the livestock sector, depleting grazing lands and animal feed resources, an increasing population of stray animals, and human-animal conflicts. To address these challenges, several organizations equipped with state-of-the-art facilities are actively engaged in research and development programmes in veterinary and animal sciences.

References

Acharya RM. 1982. Inaugural Address. In: *Proceedings of First National Seminar on Fur Animal Breeding* April 24-26, 1982. pp 8-9. ICAR-CSWRI, North Temperate Regional Station, Garsa, Kullu, Himachal Pradesh, India.

Adler J and Lawler A. 2012. How the chicken conquered the world. *Smithsonian* **43**: 40-47.

Aggarwal RA, Kour A, Gandhi RS, Niranjan SK, Paul V, Bhutia TL and Bhutia KD. 2023. Characterization of a unique Sikkimese yak population of India: a multivariate approach. *Tropical Animal Health and Production* **55**(3): 208. https://doi.org/10.21203/rs.3.rs-2047439/v1.

Agrawal R P, Budania S, Sharma P, Gupta R, Kochar DK, Panwar RB and Sahani MS. 2007. Zero prevalence of diabetes in camel milk consuming Raica community of north-west Rajasthan, India. *Diabetes Research and Clinical Practice* **76**(2): 290-296.

Agrawala VS. 1953. Fauna. In: *India As Known to Pānini (A Study of Cultural Material the Ashtādhyāyi).* pp. 218-28. University of Lucknow, Lucknow, Uttar Pradesh, India. https://ignca.gov.in/Asi_data/4695,pdf downloaded on 23-11-2023.

Ahlawat SPS. 2013. Livestock and poultry genetic resources. In: *Handbook of Animal Husbandry.* pp 19-40. Directorate of Knowledge Management in Agriculture, Indian Council of Agricultural Research, New Delhi.

Aiyadurai A, Banerjee S, Patil Y, Joshi S and Rashid KK. 2023. *Human-Bird Relations in India. A Preliminary Report.* 54p. IIT, Gandhinagar, India. https://research.iitgn.ac.in/ehrg/assets/files/Human-Birdreport050623,pdf downloaded on 18-05-2024.

Akbar MA, Sreehari S and Yadav JS. 2014. Duck rearing. *Indian Farming* **64**(5): 38-41.

Akbar MJ. 2022. *Dolally Sahib and Black Zamindar: Racism and Revenge in the British Raj.* 1st Edn pp. 74-75. Bloomsbury India, New Delhi, India.

Alexander MW and Violet W. 2012. Trade and traders of Mesopotamian Ur. *ASBBS Proceedings.* **19**(1): 12-17.

Al-Nasser A, Al-Khalaifa H, Al-Saffar A, Khalil F, Albahouh M, Ragheb G, Al-Haddad A and Mashaly M. 2007. Overview of chicken taxonomy and domestication. *World's Poultry Science Journal* **63**(2): 285-300.

Alur KR.1980. Faunal remains from the Vindhyas and the Ganga Valley In: *Beginnings of Agriculture (Epi-Palaeolithic to Neolithic): Excavations at Chopani-Mando, Mahadaha, and Mahagara.* pp.201-27. (Eds) Sharma GR, Misra VD, Mandal D, Misra BB and Pal JN. Abinash Prakashan, Allahabad, Uttar Pradesh, India.

Amills M, Capote J and Tosser-Klopp G. 2017. Goat domestication and breeding: a jigsaw of historical, biological and molecular data with missing pieces. *Animal Genetics* **48** (6): 631-44.

Anonymous. 2015. *Annual Report 2014-15.* pp.19-21. ICAR- National Research Centre on Camel, Bikaner, Rajasthan, India.

Anonymous.2019. *20th Livestock Census-2019 All India Report.* Animal Husbandry Statistic Division, Department of Animal Husbandry and Dairying Ministry of Fisheries, Animal Husbandry and Dairying, New Delhi, India https://dahd.nic.in/ahs-division/20th-livestock-census-2019-all-india-report, pdf downloaded on 23-04-2024.

Atkulwar A, Deshpande-Mukherjee A and Baig M. 2024. Ancient cattle DNA from Bhirrana: A Hakra culture/preharappan settlement of the Indus valley civilization, India. *Journal of Archaeological Science: Reports* **54**:104383.https://doi.org/10.1016/j.jasrep.2024.104383.

Baig M, Mitra B, Qu K, Peng MS, Ahmed I, Miao YW, Zan LS and Zhang YP. 2013. Mitochondrial DNA diversity and origin of *Bos frontalis*. *Current Science* **104** (1): 115-20.

Balaji G. 2018. Superstitious beliefs and supernatural powers–an ethno-archaeological study of Indian rock paintings. *Journal of Indian History and Culture* **24**: 10-24.

Baskaran N, Varma S, Sar CK and Sukumar R. 2011. Current status of Asian elephants in India. *Gajah* **35** (1-2): 47-54.

Behl R, Vij PK, Niranjan SK, Jayakumar S, Behl J and Vijh RK. 2020. Yak genetic resources of India: distribution, types and characteristics. *Indian Journal of Animal Sciences* **90**(6): 831-36.

Bharathy N, Sivakumar K, Vasanthakumar P and Sakthivadivu R. 2022. Rabbit Farming in India: An Overview. *Agricultural Reviews* **43**(2): 223-28. doi: 10.18805/ag. R-1907.

Bhasin V. 2012. Life on an edge among the Changpas of Changthang, Ladakh. *Journal of Biodiversity* **3**(2): 85-129.

Bist SS, Cheeran JV, Choudhury S, Barua P and Misra MK. 2002. The domesticated Asian elephant in India. In: *Giants on Our Hands.* pp.129-48. International Workshop on the

Domesticated Asian Elephant. 5- 10 February 2001. FAO Regional Office for Asia and the Pacific, Bangkok, (Krung Thep Maha Nakhon), Thailand.

Boivin N, Fuller D, Korisettar R and Petraglia MD.2008. First farmers in south India: the role of internal processes and external influences in the emergence of the earliest settled societies. *Pragdhara* **18:** 179-200.

Bollée W. 2020. *Gone to The Dogs in Ancient India.* (2nd Revised edn). 122 p. Cross Asia-Repository, Heidelberg, Berlin, Germany. pdf downloaded on 25-01-2023.

Borghese A and Mazzi M. 2005. Buffalo population and strategies in the world. In: *Buffalo Production and Research.* pp.1-39. (Ed.) Borgdese A., Food and Agriculture Organization of The United Nations, Rome.

Bose S. 2020. Trunk calls in antiquity: Elephant in archaeology and art. pp. 185-238. In: *Mega Mammals in Ancient India: Rhinos, Tigers, and Elephants.* Oxford University Press, Oxford, UK.

Broushaki F, Thomas MG, Link V, López S, Van Dorp L, Kirsanow K, Hofmanová Z, Diekmann Y, Cassidy LM, Díez-del-Molino D and Kousathanas A. 2016. Early Neolithic genomes from the eastern Fertile Crescent. *Science* **353**(6298): 499-503.

Chandra Y. 2021. *The Tale of the Horse: A History of India on Horseback.* 384p. Picador India, New Delhi, India.

Chatterjee RN and Rajkumar U. 2015. An overview of poultry production in India. *Indian Journal of Animal Health* **54**(2): 89-108.

Chauhan PR. 2020. Human evolution in the center of the Old World: An updated review of the South Asian Palaeolithic. In: *Pleistocene Archaeology - Migration, Technology, and Adaptation.* pp. 1-26. (Eds) Ono R and Pawlik A. IntechOpen. doi: 10.5772/intechopen.94265.

Chen N, Zhang Z, Hou J, Chen J, Gao X, Tang L, Wangdue S, Zhang X, Sinding MH, Liu X and Han J. 2023. Evidence for early domestic yak, taurine cattle, and their hybrids on the Tibetan Plateau. *Science Advances* **9**(50): eadi6857. DOI: 10.1126/sciadv. adi6857.

Chen TS and Chen PS. 2005. The death of Buddha: a medical enquiry. *Journal of Medical Biography* **13**(2):100-03. doi: 10.1177/096777200501300208. PMID: 19813312.

Clutton-Brock J. 2012. Domesticates in ancient India and Southeast Asia. In: *Animals as Domesticates: A World View Through History.* Michigan State University Press, Michigan, USA.

Danino M. 2006. The horse and the Aryan debate. *Journal of Indian History and Culture* **13:** 33-59.

Darji M, Gupta JP, Chaudhari J, Chaudhari A, Chaudhari A, Gor D, Abhi F and Urmil D. 2022. Mitochondrial DNA: A molecular and evolutionary marker. *Pharma Innovation Journal* **11**(12): 887-895.

Das PJ, Kour A, Deori S, Begum SS, Pukhrambam M, Maiti S, Sivalingam J, Paul V and Sarkar M. 2022. Characterization of Arunachali Yak: A Roadmap for Pastoral Sustainability of Yaks in India. *Sustainability* **14**(19):12655. https://doi.org/10.3390/su141912655.

Das SK, Chakurkar EB and Singh NP 2014. *Rabbit as an Alternative Source of Meat production. Technical Bulletin No 45.* 40 p. ICAR- Research Complex for Goa, Old Goa, India

Debroy B. 2008. *Sarama and Her Children.* 243p. Penguin Books, New Delhi, India.

Deshpande-Mukherjee A and Goyal P. 2022. A potential early cattle-based faunal economy from the Indus Valley civilization. In: *Cattle and People: Interdisciplinary Approaches to an Ancient Relationship.* pp.63-87. Wright E and Ginja C (Eds). Lockwood Press Columbus, GA, USA.

Devi LS, Hanah SS, Vikram R, Haque N, Khan MH, Girish PS and Mitra A. 2023. Chemical composition, fatty acids, amino acids, minerals and vitamins profiles of Mithun (*Bos frontalis*) milk reared under semi-intensive system. *Journal of Food Composition and Analysis* **124**: 105694. https://doi.org/10.1016/j.jfca.2023.105694.

Dhammika VS. 1993. *The Edicts of King Asoka- An English Rendering. The Wheel Publication No. 386/387.* 56 p. Buddhist Publication Society. Kandy, Sri Lanka.

Diwedi J, Singh AW, Ahlawat S, Sharma R, Arora R, Sharma H, Raja KN, Verma NK and Tantia MS. 2020. Comprehensive analysis of mitochondrial DNA based genetic diversity in Indian goats. *Gene* **756**: p.144910. https://doi.org/10.1016/j.gene.2020.144910.

Dolker Lamo S, Bharti VK and Chaurasia OP. 2023. Distribution and morphology of double-hump camel (*Camelus bactrianus*) in Ladakh region, India. *Indian Journal of Natural Sciences* **14** (77): 54743-52.

Dorji T, Wangdi J, Shaoliang Y, Chettri N and Wangchuk K.2021. Mithun (*Bos frontalis*): the neglected cattle species and their significance to ethnic communities in the Eastern Himalaya—A review. *Animal Bioscience*. **34**(11): 1727-38. doi: 10.5713/ab.21.0020.

Dubey-Pathak M. 2014.The rock art of the Bhimbetka area in India. *Adoranten*. 5p. https://www.rockartscandinavia.com/images/articles/a14pathak.pdf downloaded on 6-9-2023.

Dubost JM, Lamxay V, Krief S, Falshaw M, Manithip C and Deharo E. 2019. From plant selection by elephants to human and veterinary pharmacopeia of mahouts in Laos. *Journal of Ethnopharmacology* **244**: 112157. https://doi.org/10.1016/j.jep.2019.112157.

Durge A, Dhaigude V, Baby BM, Gujjalkar P, Chouraddi R, Yadav S, Singh AK, and VM, Sivaprasad MS and Nair PM. 2022. Public health threats from pet bird zoonoses. *Journal of Scientific Research and Reports* **28**(11):10-20.

Earnist S, Nawaz S, Ullah I, Bhinder MA, Imran M, Rasheed MA, Shehzad W and Zahoor MY. 2022. Mitochondrial DNA diversity and maternal origins of Pakistani donkey. *Brazilian Journal of Biology* **4**: 84: e256942. https://doi.org/10.1590/1519-6984.256942.

Eraly A. 2002. *Gem in the Lotus*. 586p. Penguin Books, Delhi, India.

Eraly A. 2014. *The First Spring: Life in the Golden Age of India Pt I.* 501p. Penguin Random House, Gurgaon, India.

Estes R. 2009. *Gayal. Encyclopedia Britannica.* https://www.britannica.com/animal/gayal.

Faye B. 2020. How many large camelids in the world? A synthetic analysis of the world camel demographic changes. *Pastoralism* **10**(1): 1-20.

Fleischer RC, Perry EA, Muralidharan K, Stevens EE and Wemmer CM. 2001. Phylogeography of the Asian elephant (*Elephas maximus*) based on mitochondrial DNA. *Evolution* **55**(9): 1882-92.

Fuller DQ and Murphy C. 2014. Overlooked but not forgotten: India as a center for agricultural domestication. *General Anthropology* **21**(2): 1-8.

Ghatani K and Tamang B. 2016. Indigenous rearing practices of Yak and its multipurpose uses in the Sikkim Himalayas. *IOSR Journal of Agriculture and Veterinary Science* **9**(3): 1-8.

Ghosh A. 1990. *An Encyclopedia of Indian Archaeology.* pp. 1-5. EJ Brill Leiden, The Netherlands.

Gill GS, Singh BB, Dhand NK, Aulakh RS, Ward MP and Brookes VJ. 2022. Stray dogs and public health: population estimation in Punjab, India. *Veterinary Sciences* **9**(2): 75. https://doi.org/10.3390/vetsci9020075.

Goluch Z and Haraf G. 2023. Goose meat as a source of dietary manganese—a systematic review. *Animals***13**(5): 840 https://doi.org/10.3390/ani13050840.

Goyal P. 2013. Multiple roles of cattle in the Harappan economy at Kanmer Gujarat. *Heritage Journal of Multidisciplinary Studies in Archaeology* **1**: 63-77.

Greene AM, Panyadee P, Inta A and Huffman MA. 2020.Asian elephant self-medication as a source of ethnoveterinary knowledge among Karen mahouts in northern Thailand. *Journal of Ethnopharmacology* **259**:112823. https://doi.org/10.1016/j.jep.2020.112823.

Hamadani H, Khan AA, Ganai TA, Banday MT and Hamadani A. 2014. Growth and production traits of domestic geese in local conditions of Kashmir, India. *Indian Journal of Animal Sciences* **84**(5): 578-79.

Han J. 2014. Yak: Domestication. In: *Encyclopedia of Global Archaeology.* pp. 7039-41. (Ed.) Smith C. Springer Science-Business Media, New York, USA.

Home C, Bhatnagar YV, Vanak AT. 2018. Canine Conundrum: domestic dogs as an invasive species and their impacts on wildlife in India. *Animal Conservation* **21**(4): 275-82.

Hoque H, Phookan A, Goswami RN, Kalita D, Das B, Das A, Hussain J and Khanikar D. 2023.Characterization and performance evaluation of indigenous geese of Assam. *Indian Journal of Animal Sciences* **93**(2): 182-86.

Jacques G, Guedes JD and Shuya Z. 2021.Yak domestication. *Ethnobiology Letters* **12**(1): 103-14.

Jadhav PV. Komatwar SJ, Channa GR and Bankar PS.2023 Donkey genetic resources of India. *International Journal of Agriculture Sciences* **15** (**6**): 12418-20.

Joshi S, Shrestha L, Bisht N, Wu N, Ismail M, Dorji T, Dangol G and Long R. 2020. Ethnic and cultural diversity amongst yak herding communities in the Asian highlands. *Sustainability* **12**(3): 957. doi:10.3390/su12030957.

Kadgaonkar SB. 2008.The role of animals and birds in ancient Indian art and culture. *Bulletin of the Deccan College Research Institute* **68-69**: 163-65. https://www.jstor.org/stable/42931202.

Kamal R, Chandran PC, Dey A, Sarma K, Padhi Mk, Giri SC and Bhatt BP.2023. Status of Indigenous duck and duck production system of India-a review. *Tropical Animal Health and Production* **55**(1). https://doi.org/10.1007/s11250-022-03401-6.

Kamalakkannan R, Kumar S, Bhavana K, Prabhu VR, Machado CB, Singha HS, Sureshgopi D, Vijay V and Nagarajan M. 2021. Evidence for independent domestication of sheep mtDNA lineage A in India and introduction of lineage B through Arabian sea route. *Scientific Reports* **11**(1): p.19733. https://doi.org/10.1038/s41598-021-97761-y.

Kamni P, Biam J K, Chamuah H, Lalzampuia L Sunitibala Devi, Vivek Joshi, Vikram R, Khan MH Hanah SS and Haque N. 2020. *Mithun (Bos frontalis): The Unique Bioresource of North East India.* ICAR-NRC on Mithun, Medziphema, Nagaland, India.

Kanakachari M, Rahman H, Chatterjee RN and Bhattacharya TK. 2022. Signature of Indian native chicken breeds: a perspective. *World's Poultry Science Journal* **78**(2): 421-45.

Khan MH and Mitra A. 2020. Mithun (*Bos frontalis*) farming: Potential threats and conservation strategies. *Indian Farming* **70**(7): 11-15.

Khan R, De S, Dewangan R, Tamboli R and Gupta R. 2023. Potential status of A1 and A2 variants of bovine beta-casein gene in milk samples of Indian cattle breeds. *Animal Biotechnology* **34**(9): 4878-84.

Kipling JL. 1904. *Beast and Man in India.* (2nd edn). Macmillan and Co. London, UK. https://archive.org/details/beastmaninindiap00kipliala/mode/1up pdf downloaded on 27-03-2024.

Koehl D. 2024. Facts about elephants in India. In*: Elephant Encyclopedia.* https://www.elephant.se/country.php?name=India, retrieved on 28-04-2024.

Köhler-Rollefson I, Rathore S, Rollefson A and Hardy K. 2013. *The Camels of Kumbhalgarh. A Biodiversity Treasure.* Lokhit Pashu-Palak Sansthan, Sadri. (http://www. lpps. org/wp-content/uploads/2013/10/Camels Of_ Kumbhalgarh_web., pdf downloaded on 17-11-2023.

Köhler-Rollefson I. 2018. *Camel Cultures of India.* https://www.sahapedia.org/camel-cultures-of-india, accessed on 17-11-2023.

Krishna N. 2010. *Sacred Animals of India.* 274 p. Penguin Random House, Gurugram, Haryana, India.

Kumar A, Misra SS, Chopra A, Narula HK, Sharma RC and Gowane GR. 2021. Sheep breeding in north-western arid and semi-arid regions of India: An overview. *Indian Journal of Small Ruminants* **27** (1):1-10.

Kumar M, Dahiya SP and Ratwan P. 2021b. Backyard poultry farming in India: A tool for nutritional security and women empowerment. *Biological Rhythm Research* **52**(10): 1476-91.

Kumar M, Dahiya SP, Ratwan P, Kumar S and Chitra A. 2019. Status, constraints and future prospects of Murrah buffaloes in India. *Indian Journal of Animal Sciences* **89** (12): 1291-1302.

Kumar RJ. 2009. *New Interpretations on Indus Valley Civilisation.* 189 p. https://sanipanhwar.com/,pdf downloaded on 25-07-2024.

Kumar S. 2023. The role of domestic goat in Harappan economy. *Journal of History, Archaeology and Architecture* **2**(1): 55-70.

Lachungpa U. 2009. Indigenous lifestyles and biodiversity conservation issues in North Sikkim. *Indian Journal of Traditional Knowledge* **8**(1): 51-55.

Lahiri-Choudhary DK.1995. History of elephants in captivity in India and their uses: An overview. *Gajah* **14:** 28-31.

Lakshminarayanan N. 2022. Elephant ecology and behaviour: Implications for captive elephant management. In: *Caring for Elephants: Managing Health and Welfare in Captivity.* pp 6-12. (Eds) Nigam P, Habib B and Pandey R. Project Elephant Division, MoEF & CC, GoI- Wildlife Institute of India, Dehradun, India.

Larson G, Liu R, Zhao X, Yuan J, Fuller D, Barton L, Dobney K, Fan Q, Gu Z, Liu XH and Luo Y. 2010. Patterns of East Asian pig domestication, migration, and turnover revealed by modern and ancient DNA. *Proceedings of the National Academy of Sciences* **107**(17): 7686-91.

Lawler A. 2016. The carnelian beard. In*: Why Did the Chicken Cross the World? The Epic Saga of the Bird that Powers Civilization.* pp. 28-52. Atria Paperback, New Delhi.

Locke P. 2013. Explorations in ethnoelephantology: Social, historical, and ecological intersections between Asian elephants and humans. *Environment and Society* **4(**1): 79-97.

Locke P. 2014. The anomalous elephant: Terminological dilemmas and the incalcitrant domestication debate. *Gajah* **41**: 12-19.

Lv FH, Peng WF, Yang J, Zhao YX, Li WR, Liu MJ, Ma YH, Zhao QJ, Yang GL, Wang F and Li JQ. 2015. Mitogenomic meta-analysis identifies two phases of migration in the history of eastern Eurasian sheep. *Molecular Biology and Evolution* **32**(10): 2515-33.

Macdonell AA. 1899. *A History of Sanskrit Literature.* William Heinmann, London, UK. pdf downloaded from Google Books on 27-03-2024.

Mahajan JM. 1987. Status of research development and constraints of breeding rabbits for meat and fur skins in India. In: *Short Course on Advances in Rabbit Production.* pp. 11-24. DFAB (CSWRI). Garsa, HP, India. 29 June-5 July, 1987. Central Sheep and Wool Research Institute, Garsa, Himachal Pradesh, India.

Majumder PP and Basu A. 2015. A genomic view of the peopling and population structure of India. *Cold Spring Harbor Perspectives in Biology* **7** (4): a008540. doi: 10.1101/cshperspect. a008540.

Manoharan NS. 2022. Occupational hazards and welfare of mahouts and elephant handers. In: *Caring for Elephants: Managing Health and Welfare in Captivity.* pp.196-200. (Eds) Nigam P, Habib B and Pandey R. Project Elephant Division, MoEF&CC, GoI- Wildlife Institute of India, Dehradun, India.

Mariyapillai MM, Paranthaman G, Napoleon K and Abbas R. 2021. A re-reading on vibrant mural paintings of Sittanavasal cave temples. *International Journal of Mechanical Engineering* **6** (Spl. Issue): 1619-23. DOI: https://doi.org/10.56452/220.

Mathpal Y. 1984. *Prehistoric Rock Paintings of Bhimbetka, Central India.* 236p. Abhinav Publications, New Delhi, India.

Meadows JRS, Hiendleder S and Kijas JW. 2011. Haplogroup relationships between domestic and wild sheep resolved using a mitogenome panel. *Heredity* **106** (4): 700–6. https://doi.org/10.1038/hdy. 2010.122.

Mehra KL. 2007. Agricultural foundation of Indus-Saraswati civilization. In: *Glimpses of the Agricultural Heritage of India.* pp 11-27. Asian Agri-History Foundation, Secunderabad, India.

Mehta SC and Bhattacharya TK.2023. *Rewal Chaal*: Equestrian sports for sustenance of indigenous horses. *Agriculture World* **9** (7): 60-62.

Mehta SC, Kumar R and Bhattacharya TK.2024. *Standards for Identification of Indigenous Horse Breeds.* ICAR-National Research Centre on Equines, Hisar, Haryana, India.

Menon N. 2019. Jumbo exports: India's history of elephant diplomacy. *Caravan* **March 2019**: 8–10.

Menon SM and Sinha A. 2023. The elephant in the Buddhist art of Kanaganahalli, southern India. In: *Composing Worlds with Elephants: Interdisciplinary Dialogues.* pp. 123-35 (Eds) Lainé N, Keil PG and Rahmat K. IRD Éditions, Montpellier, France.

Minervino AH, Zava M, Vecchio D and Borghese A 2020. *Bubalus bubalis*: A short story. *Frontiers in Veterinary Science* **7:** 570413. doi: 10.3389/fvets.2020.570413.

Mishra BP and Niranjan SK. 2022. Animal genetic resources (AnGR) diversity in India. *Indian Journal of Plant Genetic Resources* **35**(3): 223-28. DOI: 10.5958/0976-1926.2022.00073.0.

Misra VD. 2008. Beginnings of agriculture in the Vindhya- Ganga region. In: *History of Science, Philosophy, and Culture in Indian Civilization.* pp. 19-30. Gopal L and Srivastava VC (Eds). Concept Publishing Company, Delhi, India.

Mitchell P. 2018. *The Donkey in Human History: An Archaeological Perspective.* pp. 1-13, 72-107. Oxford University Press, Oxford, UK.

Mukherjee S, Mukherjee A, Kumar S, Verma H, Bhardwaj S, Togla O, Joardar SN, Longkumer I, Mech M, Khate K and Vupru K. 2022. Genetic characterization of endangered Indian Mithun (*Bos frontalis*), Indian Bison/Wild Gaur (*Bos gaurus)* and Tho-tho cattle (*Bos indicus*) populations using SSR markers reveals their diversity and unique phylogenetic status. Diversity**14**(7): 548. https://doi.org/10.3390/d14070548.

Murphy CA and Fuller DQ. 2016. The transition to agricultural production in India: South Asian entanglements of domestication. In: *A Companion to South Asia in the Past.* pp. 344-57. (Eds) Schug GR and Walimbe SR. John Wiley & Sons Inc. Online Library. DOI:10.1002/9781119055280.

Naderi S, Rezaei HR, Pompanon F, Blum MG, Negrini R, Naghash HR, Balkız Ö, Mashkour M, Gaggiotti OE, Ajmone-Marsan P and Kence A. 2008. The goat domestication process inferred from large-scale mitochondrial DNA analysis of wild and domestic individuals. *Proceedings of the National Academy of Sciences* **105**(46):17659-64.

Naik PK, Swain BK and Beura CK. 2022. Duck production in India-a review. *Indian Journal of Animal Sciences* **92(**8): 917–26.

Ncube KT, Modiba MC, Mpofu TJ, Mtileni B and Nephawe KA. 2024. Genomic tools for medicinal properties of goat's milk for cosmetic and health benefits. A review. *Preprints: Preprints.Org* 2024041662. https://doi.org/10.20944/preprints202404.1662.v1.

Niranjan SK, Behl R, Mukesh M, Bharti VK and Mishra BP. 2024. *Donkey Genetic Resources od India: Ladakhi Donkey*. 31 p. ICAR-National Bureau of Genetic Resources, Karnal, Haryana, India.

Padhi M and Giri S. 2024. Status of duck breeding in India. *Indian Journal of Animal Sciences* **94** (1): 3–10.

Pal Y, Legha RA, Bhardwaj A, and Tripathi BN. 2020. Status and conservation of equine biodiversity in India. *Indian Journal of Comparative Microbiology, Immunology and Infectious Diseases* **41**(2): 174-84.

Pandey NK, Somvanshi SP, Kumar S, Prakash B and Singh CK. 2020. Yak rearing practices by (Brokpa) pastoralist of Tawang Arunachal Pradesh. *Journal of Entomology and Zoology Studies* **8**(3): 1067-71.

Pandya AJ, Mohamed M and Khan H. 2006. Traditional Indian dairy products. In: *Handbook of Milk of Non-Bovine Mammals*. pp. 257-73. (Eds) Park YW, Haenlein GF and Wendorff WL. Blackwell Publishing https://doi.org/10.1002/9780470999738.ch10, pdf downloaded on 31-10-2023.

Peters C, Richter KK, Wilkin S, Stark S, Mir-Makhamad B, Fernandes R, Maksudov F, Mirzaakhmedov S, Rahmonov H, Schirmer S and Ashastina K. 2024. Archaeological and molecular evidence for ancient chickens in Central Asia. *Nature Communications***15**(1): 2697: https://doi.org/10.1038/s41467-024-46093-2.

Peters J, Lebrasseur O, Irving-Pease EK, Paxinos PD, Best J, Smallman R, Callou C, Gardeisen A, Trixl S, Frantz L and Sykes N . 2022. The biocultural origins and dispersal of domestic chickens. *Proceedings of the National Academy of Sciences* **119** (24): 1-9, p.e2121978119: https://doi.org/10.1073/pnas.2121978119.

Prabhu VR, Arjun MS, Bhavana K, Kamalakkannan R and Nagarajan M. 2019. Complete mitochondrial genome of Indian mithun, *Bos frontalis* and its phylogenetic implications. *Molecular Biology Reports* **46** (2): 2561-66.

Prakash V, Jyotsana B, Suthar S, Nath K, Ranjan R and Sawal RK. 2021. Molecular characterisation of growth hormone (GH) gene in Indian dromedary and Bactrian camel. *Journal of Camel Practice and Research* **28** (1): 47-51.

Rajkhowa S, Rajkhowa C, Rahman H and Bujarbaruah KM. 2004. Seroprevalence of infectious bovine rhinotracheitis in Mithun (*Bos frontalis*) in India. *Revue Scientifique et Technique - Office International des Epizooties* **23** (3): 821-29.

Ramakrishnan B, Ilakkia M, Karthick S and Veeramani A. 2018. The role of elephants in the forest ecosystem and its conservation problems in southern India. In: *Indian Hotspots: Vertebrate Faunal Diversity, Conservation and Management Volume 1*. pp. 317-43. (Eds) Sivaperuman C and Venkataraman K. Springer Nature Singapore Pvt. Ltd. eBook, https://doi.org/10.1007/978-981-10-6605-4 pdf downloaded on 30-04-2024.

Ramesha KP, Bora M, Kandeepan G and Chakravarty P. 2009. *Indigenous Traditional Knowledge of Yak Rearers*. 27p. National Research Centre on Yak, Dirang, India.

Randhawa MS. 1980. *A History of Agriculture in India. Vol I, II, II, IV.* Indian Council of Agricultural Research, New Delhi, India.

Ravichandran T, Perumal RK, Kennady V, Baltenweck I, Wright I, Burden F and Rahman H. 2023. *Mapping the Indian Donkey and Mule Population and Potential Intervention Strategies and Partners*. 31p. ILRI Research Report 115. International Livestock Research Institute (ILRI), Nairobi, Kenya.

Raviv L, Jacobson SL, Plotnik JM, Bowman J, Lynch V and Benítez-Burraco A. 2023. Elephants as an animal model for self-domestication. *Proceedings of the National Academy of Sciences* **120**(15): e2208607120. https://doi.org/10.1073/pnas.2208607120.

Risam KS, Das GK and Bhasin V. 2005. Rabbit for meat and wool production in India: A review. *Indian Journal of Animal Sciences* **75**(3): 365-82.

Rissman P. 1989. The status of research on animal domestication in India and its cultural context. In: *Early Animal Domestication and Its Cultural Context*: Vol. 6. pp. 14-23. (Eds) Crabtree PJ, Campana DV and Ryan KU. The University Museum of Archaeology and Anthropology, University of Pennsylvania, Philadelphia, USA.

Sarkar A. 2021. Indian Neolithization: Reassessment from cultural landscape context. In: *Culture, Tradition and Continuity: Disquisitions in Honour of Prof Vasant Shinde. Vol. I.* pp. 67-80. (Eds) Shirvalkar P and Prasad E. BR Publishing Corporation, New Delhi, India.

Sarma KK. 2022. Musth and its management in captive elephants. In: *Implications for captive elephant management. In: Caring for Elephants: Managing Health and Welfare in Captivity.* pp.141-53. (Eds) Nigam P, Habib B and Pandey R. Project Elephant Division, MoEF&CC, GoI- Wildlife Institute of India, Dehradun, India.

Scanes CG. 2018. The neolithic revolution, animal domestication, and early forms of animal agriculture. *Animals and Human Society.* pp. 103-31. (Eds) Scanes C.G. and Toukhsati, S. Academic Press. London, UK. doi.org/10.1016/B978-0-12-805247-1.00006-X.

Selvaramesh AS and Narmatha N. 2024. Identification of B casein gene for A1 and A2 allelic variants in Pulikulam cattle of Tamil Nadu. *International Journal of Veterinary Science and Animal Husbandry* **SP-9** (93): 8-11.

Shamasastry R (Trans.).1951. *Kautilya's Arthaśāstra.* 4th edn. 518p. Shri Raghuveer Printing Press, Mysore, Inida https://archive.org/details/in.gov.ignca.900, pdf downloaded on 09-10-2023.

Shannon LM, Boyko RH, Castelhano M, Corey E, Hayward JJ, McLean C, White ME, Abi Said M, Anita BA, Bondjengo NI and Calero J. 2015. Genetic structure in village dogs reveals a Central Asian domestication origin. *Proceedings of the National Academy of Sciences* **112**(44): 13639-44.

Shannon LM, Boyko RH, Castelhano M, Corey E, Hayward JJ, McLean C, White ME, Abi Said M, Anita BA, Sharma DK, Maldonado JE, Jhala YV and Fleischer RC. 2004. Ancient wolf lineages in India. *Proceedings of the Royal Society of London. Series B: Biological Sciences* **271**(Suppl. 3): S1-4.

Sharma TR (Trans.). 2013. *Atharva-Veda Vol. I.* Vijaykumar Govindram Hansnand, New Delhi, (Digital Distributer Agniveer). https://archive.org/details/atharva-veda-vol-2-of-2, pdf downloaded on 05-06-2023.

Sheshadri KG. 2014. Sheep in ancient Indian literature and culture. *Annals of the Bhandarkar Oriental Research Institute* **95**: 24-49.

Shinde AK and Naqvi SMK. 2015. Prospects of dairy sheep farming in India: An overview. *Indian Journal of Small Ruminants* **21** (2): 180-95.

Singh A, Pal Y, Kumar R, Kumar S, Bhardwaj A, Rani K and Ana R. 2022. Equine husbandry based agri-entrepreneurship-an overview. *Journal of Community Mobilization and Sustainable Development* **3** (Seminar Special Issue): 697-704.

Singh MK and Yadav MP. 2004. The Marwari horse: Pride of India. *Livestock International* **8**: 19–22.

Singh P. 2008. Origin of agriculture in the Vindhyas (North Central India). In: *History of Science, Philosophy, and Culture in Indian Civilization.* pp. 3-18. Gopal L and Srivastava VC (Eds). Concept Publishing Company, Delhi, India.

Singh S, Kumar S Jr, Kolte AP and Kumar S. 2013. Extensive variation and sub-structuring in lineage A mtDNA in Indian sheep: genetic evidence for domestication of sheep in India. *PLoS One* **8**(11): e77858. doi: 10.1371/journal.pone.0077858. PMID: 24244282; PMCID: PMC3823876.

Sundarapandian M and Raman P. 2023. Distribution of House Sparrows, *Passer domesticus indicus*, in Coimbatore District, Tamil Nadu, India. In: *Birds - Conservation, Research and Ecology.* pp.1-17 (Ed.) Mikkola H. IntechOpen. Available at: http://dx.doi.org/10.5772/intechopen.1002009.

Suryanarayan A, Cubas M, Craig OE, Heron CP, Shinde VS, Singh RN, O'Connell TC and Petrie CA. 2020. Lipid residues in pottery from the Indus Civilisation in northwest India. *Journal of Archaeological Science* **125:** 105291. https://doi.org/10.1016/j.jas.2020.105291.

Swinny NJ. 2019. *Horses and Ponies for Ever.* QEB Publishing Lake Forest, CA,USA.

Talokar OW, Belge AR and Belge RS. 2013. Clinical evaluation of cow-urine extract special reference to Arsha (Hemmorrhoids). *International Journal of Pharmaceutical Science Invention* **2**(3): 5-8.

Thomas PK, Joglekar PP, Matsushima Y, Pawankar SJ and Deshpande A.1997. Subsistence based on animals in the Harappan culture of Gujarat. *Anthropozoologica* **25-26**: 769-76.

Tiwari SK. 2000. *Riddles of Indian Rockshelter Paintings*. 1st edn. 280 p. Sarup & Sons, New Delhi, India.

Vajira S and Story F. 1998 M*aha-parinibbana Sutta: Last days of the Buddha*. https://www.accesstoinsight.org/tipitaka/dn/dn.16.1-6.vaji.html, pdf downloaded on 16-04-2024.

van der Geer A. 2008. *Animals in Stone*: *Indian Mammals Sculptured through Time.* Brill NV, Leiden, The Netherland. Downloaded from Brill.com on 01-04-2024.

Wang MS, Thakur M, Peng MS, Jiang YU, Frantz LA, Li M, Zhang JJ, Wang S, Peters J, Otecko NO and Suwannapoom C. 2020. 863 genomes reveal the origin and domestication of chicken. *Cell Research* **30** (8): 693-701.

Wani AY, Khan AA, Hamadani H, Sheikh IU, Banday MT, Akand AH, Shanaz S and Baba SH. 2022. Yak population trends and their breeding status in the UT of Ladakh. *Pharma Innovation Journal* **11**(12): 2411-13.

Zeder M A. 2012. The domestication of animals. *Journal of Anthropological Research* **68**(2): 161-90.

Zhang Y, Colli L and Barker JS. 2020. Asian water buffalo: domestication, history and genetics. *Animal Genetics* **51**(2): 177-91.

3

Traditional Animal Husbandry Practices in India

Aruna T. Kumar and R. Somvanshi

Eha yantu paśavo ye pareyurvāyuryesām sahacāram jujosa. Tvastā yesām rūpadheyāni vedāsmintāngosthe savitā ni yacchatu.
Let the animals come back to the stalls, all those that had gone out over the forest meadows. The air, the breeze, the winds refresh them as friends. Tvashta, the development expert, knows their breeds and qualities. Let Savita, the inspirer, keeper, keep them properly in the stalls for good health.

(Atharva Veda 2.26.1; translation by Sharma 2013)

1. Introduction
2. Livestock Production Systems in India
3. Traditional Animal Husbandry
   - Dairy Cattle and Buffalo Husbandry
     - Cattle
     - Buffalo
   - Sheep and Goat farming
   - Pig Farming
4. Ancient Indian Animal Husbandry Practices-Scientific Relevance
   - Animal Breeding
   - Animal Nutrition
   - Animal Management
   - Animal Housing
5. Traditional Husbandry: Challenges and Limitations
6. New Horizon
7. Conclusion

Introduction

The existence of humans and livestock is entwined. Humans followed sheep for greener pastures that led to newer civilizations. Cattle, sheep, and goat gave them food; horses gave them speed, elephants gave them power; camels helped them cross the deserts; and fish was with them while crossing rivers, oceans and even cold hilly streams. Livestock provides food, draught power and is a definite source of ready cash round the year globally. Animal produce, as well as, their waste are important for human society. With changing times, animal rearing practices have evolved. The harvesting of animal produce has also changed. The marketing of animal produce has transformed the value addition and supply chains, in a way that were unimaginable a few decades ago. Like any other enterprise, livestock farming is fundamentally driven by return on investment. In this sector, the inputs are: animal, animal food (nutrition), animal health, value addition, manpower and animal housing. The outputs include animal produce, animal power, animal waste. Besides this, being a living organism, the animal interaction with ecosystem is another aspect, which has to be taken care of before adopting an animal breed or any rearing system. The return-on-investment will depend on quantity of produce per unit input. The lower the investment on input, and the higher the quality output, the larger the profit. The safer the animal, the safer the environment. A sick animal will become the vector for problematic health issues for both human and animal populations. The livestock, farming researcher needs to understand that every ecosystem has its own set of livestock well adapted to the local food and climate, and that sustainable improvement is possible by manipulating these factors rather than introducing new breeds or nutritional interventions without proper study of their potential and economics an altered ecosystem.

Animal husbandry and livestock production play a vital role in Indian economy, rural livelihoods, and cultural practices. These sectors contribute significantly to agricultural GDP and provide employment to millions of people, particularly in rural areas, which drives the national economic growth. Animal husbandry provides livelihood opportunities to over 20 million farmers, many of whom are smallholders and landless labourers. It offers a stable source of income through the production of milk, meat, eggs, wool, and other animal products. In drought-prone or arid regions, livestock acts as an economic buffer for farmers when crop production is unreliable due to climate fluctuations.

The livestock production contributed 30.19% to the total agriculture Gross Value Added (GVA) in 2021-22. India is the seventh-largest country with an area of 328 million hectares, harbours the world's largest livestock (and poultry) inventory with 1.43 billion (1428.6 million) heads. It is home to huge genetic diversity vis-à-vis farm animal species with a total of 536.76 million livestock heads enumerated in the latest Livestock Census (Anonymous 2019). Dairy farming is especially important, with India being the world's largest milk producer. In terms of small ruminant production system, the country ranks second globally with approximately 74.26 million sheep and 148.88 million goat populations. India, with an overall poultry population (851.81million) is also one of the world's largest producers of poultry meat and eggs, with the industry being a major source of income for both small-scale farmers and large commercial producers. In India, the livestock production system is primarily traditional, consisting of mixed farming and pastoral systems). Resource-poor farming systems may aim at the improved management of the various livestock species in backyards. Thess systems have been classified according to a number of criteria, the main ones being integration with crop production, the animal-land relationship, intensity of production, and type of product.

Box 3.1. Global Livestock Production Systems: FAO

Livestock production systems utilizing global rangelands provide the ability for humans to effectively harvest animal protein from plants. These systems, which occur on six of the seven continents (Antarctica is the exception), are highly diverse, ranging from low-input, pastoral production systems located in arid and semiarid environments on communally owned lands to highly intensive production systems in more mesic environments which can integrate livestock-crop-forage systems to improve feed efficiency and reduce time from birth to harvest. The Food and Agriculture Organization (Seré et al. 1996) provided a comprehensive classification of livestock production systems.

Solely Livestock Systems: *Involve livestock production where*

- *More than 90% of the dry matter fed to animals comes from rangelands, pastures, annual forages, and purchased feeds.*
- *Less than 10% of the total value of production is derived from non-livestock farming activities.*

Landless Livestock Production Systems: *A subset of solely livestock systems characterized by:*

- *Less than 10% of the dry matter fed to animals being farm-produced.*
- *Annual average stocking rates exceeding 10 livestock units (LU) per hectare of agricultural land.*

Further Subdivisions

- ***Landless Monogastric Systems:*** *Where the value of production from pig or poultry enterprises surpasses that of ruminant enterprises.*
- ***Landless Ruminant Systems:*** *In these systems, the value of production from ruminant enterprises exceeds that of pig or poultry enterprises.*

Grassland-Based Systems: *A subset of solely livestock systems defined by:*

- *More than 10% of the dry matter fed to animals being farm-produced.*
- *Annual average stocking rates of less than 10 LU per hectare of agricultural land.*

Further Classifications of Grassland-Based Systems

- ***Temperate and Tropical Highland:*** *Systems located in temperate and highland regions.*
- ***Humid/Sub-Humid Tropics and Sub-Tropics:*** *Systems found in regions with humid or sub-humid climates.*
- ***Arid/Semi-Arid Tropics and Sub-Tropics:*** *Systems operating in arid or semi-arid tropical climates.*

Livestock Production Systems in India

Livestock production systems are considered a subset of farming. They can either be a component of a mixed crop-livestock farming system or an entirely livestock-based pastoral system. These systems are classified based on several criteria, including integration with crop production, the animal-land relationship, agro-geoclimatic zones, production intensity, and type of products (Box 3.1). Solely livestock production systems can be landless or grassland based. The mixed farming systems can be rainfed or irrigated production systems. There are landless livestock production systems including monogastric production and ruminant production systems. Based on production factors, livestock production systems are categorized as modern or traditional (Seré *et al.* 1996). The modern production system requires large capital investment and employs substantial amounts of hired labor, while traditional systems are low-input, relying mainly on family labour and extensive use of community land. In India, the traditional livestock production system primarily consists of mixed farming and pastoral systems (Deb 2015). Traditional sheep, goat, pig, donkey, mule, and backyard poultry farmers in rural India are mostly landless and resource-poor, relying on livestock production as a vital source of their livelihood.

Traditional production systems include grassland-based and mixed or integrated farming systems. In the Mixed Farming Systems, more than 10 percent of the dry matter fed to animals comes from crop by-products, stubble or more than 10 percent of the total value of production comes from non-livestock farming activities. The Landless Livestock Production System is defined as a subset of the solely livestock systems in which less than 10 percent of the dry matter fed to animals is farm produced and in which annual average stocking rates are above ten livestock units (LU) per hectare of agricultural land (Seré *et al.* 1996). Grassland-based systems consist of traditional pastoral and agro-pastoral systems, which are mainly prevalent in dry regions of the country that receive low or medium annual rainfall. Typical pastoral systems, based solely on livestock, are mainly found in the arid and semi-arid zones of Rajasthan, Gujarat, Haryana, and the Ladakh region, as well as in the humid and sub-humid zones of the Himalayas, including the North Eastern hills, where cropping is not feasible. It is reported that nearly 4% of agricultural land in India is under this system providing livelihood to marginal communities (Birthal *et al.* 2006).

Traditional agro-pastoral systems are practiced in arid and semi-arid areas with medium annual rainfall, where rainfed crops such as millet and sorghum are grown. Nomadic pastoralism is a pure pastoral system, characterized by minimal or no agriculture, and high mobility of people and animals in search of grazing and water. This system primarily involves rearing small ruminants. Transhumant pastoralism is based on more or less regular seasonal migrations from a permanent home and includes the rearing of sheep, yak, and mithun. Agro-pastoralism is associated with dryland or rainfed cropping, where animals are managed by village-based herders within a relatively limited rangeland. Although these herders also practice crop farming, it usually remains secondary to pastoralism for household income. The most commonly kept species in agro-pastoral systems include cattle, buffaloes, camels, sheep, and goats (Deb 2015).

Mixed or Integrated Farming System is the most prevalent livestock rearing system in India. The mixed farming systems is environmentally most sustainable because of relationship between crop and livestock production. Feed–fodder requirement of animals is fulfilled from crop residues and by-products, and animals provide draught power and dung manure for crop production. In India mixed rainfed system is practised on 46% of land and mixed irrigated system on 37% land. The mixed crop–livestock systems are characterized by considerable heterogeneity in terms of species, production efficiency, management practices and commercialization (Birthal *et al.* 2006). This heterogeneity is delineated in 15 crop–livestock systems, having cattle or buffalo as the second or third largest economic activity in most of these systems (Rao *et al.* 2004).

Traditional Animal Husbandry (TAH)

India has a rich history of animal husbandry, and rearing animals plays a crucial role in the rural economy. Deeply rooted in rural lifestyles and cultural practices, the TAH involves raising livestock such as cows, buffaloes, goats, sheep, pigs, poultry, and camels for milk, meat, wool, transportation, and agricultural assistance using indigenous resources and knowledge. These practices are closely linked to the agrarian economy and the social fabric of rural communities. Some of the main features and merits of TAH are discussed here:

Integrated Farming Systems: The livestock production system in India is primarily traditional, consisting of mixed farming and pastoral systems. Traditional animal husbandry is often combined with crop cultivation (mixed farming), creating an integrated farming system. In this system, livestock not only provide draught power but also produce farm manure, which enhances soil fertility and reduces the need for chemical fertilizers.

Cultural Integration: In India, the animal husbandry is not merely a profession, as it is in many Western countries, but a way of life that is deeply intertwined with the cultural and social fabric of rural communities. Animals are traditionally raised not only for economic reasons but also for socio-religious functions and as symbols of social status. Many owners develop a deep attachment to their animals. Animal husbandry is integrated into religious and social practices, making it a sustainable part of rural life. For example, cows hold a central role in religious ceremonies and rituals, while rams, bucks, mithun, and chickens are often sacrificed during festive occasions. Additionally, both wild and domesticated animals play a significant role in religious expression and can be seen in tourism, agriculture, and industry. Sacred animals and plant species are highly visible in everyday life, as they are venerated in Indian tradition. This unique cultural reverence has contributed to the protection of many animal and plant species. Traditional methods rely on locally available feed, natural grazing, and indigenous breeds, which require less external input.

Indigenous Breeds

India is home to 230 registered breeds of domestic animals (Figs. 3.1-3.6), which have evolved in response to varied conditions across different ago-climatic zones. Genetic diversity in Indian livestock is also a result of complex evolutionary phenomena and varied intensities of domestication applied under organized and unorganized (field) conditions as available to farmers. India boasts 77 registered bovine breeds, with contributions from cattle (54), buffalo (21), and yak (2). Native breeds are often well-adapted to local environmental conditions, showing better resistance to diseases and extreme weather. There are dual purpose indigenous breeds of livestock providing more than one animal products. Owing to these traits and low input cost, the Indian livestock and poultry breeds are very important from the utility point of view.

Studies conducted by Anthra (2006) explored the role of local breeds; description of the local breed according to farmers' perception (phenotypic, productive and reproductive); selection choice; and factors conducive to or endangering the continued rearing of a breed. Significant observations were:

- **Local breeds or Ecotypes:** Farmers knew that which breeds are reared for specific purpose and production goals.
- **Animal Selection:** Farmers select an animal keeping the production goals in mind as also in context of local conditions and resources for specific species.
- **Adaptation in Local Breeds:** Local breeds are better adapted to cope with the vagaries of weather, locally prevalent diseases and seasonal shortages for food and water.
- **Threatened Breeds:** But many breeds are threatened due to crossbreeding; mechanization of agriculture resulting in replacement of draught animals, loss of grazing lands and watering sources emergent diseases and natural calamities.
- **Organic Farming Practices:** Many traditional methods are organic, relying on natural fertilizers and feed, which promotes sustainable farming practices.
- **Biodiversity Preservation:** Indigenous breeds are preserved, contributing to biodiversity and genetic resources.

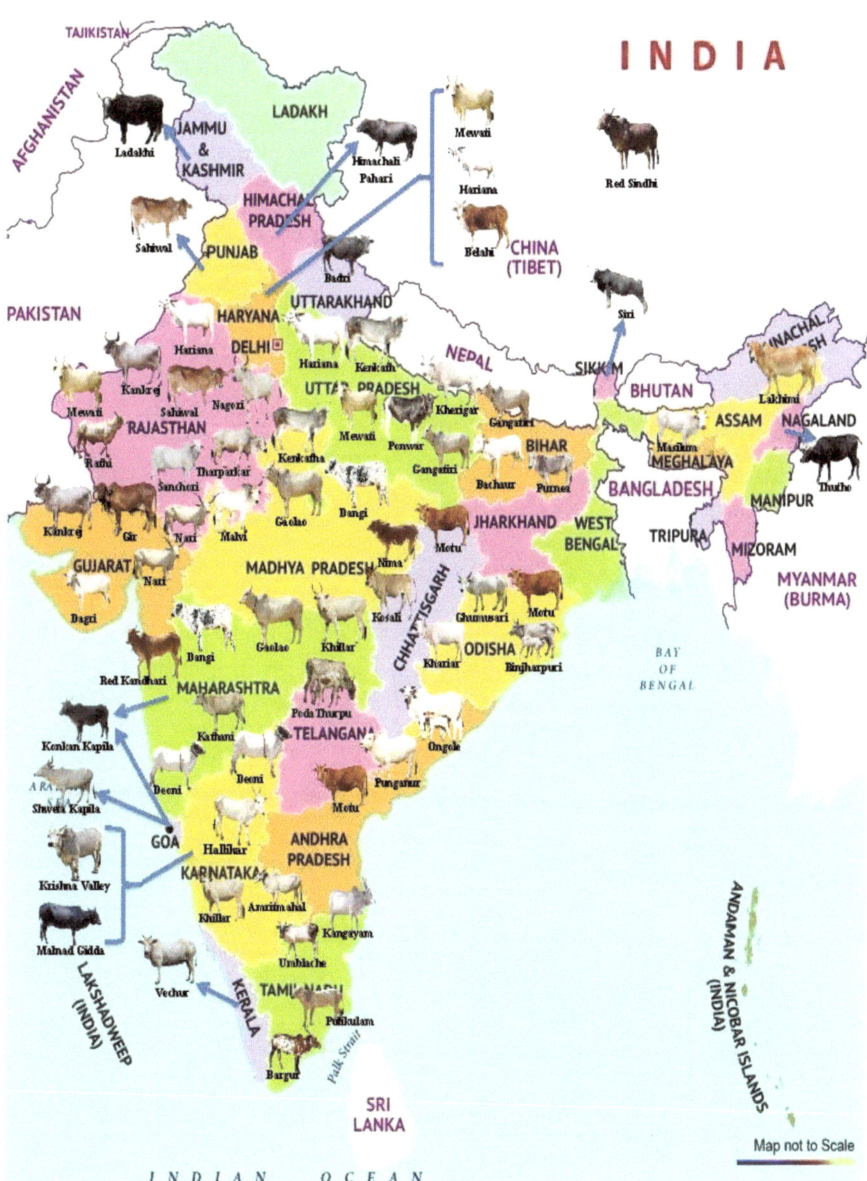

Fig. 3.1. *Distribution of indigenous registered cattle breeds in India (Indicative map courtesy of Dr. Aruna T. Kumar).*

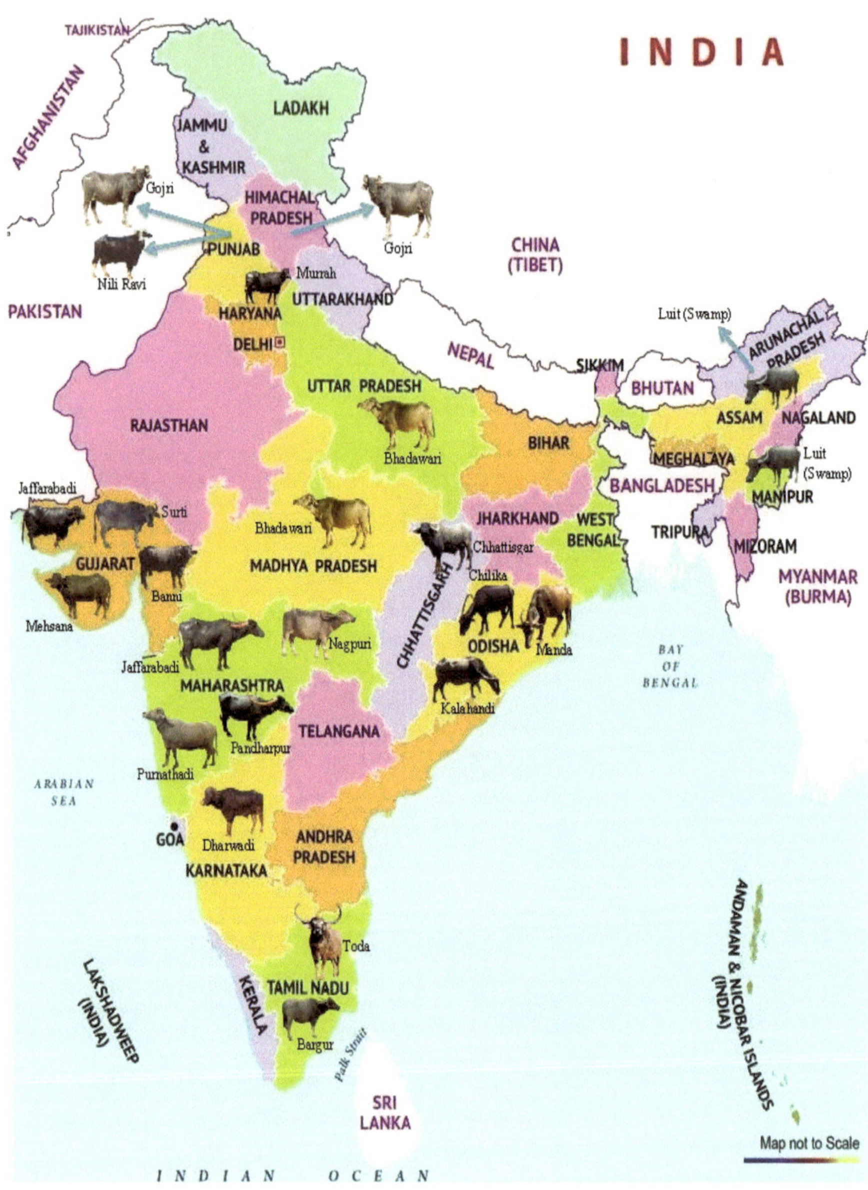

Fig. 3.2. Distribution of indigenous registered buffalo breeds in India (Indicative map courtesy of Dr. Aruna T. Kumar).

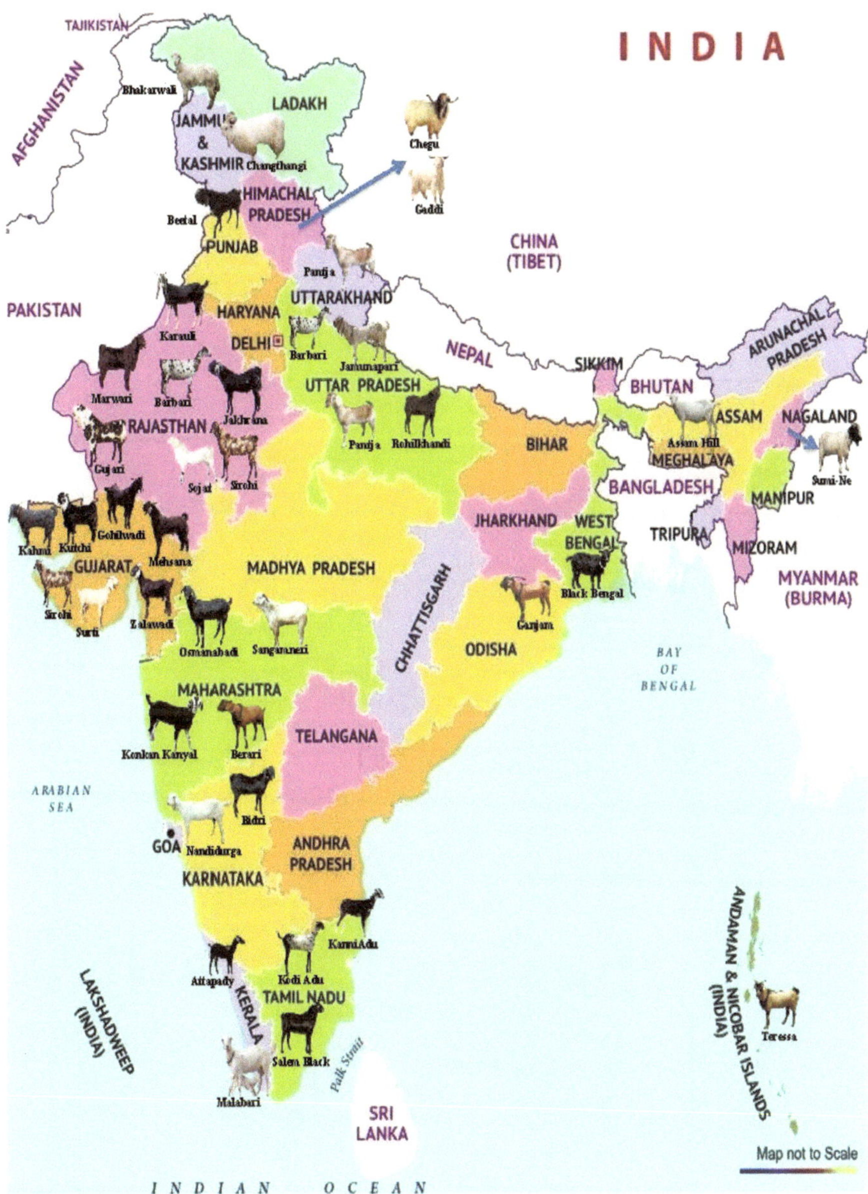

Fig. 3.3. *Distribution of indigenous registered goat breeds in India (Indicative map courtesy of Dr. Aruna T. Kumar).*

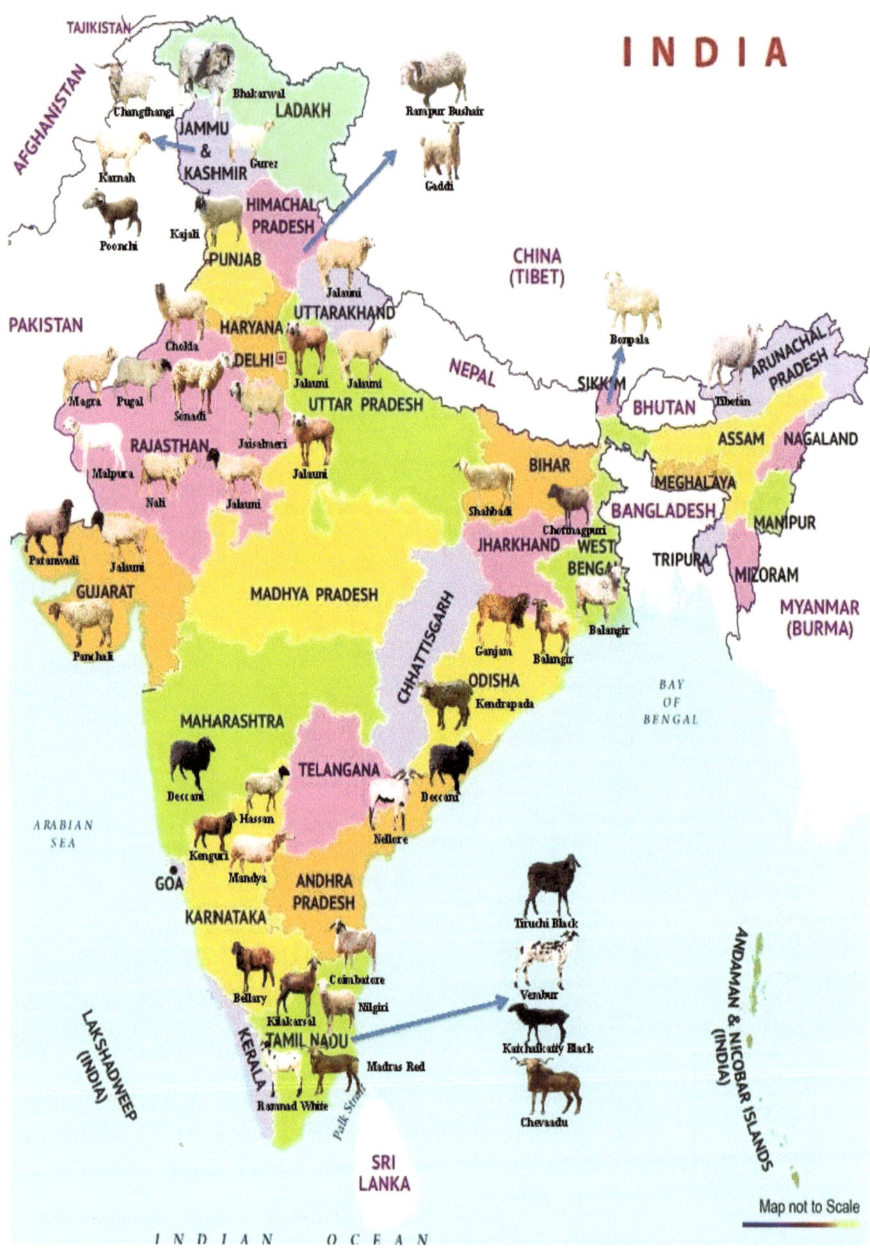

Fig. 3.4. Distribution of registered indigenous breeds of sheep in India (Indicative map courtesy of Dr. Aruna T. Kumar).

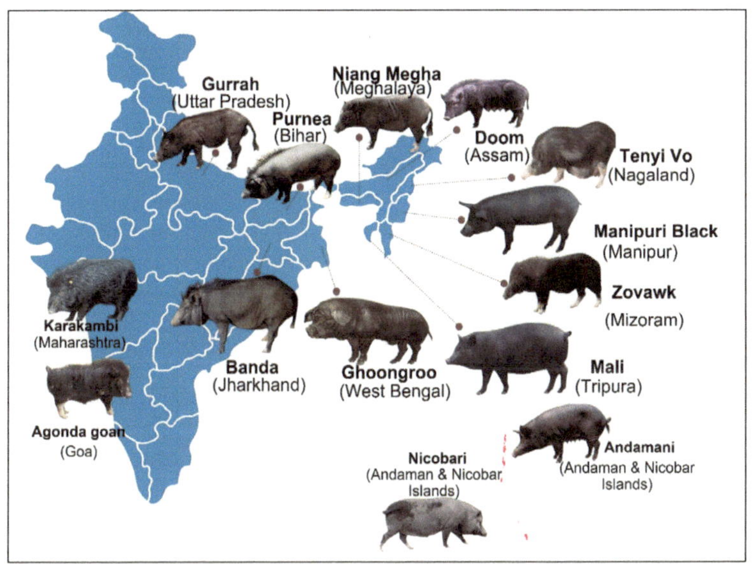

Fig. 3.5. Distribution of indigenous pig breeds (Indicative map courtesy of Dr. V.K. Gupta, ICAR- NRC on Pig).

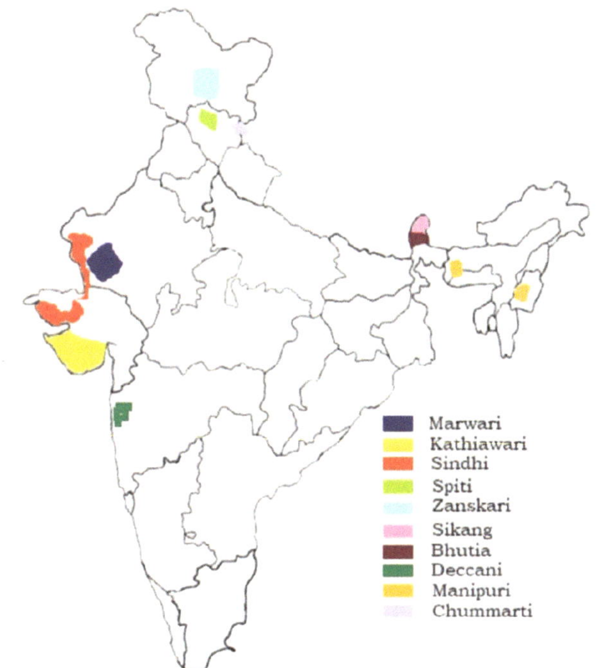

Fig. 3.6. Distribution of indigenous horse breeds (Indicative map courtesy of Dr. S.C. Mehta, ICAR-NRC on Equines, Bikaner).

Box 3.2. Concept of Organic Livestock Farming

Animal production systems—namely traditional, conventional, and organic—each possess distinct characteristics. While traditional and conventional production systems are well established, the organic animal husbandry system is still evolving. Notably, organic animal husbandry is not the same as the traditional animal husbandry practiced in India for centuries (Chander and Mukherjee 2005). It is a highly sophisticated and knowledge-intensive system of animal production designed to address human health, animal welfare, and environmental sustainability as an integrated whole. Consequently, it is crucial to develop a clear understanding of organic farming, particularly organic animal husbandry.

The global market for organically produced foods is expanding rapidly, creating significant export opportunities for developing countries. Domestic consumers are also increasingly seeking higher-quality food products. Organic certification has become synonymous with purity and quality, particularly when accredited by recognized certification agencies. In India, 11 certification agencies are currently accredited by the Agricultural and Processed Food Products Export Development Authority (APEDA) for the inspection and certification of organic agricultural products. This highlights the need for focused efforts to boost organic production and meet the growing demand for such products. With the right strategies, India stands to gain significantly from the export of organic foods but must prioritize market intelligence to fully exploit these opportunities.

The Government of India (GoI) has rightly identified organic farming as a priority area in various development plans, allocating substantial financial resources to its promotion. The Indian Council of Agricultural Research (ICAR) has also recognized organic farming as a viable agricultural system, particularly in regions with strong potential for organic practices. Livestock is central to organic farming, as sustainable organic agriculture is virtually impossible without the integration of animals into organic holdings.

Despite this importance, very little progress has been made in the field of organic animal husbandry in India. This calls for urgent attention from policymakers, research institutions, State Agricultural Universities (SAUs), and other development agencies involved in the research and development of organic farming. Concerted efforts are needed to advance organic animal husbandry in India and ensure its sustainable growth.

Dairy Cattle and Buffalo Husbandry

Traditional animal husbandry practices in India have primarily focused on dairy animals, particularly involving cattle and buffalo. The two species have been bred for milk production since the time immemorial. In rural areas, the possession of cattle and buffalo is still considered a measure of economic wealth and prosperity for individuals and families.

Dairy Cattle: Cattle rearing plays a crucial role in the rural landscape, offering direct and indirect benefits that ensure the livelihood of the poorest sections of society. These benefits are associated with nutrition, health, employment generation, and supplementary income. Some of the finest indigenous breeds of dairy and draught cattle include the Gir, Sahiwal, Red Sindhi, Ongole, and Deoni. Additionally, the dual-purpose breeds such as Hariana, Kankrej, Malvi, Mewati, Dangi, Khillari, and Nari have been traditionally reared for both milk production and draught power. Multiple scientific studies have pointed out the tolerance of indigenous cattle against pathogens, especially ticks.

Indigenous cattle are more adapted to heat stress, feed shortage, low input production systems and stressful conditions. They can produce even under low-input conditions with abundant roughage and low concentrate feed support. Desi cattle and buffaloes are comparatively more resilient to stressful stimuli and can recover early on the return of neutral conditions (Saravanan *et al.* 2022). Indigenous cattle with small teats and tight sheaths are better able to avoid injuries during grazing. Peculiar body conformation and sloppy rumps make zebu breeds suitable for intense draught work in the fields. Most of the desi cattle breeds are having light coat-colour helping in reflecting the sunlight besides preventing attacks/ bites from insects. The performance of desi cattle in case of functional traits is better than exotic or crossbred counterparts. The desi breeds are better in mothering ability, greater resistance to dystocia and mastitis and enhanced longevity compared to contemporary exotic or crossbred animals. Indicine cattle respond better to heat stress and are more thermo-tolerant than taurine breeds owing to their unique genetic makeup that may be associated with regulation of gene expression or protein function. For instance, the Vechur and Kasargode dwarf cows carry a different gene-pool due to which they can tolerate high temperatures and are less vulnerable to mastitis (Dash *et al.* 2016).

The role of A1 and A2 beta-casein milk variants in human health has garnered significant attention from the scientific community. Research has hypothesized that high consumption of A1 beta-casein may increase the risk of various diseases, including heart disease, type 1 diabetes, autism, and schizophrenia. This hypothesis is intriguing for both basic and applied studies and holds considerable implications for public health. Epidemiological evidence highlights a strong association between countries with high A1 milk consumption and a higher incidence of type 1 diabetes and heart disease (Woodford 2007). Furthermore, a double-blind, randomized, controlled human study demonstrated that consuming milk containing only A2 β-casein was linked to a significant increase in plasma glutathione levels compared to consuming milk with a combination of A1 and A2 β-casein. This finding suggests that A2 β-casein milk may have a potential advantage in promoting the production of the antioxidant glutathione in humans (Deth *et al.* 2016). In India, milk from native cattle breeds predominantly contains the A2 allele, whereas exotic breeds typically carry the A1-casein gene. A study on the status of milk protein, specifically the β-casein (A1:A2 frequency) in Indian dairy animals, revealed a predominance of the A2 variant (0.987) in zebu cattle breeds. Additionally, milk from river buffaloes exclusively contains the A2 milk type (Mishra *et al.* 2009).

Buffalo Farming: Traditional buffalo farming is a vital component of India's rural economy, contributing significantly to both milk production and other purposes such as meat and draught power. Buffalo milk commands a higher market price due to its high-fat content, ranging from 7 to 7.5%, nearly double that of cow milk. Additionally, buffaloes are highly efficient at converting low-quality feeds and coarse fodder into valuable products, making them indispensable in mixed farming systems. Their resilience to harsh climatic conditions and ability to thrive on crop residues and green forage add to their utility. India is renowned as a global hub for buffalo germplasm, hosting all recognized high-producing breeds of this species. Some prominent Indian dairy buffalo breeds include- Murrah, Nili Ravi, Surti, Mehsana, Bhadawari, Jaffarabadi, Nagpuri, Godavari, Toda, Padharpuri etc. known for their unique traits. These breeds collectively account for nearly 56% of the world's buffalo population, underlining India's pivotal role in global buffalo farming.

Buffaloes are a cornerstone of Indian dairy industry, which is undergoing a transformational shift. The buffalo sector contributes an impressive 66.3% of the total global volume of buffalo milk, highlighting its importance in the nation's milk production landscape. The high productivity and adaptability of Indian buffaloes make them an invaluable asset to the dairy industry. Buffalo farming has evolved into a sustainable livelihood and income-generating enterprise for farmers across diverse socioeconomic strata. It plays a crucial role in poverty alleviation and employment generation to rural households. As India continues to modernize its dairy industry, buffalo farming remains a key driver of growth and sustainability. With strategic investments in breeding, feed optimization, and healthcare, buffalo farming has the potential to further enhance its contributions to rural livelihoods, national milk production, and global dairy markets.

Sheep and Goat Farming

Sheep and goat husbandry in India dates back to the Neolithic period. These small ruminants were reared not only for meat but also for their valuable secondary products, including wool, hair, skin, and milk. Currently, India ranks second globally in sheep population, with approximately 74.26 million sheep, which constitute around 13.8% of the country's total livestock population. There are also 148.88 million goats, representing 41 recognized breeds along with numerous non-descript populations. Traditionally reared by resource-poor communities, sheep and goats are essential components of smallholder production systems and play a crucial role in the economy of India's extensive dryland regions, including arid, semi-arid, and dry sub-humid areas. These regions span across states such as Rajasthan, Madhya Pradesh, Maharashtra, Gujarat, Chhattisgarh, Jharkhand, Andhra Pradesh, Telangana, Karnataka, and Tamil Nadu. The multi-faceted benefits of sheep and goats—providing meat, milk, wool, skin, and manure—make them valuable contributors to the rural economy, especially in these dry areas (Kumar *et al.* 2021). The main advantages of small ruminant husbandry include:

- Adaptability to a wide range of climatic conditions, allowing them to thrive on pastures and degraded lands unsuitable for crop cultivation. They possess better thermoregulation, disease resistance, higher feed conversion rates, and endurance for long-distance grazing.
- Lower cost of purchase and maintenance, resulting in minimal financial risk.
- Flexibility for farmers in terms of capital investment, including space, feed, and management.
- Ability to be sold at any time, providing a steady source of income.
- Acting as a form of insurance and providing crucial support during natural disasters like droughts and floods.
- High reproductive capacity, short gestation periods, high prolificacy, and rapid turnover.
- Compatibility with existing farming systems without competing with traditional large livestock rearing.
- Complementarity with other husbandry practices due to their unique physical, physiological, behavioural, and economic traits.
- Small ruminants are more popular among resource-poor farmers due to its low input costs with better output. The infrastructural requirements are minimum and like poultry small units of goats are raised in backyard.
- In rangeland conditions, particularly in desert areas, goats are often more economical than other livestock. A small flock of five goats can yield higher profits compared to a single buffalo. Rearing a small flock of 1-5 goats

can generate a net annual income of approximately ₹ 3,138 per goat per household (Khadda *et al.* 2018)

- Small ruminants are like mobile banks or ATMs, serving as a primary means of investment for many marginal and small-scale farmers as well as landless people.

Despite the recent rise of commercial sheep and goat farming, the rearing of small ruminants remains predominantly traditional. Unlike dairy cattle, modern technological interventions such as artificial insemination and crossbreeding with exotic breeds are limited in sheep and goat rearing. Traditional management systems continue to play a crucial role in small ruminant production in the country. Sheep farming is generally nomadic, while goat rearing tends to be specific to certain regions. Herders often rely on traditional knowledge for the management and healthcare of their animals (Manivannan *et al.* 2018). For example, a study on traditional methods of rearing Kanni Adu goats in their native region found that goats are typically managed in flocks and only housed at night. The housing structures include open pens, half-open sheds, and closed sheds, located either near the owner's dwelling or as part of their residence. Farmers, when possible, keep breeding bucks within the flock throughout the year, with mating occurring naturally and without controlled breeding (Thiruvenkadan 2005). Another study from Tamil Nadu reported that sheep herders relied on indigenous methods to construct lamb huts for housing newborn lambs. These huts were made from locally available materials, with tender fodder leaves hung inside for young lambs. Herders avoided using ectoparasitic drugs, instead manually removing external parasites by rubbing and bathing the animals. Traditional methods for selecting breeding rams included identifying healthy, strong, and sound animals within the flock. Traditional veterinary practices, such as using turmeric powder and neem oil for treating wounds, were common. Similarly, small shelters made of bamboo were used to protect young kids. Additionally, sheep and goat herders often used animal behaviour to predict rainfall (Manivannan *et al.* 2018).

The major animal-rearing communities in the Wayanad district of Kerala—namely the Adiyan, Kuruma, Urali, and Kattunaykka tribes—primarily rely on traditional knowledge for managing, housing, and feeding their domestic animals, especially cattle and goats. The animal shelters are built using locally available materials such as areca nut wood, bamboo, paddy straw, coconut leaves, and mud. Goat sheds are typically constructed on elevated platforms, and the Urali tribe often uses tarpaulin sheets over the roofs of these sheds to make them waterproof. These tribes usually rely on forest resources and household waste to feed their goats, with commercial feed and concentrates rarely used. For example, goats are often allowed to graze or browse in paddy fields or forests during the day, then brought back to the sheds in the evening, where they are provided with water and fed jackfruit leaves at night (Abhiram and Rathish 2020).

Box 3.3. Traditional Husbandry Practices and Disease Preventive Measures

The grazing practices developed by many traditional pastoralist communities are based on their observational experience and knowledge of animals' selective foraging behaviour, including self-medication and the avoidance of toxic plants. These practices can effectively prevent worm infestations and plant toxicities. For example, farmers in West Java, Indonesia, raise their goats and sheep in elevated sheds with slatted floors (Fig. 3.7) and feed them cut fodder, resulting in fewer intestinal worms. Similarly, goat keepers in certain areas of Assam, Kerala, Gujarat and other parts in India also house their animals in traditional raised-platform goat houses. Interestingly, multitier goat houses with raised floors at ground level have been developed commercially and are gaining popularity among commercial goat farmers in India.

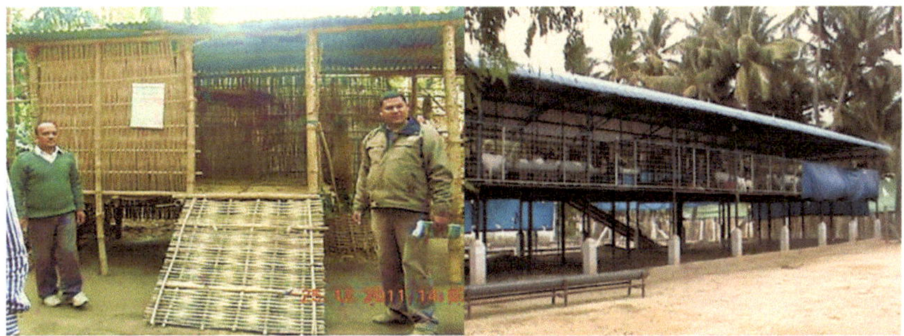

***Fig. 3.7.** A slated platform goat-pen made of indigenous material being used by Assam farmers (Left) and a commercial multitier goat-house (right) (Photo source: AICRP on Goat, AAU Guwahati, and Dr. D. Swarup).*

Pig Farming: India is recognized as one of the world's major centres of pig genetic diversity, home to a rich variety of indigenous breeds. These pigs play a dual role—deeply embedded in the socio-cultural traditions of many indigenous communities, especially in Northeast India, and serving as a crucial means of economic empowerment for marginalized populations. Compared to other livestock, pig rearing offers greater economic potential for small and marginal farmers, particularly those from lower socio-economic strata. Indigenous pigs are typically raised in traditional, small-scale, subsistence-oriented systems. These systems offer accessible and low-cost livelihood opportunities for tribal communities, scheduled castes, and resource-poor farmers by converting household waste and agricultural by-products into valuable animal protein. Smallholder pig farming significantly contributes to livelihood improvement and food security among the rural poor. In addition to supplying protein for household consumption, pigs are a key source of cash income and provide manure for crop production. They also act as a financial buffer in times of crisis and hold cultural significance in many rural societies. Among tribal communities, pig rearing supports nutritional needs, enhances income generation, and enables the recycling of domestic waste into organic fertilizer. However, traditional pigsties, often located in household backyards, are frequently unhygienic and can predispose animals to disease outbreaks Meanwhile, commercial pig production—characterized by confined rearing of improved crossbred or exotic breeds—is gaining popularity in India. This system offers greater productivity and supports growing demand in both rural and urban markets, contributing to improved food security and household income, particularly in urban and peri-urban areas (Chauhan *et al.* 2016, Gupta 2025).

Ancient Indian Animal Husbandry Practices: Scientific Relevance

The presence of numerous animal figurines and seals depicting animals from excavations at various Indus Valley sites, along with repeated references to domestic animals and their welfare in Vedic and post-Vedic scriptures—including the Vedas, Smritis, Sutras, Puranas, and epics such as the Mahabharata, Ramayana, and the Arthashastra—provides ample evidence of the significance of animal husbandry in the daily life of ancient India. Although the Mahabharata is not primarily an agricultural text, Indian sages emphasized the protection of *Varta* (agriculture, animal husbandry, and trade) in their instructions to kings. In advising Yudhishthira on ideal statesmanship and governance, Bhishma, the grandfather of both the Kauravas and Pandavas, stated, 'Agriculture, animal husbandry, and trade are the very life of the people'. According to the Arthashastra, the principles of righteousness and unrighteousness (*Dharmadharmau*) are learned from the three Vedas, while wealth and economic activities are derived from *Varta* (which includes agriculture, cattle-breeding, and trade). In defining the duties of a king, the Arthashastra specifies that during the eighth division of the night, the king should receive blessings from sacrificial priests, teachers, and the high priest. After consulting his physician, chief cook, and astrologer, he should pay respects to a cow with its calf and a bull by circumambulating them before entering his court. In court, he is then expected to personally attend to matters concerning the gods, heretics, Brahmins learned in the Vedas, cattle, sacred places, minors, the elderly, the afflicted, the helpless, and women—either in the order of priority or based on the urgency of each matter (Shamasastry 1951). Due to the importance of domestic animals, particularly in cattle and equine breeding, ancient India developed advanced practices and technologies in breeding, feeding, housing, management, and healthcare. Scholars and sages documented their knowledge, which was then passed on to their disciples. These disciples shared their teachings with learned Brahmins and priests, who, in turn, disseminated the knowledge to the common people, most of whom were farmers (Nene 2012). The information about animal husbandry given in our ancient literature is mainly on (i) relationship between phenotypic and economic traits (identifying economically important animals); (ii) use of local feed resources and quantity as per physiological state of animal; and (iii) housing as per the local climate and using local resources. This ancient information can help farmers and researchers in breeding, nutrition and housing at low cost (Kumar 2003).

Animal Breeding

Breeding Practices: Early Vedic literature notes specific cattle traits. For example, Maitrāyaṇī Saṃhitā (Maitrayani Samhita) mentions *sthunakarṇa*—post-shaped ears—and *vistṛtakarṇa*, broad ears—as auspicious signs linked to prosperity and cattle wealth. Such references suggest that ear morphology was valued not only symbolically but also in animal breeding, where these traits guided the selection of suitable bulls for breeding. Dedication of bulls for breeding purpose was a great ceremony. There were certain rules and regulations for selection of the animals for such purpose, as mentioned in Vishnu Purana. According to the Manusmṛti, bulls that are *hīnāga* (deformed), *vyādhita* (diseased), *klìva* (impotent), *ksudita* (hungry), *trista* (thirsty), and *śrānta* (fatigued) should be avoided for breeding purposes (Majumdar and Banerji 1960). Modern researchers have emphasized the importance of selecting and managing breeding bulls to achieve genetic improvements in dairy animals, thereby enhancing their milk production capacity (Dahiya 2005).

Modern Animal Breeding Literature Corroborating the Ancient Literature

Importance of Breeding and Phenomics: Animal breeding involves the selective breeding of domestic animals to improve desirable and heritable qualities in the next generation. Mankind started to create breeds accompanied with artificial selection 250 years ago. The decision to adopt improved genetics is an investment into future productivity based on current conditions including productivity of the animals. Nowadays, breeding of high productive farm animals, like cattle, pigs and poultry requires a heavy investment in state-of-the-art breeding programs (Ioan *et al.* 2020). Animal breeding improves animals by changing their genetic abilities to develop important traits that are based on the requirements of a society, which keep on changing with time. Population, quantitative and molecular genetics are influencing the trends in animal breeding. A breeding program is a circular activity in a generation the program is started with a breeding goal and ends with an evaluation of the results obtained in the next generation, and it might change the breeding goal for the next selection programme.

Elements of Animal Breeding: Breeding decisions depend upon a long process. Only the best parents are used for breeding and the average performance of the next generation will be better than that of the previous. Five very important aspects pertaining to animal breeding for consideration are: (i) the trait under selection is heritable (e.g. milk production or coat colour), (ii) animals must be from different genetic backgrounds to make selection possible, (iii) breeders decide the direction of selection, i.e., which animals are allowed to mate and to produce the next generation, (iv) success of animal breeding is judged by observing a shift in population average phenotype from one generation to the next and (v) success of animal breeding can be measured after the cumulative result of multiple generations of selection animal breeding works at population level, not automatically at individual level. In natural selection the animals that are better adapted to their environment have higher chances of survival than less adapted animals, and produce next generation, which is more adapted than the parents.

Utility of Linear Traits: Linear type traits describe the biological extremes of various visual characteristics of an animal. These traits are critical in the dairy industry due to their association with production, longevity, and profitability. The International Committee for Animal Recording (ICAR) has established a classification system for dairy cows based on these linear traits, which are of particular interest to breeders. Research has shown moderate to strong genetic correlations between certain type of traits and key indicators such as fertility measures and somatic cell count, offering opportunities for indirect selection to improve animal fertility and health within a selection index (Berry *et al.* 2004). Selecting animals based on linear traits has been associated with improvements in enhancing strength, stamina, survival and productivity in dairy cows (Boettcher *et al.* 1997, Cruickshank *et al.* 2002). Higher-yielding heifers tend to be more angular and have deeper udders (Brotherstone 2010). Lifetime production efficiency has significant relationships with conformation traits such as overall type, udder, legs, and feet (Tscharke and Banhazi 2016). Yield traits show positive correlations with rear udder height and rear udder width, but negative correlations with udder depth and attachment (Gibson *et al.* 2018). Positive and significant correlations between milk yield and udder measurements (length, width, and depth) have been observed in crossbreed cows (Patel *et al.* 2016). Modern machine vision technologies provide a revolutionary approach to classifying animals based on linear traits. These technologies can automatically analyse digital images of animals, potentially surpassing human expertise in precision and efficiency. The evidence underscores the pivotal role of linear type traits in improving the classification, selection, and management of dairy cows. By leveraging genetic insights and modern technologies, breeders can enhance the productivity, health, and profitability of dairy systems.

Animal Nutrition

Nutritional Practices: Ancient India has provided the most concrete identification of the art of feeding and management of animals for the economic benefit of man. The nutritional requirements of animals were met both from grazing and stall feeding. Scientific studies from Harappan sites in Gujarat indicate that animals were well-fed, with provisions made for year-round fodder availability, including green millet for cattle, buffaloes, and sheep and goats (Chakraborty *et al.* 2018,

Suryanarayan 2023). Barley was one of the most important grains during the Rigvedic period, and several references indicate that its cultivation was regarded as a significant agricultural activity. The Rig Veda explicitly mentions 'ploughing and sowing barley' (1.117.21) and invokes prosperity through barley in the prayer, 'Fill my hand, O Maghavan, with all that it can hold of barley, cut or gathered' (10.131.2). Importantly, barley also formed part of cattle feed, as reflected in the verse, 'The freed Kine eat the barley of the pious; I saw them as they wandered with the herdsman'(10.27.8). Sugarcane is also mentioned, and sesame residues after oil extraction served as fodder when animals were confined. The primarily pastoral Aryans settled in Punjab by clearing jungles, grazing cattle, and planting barley near villages for protection. Like the Gujjars of Jammu and Kashmir, they migrated long distances for pastures but returned home with their herds.

Animal Feeding: Apart from grass, straw and water (Panini 4.2.96), several vegetable substances, animal products, oil and oil-cake, rock-salt, sugar, etc., were used as animal diet giving nourishment to cattle, horse, mule, donkey and camel. Butter-milk was also used in diets of pig and dog (Arthshastra 2.24). According to Arthashastra, the king shall protect farmers from the molestation of oppressive fines, forced labour and taxes, and herds of cattle from thieves, tigers, poisonous creatures and cattle disease. The manner of the stock feeding was most important. The feeding depended upon breed and was done with definite rules. For bulls and horses in speed and working capacity, half a *bhara* (maund) of meadow grass, one *bhara* ordinary grass, one *tula* (100 palas) oil cake, ten *adhakas* bran, five *palas* salt, one *kudumba* oil for rubbing over the nose, one *drona* of barley or cooked black gram, one *drona* of milk, half *adhaka sura* (liquor), one *prastha* oil/ghee, ten *palas* sugar and one *palas* fruit were recommended. In general, 3/4 of all the above would form the food for mules, cows, and asses, and twice the quantity for buffaloes and camels (Krishnaswamy 1937a, b). Rations were provided on generous scale. The draught oxen and cows in milk were to be provided with food according to work load, and quantity of milk produced. All cattle should be provided with abundance of fodder and water. For bullocks, one *drona* of *masa* (*Phaselus radiatus*) or cooked barley along with other things prescribed for horses are the requisite quantity besides the additional provision of one *tula* oilcake or ten *adhakas* of bran (Krishnaswamy 1937c).

In Arthasastra, there is separate mention of straw *(trina)* and green grasses *(yavasa)*. Thus, there was a clear concept about green and dry fodder in the feeding of animals. Arthasastra has also recommended feeding of oil cakes. Ration for cows, buffaloes, mules, camels etc. have been described separately at several places. It states 'Bulls which are provided with nose strings and which are equal to horses in speed and carrying loads, are to be given half a *bhara* of meadow grass, twice the above quantity of ordinary grass *(trina)*, one *tula* (100 *palas*) of oil cakes, ten *adhikas* of bran, five *palas* of salt, one *kudumba* of oil for rubbing over the nose, one *prastha* of drink *(pana)*, one *tula* of flesh, one *adhika* of curd, one *drona* of barley or of cooked *urd (Vigna radiata)*, one drona of milk. or half an *adhika* of *sura* (liquor), one *prastha* of oil or ghee, ten palas of sugar or jaggery. One *pala* of fruit of *sringibera* (ginger) may be substituted for milk'. For cows, mules and asses, the diet was of the same commodities less by one quarter each. For buffaloes and camels, it was twice the quantity. Buttermilk (whey) was given as a drink to dogs and hogs. Moreover, all cattle were supplied with abundance of fodder and water. The quantity of the feed to be given was in proportion to the quantity of milk yielded by the cows or the duration of work in the case of bullocks (Shamasastry 1951). Arthashastra indicates that yield of milk and butter depends upon the nature of feed, soil and the quality of fodders. It is advocated that to increase the yield of milk, the cow should be given a few morsels composed of several sticks of *asvagandha* and sesame. Kalidasa, in his *Raghuvamsam sloka* 73, says that a piece of rock salt should always be kept in stable for horses and this is being practiced even to-day (Krishnaswamy 1937d). The Arthashastra recognizes the difference between straw and grass and the two are separately specified in the feed to be given to cattle, as *yavasa* (meadow or green grass) and *trina* (ordinary dry straw). Thorough-bred horses were recommended parched rice, drippings, minced meat, red rice-powder and grasses.

Drinking Water and Its Sources: Water was revered as a life-giver and valued as a healing and purifying agent in ancient Indian culture, as early as the Indus Valley Civilization. The Vedas, especially the Rig Veda, praise its medicinal and sustaining qualities: 'Amrta is in the waters; in the waters there is healing balm' and 'O Waters, teem with medicine to keep my body safe from harm' (1.23.19–21). Clean drinking water was procured for both people and livestock, as indicated in the Rig Veda: 'O Cow, at every season, and coming hitherward drink limpid water' (1.164.40). Sources included natural springs, rivers, lakes, and ponds, as well as man-made tanks and wells. Vedic texts classify water (*āpaḥ*) into forms such as rainwater (*divya*), flowing springs (*sravanti*), rivers, lakes, and dug-out waters (*khanitrimāḥ*), including wells (*kūpa*). Wells were vital for drinking and irrigation, often described metaphorically in Rig Veda hymns (1.130.2; 10.143.6). Safety concerns led to prayers for the protection of cattle from dangerous water sources, and to occasional well coverings (Rig Veda 1.88.4). Panini refers to watering places for cattle as *nipāna* and *ābhāva* (3.3.74), likely associated with wells, as was common in his time and remains so today (Agrawala 1953). Constructing ponds and wells was considered a meritorious act (*puṇya karma*), with kings and wealthy patrons often providing roadside wells for travellers and animals. This tradition endured into historical times, as recorded in Emperor Aśoka's Rock Edict II, which documents state-supported water facilities for humans and animals.

Pastures: Grazing on natural pastures constituted the principal feeding practice for livestock in ancient India. References in the Rig Veda and Atharva Veda indicate the regular practice of taking cattle to pasture fields. The Rig Veda (10.94.3; 10.102.5) refers to 'well-pastured bulls' and describes Mudgala as winning contests involving hundreds and thousands of cattle, underscoring the economic and ritual importance of wellmanaged grazing. Although cattle generally belonged to individual householders, pasture lands were commonly shared rather than privately owned. The Manusmriti reflects recognition of communal lands adjoining villages reserved for non-cultivated and common uses, where cattle could graze freely, indicating acceptance of shared grazing spaces rather than formally demarcated pastures. Kings were expected to make adequate provision for such communal lands while establishing villages, thereby supporting livestock-based rural economies. Buddhist literature also indicates the prevalence of pastoral practices. In the *Aṅguttara Nikāya*, particularly in the *Gopālaka Sutta*, the figure of the cowherd (*gopāla*) and references to suitable pasture (*gocara*), protection of cattle, and knowledge of seasonal conditions are employed as familiar analogies. The Arthashastra clearly outlines the organization of grazing resources. The king was to allocate uncultivable tracts as pasture grounds and uphold common grazing rights (2.2). It further prescribes specially designated forests, including royal game reserves and frontier public forests, reflecting systematic landuse planning. Village level administration was entrusted to the *gopa* (village accountant), responsible for recording boundaries and maintaining pasture registers (2.35–36). Destruction of pasture, such as by fire, was a punishable offence (4.11). Pastures, plains, and forests were open for cattle grazing, but owners were penalized if cattle strayed there after grazing or were maintained near pasture grounds (3.10). The cultivation of fodder crops and their preservation, including early forms of fodder conservation, are referenced in Vedic literature. Seasonal movement of herds between pastures enabled sustainable use of grazing resources. Vedic hymns addressed to Indra frequently invoke open pastures, abundant rainfall, and prosperity through cattle, underscoring the close relationship between grazing, divine favour, and agrarian livelihoods. Notably, communal grazing practices described in these ancient sources continue, in modified form, in several regions of modern India.

Graziers and Pasture Management: Grazing operations were overseen by graziers or cowherds (*gopāla*), employed by herd owners or village communities either on wages or a share of produce. They were responsible for animal identification, health, and safety. During musters, cattle were grouped by colour and marked with brand symbols, as noted in the Arthashastra (2.29). The Ashtadhyayi of Panini (4.3) refers to a drove of cattle (*samāja*) and a drive to pasture (*gochara, udaja*). Herds of cows and bulls grazing together were termed *gavāh*. Land once used for grazing but later abandoned was called *gauṣṭhina*, also referred to as *bhūtapūrva gauṣṭha*. The son of a cowherd who had attained the age to take cows out for grazing was called *anugavīna* This designation marked his readiness for pastoral responsibility and was analogous to *kavacabhara*—a term used for a *Kṣatriya* boy reaching maturity (Agrawala, 1953). After harvest, animals grazed freely in fields, while during crop growth, they were taken to designated grazing areas under a village-appointed herdsman. Graziers had to protect livestock from numerous natural dangers—quagmires, steep falls, drowning, lightning, predators such as tigers and crocodiles, snakebites, and forest fires. The Arthaśhāstra also cautions graziers to let cattle drink only from rivers or lakes that were uniformly deep, broad, and free of mire and crocodiles. Herdsmen were trained to identify individual cattle, treat wounds, protect animals from pests, manage pastures, recognize breeding bulls, and apply correct milking practices. They were advised to attach bells to the cattle's necks—to deter wild animals and help locate lost animals. Cowherds also ensured that some milk remained in the udder after milking, maintaining calf nourishment and udder health. In the event of an animal's death, the herdsman was required to return its skin, fat, bile, marrow, teeth, hooves, horns, and bones to the owner. For their services, Manu prescribed a heifer per year as wages for tending 100 cows, and for managing 200 milch cows, the herdsman was entitled to milk the herd once every eight days (Krishnaswamy 1937a, d).

Modern Animal Nutrition Literature Corroborating the Ancient Ideas

Nutrition: Important guidelines in the field of animal nutrition in the ancient literature are as follows:

- Green grasses and water were considered most nourishing feed for cattle to increase the milk-yield, and barley was the other important food for cattle (Rig Veda 1. 18-21, 135 ;10. 27).
- The other crop described in Rig Veda as fodder for animals is sugarcane. Leftovers of sesame *(til)* after extraction of oil were also used as feed, when animals were confined to home.
- It has been mentioned that cattle should graze freely so that they achieve a successful mating too and their further breeding (*Asva-Ayurveda* 11:26:1).
- All cattle were supplied with abundance of fodder and water. The quantity of the feed to be given was in proportion to the quantity of milk yielded by the cows.
- Kalidasa, in his Raghuvamsam sloka 73, says that a piece of rock salt should always be kept in stable for horses and this is being practiced even to-day (Krishnaswamy 1937 c).
- Common rights in pasture were recognized by states as per directions of Arthashastra.
- Feeding of chopped green sugarcane tops with concentrate mixture provided sufficient nutrients for maintenance and for moderate growth rate (Gendley *et al.* 2003).
- Sugarcane tops enriched with molasses can be fed to bulls in sugarcane growing areas for better intake and digestibility of nutrients (Huque and Rahman 2002).

- Daily weight gains were higher in rain tree *(Samanea saman)* pod-fed cattle (Hosamani *et al.* 2001).

- The most commonly fed tree leaves for livestock include jackfruit (*Artocarpus heterophyllus*), mango (*Mangifera indica*), *gular* (*Ficus racemosa*), *peepal* (*Ficus religiosa*), *mahua* (*Madhuca longifolia*), and *babul* (*Vachellia nilotica*). Additionally, nutritious fodder tree leaves from *ardu* (*Ailanthus excelsa*) and *siris* (*Albizia lebbeck*) are abundantly available in the region. However, these resources remain underutilized by farmers, despite their potential to provide a cost-effective feeding solution (Pandey 1997).

- Leaves from fodder tree species such as *anjan* (*Hardwickia binata*), *babul* (*Acacia nilotica*), *kardhai* (*Anogeissus latifolia*), *mahaneem* (*Melia azedarach*), and *siris* (*Albizia lebbeck*) are rich in nutrients for ruminants. These leaves are particularly suitable as supplements due to their favorable rumen degradability of dry matter, organic matter, and nitrogen (Singh *et al.* 1998).

- It has also been reported that cows, buffaloes, and draught animals are fed on *Albizia lebbeck* and Kharanu (*Carissa spinarum)*. The most common feeding practice involves mixing wheat, gram, and barley straw with green fodder or fresh stalks of maize, sorghum, pearl millet, and seasonal grasses such as *Dichanthium annulatum* and *Heteropogon contortus*. Additionally, cakes made from groundnut, mustard, castor, and linseed are commonly added to the feed of milch animals (Singh *et al.* 2003).

- Adult sheep grazing on semi-arid rangelands can maintain their body weight during the lean season by replacing concentrate mixtures with tree leaves from *Ailanthus excelsa*, *Azadirachta indica*, and *Bauhinia racemosa*. Supplementing with tree leaves offers advantages in nitrogen utilization due to the presence of condensed tannins. Additionally, using tree leaves such as *Prosopis cineraria*, *Acacia nilotica*, and *Albizia lebbeck* as supplements, rather than as sole feed, promotes better rumen fermentation patterns by minimizing excessive nitrogen loss (Bhatta *et al.* 2005a, 2005b). Supplementation of a mineral mixture and the leaves of *A. catechu, T. indica* and *L. leucocephala* in goat feeding for better health (Dhok *et al.* 2005).

- Tree leaves are an excellent source of crude protein and total digestible nutrients, making them well-suited to meet the dietary requirements of goats. For instance, *Ailanthus excelsa* can fully satisfy the maintenance needs of goats, while *Morus alba* is highly suitable for sheep. Additionally, the leaves of *Ficus benghalensis* are consumed in greater quantities by goats than by bulls (Mandal 1997). Given that tree leaves are often available at little to no cost, greater emphasis should be placed on their utilization for goat rearing—a practice advocated in ancient Indian literature.

Pasture: The feeding habits of cattle (calves, cows, and bullocks) and goats are significantly influenced by seasonal variations. Studies conducted on continuously grazed open grasslands dominated by *Cymbopogon distans* (lemon grass) with scattered *Quercus leucotrichophora* (banj or oak) trees in the Kumaun Himalayas revealed that grasses are the primary feed source during the wet season, while dead herbaceous biomass dominates in the dry season. Goats primarily rely on woody plants and tall forbs, which constitute 31–73% of their diet in both seasons. Uncontrolled livestock grazing and local land exploitation have led to the degradation of grazing lands and forests. To address this, the introduction of leguminous species is considered an effective strategy, along with the use of leaf fodder as a supplement to grasses. Planting various tree species and reclaiming *Usar* (barren) areas for pastures and fodder trees are also recommended measures to enhance fodder security for livestock (Shrivastava *et al.* 1995). Contemporary studies have shown that smaller households rely more heavily on common property resources (CPRs) for green fodder. Among bovines, local cattle make the most extensive use of CPRs (Dixit *et al.* 2001).

Animal Management in Ancient India

Ancient Indian civilization exhibited sophisticated and humane animal management practices, reflecting the profound cultural, religious, and economic significance of livestock. These practices were supported by a well-developed system of classification and a rich vocabulary that addressed various aspects of herd management. Animal welfare, including healthcare, was emphasized across all categories.

Animal Classification and Vocabulary: A rich and precise vocabulary was employed to distinguish among various classes and developmental stages of animals, reflecting the advanced understanding of animal husbandry in ancient India. Animals were systematically classified based on age, physiological condition, breed, coat colour, and intended purpose. Age was determined using specific physical markers such as the number of teeth, horn development, and the size of the hump. For example, a young calf with two teeth was referred to as *dvidan*, while one with a horn approximately one *aṅgula* in length (about 1.763 cm) was called *aṅgula-śṛṅga*. Heifer cows that had reached puberty were termed *upasaryā*, and grammarian referred to a superior-quality cow as *mahāgṛṣṭhi* (Agrawala, 1953). Cattle were further classified by coat colour—such as red, black, dappled, and light-coloured—and by their utility in tasks like ploughing, milking, or breeding. Herds were also managed using distinctive ear notches for each animal, allowing for accurate record-keeping and individual identification.

Neonatal Care: Care of a newly born calf and its mother is also mentioned in ancient literature. The neonate shall be washed as soon as it comes out. The udder of the mother is also washed and the young one is allowed to suck. If the young remain attached to the uterus, treatment for the expulsion of foetus and placenta may be given. The treatment comprised *sidhu* two seer, *trikatu* half *paav* and honey half *seer*. Food should be given after parturition. Because of the parturition, the abdominal cavity of a mare gets disturbed, hence it should be given half seer ghee together with fresh food like barley, *doob* grass, and *kulthi*. Mare and foal should be bathed on the tenth day. The colt shall be given a mixture of fresh butter and honey to lick till it is one month old (honey 250 g and butter 50 g). The feed consists of washed wheat, honey, and *ghee* (Krishnaswamy 1937a, d).

Dentition: Age of animals was judged by the condition of teeth. For example, young cows and bulls with two permanent teeth were approximately 2–2.5 years old; those with four teeth about 3 years; six teeth about 3.5 years; and eight teeth about 4 years. The chapter on the age of horses in the '*Saloter*' commences with the following rhyme-

'Examine well their teeth with caution sage, that thence you may determine what their age.'

The natural life of a horse is 32 years, during the first five of which he sheds his teeth and they grow, again...... The *Sukraniti* tells how to judge a bull's age from its teeth.

Castration: A young bull selected for draught purposes (*balivarda*) was fitted with a nose ring, tamed, and castrated (*damya*) at the age of three years (Ashtadhyayi 3.2.25, Agrawala). Castration of sheep and stallion is mentioned in the Rig Veda, and that of cattle is found in the Yajur Veda (Tatriya Samhita).

Milk and Milking: According to Arthashastra, the cowherd was responsible for milking cows. Milking was done either once in the morning (summer and spring) or twice i.e. in the morning and evening (rains, autumn and first part of winter). This was done because there was plenty of grass in the pastures in the rainy season and early winter, and in summer the pastures dried up. Apart from milk of bovine species, goat and sheep-milk also formed a part of dairy products (Arthashastra 1. 29). Ghee was included in animal rations, with elephants in particular receiving three *prasthas* of ghee per day along with other feed articles. in animal rations, with elephants in particular receiving three *prasthas* of ghee per day along with other feed articles.

Cattle Husbandry: In Rig Veda clear instructions are given on animal nourishment and feeding practices. Green grasses and water were regarded as the most nourishing provisions for cattle, contributing to increased milk yield, while barley was considered another preferred feed for milch cows. As stated, 'at once the cows yield milk; the barley meal is prepared for thee' (Rig Veda 1.135.8). Panning was another important step of rearing. Two types of abodes were built for cattle, open pasturage *(gostha)* and cow stall *(gosala)*. At night and in the heat of the day the cows seem to have been kept in the fold; while for the rest of the day they were allowed to wander at will. Bulls' horns were cast off (Panini 1.2.25). Cows were milked three times a day as reflected in Rig Veda (1.76. 3), 'Yea, come at milking time, at early morning, at noon of day and when the Sun is setting.' Prosperity in cows and calves was blessed with the expression *svasti bhavate sagave savalsaya* (*Kātyāyana* 6.3.83, Agrawala 1953). There was capital punishment for stealing a cow or hurting one. The Arthashastra ordains, 'Whoever hurts or causes another to hurt, or steals or causes another to steal a cow, should be slain.'

Care of Draught Cattle: Oxen were used for the normal purposes of ploughing and farm transport. The rains have fallen, and the ploughing of fields begins. The first ploughing of the season was inaugurated amidst much ritual. Here are hymns addressed to Shuna, Sita and Shunashira. Addressed to Shuna: 'May the oxen draw happily; the men labour happily; the plough furrow happily; may the traces bind happily; wield the goad happily.' Addressed to Sita (the earth goddess): 'Auspicious Sita, be present, we glorify thee; that thou mayest be propitious to us; that thou mayest yield us abundant fruit. May Indra take hold of Sita; may Pushan guide her; may she, well-stored with water; yield it as milk year after year.' Addressed to Shunashira: 'May the plough-shares break up our land happily; may the plough go happily with the oxen; may Parjanya water the earth with sweet showers happily; grant, Shuna and Shira, prosperity to us'. Here is reference to ploughs and ploughing. 'Our auspicious ploughs with their ornamental handles, and their sharp-pointed shares, cleave the ground to the happiness of cows, sheep and well-grown maidens' (Krishnaswamy 1937a). The ploughs were wooden and so were the ploughshares. The *Perumpanatrupadai,* another ancient Tamil poem of the Sangam Age (Before Second Century BCE), also describes the ploughing with bullocks. 'The land is ploughed with the aid of bullocks and male buffaloes. The surplus produce is sent by carts to be sold in different parts of the country. Carts carrying imported goods are also much in evidence. Because of this trade the peasants are enriched and live a happy life.'

Literary and legal sources indicate that only healthy cattle were yoked, while hungry, thirsty, tired, deformed, or diseased animals were avoided. When eight oxen were employed for a plough, they were worked for a full day; when four were used, work was limited to half a day; and when only two were available, to a quarter of a day. Causing a bull belonging to a herd to fight with another bull attracted a fine, and injury to a bull resulted in heavier penalties. The perceived usefulness of an animal largely determined whether it was regarded as sacred or otherwise. The nature of punishment also varied with the physiological and health status of animals. Cattle had fully proved their usefulness in the Mauryan age by the milk they provided to the people, and their draught power in cultivation.

***Superintendent of Cows* (*Go-Adhyaksha*):** The *Go-Adhyaksha* was responsible for overseeing milch cattle herds and managing the storage of milk and ghee. He supervised cowherds, buffalo herdsmen, milkers, churners, and hunters, ensuring that calves received sufficient milk. Herds were maintained with a balanced mix of milch cows, pregnant cows, aged cows, heifers, and calves, while special groups included crippled or difficult-to-milk cows. The superintendent branded all cattle—including calves over two months old and unclaimed strays—and registered them, noting natural markings, colour, and horn spacing.

Buffalo Cult in Indian Tradition: Ancient Hindu, Buddhist and Jain scriptures are full of reverence to nature and link many animals to spiritualty and symbolism. Devine elephant (*Airāwat*), horse (*Uchaisravā*), and cow (*Kamdhenu*) are produced as part of 14 gems during the churning of the cosmic ocean. All of these achieved the status of divine deity companions and were thus regarded as important parts of both the human and spiritual worlds. In Hindu religion, Lord Shiva is described as the master and protector of animals (*Pashupati*). According to the Arthashastra, cows were sacred animals, and killing of them was considered a grave sin. One of a king's primary duties was to worship a cow, her calf, and a bull by circling around them before attending court. By this time, buffaloes had also gained recognition as dairy animals. A Sanchi sculpture illustrating a *Jataka* tale depicts two buffaloes swimming in a pool near a hermitage. Mahiṣī refers to the buffalo, whose milk is traditionally used in Ayurveda for treating snake bites. According to the *Vṛkṣāyurveda* by Sūrapāla (ca. 1000 CE), buffalo (Mahiṣī) dung is utilized in specific bio-organic recipes for inducing plant mutagenesis (https://www.wisdomlib.org/definition/mahisi, accessed on 6-1-2025). In mythology, *Mahiṣa* a buffalo-headed man (Fig. 3.8), was a demi-god revered by indigenous pastoral communities known for their milk production and grazing practices. Mahiṣa was believed to possess the extraordinary ability to transform between human and buffalo forms. The cult of Mahiṣa continues to thrive in various forms among pastoral tribes in India, such e.g., Gonds and Maria Gonds tribes in central India, the *Katkaris* of western India, and the Todas of the Nilgiri Hills. The city of Mysore in Karnataka is said to derive its name from Mahisa (*Mahisa-ur*).

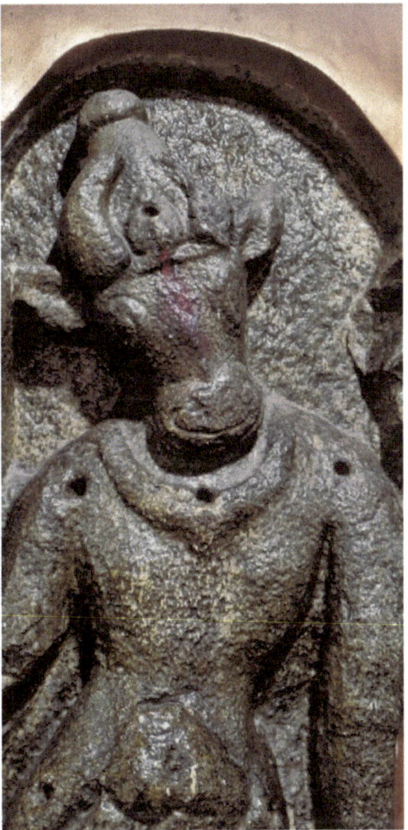

***Fig. 3.8.** Stone sculpture of a buffalo at Kamakhya Devi Temple, Guwahati, Assam (Photo courtesy of Dr. R. Somvanshi).*

Interestingly, a tribal community called Mahiṣī still exists in Karnataka (Krishna 2010), maintaining ties to this rich cultural heritage.

Animal Husbandry and Animal Welfare Guidelines and Rules: Several measures were instituted for the preservation of animal life, including prohibitions on slaughter, unethical injury, and the killing of animals. The infliction of physical harm on livestock attracted strict penalties. *Dharmaśāstra* (Dharmashastras) literature, including the Parashar Samhita (Parāśara Saṁhitā 9.1–50, Dutta 1908), enumerates acts detrimental to animal welfare and prescribes corresponding punishments. Offences included killing a cow or bullock, causing injury through negligence, branding that resulted in burns, overloading, beating, or driving animals into inaccessible terrain. However, restraint for legitimate purposes—such as ensuring safety, administering medical or surgical treatment, or managing dystocia—was not penalised, reflecting a nuanced understanding of animal management. Regulations also addressed housing, feeding, and humane handling practices. Soft ropes made of *kuśa* grass were recommended for tethering cows, whereas harsher materials, such as iron chains, were discouraged. For goading cattle, only a twig of prescribed dimensions—equal to the width of a thumb in girth, a cubit in length, and tipped with fresh, undried leaves—was permitted; the use of any other instrument was considered sinful, underscoring the ethical emphasis on minimising pain and cruelty. Beyond agrarian animals, war animals such as horses and elephants received careful management and protection. They were equipped with protective armour—chain mail and plate coverings—to safeguard vulnerable body parts during battle.

Detailed provisions governed work and production practices. Load limits were specified for draught animals, and milking frequencies were regulated according to season. Seasonal schedules were also prescribed for shearing sheep and goats. Plough oxen could work throughout the day provided adequate numbers were assigned per plough, whereas smaller teams were required to receive periodic rest. Draught horses were worked according to their capacity and were not employed immediately after feeding in order to prevent illness. The Arthashastra further elaborates administrative measures for the supervision, care, and health management of state-owned animals. Non-compliance with these provisions, or acts of cruelty towards animals, could result in severe penalties.

Elephant Husbandry: In ancient India, elephant husbandry held great cultural, religious, and economic significance, with elephants being meticulously captured, trained, and managed for use in warfare, royal processions, ceremonial rituals, and heavy-duty tasks, as described in texts like the Arthashastra and *Gajaśāstra*. According to the Arthashastra, whoever killed an elephant was sentenced to death. Whoever brought tusks of an elephant from an animal died naturally, was duly rewarded. Males above 20 years of age were captured. Female and young elephants were not captured. Procedure of capturing of elephants stipulated in Arthashastra was as follows: Guards of elephant forests, assisted by those who rear elephants, those who enchain the legs of elephants, those who guard the boundaries, those who live in forests, as well as by those who nurse elephants, shall, with the help of five or seven female elephants, help in tethering wild ones. Trace the whereabouts of herds of elephants following the course of urine and dung passed by them. They shall also precisely ascertain whether any mark is due to the movement of elephants in herds, elephant roaming single, stray elephant, leader of herds, tusker, rogue elephant, elephant in rut, young elephant or elephant that has escaped from the cage. Experts in catching elephants shall follow the instructions given to them by the elephant doctor *(anikastha)*, and catch such elephants as are possessed of auspicious characteristics and good character. The captured elephants were given military training of seven kinds, viz. drill, turning, advancing, trampling down and killing, fighting with other elephants, attacking forts and cities and warfare. The elephants under training were provided with collars and were made to work in company with trained elephants (Shamasastry 1951).

Horse Keeping and Equine Husbandry: The horse was a multipurpose animal of exceptional socio-economic, military, and political importance in ancient India. Early Vedic literature associates the horse (*aśva*) with speed, endurance, vitality, and martial strength. The Rig Veda praises swift and well-trained horses as essential to chariot warfare, sports, and ritual processions, often likening the movement of gods and warriors to powerful steeds. Horses formed the backbone of *ratha* (chariot) warfare, and a chariot driven by trained horses constituted a formidable force on the battlefield, as reflected in the Rig Veda (1.5.4): 'Whose pair of tawny horses, yoked in battles, foemen challenge not'. Horses harnessed to chariots are frequently described in Vedic and Epic texts as responding to reins, voice commands, and battlefield stimuli, indicating advanced training and close human–animal coordination. References in the Mahabharata, the Asthadhyayi, the Puranas, the works attributed to Shalihotra, and the Arthashastra distinguish superior from inferior horses on the basis of physical traits, performance, and temperament, reflecting early concepts of selective breeding, quality assessment, and systematic training.

The Arthashastra (2.30) codifies equine husbandry as a regulated state function and provides detailed guidelines for housing, feeding, and training. Royal horses were placed under the charge of a Superintendent of Horses (*Aśvādhayakṣa*), who maintained records of breed, age, colour, and place of origin. Horses were kept in well-planned stables, with steeds, stallions, and colts housed separately to ensure effective control, safety, and breeding management. Individual stalls were proportionate to the size of the animal, with smooth flooring to facilitate comfort and rolling, separate fodder compartments (*khādanakoṣṭhakam*), and efficient drainage for waste removal, reflecting an advanced understanding of hygiene and animal welfare. Stable entrances facing north or east suggest careful consideration of ventilation, climatic suitability, and environmental comfort. Training and conditioning were integral to equine management, and equal emphasis was placed on regulated feeding and healthcare, particularly during physiologically sensitive periods. The Arthashastra prescribes special post-partum care for mares, recommending energy-rich and medicinal diets immediately after foaling, followed by a gradual transition to cooked grains, meadow grass, and seasonally appropriate fodder. This indicates an empirical understanding of nutrition, recovery, and reproductive management. Horses underwent systematic exercises involving slow and circular movements, jumping, galloping, and various forms of riding to enhance strength, coordination, and battlefield manoeuvrability. Controlled grazing through tethering or hobbling, selective gelding of stallions to improve tractability, and the use of mares as draught animals for chariots demonstrate functional differentiation based on temperament and utility.

Animal Housing

Several ancient Indian texts, such as Kautilya's Arthashastra and Puranic literature—most notably the Agni Purana, Garuda Purana, and Matsya Purana—provide guidelines on animal housing and management. The *Kṛṣi-Saṃgraha* (Krishi Samagraha), a medieval Sanskrit compilation that consolidates ancient agronomic wisdom into a single manual on agriculture, is traditionally attributed to Kṛṣṇarāja (Krishnaraja) and dated to around the 12th–13th century CE. This text outlines detailed rules for the construction and sanitation of cattle sheds, the employment of cattle, and hygienic practices. It recommends cattle sheds measuring 55 cubits square, with due consideration of solar orientation, regular removal of dung to maintain animal health, separate housing for goats and cattle, and avoidance of storing cotton, husk, tools, or stale food in cowsheds. Periodic fumigation with deodar (*Cedrus deodara*), asafoetida (*Ferula asafoetida*), and mustard seeds, as well as planting an asafoetida tree near the shed, is advised to improve sanitation (Krishnaswamy 1937c, d).

Housing varied across different agro-ecological regions, utilizing locally available, low-cost materials for constructing animal shelters. Each shelter's design was adapted to the local environment and the specific species and types of animals being housed. Special accommodations were made for young and pregnant animals to ensure their safety. Additionally, region-specific plantations of beneficial trees and plants were done around the animal shelters. The animal welfare and husbandry and housing considered as the earliest known treatise on agriculture, also provides insight on farming practices including animal husbandry, animal welfare and guidelines for animal housing (Box 3.4). Many of these practices are relevant to this date.

Box 3.4. *Krishi Parashara (Krsi-Parāśara) and Guidance on Animal Husbandry*

Attributed to the sage Parashara (4th century BCE–4th century CE), Krishi Parashara is a foundational Sanskrit text on Indian agricultural science. Though brief, with about 243 verses in a single chapter, it offers valuable insights into seasonal farming, environmental awareness, and sustainable practices. It emphasizes harmony between nature and agriculture, making it a key part of India's traditional agrarian heritage. The text includes over 30 verses on animal husbandry, highlighting the ethical use, care, feeding, housing, and welfare of draught animals, especially bullocks. It advocates humane treatment, condemns the exploitation of animals, and links animal well-being with agricultural success. Essene of select verses based on English translation (Majumdar and Banerji, 1960) include:

- *A diligent farmer who treats cows kindly, goes regularly to fields, sows in season, and avoids idleness prospers in all crops (v.83).*
- *Farming should not cause pain to draught animals; grains obtained through their suffering is unfit for rituals (v.84).*
- *Corns earned through animal cruelty are doomed to perish (v.85).*
- *Proper nourishment, morning and evening grazing, and the use of molasses, fodder and smoke keep draught animals healthy (v.86).*
- *Well-constructed, clean sheds promote animal health, even with minimal feeding (v.87).*
- *Hygiene is ineffective where animals are routinely covered in dung and urine (v.88).*
- *Use of cow urine for cleaning excrements worsens conditions for draught animals (v.92).*
- *Cows avoid dark, unclean shelters devoid of prosperity (v.94).*
- *Using only two bulls for ploughing is condemned; a proper plough team should consist of at least six bulls (v.96).*
- *Pairs of black, red, or black-and-red bulls are ideal for ploughing; their faces should be anointed with ghee (v.134).*

Scientific Relevance of Animal Management in Ancient Indian Literature

Housing: Important instructions on animal management available in ancient Indian literature were compiled by Krishnaswamy (1937 c, d).

- Housing is different for different agro-ecological regions depending upon the climate of the area.
- Special practices e.g. planting of specific trees/plants around the shelter and their benefits etc. are also region-specific.

- Locally available low-cost housing material is the most appropriate material for making animal houses.
- The local environment and the animal species to be cared decide the housing design.
- Young and pregnant animals need special housing design.

Farmers in Andhra Pradesh employ innovative designs to construct goat shelters that balance protection, utility, and sustainability. Shelters are built on stilts and covered with bamboo mats. The roofs are made of bamboo and overlaid with wild grass. This design effectively protects goats from predators. Slatted bamboo flooring allows goat faeces to fall directly onto the field, enhancing soil fertility. Sheep and goat pens are commonly set up on farmland to house the animals during the day or night. In Maharashtra, bovine shelters are specifically designed to suit the local climate across different seasons. During the monsoon and winter, these shelters provide adequate protection, while for summer, roofs and walls are constructed using locally sourced materials, ensuring comfort for the animals in hot conditions (Anthra 2006).

Scientists have found effects of flooring material on growth rate in goats. Goats housed on cement flooring exhibited the lowest weight gain across all age groups, while those on sand flooring demonstrated the highest growth rates, particularly in the 15-day age group. Conversely, goats in the 5-month age group on cement flooring showed the slowest growth (Panigrahi 2005). A *kuccha* floor with a thatched roof shed offers practical economic benefits and provides a more suitable environment for female kids compared to a concrete floor with a concrete roof (Champak and Nagpaul, 2005). Also, the microenvironment of shelters significantly influences the physiological responses of goats. For hot-dry climates, an east-west orientation is recommended (Kumar *et al.* 1993). Overall, proper housing plays a crucial role in enhancing productivity and profitability in goat farming. The type of shelter significantly affects the behavior of dairy cattle. Studies show that cows are more comfortable in loose housing during summer and the rainy season, while a loose housing system with a central shed is preferable during winter (Sharma and Singh 2002).

Traditional Husbandry: Challenges and Limitations

In the modern era, India faces a twin challenge of sustainable management of its huge cattle inventory while improving the productivity of animals and profitability of farmers within the minimum possible time. This is coupled with other challenges and hindrances in terms of the limited resources and the ever-looming threat of climate change. Various other hindrances potentially hamper the efficient usage of available genetic resources. The low productivity of indigenous milch cattle is mainly due to the non-availability of improved breeds, besides many other factors. The recent improvement in the milk production status of India points towards the scope for possible genetic improvement in indigenous cattle. Therefore, there is a need to improve their productivity using modern genetic approaches coupled with improvement in different facets of breeding, feeding and healthcare management.

Factors affecting the optimal profitability and productivity of Indian livestock, especially under traditional dairy production system include large non-descript and uncharacterized population; crossbreeding by non-tested bulls, semen and artificial insemination (AI) facility; lower conception rate using AI; most of the marginal farmers with a minimal herd size of 1-2 cattle along with their scattered distribution; low productivity; survivability stress due to agricultural mechanization; disease outbreaks limiting the reproduction as well as production performance; climate change; inadequate natural resource base; fluctuating market support; low prices of by-products; and competition for feed resources with humans, to cite a few. Climate change in India is posing immense challenges to cattle husbandry. Cattle rearing sub-sector is largely unorganized due to poor or absence of critical resources and services, and inadequate market-supply chain. In most Indian states, livestock keeping is based on traditional practices with local social conditions and mainly on feeding local food resources like straw (rice and wheat). The cattle production systems are to be developed for improving the productivity of animals and the income of farmers involved in cattle farming.

According to 20th Livestock Census, about 74% of India's cattle are local breeds or nondescript types, generally yielding less milk than crossbreeds, largely due to limited genetic improvement, breeding strategies, nutrition, and herd management rather than inherent economic weakness Milk yield varies widely across states and production systems, with management intensity being a key factor (Kale *et al.* 2018). Indigenous cattle also show later first calving, longer dry periods, and extended calving intervals under traditional systems, further reducing lifetime productivity. Other common concerns affecting the traditional animal husbandry in the country are:

- **Lack of proper veterinary care**: Traditional practices often lack access to modern veterinary services, resulting in higher mortality and disease rates among livestock.
- **Overgrazing and environmental degradation**: In some areas, overgrazing leads to land degradation and loss of biodiversity, especially with limited land management strategies.
- **Limited market access**: Farmers engaged in traditional practices may face difficulties accessing commercial markets and value chains, limiting their economic benefits.
- **Pressure of modernization**: With the push for modernization, traditional practices are often neglected, leading to a loss of indigenous knowledge and practices.

New Horizon

In the modern era, India faces a dual challenge: sustainably managing its vast cattle population while simultaneously enhancing animal productivity and farmer profitability within a minimal timeframe. These challenges are compounded by limited resources and the persistent threat of climate change. Several obstacles also hinder the efficient utilization of available genetic resources. The low productivity of indigenous milch cattle is primarily attributed to the lack of improved breeds, among other factors. However, recent advancements in milk production in India highlight the potential for genetic improvement in indigenous cattle. To address these issues, modern genetic approaches, combined with advancements in breeding, feeding, and healthcare management, are essential.

Documentation

India comprises 120 agro-ecoregions, each supporting livestock well-adapted to its specific climate, nutritional resources, and management practices. Traditional farmer knowledge, rooted in centuries-old practices, plays a crucial role in sustaining these systems. Today, farmers need access to best practices, including selecting superior animals for profitable dairy enterprises. Historically, farmers have relied on visual inspection of prominent animal features to determine good dairy characteristics. Over time, this practice evolved into a classification system based on morphological traits, also known as linear type traits. Animal breeders have developed scientific methods to assess these traits for selecting the best animals. According to the International Committee for Animal Recording (ICAR), dairy cows are graded as excellent, very good, good plus, good, fair, poor, or insufficient based on individual scores derived from both general characteristics and composite traits. The primary composite traits used for evaluating dairy cattle include frame (including rump structure), dairy strength, mammary system, and legs and feet (ICAR Conformation Recording Guidelines, accessed on 06-09-2025). These traits are strongly correlated with performance traits, as documented by ICAR. However, measuring and scoring these traits in Indian dairy cattle can be challenging, time-consuming, and stressful for the animals. Consequently, experienced farmers or experts often classify dairy animals visually, focusing on two or three traits, such as hip bone structure, to judge an animal's health. This approach becomes more complex when classification involves multiple traits.

Applications of Artificial Intelligence and Machine Vision in Animal Science

The advent of artificial intelligence (AI) has transformed livestock farm management. AI technology, leveraging sensors, IoT devices, and data analytics, enables real-time monitoring and analysis of animal behavior, health, and production performance (Hamadani *et al.* 2024). This technology facilitates early disease detection, precise feeding schedules, and optimized resource allocation, improving animal welfare, productivity, and cost-effectiveness.

In animal breeding, AI has revolutionized genetic selection and optimization. Machine learning algorithms process vast amounts of genetic data, allowing breeders to identify desirable traits and predict breeding outcomes with precision. This enables the selection of superior animals, preservation of genetic diversity, and the development of healthier, more productive livestock. AI's ability to analyse real-time data significantly enhances decision-making, operational efficiency, and animal welfare.

Advances in computer vision and machine learning have further expanded the capabilities of AI in animal science. These technologies can automatically analyse images of morphological traits for classifying animals. Databases of morphological trait images are used to train and test deep learning algorithms. Applications of machine vision in animal science include breed classification, body condition scoring, unique identification, behaviour analysis, disease diagnosis, and precision dairy farming. Despite these advancements, classifying the dairyness of animals based on linear type traits remains a significant challenge.

Breeding

Estimating linear type traits or morphological characteristics for evaluating a cow's dairyness is a common practice in modern dairy farms developed in America in 1980s. Automatic measurement of morphological traits through image analysis is found to replace manual appraisal. Automated systems are swift, more convenient, and risk-free, making them a viable replacement for manual appraisal. Key morphological traits such as strength, body depth, dairy form, teat placement, stature, rump angle, and udder characteristics are crucial in determining the dairyness of cattle breeds (Qian *et al.* 2008). By employing machine learning algorithms, AI processes extensive genetic data, enabling breeders to accurately identify desirable traits and predict breeding outcomes.

Animal Nutrition

AI plays a transformative role in optimizing animal nutrition by analysing large datasets to provide insights into feeding habits. This helps farmers tailor feeding practices to meet specific nutritional requirements, improving animal health and productivity while reducing costs and environmental impact. AI-driven feeding systems can calculate and dispense precise feed quantities tailored to individual animals (Saar *et al.* 2022, Wang *et al.* 2023). Algorithms analyse factors such as weight, body condition, and growth rate to create customized feeding plans minimize overfeeding and underfeeding, promoting optimal growth and reducing nutritional wastes (Qiao *et al.* 2021). Incorporating visual algorithms and Red Green Blue – Depth (RGBD) cameras, facilitate the accurate collection of feed intake data eanabling their meticulously analysis (Muir *et al.* 2020). These systems hold significant potential for tailoring feeding plans based on traditional knowledge and local feeds.

Animal Living Environment Management

The integration of AI into animal welfare management represents a significant advancement. AI-driven systems regularly monitor key environmental factors such as temperature, humidity, and air quality, ensuring optimal living conditions for animals (Patel *et al.,* 2022). These systems automatically adjust ventilation, heating, or cooling parameters to maintain a comfortable environment, reducing stress and disease prevalence while improving productivity. Earlier efforts in environmental monitoring focused on managing ammonia levels, but recent advancements also include monitoring carbon dioxide, sulphur dioxide, and nitrogen dioxide. Models are developed to predict levels of various gases and particulate matter using AI algorithms integrated with observational data and sensors (Almalawi *et al.* 2022). This real-time forecasting enhances living conditions, supporting healthier and more productive animals.

Conclusion

Traditional animal husbandry in India has been practiced for centuries, deeply rooted in the country's agrarian culture. It primarily involved small-scale, family-owned farms where livestock was raised for milk, meat, and labour. Indigenous breeds were well-adapted to local conditions, and practices were largely sustainable, relying on natural resources and traditional knowledge passed down through generations. Today, traditional animal husbandry coexists with modern and conventional systems. While many small-scale farmers still rely on traditional methods, there has been a shift towards more intensive and commercialized practices. The focus has expanded to include improved breeding techniques, better feed and nutrition, and enhanced veterinary care. There is a growing emphasis on organic and eco-friendly farming methods, which align with traditional practices. Efforts are being made to preserve indigenous breeds and promote their unique qualities. Additionally, government initiatives and policies aim to support small-scale farmers, improve infrastructure, and provide access to markets and technology. The future holds potential for a more resilient and sustainable animal husbandry system that benefits both farmers and the environment. However, challenges such as low productivity of indigenous breeds, limited access to resources, climate change, and market fluctuations continue to impact traditional farmers.

The modern observations that phenotypic traits could be used through machine learning proves the utility of phenotypic traits, which is an age-old tradition. The information given in our ancient literature is mainly on (i) relationship between phenotypic and economic traits (identifying economically important animals);

(ii) use of local feed resources and quantity as per physiological state of animal; and (iii) housing as per the local climate and using local resources. This ancient information can help farmers and researchers in breeding, nutrition and housing at low cost (Kumar 2003). The application of AI and machine vision in traditional animal husbandry opens new horizons for sustainable livestock management. These technologies enable precise genetic selection, optimized feeding, and enhanced environmental control, contributing to improved animal welfare and productivity.

Despite limited scientific evidence, A2 milk protein is widely believed to be more easily digestible and to offer various health benefits compared to A1 milk protein. Notably, human breast milk predominantly contains β-casein of the A2 type. Some researchers suggest that A2 milk is gentler on the human digestive system because it lacks A1 β-casein, which is associated with β-casomorphin-7 (BCM7)—a compound that may cause inflammation and digestive discomfort. In 2016, a double-blind, randomized, controlled crossover study investigated plasma glutathione concentrations in healthy individuals. The study revealed a significant increase in plasma glutathione levels following the consumption of milk containing only A2 β-casein. In contrast, no such increase was observed after consuming milk with a combination of A1 and A2 β-casein. This finding suggests that A2 β-casein milk may have a unique advantage in promoting glutathione production, a key antioxidant in the human body. The global A2 milk market has experienced steady growth in recent years, particularly in the fast-expanding Asian market, where dairy consumption is on the rise. Increased consumer awareness of the potential health benefits of A2 milk has been a major driver of this market growth (Jeong *et al.*2024). Majority of Indian zebu cattle and riverine buffalo breeds have A1/A2 milk variant. This unique trait of Indian cattle and buffaloes should be validated using rigorous clinical studies to boost income of traditional dairy farmers and conservation of indigenous bovine germ plasm.

In ancient times, bulls held great significance for breeding purposes. Modern research reinforces the importance of selecting and managing breeding bulls to achieve genetic improvements in dairy animals, thereby enhancing their milk production capacity. The ancient knowledge of animal husbandry offers cost-effective solutions to many prevalent challenges in the livestock sector, particularly when adapted to the specific needs of local areas. Understanding traditional Indian practices related to breeding, nutrition, and livestock management can contribute to the development of technologies that are both appropriate and widely accepted within local farming systems. Such an approach can support sustainable farming and cost-effective veterinary solutions, especially in compliance with Sanitary and Phytosanitary (SPS) and Hazard Analysis and Critical Control Point (HACCP) regulations.

The digitization of ancient knowledge on animal sciences is crucial for modern applications. The livestock sector, vital for rural development, requires low-cost inputs and technologies tailored to local conditions. Ancient Indian literature contains such valuable insights, which need to be systematically collected, analyzed, and compared with modern scientific findings. To achieve this, policies must be established for the subject coverage of databases, data collection, acquisition of relevant materials, and literature selection criteria. This database would not only preserve traditional knowledge but also address future intellectual property rights issues. The Vedas highlight the significance of livestock, with hymns stating: 'May we escape poverty by means of cattle.' As demand for livestock products increases, it is expected to improve the income of those involved in the livestock sector. Ancient texts also emphasize the value of cows, referring to them as '*Dhenuh sadanam rayinam*' or 'the cow is the mine of wealth.' By integrating modern innovations with traditional knowledge, India can effectively tackle the dual challenges of sustainable livestock management and improved profitability. This synergy can pave the way for a more efficient and sustainable future in animal husbandry. Ultimately, the future of traditional animal husbandry in India lies in combining sustainable practices with modern advancements to ensure long-term benefits for the sector.

References

Abhiram MJ and Rathish RL. 2020. A comparative study on the indigenous traditional animal husbandry practices among four major animal rearing tribal population of Wayanad district, Kerala. *Asian Journal of Agricultural Extension, Economics and Sociology* **38**(8):162-72.

Agrawala VS. 1953. Fauna. In: *India Known to Pānini (A Study of Cultural Material the Ashtādhyāyi)* pp. 218-28. University of Lucknow, Lucknow https://ignca.gov.in/Asi_data/4695.pdf retrieved on 23-11-2023.

Almalawi A, Alsolami F, Khan AI, Alkhathlan A, Fahad A, Irshad K, Qaiyum S and Alfakeeh AS. 2022. An IoT based system for magnify air pollution monitoring and prognosis using hybrid artificial intelligence technique. *Environmental Research* **206:**112576. https://doi.org/10.1016/j.envres.2021.112576.

Anonymous. 2019. *20th Livestock Census-2019: All India Report.* Animal Husbandry Statistic Division, Department of Animal Husbandry and Dairying Ministry of Fisheries, Animal Husbandry and Dairying, New Delhi, India. https://dahd.nic.in/ahs-division/20th-livestock-census-2019-all-india-report, pdf downloaded on 23-04-2024.

Anthra. 2006. *Proceedings of National Workshop on Indigenous Knowledge Application for Livestock Care.* 14-17 September 2004. Anthra, Secunderabad, Andhra Pradesh, India.

Berry DP, Buckley F, Dillon P, Evans RD and Veerkamp RF. 2004. Genetic relationships among linear type traits, milk yield, body weight, fertility and somatic cell count in primiparous dairy cows. *Irish Journal of Agricultural and Food Research* **43**:161-76.

Bhatta R, Vaithiyanathan S, Singh NP, Shinde AK and Verma DL. 2005a. Effect of feeding tree leaves as supplements on the nutrient digestion and rumen fermentation pattern in sheep grazing on semi-arid range of India. *Small Ruminant Research* **60**(3): 273-80.

Bhatta R, Vaithiyanathan S, Singh NP, Shinde AK and Verma DL. 2005b. Effect of tree leaf as supplementation on nutrient digestion and rumen fermentation pattern in sheep grazing semi-arid range of India - II. *Small Ruminant Research* **60**(3): 281-88.

Birthal PS, Taneja VK and Thorpe W. 2006. Smallholder livestock production in India: Opportunities and challenges. In: *Proceedings of National Centre for Agricultural Economics and Policy Research- Indian Council of Agricultural Research and International Livestock Research Institute 31 January–1 February 2006.* pp.1-126. National Agricultural Science Complex, New Delhi, India

Boettcher PJ, Jairath LK, Koots KR and Dekkers JC. 1997. Effects of interactions between type and milk production on survival traits of Canadian Holsteins. *Journal of Dairy Science* **80** (11): 2984-95.

Brotherstone S. 2010. Genetic and phenotypic correlations between linear type traits and production traits in Holstein-Friesian dairy cattle. *Animal Production* **75:**18-21.

Chakraborty KS, Chakraborty S, Le Roux P, Miller HM, Shirvalkar P and Rawat Y. 2018. Enamel isotopic data from the domesticated animals at Kotada Bhadli, Gujarat, reveals specialized animal husbandry during the Indus Civilization. *Journal of Archaeological Science: Reports* **21**:183-99.

Champak B and Nagpaul PK. 2005. Effect of housing systems on the growth performance of crossbred goats. *Indian Journal of Animal Sciences* **75**(1): 69-73.

Chander Mahesh and Mukherjee Reena. 2005. Organic animal husbandry: Concept, status and possibilities– A review. *Indian Journal of Animal Sciences* **75** (12): 1460-169.

Chauhan A, Patel BH, Maurya R, Kumar S, Shukla S and Kumar S. 2016. Pig production system as a source of livelihood in Indian scenario: An overview. *International Journal of Science, Environment and Technology* **5**(4):2089-96.

Cruickshank J, Weigel KA, Dentine MR and Kirkpatrick BW. 2002. Indirect prediction of herd life in Guernsey dairy cattle. *Journal of Dairy Science* **85** (5): 1307-13.

Dahiya SP. 2005. Selection of breeding bull for genetic improvement of dairy animals. *Livestock International* **9**(6): 8-10.

Dash S, Singh A, Dixit SP and Gandhi RS. 2016.Genome-wide diversity: A tool for conservation of Indian animal genetic resources. *Indian Dairyman* **68** (1): 64-69.

Deb SM. 2015. Traditional livestock production and growth opportunities in India. In: *Sustainable Use of Grassland Resources for Forage Production, Biodiversity and Environmental Protection*: pp 69-78. (Eds) Srivastava MK Gupta CK Malaviya DR, Roy MM, Mahanta SK, Singh JB, Maity A and Ghosh PK. Proceedings of 23rd International Grassland Congress, November 20 - 24, 2015.Range Management Society of India, Jhansi, India.

Deth R, Clarke A, Ni J and Trivedi M. 2016. Clinical evaluation of glutathione concentrations after consumption of milk containing different subtypes of β-casein: results from a randomized, cross-over clinical trial. *Nutrition Journal* **15:**1-6. DOI 10.1186/s12937-016-0201-x.

Dhok AP, Rekhate DH and Wankhade SG. 2005. Mineral status of goats in relation to common tree leaves fed in the Akola district. *Indian Journal of Animal Sciences* **75**(1): 77-80.

Dixit PK, Singh RV and Dhaka JP. 2001. Common property resources and dairy farming - a study in Mandya District Karnataka State. *Indian Journal of Dairy and Biosciences* **12**: 55-62.

Dutt MN. 1908. *Parasara Samhita*. Elysium Press, 3, Furiapukur Street, Calcutta, India.

FAO. 1996. *World Livestock Production System: Current Status, Issues and Trends*. 82 p. Rome, Italy.

Gendley MK, Singh P and Garg AK. 2003. Performance of crossbred cattle fed solely on chopped green sugarcane tops supplemented with concentrate mixture or urea molasses liquid diet. *Indian Journal of Animal Science* **73** (9): 1061-65.

Gibson KD and Dechow CD. 2018. Genetic parameters for yield, fitness, and type traits in US Brown Swiss dairy cattle. *Journal of Dairy Science* **101**(2): 1251-57.

Gupta VK.2025. Indigenous pig breeds: cultural and socio-economic role in India. Personal Communication.

Hamadani H, Hamadani A and Shabir S. 2024. Artificial intelligence in animal farms for management and breeding. In*: A Biologists Guide to Artificial Intelligence.* pp.167-82. (Eds) Hamadani A, Ganai NA, Hamadani H, and Bashir J. Academic Press. https://doi.org/10.1016/B978-0-443-24001-0.00011-7.

Hosamani SV Pugashetti BK and Kulkarni VS. 2001. Effect of supplementation of rain tree (*Samanea saman*) pods on the performance of HF × Deoni heifers. *Indian Journal of Animal Sciences* **71**(1): 66-68.

Huque KS and Rahman MM. 2002. Study on voluntary intake and digestibility of banana foliage as a cattle feed. *Journal of Biology Science* **2** (1): 49-52.

Ioan H. 2020. Introduction to Animal Breeding. In. *Animal Breeding and Husbandry.* pp. 133-55. (Eds) Timisoara. Hutu I, Oldenbroek K and van der Waaij L. USAB, Agroprint, Romania.

Jeong H, Park YS and Yoon SS. 2024. A2 milk consumption and its health benefits: an update. *Food Science and Biotechnology* **33**(3): 491-503.

Kale RB, Ponnusamy K, Chakravarty AK, Mohammad A and Sendhil R. 2018. Productive and reproductive performance of cattle and buffaloes reared under farmers' management in differential dairy progressive states in India. *Indian Journal of Animal Research* **52**(10):1513-17.

Khadda BS, Singh B, Singh DV, Singh SK and Singh CB. 2018. Economics of goat farming under traditional system of management in Uttarakhand. *Indian Journal of Traditional Knowledge* **17** (4): 802-06.

Krishna N.2010. Buffalo In. *Sacred Animals of India.* pp58-63. Penguin Books, India.

Krishnaswamy A. 1937a. Animal husbandry in ancient India-I. *Indian Farming* **2**: 459-60.

Krishnaswamy A. 1937b. Animal husbandry in ancient India-II. *Indian Farming* **2**: 527-29.

Krishnaswamy A. 1937c. Animal husbandry in ancient India-III. *Indian Farming,* **2**: 579-81.

Krishnaswamy A. 1937d. Authors on Indian veterinary science: Their works, age and antiquity. *Indian Journal of Veterinary Science and Animal Husbandry* **11**: 107-12.

Kumar A, Misra SS, Chauhan IS, Gowane GR and Shinde AK. 2021 Small ruminant production in dryland regions of India: Status, challenges and opportunities. *Indian Journal of Animal Sciences* **91**(5): 350-59.

Kumar Aruna T. 2003. Ayurveda in ancient literature. *National Symposium on Historical overview on Veterinary Sciences and Animal Husbandry in Ancient India.*16 April 2002. IVRI, Izatnagar, UP., India.

Kumar P, Saini AL, Sood SB and Singh K.1993. Micro-environment in east-west and north-south oriented sheds and its impact on physiological responses in goats in hot-dry environments. *Indian Journal of Animal Sciences* **63**(6): 674-78.

Majumdar GP and Banerji SC (Ed). 1960. *Krsi-Parāśara.* 163p. The Asiatic Society Calcutta. https://archive.org/download/Bibliotheca_Indica_Series/KrishiParasara-pdf downloaded on 13-09-2024.

Mandal L.1997. Nutritive values of tree leaves of some tropical species for goats. *Small Ruminant Research* **24** (2): 95-105.

Manivannan A, Mathialagan P, Narmatha N and Mohan B. 2018. Indigenous Knowledge in Sheep and Goat Farming Systems in Tamil Nadu India. *Asian Agri-History* **22**(2): 99-106.

Mishra B, Mukesh M, Prakash B, Sodhi M, Kapila R, Kishore A, Kataria R, Joshi BK, Bhasin V, Rasool T J and Bujarbaruah KM. 2009. Status of milk protein, beta-casein variants among Indian milch animals. *Indian Journal of Animal Sciences* **79** (7): 850-59.

Muir SK, Linden NP, Kennedy A, Calder G, Kearney G, Roberts R, Knight MI and Behrendt R. 2020. Technical note: Validation of an automated feeding system for measuring individual animal feed intake in sheep housed in groups. *Translational Animal Science* **4**(2): 1006–1016. https://doi.org/10.1093/tas/txaa007.

Nene YL. 2012. Environment and spiritualism: integral parts of ancient Indian literature on agriculture. *Asian Agri-History* **16**(2): 123-41.

Pandey AK. 1997. Tree leaves for livestock feeding in Chotanagpur plateau. *Journal of Interacademicia* **1**(2): 134-36.

Panigrahi B Nayak GD and Mahopatra PS.2005. Effect of type of flooring on growth of goats. *Environment and Ecology* **23**(Spl-1): 99-101.

Patel H, Samad A, Hamza M, Muazzam A and Harahap MK. 2022. Role of artificial intelligence in livestock and poultry farming. *Sinkron: Jurnal Dan Penelitian Teknik Informatika* **7(4)**: 2425–2429. https://doi.org/10.33395/sinkron.v7i4.11837.

Patel YG, Trivedi MM, Rajpura RM, Savaliya FP and Parmar M. 2016. Udder and teat measurements and their relation with milk production in crossbred cows. *International Journal of Science, Environment and Technology* **5** (5): 3048-54.

Qian D, Wang W, Huo X and Tang J. 2008. Study on linear appraisal of dairy cow's conformation based on image processing. pp. 303-11. In: *Computer and Computing Technologies in Agriculture.* Volume I: First IFIP TC 12 International Conference on Computer and Computing Technologies in Agriculture (CCTA 2007), Wuyishan, China, August 18-20, 2007. Springer, US.

Qiao Y, Kong H, Clark C, Lomax S, Su D, Eiffert S. and Sukkarieh S. 2021. Intelligent perception for cattle monitoring: A review for cattle identification, body condition score evaluation, and weight estimation. *Computers and Electronics in Agriculture* **185**: 06143. https://doi. org/ 10.1016/j. compag.2021.106143.

Rao NV, Singh P, Balaguravaiah D, Dimes JP and Carberry PS. 2004. Systems modeling and farmers' participatory evaluation of cropping options to diversify peanut systems in Anantapur region, India I: APSIM simulations to analyze constraints and opportunities. In: *Proceedings of the 4th International Crop Science Congress.* Brisbane, Australia, 26 September–1 October 2004. https://agronomyaustraliaproceedings.org/images/sampledata /2004/poster/2/1/1/2072_raovn.pdf.

Rig Veda Samhita English Translation.2013. Griffith RT H, Compiled by Ninan MM. Available at: Microsoft Word - RIG VEDA.doc.

Saar M, Edan Y, Godo A, Lepar J, Parmet Y and Halachmi I. 2022. A machine vision system to predict individual cow feed intake of different feeds in a cowshed. *Animal* **16**(1):100432 .https://doi.org/10.1016/j.animal.2021.100432.

Saravanan KA, Panigrahi M, Kumar H, Nayak SS, Rajawat D, Bhushan B and Dutt T. 2022. Progress and future perspectives of livestock genomics in India: a mini-review. *Animal Biotechnology* **1:** 9. https://doi.org/10.1080/10495398.2022.2056046.

Seré C, Steinfeld H and Groenewold J. 1996. *World Livestock Production Systems.* 58 p. Food and Agriculture Organization of the United Nations, Rome, Italy.

Shamasastry R (Tr.). 1951. *Kautilya's Arthaśāstra* 4th edn. 518 p. Shri Raghuveer Printing Press, Mysore. https://archive.org/details/in.gov.ignca.900, pdf downloaded on 09-10-2023.

Sharma P and Singh K. 2002. Shelter seeking behaviour of dairy cattle in various types of housing systems. *Indian Journal of Animal Sciences* **72**(1): 91-95.

Sharma TR. 2013. *Atharva-Veda Vol. I.* Vijaykumar Govindram Hansnand, New Delhi, India (Digital Distributer Agniveer). https://archive.org/details/atharva-veda-vol-2-of-2, pdf downloaded on 05-06-2023.

Shrivastava MB, Shrivastava M and Lal CB. 1995. Grazing lands, causes of their deterioration and improvement in India. *Indian Journal of Forestry* **18**(3): 177-91.

Singh AK, Upadhyay VS, Misra AK and Singh KK. 1998. Ruminal dry matter, organic matter and nitrogen degradability of common tree leaves of Bundelkhand region. *Range Management and Agroforestry* **19**(2): 203-05.

Singh J, Balwant Singh BS, Wadhwa M, and Bakshi MPS. 2003. Effect of level of feeding on the performance of crossbred cows during pre- and post-partum periods. *Asian-Australasian Journal of Animal Sciences* **16**(12): 1749-54.

Sodhi M, Mukesh M, Kishore A, Mishra BP, Kataria RS and Joshi BK. 2013. Novel polymorphisms in UTR and coding region of inducible heat shock protein 70.1 gene in tropically adapted Indian zebu cattle *(Bos indicus)* and riverine buffalo *(Bubalus bubalis)*. *Gene* **527**: 606–15.

Suryanarayan A. 2023. Human-animal relationships in the Indus Civilisation: Challenges, opportunities and questions. In: *Animals in Archaeology: Integrating Landscapes, Environment and Humans in South Asia (A. Festschrift for Prof. P.P. Joglekar) Volume 1*. pp. 117-37. (Eds.) Goyal P, Abhayan GS and Channarayapatna S. Department of Archaeology, University of Kerala, Thiruvananthapuram, India.

Swarup D. 2004. Ethnoveterinary education to veterinary professionals. In: *National Workshop on Indigenous knowledge applications for livestock care*. Pune September 14-17 2004 pp. 82-85. Anthra, Secunderabad Andhra Pradesh, India.

Thiruvenkadan AK, Panneerselvam S and Kandasamy N. 2005. System of housing and management of Kanni Adu goats of southern Tamil Nadu. *Indian Journal of Animal Sciences* **75**(7): 827-29.

Tscharke M and Banhazi TM. 2016. A brief review of the application of machine vision in livestock behaviour analysis. *Journal of Agricultural Informatics* **7** (1): 23-42.

Wang H, Liu J, Dong Z, Song J and Zhu Z. 2023. Artificial intelligence-based metabolic energy prediction model for animal feed proportioning optimization. *Italian Journal of Animal Science* **22**(1): 942–52. https://doi.org/10.1080/1828051x.2023.2236132.

Woodford K. 2007. *Devil in the Milk*. Craig Potton Publishing, New Zealand.

4

Traditional Knowledge, Ethnoveterinary Medicine and Early Animal Healthcare Practices

D. Swarup

Knowledge gained through experience is far superior and many times more useful than bookish knowledge.

(Mahatma Gandhi; quotefancy.com)

Introduction

Knowledge, as defined by various scholars, encompasses a rich tapestry of meanings. According to the Merriam-Webster Dictionary, knowledge represents the awareness of something, gained through experience or association. It involves familiarity with scientific principles, artistic expressions, and technical know-how. Across different fields—humanities, sciences, agriculture, and more—knowledge takes on diverse forms. Traditional knowledge (TK), one significant category also referred to as indigenous knowledge or traditional ecological knowledge, is a cumulative repository of observations, oral and written knowledge along with innovations, practices, and beliefs that promote sustainability and responsible stewardship of cultural and natural resources through relationships between humans and their landscapes (Daniel *et al.* 2022). Emerging from centuries of experience accumulated by peoples with extended histories of interaction through direct contact with the natural environment, the traditional knowledge system is deeply rooted in the cultural traditions, beliefs, and experiences of rural and local communities. TK encompasses language, systems of classification, resource use practices, social interactions, rituals, and spirituality, constituting important components of the world's cultural diversity (UNESCO 2017). It forms the foundation for local-level decision-making in many fundamental aspects of daily life, including hunting, fishing, gathering, agriculture, and animal husbandry. TK guides the preparation, conservation, and distribution of food, the location, collection, and storage of water, the struggle against disease and injury, the interpretation of meteorological and climatic phenomena, the management of ecological relationships between society and nature, and adaptation to environmental and social changes (ICSU 2002). According to Convention on Biological Diversity Article 8(j) on Traditional Knowledge, Innovations and Practices, 'traditional knowledge tends to be collectively owned and takes forms of stories, songs, folklore, proverbs, cultural values, beliefs, rituals, community laws, local language, and agricultural practices, including the development of plant species and animal breeds and plays a practical role in agriculture, fisheries, health, horticulture, forestry, and environment management.' Moreover, TK is valuable not only to those who depend on it in their daily lives but also to modern industry and agriculture. Several widely used products, such as plant-based medicines, health products, and cosmetics, are derived from traditional knowledge. As such, traditional knowledge can make a significant contribution to sustainable development (https://www.cbd.int/traditional/intro.shtml, accessed on 21-06-2024).

Indigenous Technical Knowledge

Indigenous technical knowledge (ITK) is a subset of traditional knowledge (TK) that focuses on the practical, technical, and scientific aspects developed by indigenous communities. ITK is specifically concerned with the actual application of TK, often involving innovative techniques and tools customized to local environmental conditions and cultural contexts. This demonstrates a deep understanding of ecological processes and resource management. Characteristically, indigenous technologies are based on experiences that have gathered momentum through generations and are developed and improved through experience and trial and error, tested in the rigorous laboratory of local community survival. Both TK and ITK are not static but constantly changing, being produced and reproduced, discovered and lost. These forms of knowledge are holistic, eco-friendly, and sustainable, and are considered crucial for the sustainable development and resilience of local communities (Das *et al.* 2002).

Indigenous Knowledge System vs. Western Knowledge System

Both indigenous knowledge systems (IKS) and the modern science-based western knowledge system (WKS) provide technologies and practices used by modern society for a range of activities. While WKS assumes greater importance in industrialized countries, its significance is also growing in developing nations due to the adoption of modern education systems. Yet, indigenous knowledge (IK) remains popular in many countries, particularly those like India that possess a rich heritage of local knowledge and traditional practices (ITK). The concepts and practices of these two knowledge systems, however, differ considerably (Das *et al.* 2002, Swarup *et al.* 2013). Some key differences between the two systems are discussed here.

Worldview and Interdependence: IKS regards the natural world as animate, considering all life forms as interdependent. In contrast, WKS often places human life as superior, granting a moral right to control other life forms.

Environmental Impact: IK-based technologies tend to be eco-friendly and sustainable, whereas WKS technologies may promote human greed and the exploitation of natural resources.

Knowledge Generation: IK is generated and acquired by resource users over a diachronic (long-term) time scale through observations and practical experience. WKS, on the other hand, is learned and generated by specialist researchers on a synchronic (short-term) time scale, often in a context remote from its practical application.

Compatibility and Adoption: ITK systems are compatible with local contexts and rely less on external inputs. The majority of ITKs are easy to adopt. In contrast, modern technologies may or may not align with the existing situation of farmers, often requiring external input and specialized skills for field application. For instance, local communities can readily use and adopt IK-based technologies, such as applying turmeric, coconut, or mustard oil for wound treatment, rather than relying solely on WKS-based antibiotics and antiseptics.

Transmission and Characteristics: IK is primarily transmitted through oral traditions. It embodies a holistic, intuitive, qualitative, and practical approach. WKS, on the other hand, is predominantly conveyed through written words. It tends to be reductionist, quantitative, analytical, and theoretical.

Influence and Nature of Knowledge: In IKS, the nature and status of specific knowledge are influenced by socio-cultural factors, including spiritual beliefs. This knowledge is used to make informed decisions under varying conditions. In WKS, knowledge undergoes peer review, and is often held by individual specialists.

Cost-effectiveness: IK focuses on the practical application of local wisdom and experiences within a specific area. Consequently, it is generally cost-effective. WKS, however, may not always address the unique problems of a particular community or area, potentially making it less cost-effective under field conditions.

Box 4.1. Key Aspects of Traditional Knowledge (TK)

Encompassing a vast spectrum of invaluable insights in diverse fields such as herbal medicine, sustainable farming practices, and local ecosystem, TK bridges ancient wisdom with contemporary challenges. Its crucial role for achieving the Sustainable Development Goals (SDGs) and in addressing the most pressing global problems is gaining international attraction Some key aspects of TK include:

Biodiversity conservation: *Deep understanding of indigenous communities' knowledge on local ecosystems, plant species, and animal behaviour informs sustainable practices. Integrating TK with modern scientific understanding can significantly contribute to the preservation of biodiversity.*

Climate change adaptation: *TK offers valuable insights into climate patterns, local weather forecasting, and adaptation strategies, which can be crucial in addressing climate challenges and resource management.*

Agriculture and food security: *TK guides agricultural practices, crop selection, and soil management. It emphasizes diverse, resilient crops and traditional farming techniques. TK along with modern knowledge can enhance food security.*

Health and medicine: *Traditional healing practices, herbal remedies, and holistic approaches are part of TK. Incorporating these practices with Western medicine can lead to more comprehensive healthcare solutions.*

Cultural identity and revitalization: *Reviving and respecting indigenous practices helps maintain cultural diversity and fosters pride within communities.(References: UNESCO2017, UNDESA 2019, Lite-Nepal 2023)*

TK Challenges

Traditional knowledge based technologies face several challenges in the modern world. Some key challenges include:

Erosion and Loss: TK, often passed down orally or through practical experience, can erode due to changing lifestyles, migration, and urbanization in modern societies. The advent of modern scientific technologies has led to a lack of interest among younger generations, who may not value or learn traditional practices.

Intellectual Property Rights: Protecting TK from exploitation or misappropriation is challenging. Intellectual property laws often favour formal patents and copyrights, leaving traditional knowledge vulnerable to appropriation without proper recognition or compensation.

Climate Change and Adaptation: Traditional practices are often closely tied to local ecosystems and climate conditions. However, as these conditions change due to climate change, traditional knowledge may become less effective.

Globalization and Homogenization: Global markets and industrial agriculture promote standardized practices. This can marginalize or replace traditional knowledge, leading to a loss of both biodiversity and cultural diversity.

Education and Transmission: Formal education systems prioritize scientific knowledge over traditional wisdom. Consequently, fewer people learn traditional practices, widening the generational gap.

Documentation and Preservation: Recording and documenting traditional knowledge is essential. However, many practices remain undocumented, risking their disappearance. Efforts to preserve and digitize this knowledge are crucial.

Power Dynamics and Marginalization: Traditional knowledge often originates from marginalized communities. Power imbalances can lead to the exploitation and sidelining of these communities' contributions.

Conflicts with Modern Science: Traditional practices sometimes conflict with scientific recommendations. Balancing both perspectives is challenging, especially when addressing issues like crop management, pest control, soil health and human and animal health.

Access to Resources: Traditional practices often rely on local resources and community cooperation. As land ownership changes and resources become scarce, access to these essential elements becomes difficult.

Ethnoveterinary Medicine (EVM)

The ethnoveterinary medicine (EVM), sometimes also called as veterinary anthropology or traditional veterinary medicine, is an important component of indigenous traditional knowledge (ITK). It encapsulates a holistic, interdisciplinary study of local knowledge, skills, beliefs, and social structures related to animal healthcare and husbandry. The term ethnoveterinary medicine is defined as — 'the holistic interdisciplinary study of local knowledge and is associated with skills, practices, beliefs, practitioners, and social structures pertaining to the healthcare and healthful husbandry of foods, work, and other income producing animals, always with an eye to practical development applications within livestock production and livelihood systems and with the ultimate goal of increasing human well-being via increased benefits from stock raising' (McCorkle 1998). According to another comprehensive definition, EVM is a holistic tradition or local/native system of livestock health management rooted in people's cultures, customs, taboos, and traditions. It is adopted by livestock raisers worldwide in their respective environmental conditions to keep their animals healthy and productive and to treat and control diseases and livestock-related problems. This is achieved using medicines, management practices, information about diseases, animal production and breeding methods, tools and technologies, and magico-religious beliefs embodied in people's traditional and local practices for their own development and survival (Wanzala *et al.* 2005). In summary, EVM encompasses a complex system of information, knowledge, skills, methods, practices, tools, technologies, beliefs, breeds, and human and natural resources used by people for husbandry and general care of their animals often in a sustainable and environment-friendly manner, and its role extends beyond mere animal treatment (McCorkle 1986, Mathias 2001, Swarup *et al.* 2013).

Origin of Ethnoveterinary Knowledge and Veterinary Medicine

The exact time and place of origin of veterinary medicine, including traditional veterinary practices, remain unknown due to a lack of documentary evidence from the time before writing skills developed in the ancient world. However, it is argued that civilized qualities such as gentleness, caring, responsibility, compassion, non-violence, and contemplation emerged among sheep culture people, making roamer shepherds the first true humans. These humane qualities sparked interest among primitive nomads in healing, leading to the acquisition of rudimentary skills in the healing art (Schwabe 1978). Over the time, these qualities were further honed with increasing socio-economic and religious value placed on different species of animals. The knowledge of ethology, anatomy and physiology of animals like cattle and sheep, which were used for divination and appeasement of gods in the ancient cultures, was highly crucial from religious aspect. Raising superior livestock and keep them healthy were prime requirements for better production and performance. Under these circumstances, the veterinary and animal husbandry knowledge originated in different ancient civilizations in form of selective breeds and breeding, animal feeds and feeding, animal behaviour, ritualism, herbalism, spiritualism, and ethno-epidemiology of livestock diseases (Schwabe 1984, Swabe 1999, Wanzala *et al.* 2005, Swarup *et al.* 2013).

Zooarchaeological evidence suggests that early Neolithic herders possessed strong zootechnical knowledge. They adopted different livestock management strategies with different breeding, feeding and mobility patterns occurring within this archaeological short period (Sierra *et al.* 2024). Shepherd managed sheep breeding seasons, determined optimal age for slaughter to maximize meat production, and practiced culling to manage flock size (Arbuckle *et al.* 2009) Similarly, the Neolithic farmers strategically fed, and housed dairy cattle and conducted intensive post-lactation slaughter to enhance milk production. They also manipulated calving season to minimize winter calf mortality (Kamjan *et al.* 2021). It is stated that ancient breeders and animal healers were effective managers who were sensitive to the animals' well-being. Their approaches to curing animal diseases were based on experience rather than theories of disease (Bodson 1994).

Early Animal Healing Practices and Concepts of Illness

Based on theories and observations of how the animal body functions, the animal healing system can be organized into five categories: self-healing (zoopharmacognosy); mystical (religious, spiritual, or magical); empirical (therapy based on educated guess); ethnoveterinary medicine (traditional methods used by laypeople and professionals); and contemporary veterinary medicine comprising modern veterinary medicine including western professional knowledge about veterinary science, and therapeutic methods that developed during the past two centuries (Jones and Koolmees 2022). Although all pre-modern veterinary practices may not qualify as ethnoveterinary medicine, some of these are important for their contextual relevance in understanding the evolution of EVM. Further, most of the pre-modern veterinary practices are rooted in traditional knowledge, and practiced by traditional healers or professionals experienced in indigenous systems of animal healthcare and husbandry evolved in over the time in different cultures.

Changing Concept and Theories of Disease: Guided by changing concepts and beliefs about the causes of diseases, as well as the socio-economic importance of domestic animals, the evolution of veterinary knowledge and practices has undergone following five stable periods and revolutions (Thrusfield 2018):

1. The first period, which began with the initial domestication of animals and continued until the 1st century CE.
2. The second phase, spanning from the first century CE until 1762.
3. The third period, from 1762 to 1984.
4. The fourth period, lasting from 1884 to 1960.
5. The fifth phase, characterized by contemporary veterinary medicine

During the first phase until the early modern period, veterinary practices were primarily based on traditional knowledge and experience of livestock raisers and professionals. The earlier theories emerged to define causes of diseases included **Demonic Theory** (spirituality); **Divine Wrath** (displeased Supreme Being or punishment of God); **Metaphysical Medicine** (occult forces beyond the physical universe- moon, planets, stars, earthquakes, floods and comets); **The Universe of Natural Law and Miasmata Theory** (diseases caused by external forces including climate and geological factors and derangement of four humours of body associated with four properties- heat, moister, dryness and cold; local outbreaks occurring due to noxious air- miasmas); **The Contagion Theory** (diseases transmitted by contact or air-borne means being taken in via nose or mouth). The remedy for illness therefore included identifying the offending supernatural power, appeasing the angry gods, and exorcising evil spirits. Treatment practices were in their infancy and involved placation, forcible expulsion through exorcism, and evasion via ritual ceremonies and the use of material objects such as amulets, periapt, talismans, and fetishes. These objects could be carried or suspended over buildings to ward off evil spirits. Witch doctors and other special individuals also played a role. Empirical therapeutic measures including use of herbs were also practiced against certain recognized symptom complexes. However, despite these techniques, draught animals continued to die.

The loss of valuable animals in urban society led to the development of the first stable period of veterinary medicine (approximately 6000 BCE to the 1st century CE). During this period, veterinary specialists emerged, including Egyptian priest-healers and Vedic Brahmin healers known as *Salihotriyas,* who founded the first veterinary hospitals. Humoral pathology developed, and the miasmatic theory of causation evolved. Treatment techniques required careful recognition of clinical signs, following the Greek Coan-tradition (Thrusfield 2018). Herbs, minerals, organic compounds, zootherapeutic methods, and trepanning (the removal of bone discs from the skull) were also used to treat diseases in both humans and animals. Although early therapists acquired some knowledge and understanding of certain aspects of diseases, they lacked an understanding of its root cause. When treatments failed, their last resort was to use spells and incantations to appease the gods (Jones 2021). Some basic biomedical knowledge also emerged and early biomedical theories were propounded during the early phase of evolutionary period, particularly in the temple cities of Egypt. Dissections of sacrificed bulls and observations made by the Egyptian priests led them to rudimentary understanding of animal anatomy and physiology, thus, by analogy, of human anatomy and physiology. Although ancient animal healers did not achieve the same theoretical development as their human medical counterparts, Greek thinkers and physicians still significantly influenced the ideas and medical practices of future generations. In fact, the disease concept of humoral pathology—specifically the belief (espoused by Hippocrates and others) that diseases arise from imbalances in the body's fluids—remained influential in veterinary medicine until the 19th century CE (Swabe 1999).

Early Animal Healers and Veterinary Activities in Ancient Civilizations

The roots of veterinary knowledge and practice can be traced to ancient civilizations—long before 3000 BCE—in regions such as Mesopotamia, Africa, China, and India. Healers in these cultures were engaged in veterinary medicine well before any written documentation of such practices appeared. These early advancements significantly predate the emergence of veterinary practices in Greece and Rome, which later served as conduits for their spread throughout Europe. Contrary to popular belief, the Greek and Roman figures often credited as the 'Fathers of Veterinary Medicine' built upon foundations that had already been firmly established in earlier cultures (Mark 2020). In general, early animal healing practices involved various methods, including magic spells, incantations, the use of medicinal botanicals and minerals, zootherapies, and therapeutic phlebotomy (bleeding). These practices were observed in different ancient civilizations after the domestication of animals and ethical guidelines and laws were developed to protect animals and ensure their welfare.

Mesopotamia: The ancient region of southwest Asia between rivers Tigris and Euphrates is referred as Fertile Crescent and the cradle of civilization. The modern name Mesopotamia comes from the Greek *mesos* for middle and *potamos* for river, literally meaning — a country between two rivers. The Mesopotamia civilization, which began to form around the time of the Neolithic Revolution, comprised several major ancient civilizations including the Sumerian, Assyrian, Akkadian, and Babylonian civilizations. Evidence shows extensive use of technology, literature, legal codes, philosophy, religion, and architecture in these societies. The Neolithic Agricultural Revolution that consisted domestication of first four farm animals: cattle, sheep, and goat took place in this region, and much of the early knowledge on animal husbandry and veterinary art evolved in the temple cities of Mesopotamian civilization. The medical culture that arose in Mesopotamia, eventually concentrating in Babylonia was based on a belief that disease was a supernatural effect of demons, and was diagnosed by omens. Treatment was based on observable symptoms and dominated by incantations, magic and religious rites, both in medical and veterinary practices. Medication was mostly of plant-origin with some mineral and animal organs. Cassia, myrtle, belladonna, willow, asafoetida, salt (cleanser) and saltpetre (astringent) were all used. Preparations included infusions, decoctions, salves, range of embrocation, ointments, enemas and suppositories. It was recorded that oral herbal mixtures could be taken in either beer or milk to improve palatability. Fracture treatment with splints was practised. It is assumed that the practices known to the human healers were used for treatment of animals. Veterinary surgical procedures were restricted to castration and treatment of wound and fractures (Jones 2021).

The early healers were closely integrated with the powerful priest fraternity of ancient religions, which thought of gods in animal forms or with pronounced animal attributes. The priests were designated according to their jobs. *Shanga* slaughtered and offered thankfulness and supplication on behalf of community animal sacrifices. The *Baru* (a divinatory or astrological priest) declared the divine will through signs and omens. They dissected and minutely studied the visceral organs of sacrificed animals to predict future of community and its individuals and to suggest their corrective measures (Schwabe 1984). The two primary types of doctors in Mesopotamia were the *Asu* a medical doctor who treated illness or injury based on observation and physical treatment of symptoms and the *Asipu* who treated illness of man and cattle alike due to evil spirit. They were faith healers who relied on magical incantations, prayers, and herbs (Mark 2020). By the Hammurabi time, the medical and veterinary healers were known as *Asos* or *Azu* (healer or doctor). They used manual skills and available products of nature including herbs for treatment of man and animal (Jones 2021). A method called Hepatoscopy was used for Divinations. Priests examined the livers of sheep offered to the gods by the patients , cutting them open and studying them thoroughly. They believed that the liver was the seat of soul and life in both human and animal and useful for diagnosis of disease. Prognosis of the diseases of patients was good when size of liver, especially that of right lobe was large. The prognosis was bad when the liver was atrophic and malformed. Babylonians also left many clay models of sheep livers well studied anatomically (Jastrow 1908).

Urlugaledinna: A Sumerian physician, Urlugaledinna (ca. 2300 BCE) who served under Ur-Ninjitsu (r. 2121–2118 BCE), king of Lagash, son and successor of the great king Gudea (r. 2141–2122 BCE) is believed to be the first veterinarian known by name in the history (Mark 2020). A cylinder seal recovered from Mesopotamian city of Lagash shows a bovine obstetrical cord hanging from a medicinal plant and two urns for drug or fumigants. The Cuneiform text reads, ‘O God *Edenmugi* (i.e. who makes pastures safe), vizier of the God *Shakan* (means who help pregnant animals give birth), Urlugaledinna, the healer is your servant’ (Schwabe 1978). Urlugaledinna gave a particular attention to an apparatus consisting of two metal handles attached to two twisted cords with two shafts or lamina, which bend upwards at their tips representing a kind of forceps used by Sumerian obstetricians in difficult live births. It proves also that surgical instruments were used for opening abscesses and other minor surgical operations, and Sumerian surgeons used needles and threads for suturing (Al-Samarrai1972).

***Code of Hammurabi* (ca. 2100-1800 BCE):** The great Babylonian King Hammurabi introduced a code of laws and provisions to govern various customs and activities, including animal husbandry and veterinary practices. Engraved around 1750 BCE on a stele (a shaft or slab) made of black diorite and standing about seven feet high, the code was discovered by the distinguished French excavators in 1901–1902 in the city of Susa, Iran (Kelly 1995). Originally written in the Old Babylonian dialect of Akkadian, Hammurabi’s code has been translated into modern languages, including an English translation published in *Records of The Past*, Vol. II, Part III in 1903 (https://acrobat.adobe.com/id/urn:aaid:sc:AP:c4d1d52b-f713-4d37-b702-60cc45c86484 pdf downloaded 25.06.2024). The code contains an ancient set of 282 laws, out of which 24 laws (Code 7-8, 57-58, 224-225, 241 to 251 and 261 to 267) define legal aspects pertaining to rearing of livestock, provision of fee for veterinarians and compensation or penalties on loss of livestock wealth. Agricultural field and products (corn, oils), livestock and livestock products (milk) and garden and trees were the valuable assets. Vast flocks of sheep and herds of cattle, owned by individuals, were entrusted to herdsman or shepherd whose wage and responsibilities were fixed (Vincent 1904, Urch 1929, Nagarajan 2011). According to Code-261 ‘If a man has hired a herdsman, to pasture oxen, or sheep, he shall pay him eight GUR of corn yearly.’ Shepherd was responsible for all care of flocks, taking flocks to pasture, maintaining the inventory of animals, restoring value of animals on loss and breeding them satisfactorily. Defines Code-267- ‘If the herdsman has been careless, and a loss has occurred in the fold, the herdsman shall make good the loss in the fold; he shall repay the oxen, or sheep, to their owner.’ Ten-fold price of animal was the penalty for any dishonest use of the flock by shepherd. However, herdsmen were not liable for loss due to natural causes and it fell on owners. As defined under Code 266- 'If lightning has struck a fold, or a lion has made a slaughter, the herdsman shall purge himself by oath, and the owner of the fold shall bear the loss of the fold.' Shepherder also treated animals. It is not known if there were separate doctors exclusively for animals. However, the code refers to treatments of oxen by veterinary doctors and defines fee to be paid to doctors of oxen or asses or penalty to be levied from him. Cites the code 'if a doctor of beeves (oxen) or asses has treated either ox or ass for a severe illness, and cured it, the owner of the ox or ass shall give to the doctor one-sixth of a shekel of silver as his fee' (code 224) and 'if he performs a serious operation on an ass or ox, and kills it, he shall pay the owner one-fourth of its value' (code 225). The monetary value of veterinary fees in ancient times can be compared with other wages. For instance, an ordinary craftsman received 1/50 silver shekel as daily pay, while a builder earned two shekels for each *sar* (floor?) constructed in a building. A good middle-class dwelling could be rented for five shekels per year. However, the fees prescribed for veterinary doctors were much lower than those stipulated for human physicians and surgeons, which ranged from 2 to 10 shekels. Notably, the Hammurabi Code (Fig. 4.1), one of the earliest and most complete legal written codes, addressed veterinary fees and also imposed fines for malpractice. This Code provided valuable insight into ethical and professional dimensions of veterinary practice in the ancient world.

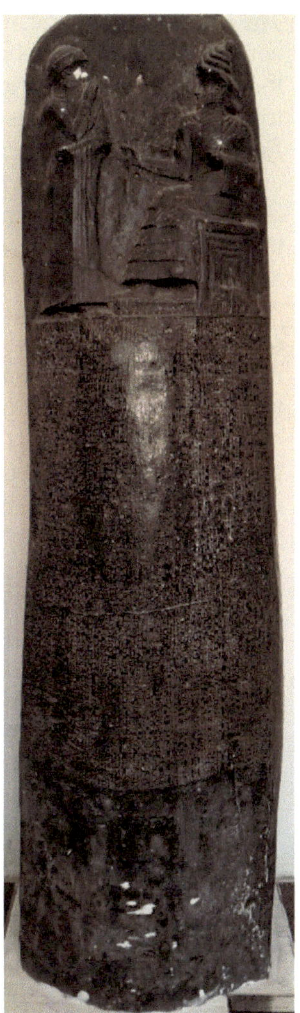

Fig. 4.1. *Replica of code of Hammurabi displayed at National Museum New Delhi (Photo by the Author).*

Ugaritic Hippiatric (Veterinary) Texts: Ugarit, located in what is now modern-day Syria, was one of the city-states that emerged in the Eastern Mediterranean during the 2nd millennium BCE. The site has been continuously inhabited since the Early Neolithic period (around 6500–6000 BCE). The modern name of the place is Ras Shamra (Cape Fennel). The site has been excavated since 1929 yielding numerous cuneiform tablets in Ugaritic, Akkadian, Sumerian, Hurrian, and Hittite languages in the archives of Ugarit. The overwhelming majority of these cuneiform texts are related to economics, literature, and religion (Zemánek 1996, Tropper and Vita 2019). Among them, some tablets contain hippiatric/medical texts, which provide insights into the treatment of diseases in horses.

The Ugaritic Hippiatric Texts (UHT) are therapeutic texts focusing on curing sick horses, and differ from *Akkadian* and *Hittite Hippiatric Texts*, which deal with the training of (healthy) chariot horses. The latter are more akin to hippology texts. The tripartite structure of all sections in the UHT resembles a modern therapeutic index. Each section has a main heading, individual descriptions of symptoms (protasis), and corresponding remedies (apodosis). These remedies include professional instructions for preparation, along with a ritual element. The instructions specify the dosage of the drug per horse and how to administer it, concluding with an assertion that the horse will recover. The remedial preparations in the UHT include whole or parts of plants, salt, and certain animal products. Honey, oil, and beer serve as vehicles for mixing medicinal constituents into the regular diet of horses. Additionally, stomach tubes are used to force-feed sick horses by introducing the mixture through the nostrils. Leather enema bags are used for administering drug preparations in both horses and humans. Interestingly, specific medical prescriptions in higher doses are used for the same ailments in horses. Common ingredients in both human and horse prescriptions include resins, figs, cinnamon, wormwood, cedar cypress, juniper, box-tree, elder tree, and aromatic plants. Salt and aromatic substances are also frequently used. The Neo-Assyrian Akkadian Medical Text BAM 159 contains prescriptions and descriptions of various pathological symptoms in humans, including two dealing with sick horses (Cohen 1983). This unique finding suggests that medical and equine medicine knowledge evolved cohesively in Mesopotamian civilization. The diagnostic approach to human and horse sickness, as mentioned in BAM 159, follows a similar structure, usually defined by signs/symptoms, illness, prognosis, and treatment. This unique finding suggests that medical and equine medicine knowledge evolved in tandem within Mesopotamian civilization. The diagnostic approaches for human and horse illnesses, as mentioned in BAM 159, were similar. These approaches typically involved four components: signs/symptoms, illness, prognosis, and treatment. They relied on hypothetical-deductive reasoning, akin to the modern method of disease diagnosis known as abduction, which is based on ignorance-preserving reasoning. Also, the analysis of Akkadian medical and *hippiatric* texts reveals that medical and veterinary knowledge coexisted in ancient Mesopotamia (Gómez 2021). Interestingly the Hippiatric Texts provide clear evidence of a non-magical pharmacopoeia that prescribe use of herbs, minerals and animal products like honey and milk in veterinary practice with proper professional instructions.

Hittite Training Texts for Chariot Horses: Introduced into the Near East by Indo-Europeans, horses and horse-driven chariots became highly valuable in ancient Mesopotamian society. The rise of Hittite power and the expansion of their empire were partly due to the large-scale use of fast, light horse chariots with two spoked wheels. Specialized knowledge was required to raise horses and train them in new habitats. The Hittites developed instructions and veterinary protocols for training, management, and healthcare of horses. These Hittite training texts for chariot horses were discovered during excavations in Boğazkale and Ḫattuša in

1906-1907 (Fig. 4.2). They are written in the Hittite language on four extant clay tablets, using Hittite cuneiform signs. Kikkuli, a master horse trainer (*assussanni*) from Mittani (a Hurrian state in northern Mesopotamia and Syria), along with his colleagues, authored these texts. Additional tablets came to light in the layers excavated under Kurt Bittel (1907-1991) in the 1930s, and they were named the New Hittite Horse Texts. One of these texts describes training instructions, while other purely contains Hittite training (Raulwing 2009).

Composed in the 2nd millennium BCE, approximately 3,500 years ago, the Kikkuli text is probably the earliest known written record on equine management and training. The text provides first hand information on the training and care of chariot horses. The instructions include daily routines, systematic conditioning, grain feeding, and warm-ups for horses, ensuring their efficient use in warfare (McMiken 1990, Walter 2014). The text also covers swimming, massages, blanketing, clipping, and turning out to paddocks—elements well-known to modern horse trainers. Dietary instructions involve feeding a limited portion of grass and legume plants, as well as cereals like barley (sometimes boiled), and allowing pasture grazing at specific periods of the day or night. Notably, the author demonstrates awareness of electrolytes' importance by providing instructions for giving horses salted or malt water after strenuous exercise. In the 1990s, the *Kikkuli* training method was tested on Arabian horses by Australian Hittitologist A. Nyland, who authored the book *The Kikkuli Method of Horse Training* based on her trial (revised edition published by CreateSpace Independent Publishers in 2009). Nyland reported that the endurance improvement achieved using the Kikkuli method was incomparable to any modern interval training program. Following the old rules can be beneficial, especially for trainers seeking to improve endurance of horses while maintaining their welfare (Klecel and

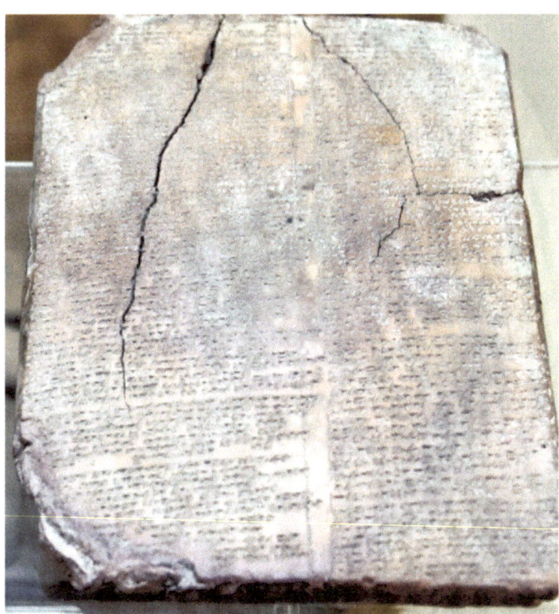

Fig. 4.2. *Training Horses Tablet from Hattusa. Lines 31-42 of this clay tablet describes the methods used by Kikkuli of the Mittani for training horses (Source: Amin OSM. 2018, September 10. Training Horses Tablet from Hattusa. World History Encyclopedia. Retrieved from https://www.worldhistory.org/image/9175/training-horses-tablet-from-hattusa/ on 10-07-2024).*

Martyniuk 2021). Interestingly, a series of numerals found in the Kikkuli text, such as *aika* (Sanskrit *eka* for one) and *panza* (Sanskrit *pañca* for five), have Indian origins. These numerals also appear in compounds with the noun *wartanna* (Sanskrit *vartana* for turn or ring), such as *-aika-uartanna-* (Lazzeroni 1998). This finding represents one of the earliest records of the relationship between Mesopotamia and Indian culture and their equine expertise (Jones 2021).

Ancient Egypt: Although ancient Egyptians raised all the major livestock species from Neolithic times, cattle herding was their most important preoccupation due to its significant socio-economic and cultural value. People relied on cattle for draught power, secondary products, and meat, which elevated these animals to a position of importance. Cattle symbolized wealth, power, and fertility, leading to their reverence, anthropomorphism, and even worship. Oxen, in particular, were seen as mighty symbols, and the Pharaohs of Egypt referred to themselves as mighty bulls. Egyptians developed various cattle breeds, including a large African breed with horns for fattening, a generally hornless smaller breed, and wild long-horned cattle. To make cattle more docile, they used several techniques that are prevailing even today. Unwanted horn growth was controlled by burning or scraping off budding horns or clipping them. The cattle's noses were pierced, and their heads were roped. Farmers housed their cattle in pens made of tree branches and fed them cut fodder during the inundation season when grazing areas were scarce. Specialized farms focused on fattening cattle for meat purpose. These animals grazed during the day and returned to the sheds in the evening, where they were fed corn pellets or mash (Schwabe 1984, Swabe 1999).

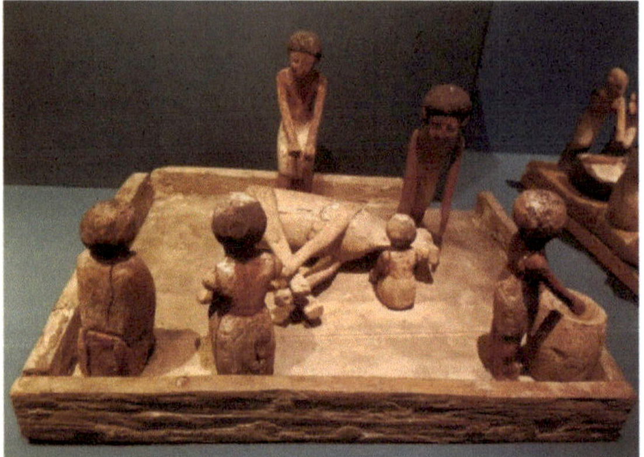

***Fig. 4.3.** Twelfth Dynasty (1985-1795 BCE) Wooden funerary model (1985-1795 BCE) representing the slaughtering of a bull, enabling it to be sacrificed for eternity in the afterlife. Bull's foreleg, was a typical offering. (Source: Miate L. 2017 A Bull's Slaughter Wooden Funerary Model. World History Encyclopedia. Retrieved on 16-08-2023 from. https://www.worldhistory.org/image/6590/a-bulls-slaughter-wooden-funerary-model/).*

From earliest time, Egyptians forbade eating cow meat and only ritual sacrifices were made of steers and bulls (Fig. 4.3). Drinking cow milk by ancient peoples, especially as portrayed by the adult pharaoh kneeling at the side of the cow goddess Hathor and sucking directly from her teat, was associated with early beliefs in the cow as the mother of humankind. The cow and bull (bovine animals) together were called *ka*. All mankind was referred to cattle of *Ra* (Schwabe 1978). Besides being source of capital that led to accumulation of wealth, cattle played a central role in the beginning of rational medicine as ancient ritual cattle sacrifice in Egypt led to a rudimentary understanding of animal anatomy and physiology, which was then applied to humans. Some of the Egyptian hieroglyphs for internal organs and many external organs (such as the heart, throat, head, and womb) are derived from those of animals, chiefly cattle, rather than from human organs. The hierographic sign for life- *Ankh* is a representation of a thoracic vertebra from a bull when viewed from the front. Additionally, the first two biomedical theories—life as movement (especially observed in the fasciolations of excised limbs, where muscle fascicles and intact muscles from sacrificial bulls can be stimulated to contract for a considerable period after the animal's death), and the male's role in reproduction—were developed based on inferences drawn from animal dissections, particularly of cattle. It seems reasonable that the Egyptians were not merely resorting to random trial and error or purely magical analogy; rather they had taken consequential steps in the development of an orderly process of comparative inquiry, especially in relation to biomedical understandings (Schwabe 1994, Gordon and Schwabe 2004). Probably the medicine and veterinary medicine originated concurrently soon after domestication, and the two areas gradually separated as Egyptian bureaucracy and technology advanced. However, some similarities observed in ancient papyri suggest a once-close association between human and animal care knowledge and practices (Lord 2016).

In ancient Egypt, environmental conditions significantly influenced both human and animal health. Although precise details about animal diseases remain scarce, it is likely that the close interaction between humans and animals facilitated disease transmission. People suffered from zoonotic bacterial, fungal, and parasitic infections. Tuberculosis, schistosomiasis, trichinosis, and trypanosomiasis (sleeping sickness) were among the diseases that might have been transmitted from animals due to frequent contact. The harsh environmental conditions, characterized by frequent dust storms and intense sunlight, likely contributed to high incidences of ophthalmic conditions in both humans and livestock. Additionally, wounds, fractures, and bites from snakes and scorpions were common occurrences (Lord 2016). Zoonotic infections were undoubtedly a scourge on the lives of ancient Egyptians and their valuable animals. Some scholars even suggest that the outbreak of anthrax—one of the oldest known zoonotic diseases—could have been one of the seven plagues that devastated Egyptians and their livestock (Swabe 1999). As a result, ancient Egyptian likely acted proactively to prevent animal diseases and safeguard their own lives and economically important livestock wealth, particularly when it came to protecting highly valuable cattle. In fact, some scholars have argued that veterinary practice in Egypt is among the earliest in the world, dating back at least to the time of the Old Kingdom (ca. 2613-2181 BCE) if not earlier (Mark 2020).

Egyptian Priest Healers: The early Egyptians' knowledge of veterinary care was intricately intertwined with spiritual beliefs and religious rituals. The priests, who held technical roles in the temple, were the individuals of great authority, piety, learning, and wisdom, constituting a highly revered hereditary institution of priesthood. Similar to ancient Mesopotamia, there was a division of labour among different types of priests based on their duties. One class of priests was responsible for animal care, particularly regarding sacrificial cattle, and they learned the art of healing and animal healthcare. Both human and animal diseases were attributed to supernatural causes, and priests acted to appease these supernatural powers. Their primary goal was to prevent or control plagues among people or their sacred, economically valuable animals (Schwabe 1978). A separate order of lesser priests *pastophore* (*pastophori*), originally served as doorkeepers to temples, existed from the Third Dynasty (ca. 2686–ca. 2613 BCE). They were responsible for guarding sacred symbols and caring designated holy animals and birds. *Pastophori* priests observed the behaviour patterns of these animals for prophecy and participated in processions where they, carried the gods. They were experts in the diseases of the animals they cared for, and were said to cure ailing animal gods when needed and divided into specialist groups for different types and species of holy animals and birds. They also examined the meat of slaughtered animals, banning the consumption of meat they considered objectionable, including saltwater species (Jones 2021). There were numerous *Wab* priests (also known as washed or purified ones) who examined animals to ensure they were free from blemishes. These priests used animal entrails for divination purposes. Through their duties, they acquired knowledge of veterinary physiology, anatomy, pathology and medicine. The high priests, called *hem-netjer* (servants of the god), and females, known as *hemet-netjer,* were scholarly individuals responsible for caring for sacred animal gods in the temple. A select few held the highest priestly rank as prophets. These scholarly priests authored papyri based on their knowledge of various subjects, including human and veterinary medicine (Schwabe 1978).

The *wab* priests of the goddess Sekhmet were ritualists closely associated with the *Houses of Life.* The title *Head of the Pure Priests of Sekhmet* could be earned or inherited, often passed down within families or castes. In addition to their expertise in calming the goddess Sekhmet and safeguarding the country, wab priests had other responsibilities. They practiced medicine, diagnosing illnesses by observing blood circulation, and also served as stable veterinarians, ensuring the well-being of temple bull herds. These priests also held the title *mr ihw* (Director of the Bulls). Ancient texts, including the Edwin Smith and Ebers medical papyri, highlight *wab* priests as specialists in diagnosing human ailments, alongside other practitioners like the *swnw* and the *sa-srkt* (Benezet 2021). Interestingly, ancient records suggest that there was no clear distinction between physicians and veterinarians; both were equally respected. Medicine was an art that was applied to both humans and animals. Priests and physicians, including surgeons, constituted an elite segment of the civil service hierarchy that operated across the country. They held official titles denoting their status and were assisted by individuals of varying ranks. These experts transmitted their knowledge to family members or within their caste. They did not charge any fees; instead, their compensation came in the form of food and clothing. Among them, some were categorized as doctor-priests, while others were known as doctor-magicians (Jones 2021).

Lay Healers of Ancient Egypt: Like other contemporary civilizations, the disease in the ancient Egypt was believed to have supernatural origins. The owners of animals would urge priests to seek communication with the gods to intervene and preserve the health of ailing, though such efforts were not always successful. However, with exception of priests of Sekhmet, some of whom also functioned generally as the physician-veterinarian, there is little evidence that the priest healers served for general public. The accumulated knowledge of healing was extended to more people and to be used for cattle and other livestock species. As such, not only the priests but other classes of medical and veterinary practitioners including overseer of cattle and other animals and lay-therapists known as *swnw* emerged. It is unclear whether any hierarchical or professional relationship existed between priest-healers and *swnw*, or how they acquired their healing practices (Schwabe 1978). The ancient Egyptian word *swnw* likely has two components: *swn* (affliction) and *swnyt* (pain), referring to individuals knowledgeable in both medical and veterinary matters (Bahaaeldeen *et al.* 2019). The title *swnw* was used in Pharaonic Egypt to describe a range of medical roles and responsibilities. These included palace *swnw*, inspectors of palace *swnw*, and *swnw* specializing in eye, belly, and gastro-intestinal ailments (Lord 2016). *Swnw* were tasked with supervising cattle and inspecting sacrificial animals and their meat. Interestingly, some of these *swnw* also held the position of wab priest (Schwabe 1978). For instance, a *swnw* named Irenakhti, depicted as smelling the bloodstained hand of a butcher and proclaiming–it is pure! was undoubtedly a wab-Sekhmet priest. The practice of examining entrails and sniffing animal blood persists in modern-day Egyptian villages as a means to assess health and edibility of animals (Benezet 2021).

In addition to priests and *swnw*, there were overseers responsible for cattle, horses, and birds. These overseers performed various roles related to animal husbandry and veterinary practice. Individuals holding title as overseer of cattle were also the veterinary obstetricians. Their duties encompassed delivering calves manually, removing placenta from cows, conducting rectal and vaginal examinations, and caring for newborn calves (Swawbe 1978, Bahaaeldeen *et al.* 2019). It is likely that experienced herdsmen possessed knowledge of animal healthcare and attended to most animal needs, including the treatment of ill animals. Archaeological remains and tomb reliefs not only demonstrate the essential role animals played in ancient Egyptian agriculture but also highlight the affection pastoralists had for their animal charges. In many scenes involving herdsmen and their livestock, men are depicted making magical gestures of protection towards the animals. Since these herdsmen were mostly illiterate, any skills and knowledge they possessed would not have been written down but may well have been passed on orally or learned anew through trial and error. Similarly, the practical knowledge of herdsmen regarding animal husbandry and the basic magic involved in protection spells would have been transmitted orally from generation to generation (Lord 2016). Treatment of animals by their owners remained one of the most common affordable alternatives in Byzantine Egypt (Ashoor 2023).

Veterinary Papyrus of Kahun or El-Lahun (ca. 1900 BCE): Some of the priests involved in animal care were scholarly individuals who recorded their technical skills on steles or papyrus. A fragment of an ancient text, written by one such scholar during the Middle Kingdom, was discovered in 1889 in the ancient Egyptian temple community of El-Lahun, located to the west of the Nile. The term Kahun for El-Lahun was coined by archaeologist William Matthew Flinders Petrie, who found the medical papyrus (https://en.wikipedia.org/wiki/El_Lahun). The Kahun papyri constitute one of the largest collections of papyri ever found, and are known to be the earliest veterinary medicine records in the world (Kgasi 2021). Despite severe fragmentation, this unique papyrus provides solid evidence of animal healing practices in ancient Egypt. The main fragment measures 25 inches in length and 5.5 inches in width, containing 48 columns and 3 horizontal headings. Analysis of the papyrus reveals that the ancient Egyptians recognized animal diseases and understood the need for human intervention in certain cases. The surviving text relates to three case studies involving bulls. These descriptions outline a logical approach to animal healing, with some treatments still applicable in modern veterinary practice (Lord 2011). Of the three case studies presented in the papyrus, the longest is *Treatment for the eyes of a bull with the wind (cold).* The translated extract from the papyrus states: - ‘I see [a bull with] wind, he is with his eyes running, his forehead? uden *(wrinkled?)* the roots (gums?) of his teeth red, his neck swollen (or raised?): repeat the incantation for him. Let him be laid on his side, let him be sprinkled with cold water, let his eyes and his hoofs (?) and all his body be rubbed with gourds (?) or *khenesh* plants, let him be fumigated with gourds ……… wait herdsman ……………. be soaked ……… that it draws in soaking ………. until it dissolves into water: let him be rubbed with gourds of cucumbers. Thou shalt gash (?) him upon his nose and his tail, thou shalt say as to it, “he that has a cut either dies with it or lives with it.” If he does not recover and he is wrinkled (?) under thy fingers, and blinks (?) his eyes, thou shalt bandage his eyes with linen lighted with fire to stop the running’ (Kgasi 2021). The clinical signs described in this case are suggestive of viral infection, specifically malignant catarrh fever (MCF). MCF is characterized by high fever, profuse discharge from the eyes and nose, bilateral corneal opacity, and necrosis and erosion of the buccal epithelium. Since the bull was suffering from fever, the healer aimed to cool the animal down. The bull was forcefully cast onto its side, cooled with water, and rubbed all over the body with *khenesh* plant (Lord 2016). In addition to cattle, the papyrus fragment also briefly addresses diseases of dogs and fish, particularly those affecting the animals’ eyes. Ensuring the birth of healthy offspring was a crucial objective for profitable cattle rearing, leading to the development of knowledge in veterinary obstetrics and gynaecology among ancient Egyptians. Portions of the Kahun papyrus also contain information related to veterinary gynaecological aspects (Schwabe 1978).

Ancient Near East: Ample information on traditional knowledge on man and animal relation, and law and customs for animal care are provided in the ancient Near East and European literature including holy books- Bible and Talmud. The Biblical Jews were sheep culture people, but they also reared cows and other important farm animals. The sacred Jewish book Talmud, consisting of 6 volumes of the Mishnah and 60 chapters of the Gemara elaborates various aspects of both human and animal medicine. Mishnah mentions separate physicians (doctors for man) and veterinary surgeon (doctor for animals) with details on appropriate professional approaches, instruments, wages and specialization (Hadani and Shimshony 1994).

Several commandments exist in Torah pertaining to animal and ensuring their welfare. Saving an animal from a harmful or dangerous situation, minimizing any traumatic event, are considered obligations from the Torah (*mitzwa me-de-Oraita*). These are the basic teachings of Judaism relative to animal welfare. According to Judaism, there are two obligations–to help or save an animal (positive/active commandment), and abstain from performing harmful or painful actions on animals (negative/abstain commandment). Abstaining from any intentionally traumatic action, abstaining from any unnecessarily painful action, are considered obligations instituted by the Sages (*mitzwa me-de-Rabbanan*). Though killing of animals as source of food to man is permitted, it must be done in as much painless manner as possible. Judaism developed a highly skilled and regulated way, the *shechita*, for slaughtering animals considered for food production, aimed to be quick, precise and as painless as possible; exclusively using skilled professionals (Pozzi and Gardella Tedeschi 2023).

A complete system of slaughter of animals and inspection of carcasses from public health point of view existed in the ancient Near east. The Mishnah mentions anatomic-pathological defects for the disqualification of slaughtered animals for human consumption, which in contemporary veterinary medicine are still considered a serious threat to the public health, and are contrary to the rules of hygiene (Pipano 2022). The Talmud distinguishes three major pathological changes in the brain and spinal cord: liquid encephalopathy, soft brain, and loss (degeneration) of tissue. Veterinary experts were capable of making accurate diagnoses of clinical cases involving the central nervous system. Cows, sows, sheep, and goats were subjected to pregnancy diagnosis before slaughter, and experts charged fees for this service. According to Mishnah 'he who charges fees for pregnancy diagnosis must be an expert - like Ilah of Yavneh - in order to permit the slaughter of the animal' (Hadani and Shimshony 1994). Ilah (Illa) was a veterinarian who lived and practiced in Yavneh about 2,000 years ago. He became famous for his veterinary skills and integrity, and can be considered a model for the veterinary profession. It is interesting to note that the two of the ancient villages (Zarnuga and Doron), in which Ila practiced are known today as the modern city of Rehovot, now the site of Israel's veterinary school (Shahar and Bark 2006).

Todos is mentioned as an expert in human anatomy with knowledge of animal surgical interventions, such as hysterectomy in cows and sows. Other ancestral medical and veterinary professionals in the region included the Jewish kohanim (priests), who, in addition to their various temple roles, performed ritual slaughter of sacrificial animals. There were also Arab *derwishes*, *chatibs* (makers of amulets and tokens), *medjabars* (orthopaedists), *attars* (sellers of medical spices or herbalists), and *shepherds* (caring for animals in pastures). Traditional Bedouins (nomads and shepherds) and Fellahs (sedentary farmers) were other sources of traditional veterinary knowledge in the Near East. Bedouins, in particular, had a long tradition of experience in diagnosing and treating various ailments, predominantly using plant mixtures and fire branding. Mange in camel and sheep was one of the most common skin diseases in the ancient Near East, and various measures were suggested for its control. Commonly used traditional preparations and practices for treating mange, skin lesions, and dermatitis included smearing lesions with asphalt oil and honey, applying powdered dried leaves of *isbaat il barait* (*Plantago psyllium*), concocting leaves of *tufah sedom* (*Calotropis procera*), using sulphurous water from natural sources, and hot-iron branding of the nose in sheep. Bedouins were also aware of the zoonotic significance of sarcoptic mange (Hadani and Shimshony 1994).

Ancient Greece and Roman Civilizations: In early Greco-Roman societies, great importance was attached to domestic animals, as they were indispensable for transport, food, animal traction, and warfare. Sheep, goats, cattle, pigs, mules, horses, and chickens were the main livestock species raised for various purposes. Highly versatile cattle were considered indicators of wealth, and herds often served as barter and gifts in arranged marriages. The oxen were treated with affection and called by names such as Blondie, Dapple, Darkie, Winey and Whitefoot (Jones 2021). Horses, donkeys and mules were used for traction and military purposes, while dogs and cats were kept as pets. Beyond economic reasons, animals held significant roles in Graeco-Roman religion and rituals. The pantheon of gods exerted considerable influence on early Hellenic endeavours, and animals were seen as mediators between gods and humans. Some Greek gods had close connections with specific animals. For instance, Poseidon was associated with the power of horses, and Dionysus was believed to appear to worshippers as a bull. Sacrifices also played a role in these connections; Dionysus, for example, was known as *Taurophagos* (bull-eating) due to bull sacrifices (Bremmer 2020). Dogs were associated with mythological Goddess Hecate and were sacred to Artemis-the goddess of hunt, wilderness, wild animals, vegetation, nature and childcare. Overall, animal husbandry in Greco-Roman culture was primarily practiced by wealthy and powerful individuals who maintained large herds. Their goal was to maintain a healthy stock, achieved through managing diseased animals and preventing healthy ones from falling ill. Zeus the all-powerful, head of the pantheon, presided over many gods who possessed the power of healing and to bring about disease when angered. They could also assume human form and behave like men. Apollo was the master of the creative arts and could spell diseases if displeased. In the mythology Chiron was the son of Cronos the Titan and Philyra the Oceanid. These mythical entities might have had some origin in historical people, in particular Chiron the immortal and Asclepius (Jones 2021).

Chiron the Centaur: Practice of healing in Ancient Greece was attributed to Chiron the Centaur, a sage among the unknown horse culture people who first invaded them. Contrary to the popular myth of half-horse, half-man creatures, the Centaurs were likely tribal people. Chiron, a historic figure from the Prosomeric Period (around 1300 BCE), taught medicine to the ruling class of his time in a specially prepared cave in the Pelion Mountains (also known as the healing mountains). His knowledge combined Indo-Germanic and Asiatic traditions, addressing injuries and diseases in both humans and animal. A cave that matched the traditional and folklore description of original cave dwelling of Chiron was discovered in 1981 by Walter Hausmann in Pelion Mountain in southeastern part of Thessaly in northern Greece (Hausmann and Jöchle 1988). Chiron's expertise extended to botany, pharmacy, and medicine, making him the mentor of Asklepios (the Greek God of Medicine) and Achilles (the Trojan War Hero) who taught art of medicine to Patroclus. Chiron's legacy continued through a family of physicians who passed down the secrets of the herbs of Pelion from father to son, and healed people without charging any fees (Gorrini 2006).

Though regarded a mythical character, Chiron has fascinated the modern veterinary profession, and is upheld symbol of many veterinary associations. For example, the first logo of the United States Veterinary Medical Association featured Chiron holding a scroll inscribed with the Latin phrase *non nobis solum* (meaning not for us alone). The logo was later replaced in 1920 (https://www.avma.org/javma-news/2013-03-01/avma-replace-its-logo, accessed on 24-07-2024). However, the Chiron figure remains on the monograms and heraldic devices of Royal College of Veterinary Surgeons, and Australian Veterinary Association. The Greek representation of Chiron with a branch of lime tree over his shoulder finds place in the emblem of Veterinary History Society, established in 1962. Traditionally, the lime blossom was seen as a remedy and strips of bark were used for divination. Starting with Chiron, the medicine quickly split into two schools- the school of Chironids and the school of Asklepios dividing an originally one-medicine tradition into a medical and veterinary branch. Medically, Asclepius was the most important pupil of Chiron, becoming the god of medicine in ancient Greece. Apsyrtos, Theomnestos, Pelagonios, Columella, Chiron the Younger, and Vegetius Renatus belonged to Chiron's tradition of veterinary medicine (Hausmann and Jöchle 1988).

***Asclepius* (*Aesculapius Asklepios and Asclepios*)**: Like Chiron, Asclepius, the god of medicine and son of Apollo and Coronis (or Arsinoe in Greek mythology), is also believed to be a historic figure. Asclepius treated both humans and animals. According to legend, Apollo himself taught Asclepius many things about medicine. Later, Asclepius was sent to Chiron the Centaur for formal education, where he learned the art of healing. His healing abilities grew, and he eventually gained the power to raise the dead. However, Hades, the god of the underworld, complained to Zeus that Asclepius was depopulating his domain. As a result, Asclepius was punished with a lightning bolt for interfering with the natural order. After his death, Zeus deified Asclepius, making him the god of medicine (Hart 1965). In mythology, Asclepius had five daughters, each with a medical attribute. Hygeia taught people how to lead healthy lives (hygiene), while Panacea healed all and was the originator of medicines. Homer mentioned two sons of Asclepius: Machaon, a gifted surgeon, and Polidarius, who devoted himself to medicine (Jones 2021).

The early Greek physicians were craftsmen who travelled the countryside, carrying instruments, medicines, and a staff. They charged fees from those who could afford it but treated the poor without charge. Asclepius was their hero. Around the sixth century BCE, the physicians became Asclepiads, or sons of Asclepius. This family symbolism represents the earliest attempt by practicing physicians to band together in a group for mutual protection and advancement. By the fifth century BCE, the hero of the physicians became the god of physicians because doctors needed a deity to support and bless their difficult tasks. From this evolution emerged the Cult of Asclepius and the practice of temple medicine, establishing many temples and healing centres around the Mediterranean. The resident priests, known as Asclepiads, offered a particular type of religious medicine by invoking the inspiration and benevolence of Asclepius. They instituted and planned various worship ceremonies. Much of the treatment provided involved the use of baths, diet, light, air, and exercise—customs that are still followed in today's spas (Hart 1965, Jones 2021). An ancient cave sanctuary, identified as a healing shrine, has been discovered beneath the theatre of Miletus in western Turkey. Parts of an image of Asclepius that were on display in the sanctuary and a black marble rod encircled by a serpent (the Asklepion staff) have also been recovered from the site (Niewöhner *et al.* 2017).

Hippocrates (ca.460 -370 BCE): Also known as Hippocrates II and traditionally referred to as the Father of Modern Medicine, is credited by historians with shifting the field of medicine away from its previously supernatural and religious approach, which had been closely linked to the Greek god of healing, Asclepius. Hippocrates advocated for a modern approach based on observation, classification, cause-and-effect relationships, and disease diagnosis. He emphasized the importance of diet and exercise for maintaining a healthy body (Cartwright 2016). Hippocrates was the first Greek healer to assert that illnesses were caused by environmental factors, diet, and lifestyle, rather than being punishments from the gods or afflictions caused by evil spirits or restless souls. However, he was not the originator of this theory. The Egyptian polymath Imhotep (c. 2667-2600 BCE) had suggested a similar concept much earlier, as did Sushruta and Shalihotra in India (Mark 2020). Hippocrates' theory of humoral pathology continued to dominate medicine, including veterinary medicine, for over two millennia.

Aristotle (383–322 BCE): Considered one of the greatest philosophers and scientists of the ancient western world, Aristotle laid the basis for biology by classifying about 500 different animal species. He discussed comparative human and animal anatomy, physiology and pathology and described breeding and lifespan of horses, donkeys, and mules, as well as the castration of bulls and boar, and how these animals grow fatter. Aristotle named several animal diseases with their symptoms but mentioned only bloodletting as treatment. Bloodletting of horses after wintertime remained a regular treatment until well into the nineteenth century. Aristotelian and Hippocratic texts were augmented later by the work of the influential Greek/Roman physician Claudius Galen (Jones and Koolmees 2022). Aristotle's allusion to the opinion of the experienced (ἔμπειροι) that horses suffer from the same diseases as humans suggests that there were people specialized in horse care, but it does not make clear that they were professional horse doctors (McCabe 2007).

Hippiatrica Text: The Hippiatrica is a Byzantine compilation of ancient Greek texts, mainly incorporating excerpts from writing of Apsyrtus, Eumelus, Hierocles, Hippocrates, and Theomnestus, dedicated to the care and healing of horses. Additionally, it includes a Latin text originally written by Pelagonius but translated into Greek. The authors of the Hippiatrica cite to their classical Greek veterinary predecessors notably, Xenophon and Simon of Athens. The Hippiatrica was probably compiled in the fifth or sixth century CE by an unknown editor. The work remains a significant monument of technical literature in Greece, focusing on equine diseases. The Hippiatrica originally presented (but somewhat disorganised by later copyists) the vast work in an organized manner, ailment-by-ailment and author-by-author, concluding with lists of drug recipes. The symptoms and maladies described in the text largely persist in horses today, including lameness, cough, colic, laminitis, glanders, and parasites. However, some conditions, like affliction by the evil eye, are no longer covered in horse care manuals (though they may still be a cause for concern). Additionally, the text sheds light on other aspects of horse care, such as breeding, breaking, feeding, grooming, and stable management. No other source provides such vivid glimpses into daily life of stables as does Hippiatrica. For example, it mentions that horses were massaged with wine and oil and their stalls were strewn with bay and myrtle leaves or fumigated with myrrh. Horses were brought down to the sea to swim and their treatment prescriptions composed of exotic and expensive spices, sauna sessions in Roman baths, and the use of incantations. Magical amulets and chicken soup were also part of the regimen, reflecting the care lavished on these valuable animals. Moreover, descriptions reveal the deep affection owners felt for their horses, as well as their distress when the animals suffered (McCabe 2007).

Romans adopted Greek medical and veterinary practices, which spread throughout Europe within the confines of their empire. According to BV Jones, the procedures and medications during the Roman period are known, but it remains uncertain who used them and what their official position or status was. Professional veterinarians primarily worked with equids, and cattle used in transportation within the army. On livestock farms, herdsmen or the owners and managers were responsible for animal healthcare. Herdsmen were expected to have some veterinary knowledge, maintain health records, and likely used recipes for medications (Jones 2021). They would decide if a specialist was required, indicating the need for veterinarians in general practice. In all texts dating back to Varro and Columella certain basic principles were advocated. The fundamental approach was disease prevention through hygiene, cleanliness, proper housing, clean flooring, access to clean water and salt, quality feed, attentive care for all livestock. A mix of herbal concoction and ritual applications was also practiced to prevent disease. Garlic, frankincense, laurel leaves and leek (*Allium ampeloprasum*) were used for prevention of illness at cattle farms. Daily checks and isolation of sick animals were common practices. In disease out-breaks the sick animals were separated and sent to distant isolation; were treated with mix of herbs including panax and eryngo roots, cinnamon, myrrh, and frankincense (Akers-Campbell 2016).

Skin diseases and gastrointestinal helminthic infections were prevalent in sheep, and herbal antiparasitic were used for treatment. Pigs were highly popular farm animals. They were bred for meat and fat and also used in sacrificial rituals in ancient Rome. Ancient veterinary authors described symptoms resembling anthrax, foot-and-mouth disease, and swine fever. Various skin problems were recognized, and treatments included bleeding and herbal medicine (Jones 2021). Sows were given a separate diet based on barley or roasted wheat to increase milk production, thus ensuring the healthy development of piglets. During winter and autumn, the diet of pigs was supplemented by feeding acorns, leaves, chaff, and other items. These preferred diets not only provided nutrient-rich food but also helped maintain the animals in good shape (Bartnik 2023). Published literature highlights the significance of domestic birds, especially chickens in Roman culture. In avian medicine, emphasis was placed on hygienic measures, and adequate feed. Preventive measures included construction of perches to allow birds sleep elevated from their own manure, addition of clean bedding to nesting boxes and use of covered water trough to check contamination from manure and fumigation. Garlic, wild grape, and warm oil were fed orally to moderately sick birds (Akers-Campbell 2016).

Horse and equine medicine held a central place in veterinary activities during ancient Rome. Horse breeding and training were essential animal husbandry practices in the Roman Empire. In addition to transportation and military use, horses were widely used in chariot racing. It is likely that herds of horses kept for breeding and those used for other purposes, such as riding or circus performances, were kept separately. Horses bred for breeding purpose were primarily raised on well-off estates with the necessary resources for keeping, training, and selling them. From an early age, horses were desensitized to handling and harnesses. Colts were broken in at three year age under the saddle, and light exercise was introduced. By the age of five, circus horses underwent evaluation and were assigned to one of two chariot positions, beginning their racing careers, which sometimes lasted up to 15 years (Klecel and Martyniuk 2021). Donkeys, though categorized as lesser farm animals, were highly valued in Roman society for their sturdiness and ability to work on frugal feed. They were primarily used in mills and fields for hauling out manure, ploughing light soil, and serving as beasts of burden. Romans also bred mules (*muli*) and hinnies (*hinni*). The mules were used primarily for carting and as pack animals (Akers-Campbell 2016).

Equine medicine was well-developed in ancient Rome. General health advice included daily grooming, access to shelter, water, and exercise at appropriate times. Sick horses were well-bedded. Similar to many old-timers today, Romans believed that having a horse drink after sweating was dangerous. The most common sources of problems were fatigue, overheating, failure to pass urine, and prolonged standing before work. Pregnant mares received special care and were not used for heavy work. Foals were left untouched after birth. Breeders ensured a spacious, warm environment for the foal and mare, taking care not to let the foal's hooves become caked with manure (Akers-Campbell 2016). Bleeding from specific sites (*Diocletian, Depletura*, and *Purgationes*) was practiced to remove corrupted blood and achieve humoral balance. *Tonsurae* (clipping) to keep horses looking good, and *Aptaturae pedis* (foot care and dressing) were common procedures (Jones 2021). The treatment of equine diseases primarily relied on specific natural medicines and physiotherapy. Professional animal healers responsible for equine health were initially known as *medicus equorum* (horse doctors) and *veterinarius*, later evolving into *mulomedicus* (mule doctors) in the fourth century. The term *veterinarius*, referring to caretakers of *bestia veterina* (equines) appeared in Columella's treatise on Roman agriculture (Jones and Koolmees 2022).

The dog was a much-loved companion and performed various functions in ancient Rome. There were hunting dogs known as *canes venatici* (sporting dogs), which were categorized based on their specific hunting roles. The *sagaces* were used to track prey (hounds), the *celeres* were fast dogs used for pursuing prey, with a preference for the greyhound (*canes vertragus*), and the canes *pugnaces* were used to attack prey, particularly wild boars and other animals. Rural communities used dogs for herding and guarding villages, while *canes pastorales* (shepherd dogs) were responsible for caring for and transporting livestock. These dogs also protected livestock from predators in the fields and forests. The *canes villatici* (watchdogs) were assigned to guard homes, estates (*domus*), islands (*insulae*), villas, or workshops, alerting their owners to the presence of strangers (Tanga *et al.* 2022). Selective breeding and maintaining healthy puppies were priorities for all dog species. Weak pups were culled. Their diet primarily consisted of meat, bones, and barley bread. Skin issues such as mange, fleas, and ticks were treated with sulphur preparations. Common conditions like foot diseases (*podagra*), cough, constipation, and diarrhoea were addressed using similar medications as those used for livestock. Rabies (*lyssa*) was also recognized, and cauterizing dog bites was recommended to prevent its spread (Yeates 2018).

In ancient Rome, a notable list of writers—including Cato, Varro, Vergil, Vegetius, Columella, Pliny, and Palladius—focused on agriculture, animal husbandry, and veterinary medicine. While many of these authors drew from their own sources, the bulk of their information, whether cited or uncited, came from ancient Greek literature related to agriculture. Additionally, the text of Mago the Carthaginian served as a crucial source for Roman writers; it was translated into Latin from Punic by decree of the Senate in 146 BCE (Akers-Campbell, 2016). The Roman works dedicated entirely to veterinary medicine, include *Ars Veterinaria* by Pelagonius and *Digesta Artis Mulomedicinae* by Vegetius (Jones and Koolmees 2022). For further insights into Roman authors who wrote about veterinary and agricultural practices, *The History of Veterinary Medicine and the Animal-Human Relationship* (Jones 2021) provides concise information, and a select authors few and their work are briefly mentioned here.

***Marcus Portius Cato (234–149 BCE)*:** Cato the Elder, also known as Cato the Censor, was a Roman senator who possessed a large estate. He showed a particular interest in agriculture. His manual on running a farm, *De agri cultura* (On Agriculture), is his only surviving work. Written around 160 BC, *De agri cultura* is the earliest Roman agricultural and veterinary text. It provides insights into the state of ancient Roman agriculture and their veterinary practices. Cato's specific veterinary remedies often lack rationality, with much of the advice rooted in folklore. However, some practical recommendations stand out. For instance, he advised coating the feet of working oxen with tar: 'Smear the bottom of the hoof with liquid pitch before driving them anywhere on the road.' Cato recognized sheep scab and external parasites, recommending the use of salves and washing. Emphasizing the importance of cattle as draught animals, Cato suggested that owners should sell old work oxen and blemished cattle and sheep. He also wrote about preventive medicine and animal welfare, emphasizing the value of providing clear, clean water for livestock (Jones 2021).

***Marcus Terentius Varro (116–27 BCE)*:** One of the greatest scholars of ancient Rome, Varro was born in Reate, Italy. He studied under a prominent Latin scholar and the philosopher Antiochus of Ascalon in Athens. Although he was not drawn to a political career, Varro's immense learning and prolific writing led him to produce approximately 74 works across more than 600 books. His diverse subjects included jurisprudence, astronomy, geography, education, literary history, satires, poems, orations, and letters. Among his surviving works, the *Res Rustica* (Farm Topics) stands out (Encyclopedia Britannica. https://www.britannica.com/biography/Marcus-Terentius-Varro). This three-section work provides practical instructions on general agriculture and animal husbandry. The sections cover:

General Agriculture (Section 1); Cattle and Sheep Breeding (Section 2) and Other Animals, including Birds and Bees (Section 3). Varro emphasized the value of cattle as the foundation of wealth. Interestingly, neither cattle nor sheep were primarily considered meat animals. Instead, Varro assumed that every farmer would also raise pigs and poultry for this purpose. While veterinary practices were a minor part of Varro's writing, they shed light on the significant challenges faced in livestock farming during his time. Varro advised protecting cattle from flies during the summer. He also emphasized well-paved floors in their housing, proper drainage, and regular dung removal. Varro gives us a detailed description of the leading cause and treatment of exertional rhabdomyolysis (ER), or so-called tying-up and correctly states that it occurs when a horse is given feed or water immediately after the exercise, which causes fever and pain. The treatment proposed is to drench an animal with water, rub down with oil and wine, cover it with a blanket, and restrain it from any food. In current treatment also this procedure is almost identical (Klecel and Martyniuk 2021). Pregnant sows needed individual housing, and poultry required examination for mites. Varro recognized the importance of bees (honey being the sole sweetener). He understood bee diseases and emphasized their care. Scab prevention was essential in sheep, and affected sheep should not be sheared. Wounds from shearing were treated with liquid tar. Varro's approach to disease considered three factors: cause, symptoms, and treatment. Feeding, housing, breeding, and care were also crucial aspects of livestock management (Jones 2021). His legacy endures, and his multidisciplinary contributions continue to inspire scholars across generations, and his work has been cited widely by the ancient Roman authors.

***Lucius Junius Moderatus Columella (ca. 4–70 CE)*:** Born in southwestern Spain, Columella moved to Rome, where he owned a large agricultural farm. Columella authored *De Re Rustica* (On Agriculture), one of the most comprehensive surviving farming manuals of the ancient world. Of the twelve volumes (books) of *De Re Rustica*, four volumes (VI-IX) focus on breeding, care, and diseases of oxen, bulls, cows, horses, and mules (Vol. VI); diseases of asses, sheep, goats, pigs, and dogs (Vol. VII); poultry, fowl, geese, ducks, doves, thrushes, peacocks, fish, and fish ponds (Vol. VIII); and the management of wild animals, their diseases, pests, honey bees, and wax (Vol. IX). Columella referred to his uncle Marcus Columella as a clever man and an exceptional farmer, who had conducted experiments in sheep breeding, such as crossing colourful wild rams from Africa with domestic sheep for gladiatorial games. Columella emphasizes the care, management, and hygiene of animals, as well as good feeding practices. He suggests cause and treatment of plague in cattle using herbs including lungwort and fennel seeds with wheat flour. Remedies for cough, scab, and worm in calves are also described (Vol V). Besides treatment of different conditions, restraining cruelty of stallion is mentioned in Book VI. He recognized that certain diseases are contagious and stressed the importance of separating healthy and sick animals, with isolation of the latter (Jones 2021).

Aelius Galenus or Claudius Galenus (ca. 129–216CE): Also known as Galen of Pergamum, Gelen was one of the most famous Greek and Roman physicians. Born in Pergamum, Mysia (Anatolia, Turkey) in 129 CE, he later moved to Rome in 162 CE. Galen frequently dissected and experimented on lower animals, recognizing the similarities between human and animal physiology. He used dissections on farm animals—pigs, sheep, and goats—to develop ideas and knowledge of human anatomy, which became a cornerstone in medicine (Yeates 2018). His ability to treat patients was informed by his knowledge of anatomy derived from experiments on animals. Galen correctly assumed that what was harmful to an animal would be equally harmful to a human, and conversely, what would promote health in one would likely do so in the other (Mark 2020). Other important writings dealing with early veterinary knowledge in ancient Rome, included the *Digesta Artis Mulomedicinae*, authored by Flavius Vegetius Renatus, a late Roman military man and horse breeder (around 385 CE), and *Opus Agriculturae* by Palladius (4th–5th century CE).

In general, most of the ancient agricultural and veterinary treatises were written by individuals with extensive farming or military experience in equine care and medicine. Their focus was on disease prevention, ensuring adequate feeding, clean water, proper housing, and responsible breeding practices, including care for pregnant animals and newborns. Greek and Roman writers also recognized the importance of animal welfare. While some of the ancient veterinary practice may seem unappealing by modern standards, certain herbal remedies, feeding strategies and hygienic measures hold good even today.

Traditional Chinese Veterinary Medicine (TCVM): Chinese veterinary medicine, including acupuncture and herbal treatments, is believed to have evolved alongside the domestication of animals. According to legend, Emperor Fusi (Fuxi or Fu His) played a pivotal role in founding animal husbandry and veterinary medicine in China. He taught the Chinese ancestors how to domesticate animals and fish, thereby contributing to the advancement of civilization in the primitive society of ancient China. Fusi is revered as the forefather of Chinese culture. In Middle Eastern countries, shepherds relied on a basic understanding of medical techniques and skills to care for their dogs and other animals. For nearly two millennia, early medical practitioners in ancient China treated both humans and animals. Although the first mention of diseases and horse treatments can be traced back to the writings of the Shang Dynasty (1766–1027 BCE), a distinct branch of Traditional Chinese Veterinary Medicine (TCVM) emerged during the Zhou Dynasty (1122–770 BCE). During the Western Zhou Dynasty (1111–771 BCE), veterinary departments were integrated into the national healthcare system, emphasizing the importance of animal health alongside human health. The *Bai Le's Canon of Veterinary Medicine*, written during the 8th century by Sun Yang, is considered the earliest text on TCVM (Lin and Panzer 1994).

The fundamental concept of both Traditional Chinese Medicine (TCM) and Traditional Chinese Veterinary Medicine (TCVM), is derived from Chinese philosophical thinking, emphasizing the essential truth of health as balance. This balance extends to various aspects: within oneself, with others, in one's diet, and in harmony with nature. Chinese traditional veterinary practices encompass five major branches: **Chinese Herbal Therapy**–utilizing herbs for healing; **Acupuncture**–the practice of inserting fine needles into specific points on the body to promote balance and alleviate ailments; **Chinese Food Therapy**–Focusing on dietary adjustments to maintain health; **Tui-na**–A form of therapeutic massage and manipulation; and **Qi-gong (Chi-gong)**–incorporating energy cultivation exercises. These branches are influenced by decisive theories, such as Yin-yang theory, the five-element theory, the human body channel system, Zang-Fu organ physiology, six confirmations and four layers theory. In terms of modern Patho-physiological understandings, the traditional Chinese medical and veterinary theories could be linked to activation of humoral immunity, management of water and electrolytes via kidney, intestine and colon, and dependence of normal development on liquid substances (hormones), which, if lacking at birth, could not be replaced (Marsden 2007). Treatment approaches, tailored to signs and diagnoses included herbs, special diets, manipulation, and moxibustion (burning bits of the herb Artemesia at points on the skin to affect the body's interior), as well as external interventions such as cautery, cutting, and a type of bone-setting ((Jones and Koolmees 2022).

The Chinese possessed extensive knowledge of medicinal herbs and routinely used them for healthcare, often in conjunction with acupuncture. These herbs were classified based on their efficacy and toxicity, and polyherbal formulations were commonly used. The components within these formulations were graded according to their specific functions. The nearly 5,000-year-old *Materia Medica*, now known as the *Herbal Classics of Shen Nong (Shen Nong Ben Cao Jing*), was compiled by the ancient Chinese emperor Shen Nong, also known as the mythical divine farmer. This text, believed to have originated around 2800 BC, lists 365 substances along with their descriptions and medicinal uses. Each item is categorized into one of six classes: minerals, herbs, woods, animals, fruits and vegetables, and cereals. Additionally, substances are further classified into three grades of quality: noble (120), middle (120), and inferior (125). Noble substances are non-toxic and suitable for long-term use in disease treatment, promoting longevity. Middle-grade substances range from nontoxic to mildly toxic and are recommended for treating ailments and expelling pathogens, but not for extended periods. Highly toxic substances, sometimes violent and dangerous, are advised for infrequent usage in low doses. Despite an apparent discrepancy between the work's date of origin and its attributed author (disregarding Shen Nong's mythical nature), it is likely that the information in this text was transmitted orally until the 3rd century CE, at which point it was attributed to Shen Nong. Many of the ingredients listed in the book continue to be used in Traditional Chinese Medicine today (https://healthandfitnesshistory.com/ancient-medicine/herbal-classic-of-shen-nong/, accessed on 5-08-2024). Notably, herbs such as ephedra, ginger, rhubarb, Ginseng, and wormwood have been scientifically validated and find application in modern veterinary and medical practices. For instance, Chinese wormwood (*Artemisia annua*), described in the text as antipyretic, has been scientifically proven to possess antimalarial properties, while Ginseng remains widely used as an immunomodulator.

Acupuncture is an ancient Chinese medical practice that has been scientifically validated and is increasingly used by modern medical and veterinary practitioners. The first written medical reference on Chinese acupuncture theory and treatment dates back around two millennia. In Chinese traditional medicine, *Qi* (often pronounced as *Chee*) represents the specific type of power that sustains life. It is generated by the interplay of Yin and Yang and flows through the body along interconnected pathways that link the external body surface with internal organs. When this power is deficient, an organ may function poorly. The goal of acupuncture therapy is to facilitate the free flow of Qi, thereby maintaining the body's balance (homeostasis). Acupuncture needles, when strategically placed at specific points, activate the movement of Qi. Acupuncture is practiced in many countries, particularly China, Korea, and Japan, to address a range of chronic conditions, including chronic pain resulting from cancer or trauma. Modern scientific studies have demonstrated acupuncture's validity as a cost-effective treatment in veterinary medicine, with significant efficacy across a wide variety of diseases—even those for which conventional treatments are ineffective (Xie and Wedemeyer 2012). For example, numerous clinical studies revealed that acupuncture effectively manages pain and improves the quality of life in dogs with osteoarthritis, as well as certain neurologic and musculoskeletal disorders. It is particularly effective when used as a complementary therapy alongside other modalities such as analgesics (pain medications), laser therapy, massage, and physical therapy. These multimodal treatment protocols are beneficial for neurological and musculoskeletal diseases in dogs (Silva *et al.* 2017, Bailey 2022). Another essential branch of Traditional Chinese Veterinary Medicine (TCVM) is food therapy. Chinese medicine categorizes different food ingredients based on their cooling or warming properties and flavours, which can influence the balance of Yin and Yang and overall health. Consequently, specific food combinations are prescribed to correct imbalances in the body during disease conditions. The modern concept of functional foods and nutraceuticals aligns with this ancient Chinese perspective.

Ancient India: The origins of animal husbandry and veterinary medicine in India date back to the early Food Production Era around 7000 BCE, predating the Indus Valley Civilization. The sheep-rearing communities were the first herders in the subcontinent and possibly the earliest animal healers. These early healers likely practiced magico-religious methods and used basic knowledge of medicinal herbs to keep their animals disease-free. The subsequent domestication of other animals, particularly cattle, and the cultivation of crops, led to a rapid transition to a sedentary lifestyle, fostering socio-economic and cultural growth. This period gave rise to the Indus Valley or Harappan Civilization, the largest of the five original major civilizations of ancient times, spanning a vast territory of approximately 1,500,000 squares km with over 1,500 sites, ranging from village-farming communities and small towns to wealthy urban centres during the Mature Harappan Phase (Arnott 2024).

Indus Valley Civilization (3500–1300 BCE): Zooarchaeological evidence suggests that during the Indus Valley Civilization, domestic animals—including cattle, buffaloes, sheep, goats, pigs, and poultry—were highly valued for their socio-religious and economic roles, receiving proper care. The people of the Indus Valley likely mastered the art of taming elephants, using them for riding. They were also knowledgeable about various wild game and animal products, such as milk, meat, curd, ghee, cheese, and honey. However, unlike the numerous studies that provide valuable insights into human diseases and medical care, information on animal diseases and veterinary practices during Indus Valley Period remains scarce. Reports indicate that many infectious and non-infectious medical conditions, including zoonotic diseases like anthrax, tuberculosis, and rabies, as well as malaria, smallpox, sickle cell anaemia, metabolic disorders, occupational health hazards, traumatic injuries, dental diseases, osteoarthritis, and other degenerative bone diseases, were prevalent among the Indus Valley population. Their healing practices included healing cults, Indus Valley votives, and remedies based on plant, mineral, and animal products, along with food and drinks, surgical practices such as trepanation, and orthopaedics. The people had a high sense of sanitation, as evidenced by public health and sanitation infrastructure like the Great Bath unearthed at Mohenjo-Daro, urban drainage and sewage systems, and potable water supply (Arnott 2024).

Although the precise status of veterinary activities in the Indus Valley is unclear, studies suggest that secondary animal products, such as milk, wool, and draught power, were significant to the Harappan economy. Male cattle and buffaloes were used for breeding and as draught animals for agricultural work and cart-pulling, while cows were raised for dairying and sheep for wool. It is conceivable that maintaining healthy animals and preventing disease were not only economically important but also vital for safeguarding public health from zoonotic hazards. It is likely that some affordable healing practices used in human medicine were also applied to animals. Castration and dehorning were probably common practices to raise strong yet docile bullocks for draught purposes. Scientific studies from Harappan sites in Gujarat indicate that animals were well-fed, with provisions made for year-round fodder availability, including green millet for cattle, buffaloes, and sheep and goats (Chakraborty *et al.* 2018, Suryanarayan 2023).

Vedic India (ca.1500 – 600 BCE) : The early Aryans primarily relied on crop cultivation and livestock for their livelihood. They harnessed the power of oxen and horses for various agricultural activities and honed their horse-riding skills.

The Aryans also utilized mares for milk production. In Vedic culture, cows were revered as representations of the Earth, often associated with the goddess *Aditi.* Many tribal conflicts centered around protecting or acquiring livestock wealth. Cow's milk was considered a source of special energy, strength, and intelligence, while cow dung and urine nourished agricultural practices. In Vedic villages, children often directly suck milk from cow udders, much like they would from their mother's breast. The presence of milch cows in their homes, visible every day, contributed to the moral value of equating the cow with the mother, the son with the calf (*vatsa*), and the daughter with the she-calf (*vatsā*). Sentimental affection seems to have developed between the cows and daughters, leading to the daughters being entrusted with the task of milking the cows. This earned them the epithet of *duhitā* (milker*).* The veneration for cows was so profound that the *pañca-gav (Panchgavya)*, a mixture of five cow products (milk, curds, ghee, urine, and dung), was considered health-giving and effective for purification (Kansara 1995). The term *Godhuli*, referring to the dust raised by cows returning home during sunset, holds great auspicious significance in Hindu tradition. It symbolizes abundance, prosperity, and well-being associated with cows returning from pastures with their udders filled with milk since the Vedic period. Bullock power played a crucial role in developing agricultural techniques, including carrying heavy loads, transportation, and supporting cottage industries. Animal skins from deceased animals supported the leather industry and handicrafts. In summary, cattle husbandry held a central place in Indian lifestyle and economy during the Vedic period (Somvanshi 2006).

Vedic literature indicates the role of Gods (*Dev*) in protecting their worshippers, granting them food, large flocks, large families, and long life. The sixth *Anuvaka* of the eighth Mandala of the Rigveda is entirely related to liberal gifts in the form of horses, camels, brown mares, and cows with red patches (Rig Veda 8.6.4.22). Vedic literature also mentions the association of different gods with domestication, care, housing, safety, and treatment of animals. For example, Rudra is the creator and mentor of all four-legged animals; Indra serves as the protector, saviour, animal healer, and obstetrician; Vayu protects animals on pasture; Tvasta is involved in pairing (breeding?), and Brahaspati brings cows into *Gosthas* (domestication of wild cattle?). According to Indian mythological belief, Brahma taught the knowledge of Veda to the other gods including the Sun God and his twin sons-Ashvins (Centaur?) who became the physician of Gods and custodian of Atharva Veda. Rudra, the primary Vedic name for Shiva, is revered as the foremost doctor and healer, lauded in the Rig Veda as the supreme physician (*bhishaktamam tvā bhishajām shṛṇomi*). The sacred *Mahamrityunjaya Mantra*, which first appeared in the Rig Veda (7.59.12) is considered one of the most powerful and ancient mantras dedicated to Lord Shiva. In this mantra, which also appears in Yajur Veda, Rudra is invoked as the personification of the healing ritual, granting well-being and longevity (*Ayu*), freedom from disease, and protection from untimely death. As legend goes Brahma taught *Hayayurveda* to Shalihotra, the founder of veterinary science in the Indian tradition (Krishna *et al.* 2005, Swarup *et al.*

2013). In line with other contemporary civilizations, religious priests or sages were the earliest animal healers or veterinarians. Originally, the term Brahmin meant healer, as Brahmins constituted a class of healers (Thrusfield 2018). Numerous Vedic hymns highlight the medicinal properties of herbs, suggesting that these priests were well-versed in their use. They likely applied their medical knowledge to maintain the health of sacred cattle (Somvanshi 2006). The Vedic sages recognized the importance of human, animal, and plant health, leading to the evolution of the science of Ayurveda, which comprised not only the Ayurveda for human health, but also *Pashu* or *Mrig-Ayurveda* for the health and welfare of animals, and *Vriksha Ayurveda* for plant health. The sages of the Atharva Veda (8.7.11) state: *Apakrītāḥ sahīyasīrvīrudho yā abhiṣtutāh. Trāyantāmasmingrāme gāmaśvaṁ puruṣaṁ paśum*: 'Let herbs and plants, purchased, raised in power, and reinforced, properly assessed, adjudged, and defined, protect the people, cows, and other animals in the village' (Sharma 2013). It can be said that the Vedic sages were the first to conceptualize the idea of one-health.

Vedic texts document the use of medicinal herbs to cure human and animal ailments. Zoopharmacognosy (self-medication by animals) also finds its roots in these texts, as sages closely observed and recorded the behaviour of sick animals. The Atharva Veda (8. 7.23) mentions that a wild boar knows the herb which will cure it, as does the mongoose. Benefits of herbs and their ointments for human beings, cows, and horses are also described in Atharva Veda (4. 9.2). Surgical treatment of animal disease was very much developed during Vedic period. Skilful surgeons treated animals with precision and great perfection. Various techniques of veterinary surgical operations along with instruments have been dealt in detail in Shalihotra's and Palakapya's works. Common surgical methods used by Vedic physicians and surgeons included the application of cautery, removal of foreign bodies and obstructions, surgical grafting, and treatment of fractures, dislocations, and fistulas to cure both humans and animals. The surgeons were skilled in suturing and plastering practices, routinely applying surgical knowledge to treat sinus fistulas, burns, scalds, snakebites, fractures, ligament/tendon ailments, dystocia, and the removal of dead foetuses (Somvanshi 2006).

The dissection of animals was considered valuable for studying the human body, and procedures for animal dissection have been described in the Susrutasamhitâ, the seminal work attributed to (Sushruta) the father of surgery and the inventor of plastic surgery. Veterinarians, like surgeons, needed to be aware of vulnerable regions or vital points called *marma*. The word *marma* is derived from Sanskrit *mru* or *murr* and is defined as *maryate iti marmani*, meaning there is a likelihood of death or serious health problems upon inflicting injury on these points, hence they are called marma. These vital points are anatomically defined as areas with high vascularity, joining points of tendons, veins, arteries, and bones (joints). Ayurveda defines 107 such points in the human body, and animals may also have a similar number of *marma* points. The concept of *marma* therapy and its possible applications are discussed in Chapter 9 on Veterinary Ayurveda.

Epic Age (ca. 1000 to 600 BCE): The concept of *ahimsa* emerged in this era to prevent the practice of sacrificing animals to please the gods. Mahabharata, tells in length about merits of vegetarianism and demerits of consuming meat to solely to allude to the torture and slaughter of animals, and declares- *ahiṃsā paramo dharmas tathāhiṃsā param tapah; ahiṃsā paramaṃ satyam yato dharmah pravartate tapaḥ*- Translated as 'abstention from injury is the highest religion; it is, again, the highest penance; it is also the highest truth from which all duty proceeds.' (*Anushasana Parva*115. 23). Both the Ramayana and Mahabharata mention the uses and care of domestic and war animals, including cattle, horses, donkeys, elephants, and dogs. The cow was adored and regarded as a source of wealth, happiness, and good fortune. Two important festivals of Braj—*Gopashtami* (celebrated on the eighth lunar day of Kartik) and *Govardhan Puja* (celebrated the day after Diwali in Kartik)—are dedicated to cattle and Lord Krishna, with their origins traceable to medieval Hindu texts (Lodric 1987). The name *Govardhana* comes from Sanskrit: *go* (cow) + *vardhana* (to increase, grow, or nourish), literally meaning 'nourishment of cows', 'increasing cows' or 'cow nourisher'. *Gopashtami* derives from *gopa* (cowherd) + *aṣṭamī* (eighth lunar day), literally 'the eighth day of the cowherds.' According to legend, Krishna, as a young cowherd, was entrusted with the responsibility of tending cows—transitioning from calves to adult cattle—on this day. The myths and rituals associated with these festivals highlight Krishna's profound connection with cows, reinforcing traditional Hindu concepts and underscoring the essential role of cattle in sustaining life. Cows symbolize nourishment, selflessness, prosperity, and the nurturing energy that fosters harmony with nature. Indian philosophy also explored the mysteries of life and the universe, leading to the development of cow science (*go-vijñāna*)—a unique contribution of India to the world. Ancient Indian scholars regarded the entire cow family (*gau vansh*) as indispensable for the existence, protection, nourishment, development, and cultural foundation of humanity (Somvanshi 2006).

Lord Krishna was also an equine expert, and glimpses of his equine medicine skills can be found in the Mahabharata. He is referred to as *kuśalo hyaśvakarmaṇi*, which translates to well-skilled in grooming horses. The epic portrays Krishna performing the role of a battlefield veterinarian. Skilled in the care of horses, he relieved the steeds of exhaustion, pain, trembling, and wounds, removed embedded arrows, rubbed them with his own hands, made them walk properly, refreshed them with water, and then carefully re-yoked them to the chariot (Mahabharata, Drona Parva 100.14–15). Medicinal herbs like *arjuna* (*Terminalia arjuna*), coral swirl or *kutaja* (*Holarrhena antidysenterica*), common-bur flower tree or *kadamba* (*Anthocephalus cadamba*), Indian copal tree or *dhupa* (*Vateria indica*), margosa tree or *neem* (*Azadirachta indica*), Asok tree or *Ashoka* (*Saraca asoca*), etc., were commonly used to treat human and animal diseases. Diseases like leprosy, tuberculosis, mental disorders, etc. were described along with treatment. The herbs found in the mountains of Kanchenjunga and Kailash (now in China) are said to possess good medicinal quality (Somvanshi 2006). Other treatment methods included use of animal products, minerals and fumigation and rituals to appease the god.

Buddhist and Mauryan Period (600 – 200 BCE): This period witnessed an all-round progress in animal husbandry and healthcare of livestock, which contributed richly to state economy. The animal wealth was one of the most important state assets as cattle, buffalo, sheep, goat, horses, donkeys, elephants and camel served the society in several ways. Majority of population was agriculturists and engaged in animal husbandry. Like Vedic and epic periods, cows continued to be adored and highly protected class of animal in Buddhist text. The Suttanipāta regards cattle as givers of food (annada), beauty (vaṇṇada), and therefore deserving of protection. The period marked with development of several concepts pertaining to animal breeding, feeding, management and healthcare such as concept of feeding both green (*yavasa*) and dry fodder (*trina*) to maintain optimum health and production. Feeding of oil cakes was also recommended. Even today, the dairy farmers in India follow this feeding practice. Concept of proper milking was also developed during the Mauryan time. Cows were milked only once in morning during summer and spring months and twice daily during rest of the year. They were the main dairy animal, though buffaloes and goats were also recognized as the important source of milk.

Kautilya's Arthaśāstra (4th – 3rd century BCE): This widely acknowledged source of ancient knowledge elaborates management of different categories of livestock under the over-all supervision of cattle superintendent. Stall feeding was rarely practiced and domestic animals were commonly raised on pastures. The grazing pastures were located in the safe forest areas free from tigers, beasts and thieves. Common pasture lands, located within village boundary-walls, were maintained by village head who would charge prescribed grazing fee. Village head was also responsible to ensure that animals do not graze or enter into cultivated field or garden

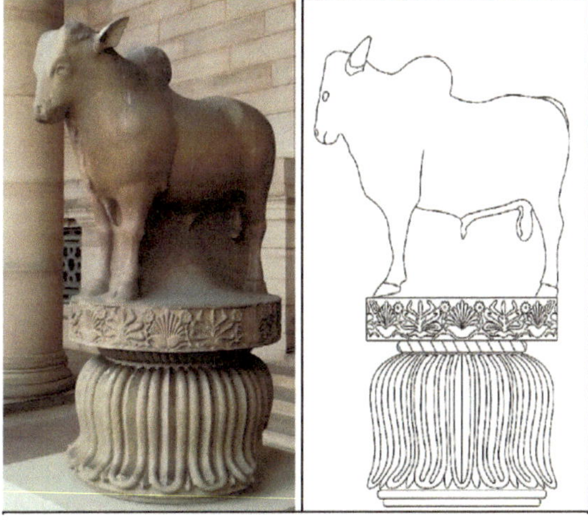

Fig.4.4. *Discovered at the Rampurva archaeological site in Bihar, the iconic Rampurva Vrishabhashirsha Stambh, or Rampurva bull capital, is one of the seven remaining animal capitals from the pillars of Ashoka. This zebu bull, standing gracefully on a pedestal with sensitive nostrils, alert ears, and strong legs, has become a significant symbol of veterinary science being used as a logo by many veterinary and animal science institutes in India (Photo and sketch image courtesy of Dr. Rameshwar Singh BASU).*

land. Alike to Hammurabi Code, provision for charging fee and fines are also defined in Arthasastra. However, bulls belonging to village temples, stud bulls and cows up to ten days post- calving were exempted from grazing charges prescribed as 1/16 -1/4 pana for sheep and goat; 1/8- ½ pana for cattle, horses, donkeys and ½ to 1 pana depending upon the type of grazing practices. Animal breeding was given special attention and an official breeder was appointed for improving the breed of animals. Arthasastra mentions that for breeding purpose, 5 stallion (donkeys and horses), 10 rams and bucks (sheep and goats) and 4 bulls (cows, buffaloes or camel) should be kept for every herd of 100 animals. More or less, the same proportion of breeding males is used by modern breeders. Kautilya's Arsthasastra also defines method of animal identification and maintaining record of identified animals and type of nutrition to be provided to animals under certain physiological conditions. Oxen and cows were provided subsistence proportionate to duration of work (draught) and quantity of milk produced. Fodder and water were provided *ad lib.* to all cattle. State funded veterinary services were introduced during the Mauryan period and the first known veterinary hospital with indoor patient facility was erected during the reign of great Ashoka (ca. 269– 232 BCE). He also established protocols for use of medicinal herbs both for human and animal treatment. Rock Edict II (Fig. 4.5) inscribes that '……everywhere has Beloved-of-the-Gods, King Piyadasi, made provision for two types of medical treatment: medical treatment for humans and medical treatment for animals. Wherever medical herbs suitable for humans or animals are not available, I have had them imported and grown. Wherever roots or fruits are not available I have had them brought and grown. Along roads I have had wells dug and trees planted for the benefit of humans and animals.' By so doing, Asoka was following the advice given by the Buddha at Saṃyutta *Nikāya* (Dhammika 1993).

In ancient India, animals received excellent medical care. Physicians who treated human beings were also trained in animal care. Indian medical treatises, such as the Charaka Samhita, Sushruta Samhita, and Harita Samhita, contain chapters or references related to the care of both diseased and healthy animals. Athrva Veda, Purāṇas, Brāhmaṇa, and epics also contain information on animal care. Perhaps the practice of animal and human treatment acquired status of separate profession during later Vedic and epic period with the emergence of prominent veterinary experts who specialized exclusively in animal care or focused on specific classes of animals. The most renowned among them was Shalihotra—the world's first known veterinarian and the father of Indian veterinary sciences (Mark 2020). In general, Indian traditional medicine practices and philosophies greatly influenced the early understanding of diseases, their pathophysiology, diagnosis and treatment in the ancient world with constant interchange of ideas. Some Hippocratic ideas can be determined in the original Indian concepts (See chapters 6 and 9 for more details).

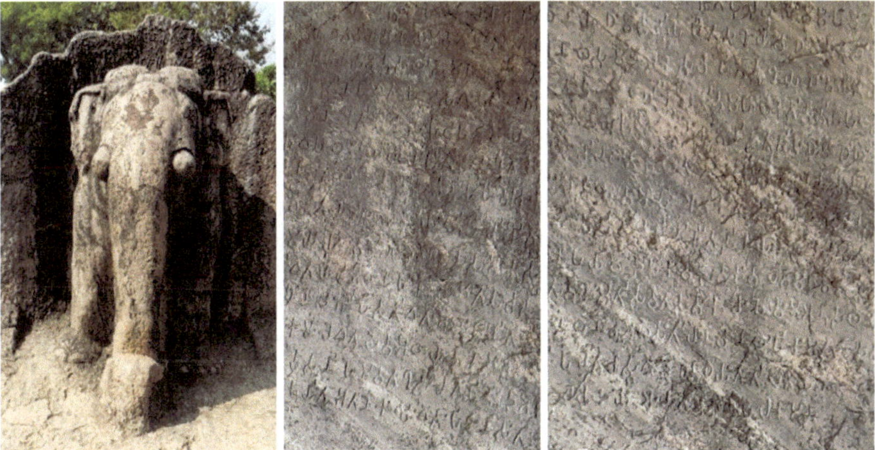

Fig.4.5. Dating back to the 3rd century BCE, the Asokan edicts are located on a small hill called Aswathama at Dhauli, near Bhubaneswar. The standard version of Rock edicts I to X and 14 are inscribed below the forepart of the rock-cut elephant-Gajatame- symbolizing the conception of Buddha (Photo by the Author).

Ethnoveterinary Medicine (EVM) Today

The role of EVM in livestock development, as a key component of complementary alternative veterinary medicine (CAVM), is increasingly recognized, particularly in countries with a rich base of traditional knowledge. CAVM is an umbrella term that encompasses various modalities used in the healing and healthcare of animals, which are not routinely included in modern Western veterinary practices. These modalities include veterinary acupuncture and acutherapy, veterinary chiropractic, veterinary physical therapy, veterinary massage therapy, veterinary homeopathy, veterinary botanical medicine, and veterinary nutraceutical medicine. CAVM also includes mineral therapy, hirudotherapy, mud therapy, vibration and sound therapy (Hare 1999, Bergh *et al.* 2021). Many of the healing practices defined in CAVM are integral to EVM and have been traditionally practiced for generations in the treatment of animals. Furthermore, EVM extends beyond mere healing approaches; it encompasses practices, beliefs, skills, tools and technologies, selection of breeds and human resources/traditional healers, beliefs, rituals, and traditional practices and technologies for better animal health and production. However, until the last quarter of the twentieth century, ethnoveterinary medicine and other ethnoknowledge systems were often viewed with suspicion and scepticism by modern veterinary researchers and practitioners. Additionally, several factors contributed to the declining popularity of EVM practices. These included the lack of scientific documentation and validation, the concealment and distortion of traditional knowledge, inadequate dissemination, the unavailability of proper raw materials, declining herbal resources, slower therapeutic responses in acute conditions, the adoption of intensive livestock production systems, and inappropriate utilization and a lack of interest among the younger generation in traditional livestock rearing. During surveys to document EVM practices, traditional healers were often found secretive and reluctant to share their knowledge openly, increasing the risk of information loss and its potential misuse. Veterinary academic curricula have also largely ignored the significance of traditional healing practices, which remained popular until the advent of modern drugs. Despite these challenges, ignorance, and scepticism, nearly 80 % of people in Afro-Asian countries still rely on traditional methods of healing and livestock management. EVM is also seen as a potential tool for overcoming the side effects of modern drugs and promoting organic farming in both developing and developed nations. For instance, the Netherlands has achieved a 70 % reduction in antibiotic use since 2009 by optimizing farm management and housing practices and by using natural products, particularly plant-based (phytogenic) health-supporting products, to maintain animal health. To make information on alternatives and their potential applications accessible to the wider public, the Dutch Ministry of Agriculture, Nature, and Food Quality has published *Barn Books* for different categories of animals (Groot *et al.* 2021).

Global Recognition of EVM: The recognition and subsequent appreciation of traditional animal healthcare practices were ignited by a resolution adopted at the 30th World Health Assembly in 1977, urging interested governments to integrate their traditional medicine systems into their national health delivery frameworks. There was also a growing realization among international livestock developers and policymakers that high-cost healthcare and husbandry practices, borrowed from developed nations, could not sustainably meet the needs of livestock raisers in developing countries. The misuse, abuse, and side effects of modern drugs, shrinking financial resources, the reluctance of private veterinarians to settle in rural areas, and increasing consumer interest in organic food products also provided significant impetus for the emergence and recognition of ethnoveterinary medicine as a cost-effective animal healthcare option—not only in developing countries but also in developed nations, including the USA and several European countries. Against the backdrop of these resolutions and realizations, traditional knowledge of animal healthcare and husbandry began attracting scientific and academic attention during the 1970s and gained momentum in the early 1980s. The term *ethnoveterinary* was introduced into academic and scientific circles in the 1980s (McCorkle 1986). This period is rightly regarded as a revolutionary era for modern-day ethnoveterinary medicine.

Previously, information on ethnoveterinary medicine was often hidden in grey literature, but since this revolutionary period, a substantial body of work has been published. This includes a series of FAO reports documenting traditional (indigenous) veterinary medicine systems for small-scale farmers in countries like India, Thailand, Nepal, Pakistan, Sri Lanka, the Philippines, and Tanzania, as well as several books, status reports, research papers, scientific reviews, conference proceedings, and workshop manuals (Wanzala *et al.* 2005). An

International Conference on Ethnoveterinary Medicine: *Alternatives for Livestock Development* was organized in 1997 in Pune, India. Additionally, a website (http://www.ethnovetweb.com) was established to share information on ethnoveterinary medicine and to guide people worldwide in keeping their animals healthy and productive. EVM programs have been supported by various national and international government and non-government agencies, including Heifer International Project-US, the Philippines-based International Institute for Rural Reconstruction (IIRR), the International Technology Development Group (ITDG)-UK, Germany's League for Pastoral People (LPP), and ANTHRA-India, among others. From the 1970s onward, an increasing number of master's and doctoral dissertations in anthropology and veterinary medicine have addressed EVM. In 2004, ANTHRA also published an annotated bibliography on Ethnoveterinary Research in India.

The last five decades have witnessed phenomenal progress in EVM, with numerous systematic studies on various aspects of ethnoveterinary medicine, particularly the scientific validation of traditional phytomedicines, conducted across the world with encouraging results. Training programs are organized by modern veterinary institutions, and many EVM-based remedies are included in the treatment guidelines of standard veterinary medicine textbooks. For example, an ethnoveterinary remedy comprising a natural soda ash solution (97 % sodium bicarbonate), honey, and finger millet flour, which was used effectively to manage foot-and-mouth disease (FMD) lesions during an outbreak on a medium-scale dairy farm in Kenya, has been included for the same purpose in the latest edition of widely referred textbook of Veterinary Medicine (Constable *et al.* 2017). A rapid healing of the lesions with the animals resuming feeding after three days vindicates the use of these low cost, locally available and easy to apply products in the management of FMD lesions (Gakuya *et al.* 2011).

Ethnoveterinary Medicine: Limitations and Challenges

Despite growing academic and scientific interest in various aspects of Ethnoveterinary Medicine (EVM), many professionals still question its usefulness, applicability, and adaptability. In the modern era of evidence-based veterinary medicine, it is argued that traditional practices often lack scientific evidence and may not be as effective as claimed. Some practices are even harmful or not readily accessible. There is no doubt that many concerns regarding EVM practices are valid to some extent. However, like other systems of medicine, EVM has both limitations and strengths. Based on the published scientific literature and author's own experience, some limitations and possible reasons for the decline of ethnoveterinary medicine with the advent of Western animal healthcare practices, are discussed here:

- Ethnoveterinary medicines are often not as fast-acting or potent as allopathic medicines, making them less suitable for controlling and treating epidemic and endemic infectious diseases. Additionally, the effectiveness of EVM practices is questionable when it comes to emerging infectious diseases.

- Many so-called effective EVM remedies may be virtually ineffective, and some are difficult to prepare or use in field situations.
- The majority of traditional animal healthcare practices are unregulated and prone to abuse and quackery due to concealment, distortions, and misleading claims. Consequently, a large proportion of conventional practitioners, whether in human or animal healthcare, are sceptical about the value of alternative practices.
- Certain EVM practices can be harmful if used improperly or without appropriate knowledge and study. Even herbal preparations that are safe for use in some animal species may be toxic to others. For example, garlic, which is recommended to reduce blood cholesterol in humans, can cause anaemia in dogs. White willow (*Salix alba*), used to treat fever, rheumatic arthritis, and headaches in humans, can be fatal to cats, as felids cannot metabolize salicylic acid, a metabolite of salicin present in willow bark. Moreover, herbal products may be contaminated or adulterated. Remedies prepared from misidentified, improperly collected, stored, or processed medicinal plants or their parts may be injurious to health.
- Lack of documentation, inadequate scientific validation, and the failure to disseminate and promote evaluated practices for field application have adversely affected the development and full utilization of EVM by end users. Without this information, particularly regarding proven clinical efficacy, field veterinarians are often hesitant to use EVM remedies to avoid the risk of treatment failure.
- The underlying science of EVM is poorly researched and understood.
- No formal degree/ diploma/ or courses on alternative system within the present academic curricula in many countries.
- The diagnosis of diseases and identification of underlying causes are often inadequate.
- Medicinal plant resources are depleting, and the availability of certain plants is seasonal, making ingredients for preparing medicine scarce. This increases the likelihood of adulteration, raises the cost of treatment, and compromises the cost-effectiveness and safety of EVM remedies.
- There is a rapid decline in experienced traditional healers and pastoralist communities. The younger generation is less inclined to use EVM, likely due to a lack of information, interest, or because of rural exodus.

Ethnoveterinary Medicine (EVM): Strength and Options

The introduction of modern practices and scientific technologies though has made it difficult for the younger generations to value and use traditional practices, a substantial number of animal owners worldwide continue to rely on ethnoveterinary practices, including the use of medicinal plants for treatment of their animals. The evaluated veterinary traditional healthcare and management practices as well as herbal and holistic medicines are globally accepted as an important alternative to address animal health problems. In general, though abuse and quackery exist, the application of traditional practices can be a pragmatic response in the areas without adequate veterinary services because of following advantages:

- Traditional knowledge has been generated and acquired by resource users in a diachronic (long term) time scale through observations and practical experience and are compatible with the local situation and less dependent on use of external inputs.
- Farmers are generally more comfortable to receive healthcare from known, trusted people (ethnovets or extension specialists) who speak same language and have better understandings of local conditions than those who are alien to their socio-cultural background.
- Most traditional practices are easy to adopt; whereas the modern technologies may or may not be compatible with the existing situation of the farmers and they may need costly external input and special skill for field application. For example, indigenous knowledge-based technology such as applying turmeric and coconut or mustard oil for treatment of wounds can be easily adopted and applied by local people; rather than using antibiotic and antiseptic treatment. Thus, acknowledgment of value of traditional knowledge empowers local herders/farmers to try to solve disease problems of their livestock in a cost-effective way.
- EVM may be a potential tool to create better understanding between vets and extension personnel and communities. It can ensure proper health and productivity of animals in the areas where modern veterinary services are not readily available.
- Validated EVM techniques may be the most realistic choice for financially poor stock raisers, who can neither afford nor may access expensive high-tech modern healthcare practices.
- In emergencies or during fast spreading epidemics, traditional healers and their treatments may be more easily available with minimum expenses on transport and opportunity costs. There are fewer chances that expired or spurious allopathic drugs are sold to uneducated animal owners when EVM options are available for treatment of diseases.

- EVM research and developments have practical applications for cost-effective ways to control several economically important health problems such as internal or external parasitism, whether related to epidemiology, diagnostics and therapy, or to comprehensive disease control methods leading to integrated pest/disease management.
- Low-cost EVM remedies may ensure freedoms from pain and diseases concerning to welfare of animals with low market value (sheep, goat, poultry). Regardless of economic status of the stock raisers, these animals are likely to suffer for want of treatment involving high-cost modern drugs.
- Proper application and adoption of EVM treatment approaches can provide a plausible answer to side effects of conventional drugs. These can limit any unnecessary use of antibiotics and other chemical drugs to overcome residue problems and the growing resistance of micro-organisms.
- The traditional animal healthcare and husbandry practices are well integrated with local environment and needs. Therefore, EVM practices and technologies are generally cost-effective, established supply chain, environmental-friendly and sustainable to a specific area. For example, traditional herd- grazing and pasture management involve practices that do not over-exploit the natural carrying capacity of the land. There are several examples when substitution of some traditional practices has resulted in serious ecological impacts.
- EVM provides a highly intricate indigenous knowledge systems pertaining to animal husbandry that have been developed by several pastoral societies to orient their animals according to their own specific breeding goals and animal utilization. For example, the indigenous strategies for safeguarding and developing their valuable genetic resources include a variety of social mechanisms such as stock-sharing arrangements to prevent inbreeding and favouring birth of upgraded offspring; careful selection of breeding males with long list of favourable traits; castration to ensure that only best male reproduces and study the genealogy of their animals.
- Traditional practices constitute a potential knowledge resource for novel ideas and hypotheses. For example, understanding of zoopharmacognosy can provide ideas for developing grazing practices to prevent disease and discovery of medicinal use of plants as well as discovery of novel drug molecules. It is reported that 25 % prescribed drugs worldwide are plant-derived, with 121 active compounds currently in use, and that 11% of the 252 drugs on the WHO's essential medicines list is plant-based (Yahoo Finance, 20 Jan. 2025, https://uk.finance.yahoo.com/news/herbal-medicine-market-valuation-projected-113000935.html). Many of these phytomedicines trace their origins to plants traditionally discovered and used by indigenous peoples.

- EVM practices may effectively prevent occurrences of diseases thereby avoiding financial loss due to treatment cost and production losses.
- Strengthening of EVM and recognition of the age-old status of healers (ethnovets) give rise to a new approach referred to as participatory epidemiology, which promises to improve epidemiological surveillance in remote areas while simultaneously encouraging community participation in disease control to exchange professional information and also document their composite knowledge and experience.
- EVM may be an effective resource for community development and to protect the right of ethnovets and owners of traditional knowledge at community level.
- EVM bridges the gap between natural resources and their human management for the future, as it characteristically promotes traditional practices and facilitates conservation, protection and propagation of floral biodiversity.
- EVM supports emerging agri-business opportunities such as organic animal husbandry and herbal farming.

Conclusion

The indigenous traditional knowledge (ITK) system has evolved over centuries, shaped by the experiences of people with long histories of direct interaction with their natural environments. This knowledge system is deeply rooted in the cultural traditions, beliefs, and experiences of rural and local communities. It encompasses language, classification systems, resource use practices, social interactions, rituals, and spirituality, forming vital components of the world's cultural diversity. Ethnoveterinary medicine (EVM) is a significant aspect of ITK, developed and utilized by animal breeders to promote the health, husbandry, and welfare of their animals over generations. In many Afro-Asian countries, and other regions where allopathic veterinary medicines are often inaccessible or unaffordable, livestock owners continue to rely on EVM while increasingly integrating modern veterinary practices into their traditional approaches. While ethnobotanical knowledge and phytomedicines remain central to EVM, its scope extends well beyond herbal therapies, encompassing a wide array of non-phytogenic practices and remedial measures related to animal healthcare and welfare. Overall, contemporary EVM represents a complex system of information, knowledge, skills, methods, practices, tools, technologies, beliefs, breeds, and human and natural resources used for animal husbandry and care, often in an environmentally sustainable manner (McCorkle 1986, Mathias 2001, Swarup *et al.* 2005). The EVM has evolved to encompass a wide range of topics, including zoopharmacognosy (exploring potential sources of EVM ideas), participatory epidemiology, gender-specific knowledge and skills in EVM, safety protocols for handling and processing food and animal products, product marketing and agri-business skills, conservation of biodiversity (including animal genetic resources), interactions between domestic and wild animals, ecosystem health (aligned with the one-health concept), EVM-related education in rural areas, and training programs for veterinary professionals and paraprofessionals. Policy, institutional, and economic analyses also play a crucial role in these areas (Lans *et al.* 2007). In the modern era of Evidence-Based Veterinary Medicine, the propagation and field application of EVM face many challenges. However, this traditional knowledge—enriched with long-term practical understanding of local ecology, livestock and wildlife behaviour, and natural resources—may lead to management interventions that are even more effective in preventing diseases. This, in turn, can reduce economic losses associated with treatment costs and production decline following disease outbreaks. The study of treatment practices across different cultures and bio-social groups may introduce new ideas, techniques, and materia medica for preventing diseases and promoting or restoring the health and welfare of both animals and people.

The revival of interest in ethnoveterinary medicine and its recognition as a legitimate field within modern veterinary practices began more than five decades ago. During this time, interest in EVM has grown considerably, and a wealth of literature has been published on various aspects of ethnoveterinary medicine and related topics worldwide. However, this increased interest has not yet led to a greater application of EVM in sustainable livestock development. To address the questions, "What is the future of EVM?" or "Where is EVM headed next?" certain concerns need to be addressed. Proper documentation, validation, and transfer of EVM practices for field use could resolve many of these issues. Promoting EVM-based, cost-effective, and environmentally friendly animal health practices could help mitigate emerging health hazards, such as antimicrobial resistance (AMR) and anthelmintic drug resistance, associated with the misuse of modern drug technologies. Furthermore, EVM is viewed as a potential tool for promoting organic farming and conserving indigenous traditional knowledge (ITK) as well as floral and faunal biodiversity.

References

Akers-Campbell H. 2016. *Farm like a Roman: Livestock in Ancient Italy.* Bachelor of Arts Thesis, Wesleyan University, Middletown, Connecticut. https://digitalcollections.wesleyan.edu/_flysystem/fedora/2023-03/24084-Original%20File.pdf.

Al-Samarrai SF. 1972. Historical review of medicine in Arab world I. Mesopotamian medicine. *Bulletin of the Society for Near Eastern Studies in Japan* **15**(1):129-134, accessed on 03-06-2024.

Arbuckle BS, Öztan A and Gülçur S. 2009. The evolution of sheep and goat husbandry in central Anatolia. *Anthropozoologica* **44**(1): 129-57.

Arnott R. 2024. *Disease and Healing in the Indus Civilisation.* 214 p. Archaeopress Publishing Ltd Summertown, Oxford,UK.

Ashoor UF. 2023. Veterinary medicine in Byzantine Egypt. *Journal of Faculty of Archaeology at Ain-Shams University* IWNW. **2**: 171-80.

Bahaaeldeen A, Elkadragy M, Sharsher A, Rashed R and ElbazT. 2019. Veterinary surgery and gynecology in the ancient Egypt. *Assiut Veterinary Medical Journal* **65** (162). 129-34.

Bailey J. 2022. Acupuncture for dogs: Whether the veterinary acupuncturist practices Traditional Chinese Medicine or Western medical acupuncture, the treatment helps, especially for dogs with arthritis or neurological problems. *Whole Dog Journal* **26**(3):12-14.

Bartnik A. 2023. Feeding pigs in ancient Rome. *Zeszyty Wiejskie* **29**:139-53.

Benezet Núria T. 2021. The pure priest of Sekhmet, between health and disease. *Proceedings of 3rd International Conference on Pharmacy and Medicine in Ancient Egypt*. October 25-26, 2018, Barcelona. pp.116-24. (Eds) Rosa Solà D, Jané G, Rosa M and Georges FM. Archaeopress, 5054852 Oxford, UK. Available at: (PDF) The Pure Priest of Sekhmet, Between Health and Disease.

Bergh A, Lund I, Boström A, Hyytiäinen H and Asplund K. A 2021. systematic review of complementary and alternative veterinary medicine: "Miscellaneous therapies". *Animals* **11**(12): 3356. https://doi.org/10.3390/ani11123356.

Bodson L. 1994. Ancient views on pests and parasites of livestock. *Argos*: *Bulletin van het Veterinair Historisch Genootschap* **10**: 303–10. (Cited by Swabe 1999).

Bremmer JN. 2020. Theriomorphism of major Greek gods. Animals in Ancient Greek Religion. pp. 102-126. (Ed). Kindt J. Routledge, London. https://doi.org/10.4324/9780429424304.

Cartwright M. 2016. *Hippocrates-World History Encyclopedia.* https://www.worldhistory.org/Hippocrates/, accessed on 27-07-2024.

Chakraborty KS, Chakraborty S, Le Roux P, Miller HM, Shirvalkar P and Rawat Y. 2018. Enamel isotopic data from the domesticated animals at Kotada Bhadli, Gujarat, reveals specialized animal husbandry during the Indus Civilization. *Journal of Archaeological Science: Reports* **21**:183-99.

Cohen C. 1983. The Ugaritic Hippiatric texts and BAM 159. *Journal of the Ancient Near Eastern Society* **15**(1): 1-12.

Constable PD, Hinchcliff KW, Done SH and Grünberg W 2017. *Veterinary Medicine: A Textbook of the Diseases of Cattle, Horses, Sheep, Pigs and Goats.* 11th edn. p. 2064. Elsevier St Louise Missouri,USA.

Daniel RA, Wilhelm TA, Case-Scott H, Goldman G and Hinzman L. 2022. What is "Indigenous Knowledge" and Why Does it matter? Integrating ancestral wisdom and approaches into federal decision-making. The White House. https://www.whitehouse.gov/ostp/news-updates/2022/12/02/, accessed on 19-06-2024.

Das SK, Arya HPS, Subba Reddy G and Mishra A. 2002. *Inventory of Indigenous Technical Knowledge in Agriculture Document 1.* 411p. Mission Unit, Division of Agriculture Extension, Indian Council of Agricultural Research, New Delhi, India.

Dhammika VS. 1993.*The Edicts of King Asoka- An English Rendering. The Wheel Publication No. 386/387*. 56 p. Buddhist Publication Society. Kandy, Sri Lanka.

Gakuya DW, Mulei CM and Wekesa SB. 2011 Use of ethnoveterinary remedies in the management of foot and mouth disease lesions in a dairy herd. *African Journal of Traditional, Complementary and Alternative medicines* **8**(2): 165-69.

Gómez, CB. 2021. An analysis of ancient medical-veterinary diagnosis. *Proceedings of the X Conference of the Spanish Society of Logic, Methodology and Philosophy of Science.* 16-19 November 2021.Salamanca, Spain pp. 30-32. (Eds) Cuevas A, Torres O Aranda V and Moldovan A. Instituto de Estudios de la Ciencia y la Tecnología, Spain. Available at researchgate.net.

Gordon A and Schwabe C W. 2004. *The Quick and the Dead: Biomedical Theory in Ancient Egypt*. Vol. 4. Brill, Styx, Leiden, Boston, USA.

Gorrini ME. 2006. Healing heroes in Thessaly: Chiron the centaur. In: *The Archaeological Work of Thessaly and Sterea Greece, Proceedings of the 1st Archaeological Symposium* **27.** https://www.academia.edu/download/18981618/chiron, pdf accessed on 24-07-2024.

Groot MJ, Berendsen BJ and Cleton NB. 2021. The next step to further decrease veterinary antibiotic applications: Phytogenic alternatives and effective monitoring; the Dutch approach. *Frontiers in Veterinary Science* 8: 709750. doi: 10.3389/fvets.2021.709750.

Hadani A and Shimshony A. 1994.Traditional veterinary medicine in the Near East: Jews, Arab Bedouins and Fellahs. *Revue Scientifique Et Technique De L Office International Des Epizooties* **13** (2): 581-97. doi: 10.20506/rst.13.2.778. PMID: 8038454.

Hare D. 1999. Complementary and alternative veterinary medicine. *The Canadian Veterinary Journal* **40**(6): 376-77.

Hart GD. 1965. Asclepius, God of medicine. *Canadian Medical Association Journal* **92**(5):232-36.

Hausmann W and Jöchle W. 1988. The discovery of Chiron's cave, a prehistoric school of medicine for animals and humans. *Canadian Veterinary Journal* **29**(10): 857-60.

ICSU. 2002. *Science and Traditional Knowledge: Report from the ICSU Study Group on Science and Traditional Knowledge. 3p. International Council for Science, Paris.*

Jastrow M. 1908. Divination through the Liver and the beginning of anatomy. *Transactions of the College of Physicians* **29**: 117-138 (Cited by Al-Samarrai 1972).

Jones BV. 2021. *The History of Veterinary Medicine and the Animal-Human Relationship*. 608 p. 5m Books Ltd., Essex, UK.

Jones SD and Koolmees PA. 2022. *A Concise History of Veterinary Medicine*. pp 1-13. Cambridge University Press., Essex, UK.

Kamjan S, de Groene D, van den Hurk Y, Zidarov P, Elenski N, Patterson WP and Çakırlar C. 2021. The emergence and evolution of Neolithic cattle farming in southeastern Europe: New zooarchaeological and stable isotope data from Džuljunica-Smărdeš, in northeastern Bulgaria (ca. 6200–5500 cal. BCE). *Journal of Archaeological Science: Reports* **36** (April 2021): 102789. https://doi.org/10.1016/j.jasrep. 2021.102789.

Kansara NM. 1995. *Animal Husbandry in the Vedas. Monograph Series-1.* 290p. Dharam Hinduja International Centre of Indic Research, Nag Publishers, Delhi, India.

Kelly JT. 1995 The Fascinating code of Hammurabi: Wow! I didn't know that! *The History Teacher* **28**(4):555-62. https://knowledgebasedsociety.com/wp-content/uploads/2021/12/494642.pdf downloaded on 03-07-2024.

Kgasi AT. 2021. Ancient veterinary practices in Africa and contextual relevance in primary animal health care pp.1-20. *Veterinary History (History Society of the South African Veterinary Association)*. Available at http://hdl.handle.net/2263/80897.

Klecel W and Martyniuk E. 2021. From the Eurasian steppes to the Roman circuses: A review of early development of horse breeding and management. *Animals* **11**(7): 1859. https://doi.org/10.3390/ani11071859.

Krishna L, Swarup D and Patra RC. 2005. An overview of prospects of ethno-veterinary medicine in India. The Indian Journal of Animal Sciences **75**(12): 1481-91.

Lans C, Khan TE, Curran MM and McCorkle CM. 2007. Ethnoveterinary medicine: potential solutions for large-scale problems? In: *Veterinary Herbal Medicine* pp. 17-32. (Eds) Wynn SG, and Fougère BJ. Mosby Elsevier, St Louis,USA.

Lazzeroni R. 1998. Sanskrit. In: *The Indo-European Languages*. pp 98-124. (Eds)Anna Giacalone Ramat AG and Ramat P. Routledge, London and New York,USA.

Lin JH and Panzer R. 1994. Use of Chinese herbal medicine in veterinary science: History and perspectives *Revue Scientifique Et Technique De L Office International Des Epizooties* **13** (2): 425-32.

Lite-Nepal. 2023. *The Significance of Traditional Knowledge*. Lite Nepal, lite-nepal.com, accessed on 24-06-2024.

Lodrick DO. 1987. Gopashtami and Govardhan Puja: Two Krishna Festivals of India. *Journal of Cultural Geography* **7** (2): 101-16. https://doi.org/10.1080/08873638709478510.

Lord C. 2011. The veterinary papyrus of Kahun. In: *Current Research in Egyptology 2009.* Proceedings of the Tenth Annual Symposium, University of Liverpool January 2009. pp.99-105. (Eds) Daniel B, Claire M and Judith C. Oxbow Books, UK. Available at Current Research in Egyptology 2009 : Proceedings of the Tenth Annual Symposium - Boatright, Daniel - Malleson, Claire - Corbelli, Judith - Oxbow Books - Torrossa.

Lord C. 2016. One and the same? An investigation into the connection between veterinary and medical practice in ancient Egypt. In: *Mummies, Magic and Medicine in Ancient Egypt. Multidisciplinary Essays for Rosalie David.* pp. 140-54. (Eds) Price C, Forshaw R, Chamberlain A and Nicholson P. Manchester University Press, Manchester, UK. https://doi.org/10.7765/9781784997502.00024.

Mahabharata. 2016 (Vikrama Samvat 2072). Hindi and Sanskrit edition. Gita Press, Gorakhpur, India. Available at: Internet Archive.

Mark JJ. 2020. A brief history of veterinary medicine. *World History Encyclopedia.* https://www.worldhistory.org/article/1549/a-brief-history-of-veterinary-medicine/, accessed on 11-01-2023.

Marsden SP. 2007. Overview of traditional Chinese medicine: The cooking pot analog. In: *Veterinary Herbal Medicine* pp. 51-58. (Eds) Wynn SG, and Fougère BJ. Mosby Elsevier, St Louis, USA.

Mathias E. 2001. *Introducing Ethnoveterinary Medicine.* October 2001. www.ethnovetweb.com.

McCabe A. 2007. *A Byzantine Encyclopaedia of Horse Medicine: The Sources, Compilation, and Transmission of the Hippiatrica.* pp. 1-17. Oxford University Press, UK.

McCorkle CM. 1986. An introduction to ethnoveterinary research and development. *Journal of Ethnobiology* **6** (1): 129-49.

McCorkle CM. 1998. Ethnoveterinary Medicine: Ethnoscience or just Anti-Science? In: *Complementary and Alternative Veterinary Medicine: Principles and Practice.* (Eds) Schoen A M and Wynn SG, St. Louis, USA.

McMiken DF. 1990. Ancient origins of horsemanship. *Equine Veterinary Journal* **22**(2): 73-78.

Nagarajan KV. 2011. The code of Hammurabi: An economic interpretation. *International Journal of Business and Social Science* **2** (8): 108-17.

Niewöhner P, Audley-Miller, Erkul E, Giese S and Huy S. 2017. An ancient cave sanctuary underneath the theatre of Miletus: beauty, mutilation and burial of ancient sculpture in Late Antiquity. *Archäologischer Anzeiger* **2016** (1): 67–156. https://ora.ox.ac.uk/objects/uuid:c46007df-405d-4f76-b6a2-17487a19f1ca.

Pipano E. 2022. One hundred years of veterinary parasitology in the land of Israel. *Israel Journal of Veterinary Medicine*. **77**:3. http://www.ijvm.org.il/sites/default/files/2pipano.pdf.

Pozzi P and Gardella Tedeschi B. 2023. Use of animals in Jewish tradition. *Israel Journal of Veterinary Medicine*. **78**:2.http://www.ijvm.org.il/sites/default/files/jewish_tradition.pdf.

Raulwing P. 2009 The Kikkuli Text (CTH 284): Some interdisciplinary remarks on Hittite Training Texts for chariot horses in the second half of the 2nd millennium BC *Irgaf. org*, pp.1—21. http://www.lrgaf.org/Peter_Raulwing_The_Kikkuli_Text_MasterFile_Dec_2009.pdf downloaded on 11-06-2021.

Schwabe CW. 1978. *Cattle, Priests and Progress in Medicine (Vol 4)*. University of Minnesota Press, Minneapolis,USA.

Schwabe CW. 1984. *Veterinary Medicine and Human Health.* 3rd edn. Williams and Wilkins, Baltimore,USA.

Schwabe CW. 1994. Animals in the ancient world. In: *Animals and Human Society Changing Perspectives.* pp.36-58. (Eds) Manning A and James Serpell J. Routledge, London, UK.

Shahar R and Bark H. 2006. Veterinary education in Israel. *Journal of Veterinary Medical Education* **33**(2): 233-37.

Sharma TR (Trans.). 2013. *Atharva-Veda Vol. I.* Vijaykumar Govindram Hansnand, New Delhi, India (Digital Distributer Agniveer). https://archive.org/details/atharva-veda-vol-2-of-2, pdf downloaded on 05-06-2023.

Sierra A, Navarrete V, Alcàntara R, Camalich MD, Martín-Socas D, Fiorillo D, McGrath K and Saña M. 2024. Shepherding the past: High-resolution data on Neolithic Southern Iberian livestock management at Cueva de El Toro (Antequera, Málaga). *PLoS ONE* **19**(4) e0299786. https://doi.org/10.1371/journal.pone.0299786.

Silva NE, Luna SP, Joaquim JG, Coutinho HD and Possebon FS. 2017. Effect of acupuncture on pain and quality of life in canine neurological and musculoskeletal diseases. *Canadian Veterinary Journal* **58**(9): 941-51.

Somvanshi R. 2006. Veterinary medicine and animal keeping in ancient India. *Asian Agri-History* **10**(2): 133-46.

Suryanarayan A. 2023. Human-animal relationships in the Indus Civilisation: Challenges, opportunities and questions. In: *Animals in Archaeology: Integrating Landscapes, Environment and Humans in South Asia (A Festschrift for Prof. P.P. Joglekar) Volume 1.* pp. 117-37. (Eds) Goyal P, Abhayan GS, and Channarayapatna S. Department of Archaeology, University of Kerala, Thiruvananthapuram, India.

Swabe J. 2005. *Animals, Disease, and Human Society: Human-Animal Relations and the Rise of Veterinary Medicine.* 192 p. Routledge, London, UK Taylor & Francis. Master e-Library, 2005, pdf downloaded on 08-02-2023.

Swarup D and Patra R.C. 2005. Perspectives of ethnoveterinary medicine in veterinary practice. In: *Proceedings of the National conference on Contemporary Relevance of Ethnoveterinary Medical Traditions of India.* pp. 8-15. Foundation for Revitalization of Local Health Traditions (FRLHT) & Dakshin Kannada Milk Union (DKMU), Udupi, October 17-18, 2005, Mangalore, Karnataka, India.

Swarup D, Dey S and Dwivedi HP. 2013. Indigenous technical knowledge in animal husbandry and ethnoveterinary medicine. *Handbook of Animal Husbandry*. pp 953-79. Directorate of Knowledge Management in Agriculture, Indian Council of Agricultural Research, New Delhi, India.

Tanga C, Remigio M and Viciano J. 2022. Transmission of zoonotic diseases in the daily life of ancient Pompeii and Herculaneum (79 CE, Italy): A review of animal–human–environment interactions through biological, historical and archaeological sources. *Animals* **12**(2): 213. https://doi.org/10.3390/ani12020213.

Thrusfield M. 2018 Development of veterinary medicine. In: *Veterinary Epidemiology.* 4th edn. pp 1-27. (Eds) Thrusfield M and Christley R. John Wiley & Sons Ltd, Oxford,UK.

Tropper J and Vita JP. 2019. Ugaritic-1. In: *The Semitic Languages*. 2nd edn. pp. 482-509. (Eds) John Huehnergard J and Pat-El Na'ama. Routledge, London. https://doi.org/10.4324/9780429025563, pdf downloaded on 04-07-2024..

UNDESA. 2019. *Traditional Knowledge – An Answer to the Most Pressing Global Problems*? UN DESA | United Nations Department of Economic and Social Affairs, accessed on 24-06-2024.

UNESCO. 2017. *Local Knowledge, Global Goals.* 48p. UNESCO, Paris, France.

Urch EJ. 1929. The law code of Hammurabi. *American Bar Association Journal* **15**(7): 437-441. https://www.jstor.org/stable/25707711, pdf downloaded on 04-07-2024.

Vincent GE. 1904. The laws of Hammurabi. *American Journal of Sociology* **9**(6): 737-54.

Walter C. 2014. *Horse and Rider Figurines from Ancient Marion.* Master of Arts Thesis. 93 p. Arizona State University, USA.

Wanzala W, Zessin KH, Kyule NM, Baumann MPO, Mathias E and Hassanali A. 2005. Ethnoveterinary medicine: a critical review of its evolution, perception, understanding and the way forward. *Livestock Research for Rural Development* **17:** 1-31.

Xie H and Wedemeyer L. 2012. The validity of acupuncture in veterinary medicine. *American Journal of Traditional Chinese Veterinary Medicine* **7** (1): 35-43.

Yeates J. 2018. *Veterinary Science: A Very Short Introduction.* Oxford University Press, UK.

Zemánek P. 1996. Language and State in Ancient Near East: The case of Ugarit. In: *L'État, le pouvoir, les prestations et leurs formes en Mésopotamie ancienne*. pp129-136. Univerzita Karlova v Praze Filozofická fakulta, France. pdf downloaded on 4-07-2024.

5

Zoopharmacognosy and Ethnoveterinary Materia Medica

D. Swarup

Simhasyeva stanathoh sam vijante'gneriva vijanta ābhṛtābhyaḥ. Gavāṁ yakṣmaḥ puruṣāṇām vīrudbhiratinutto nāvyā etu srotyāh.

As deer from the lion's roar and cold from the heat of fire, so do ailments run off from the force of herbs and medications when they are brought for the sick and suffering. Let the consumptive and cancerous diseases of cows and people go away by herbal medications beyond the navigable streams.

(Atharva Veda 8.7.15; translation by Sharma 2013)

1. Introduction
2. Zoopharmacognosy (Self-healing Behaviours in Animals)
   - Early Roots of Zoopharmacognosy
   - Zoopharmacognosy and Traditional Medicine
   - Methods and Mechanisms
3. Ethnoveterinary Materia Medica
   - Natural products- Medicinal Plants and their Products, Animals and Animal Products, Minerals, Clay and Other Natural Substances
   - Acupuncture
   - Surgical Practices
   - Disease Preventive Practices
4. Ethnoveterinary Pharmacy Preparations
5. Conclusion

Introduction

Humans have lived alongside animals for centuries, and it is likely that early interactions included attempts to treat animals when they were ill, leading to the development of veterinary medicine. Veterinary medicine is the science focused on diagnosing, treating, and preventing diseases and injuries in animals. Historically, the term *veterinary* originates from the Latin word *veterinarius*, meaning of or pertaining to beasts of burden, with *veterinae* referring to a cattle doctor. The root word *vetus*, meaning old or experienced, may also signify animals mature enough for work (Veterinarian - Etymology, Origin & Meaning, accessed on 15-11-2024). In modern times, veterinary medicine has evolved to encompass a wide range of disciplines, technical skills, and practices. Over the centuries, various healers—including formally educated veterinarians, botanists, disease specialists, castrators, and even animal owners—have contributed to animal care and welfare practices. The evolutionary history of animal healing practices has been classified into five broad stages, each reflecting distinct theories of disease and corresponding therapeutic approaches developed over time. Among these, zoopharmacognosy—referring to instinctive behaviours through which animals self-medicate by selecting and utilizing natural substances such as specific plants, minerals, or soils to alleviate ailments—is considered as the first healing approach (Jones and Koolmees 2022).

Ethnoveterinary medicine is defined as the knowledge, skills, methods, practices, and beliefs that people use in caring for their animals. The *Ethnoveterinary Materia Medica* encompasses natural products (e.g., medicinal plants, animal products, minerals), spiritual appeals, physical manipulations, and surgeries (Toyang *et al.* 2007), as well as husbandry practices such as selective grazing, pasture management, and housing for disease prevention (McCorkle 1986, Wanzala *et al.* 2005). Additionally, the observation of animals' self-medication behaviours has contributed traditional knowledge about the medicinal use of plants in both human and animal healthcare. This chapter will explore these practices, including animal self-healing behaviour, the use of natural products, traditional surgical methods, and other ethnoveterinary methods.

Zoopharmacognosy (Self-healing Behaviours in Animals)

The term *zoopharmacognosy* is derived from the Greek-*zoo* (meaning animal), *pharmacon* (meaning drug or medicine), and *gnosy* (meaning knowing). It was coined by anthropologists Eloy Rodriguez and Robert Wrangham to describe the process by which wild animals actively select and use specific plants or other natural substances with medicinal properties to treat or prevent disease. The pharmacognosy was to refer to the scientific study of the interactions between chemicals being investigated as potential drugs and the biological systems of the organisms that consume them. It requires an understanding of chemistry, chemical techniques, and the anatomy and physiology of the animals receiving the drugs (Rodriguez and Wrangham1993). The term has gained popularity from academic works and is used to study self-medication behaviour both in wild and domestic animals.

The self- medication behaviours are observed in various species of animals including mammals, birds and insects as a primary line of defence against physical and psychological stressors. When left undisturbed, animals use natural materials or chemical substances to influence their behaviour or modify their body's response to parasites, pathogens, or other causes of illness. For instance, the first instinctive response of injured or sick animals is often to hide and rest. Overheated animals seek cooler areas, dehydrated animals search for water, and anxious animals move to safer environments. In the wild, chimpanzees with gastrointestinal issues, such as diarrhoea, have been observed consuming termite mound soil or scraping subsoils from exposed cliff faces or riverbanks to alleviate their symptoms (Engel 2007). When faced with illness induced by consuming tannin-rich food, domestic sheep have been shown to self-medicate. They selectively consume substances such as sodium bentonite, polyethylene glycol, and dicalcium phosphate, which aid in recovery from conditions caused by excessive intake of grain, tannins, or oxalic acid (Villalba and Provenza 2007).

Early Roots of Zoopharmacognosy

Although the term zoopharmacognosy and modern research in this fascinating field are relatively recent, the awe-inspiring ability of animals to self-medicate is anything but new. Humans have marvelled at and drawn inspiration from this phenomenon for millennia. Evidence of an ancient understanding of self-medication, both in its practical application and its profound implications for human and animal health, shines through the verses of the Atharva Veda. The Vedic sages—wisdom-packed pioneers of observation—immortalized this knowledge in poetic hymns, offering glimpses of a world where animals served as nature's pharmacologists. Recognizing the importance of the self-medication behaviours of different animal species, Sage Atharva sings:

> *Varāho veda vīrudhaṁ nakulo veda bhesjīm. Sarpā gandharvā yā vidustā asmā avase huve* (Atharva Veda 8.7.23).

- 'The wild boar knows the herb; the mongoose knows the medicinal herb for itself. Of these, what the snakes and other wild creatures of the earth, know, I invoke and administer for the cure of this patient' (Sharma 2013).

  Sage Atharva further elaborates on this universal pharmacy:

> *Yāh suparṇā āngirasardivyā yā raghaao viduh Vayāmsi hamsā yā viduryāśca sarvepatattriṇah. Mṛgaāg yā vidurosadhīstā asmāavase huve* (Atharva Veda 8.7.24).

- 'The life-giving herbs which the eagle knows and recognises, the divine herbs which the sparrows know and recognise, those that the swans, other such and all birds know and recognise, and those which the deer know and recognise, all those herbs I take up and administer for the cure of this patient' (Sharma 2013).

Yāvatīnāmosadhīnām gāvaḥ prāśnantyaghnyā yāvatīnāmajāvayah. Tāvatīstubhyamosadhīh śarma yacchantvābhṛtāḥ (Atharva Veda 8.7.25).

- 'As many herbs as inviolable cows eat, as many as sheep and goats eat, those many herbs, selected and collected for you, O man, may give you good health, peace and comfort at heart' (Sharma 2013).

These poetic expressions by the Vedic sages reflect not only their knowledge of zoopharmacognosy but also their wisdom in channelling the instinctive pharmacy of animals—such as wild boars, mongooses, serpents, eagles, sparrows, swans, and deer—into human healing. The sages' insights extended beyond wild creatures to include domesticated animals, recognizing their inherent knowledge of medicinal plants. These observations were far from simple pastoral musings—they laid the groundwork for advances in pharmacology and veterinary medicine long before modern science claimed credit.

Early references to animal self-medication also appear in Book VIII of Aristotle's *Historia Animalium.* Aristotle described how wolves (*Canis lupus*), when experiencing extreme hunger, consume a certain type of earth—a behaviour now known as geophagy, observed in both humans and animals. He also wrote about the grass-eating habits of dogs, explaining that carnivorous animals only eat grass when unwell. Dogs, for example, consume grass to induce vomiting, likely as a method of purging and deworming. Additionally, Aristotle noted that bears, after hibernation, consume arum (a type of lily) to open and distend their gut. In his work *Naturalis Historia* (*Natural History*), Pliny the Elder also described geophagy in animals such as wolves and elephants (Álvaro *et al.* 2019). Pliny further explained that the use of dittany (*Origanum dictamnus*) to treat arrow wounds likely originated from observing wounded stags grazing on this herb. Aristotle and Dioscorides credited wild goats with the discovery of certain medicinal plants, as humans often learned self-medication by observing animals (*How Humans Learned to Self-Medicate with Certain Plants by Observing Animals*, PBS News, accessed 19-11-2024). Dittany, an endemic plant of the Greek island of Crete, is widely used in traditional medicine across Europe. Recent studies have identified several bioactive compounds in dittany, including flavonoids, lipids, and terpenoids (primarily carvacrol and thymol). These findings strongly support its traditional medicinal uses in treating ailments such as sore throats, coughs, and gastric ulcers (Liolios *et al.* 2010).

Zoopharmacognosy and Traditional Medicine

Self-medication behaviours of animals has significantly contributed to traditional healing practices and the discovery of novel drug compounds used in modern medicine. Scholars argue that a large number of medicinal plants used in modern drugs were first discovered by Indigenous peoples and past cultures who observed animals employing plants and emulated them. For instance, strong similarities are reported in plant selection criteria among the African great apes in response to parasitic infection and gastrointestinal upset, and the common use of some plants by humans to treat such illnesses. Many wild animals employ mechanical scouring to eliminate worm infestations, a technique also adopted by traditional herbalists for worm control. Great apes exhibit two forms of self-medicative behaviour to manage parasitic infestations, particularly before the rainy season: bitter-pith chewing and leaf swallowing. One notable medicinal plant involved in this behaviour is bitter leaf (*Vernonia amygdalina*), a putative medicinal plant, which is widely distributed across tropical sub-Saharan Africa. Chimpanzees carefully strip the outer bark and leaves from young *V. amygdalina* shoots, exposing the pith. They then chew on this pith to extract its extremely bitter juice along with residual fibres. The ingestion of this bitter pith has been observed to reduce the reproductive output of nodular worms and alleviate associated gastrointestinal symptoms. When experiencing symptoms of nodular worm infestation—such as diarrhoea, malaise, and abdominal pain—great apes also swallow leaves from a variety of herbs, trees, vines, and shrubs. The coarse texture of these leaves acts as a mechanical cleanser, scraping intestinal worms from the gut lining (Huffman 2001). Observations from Mahale Mountains National Park in Tanzania reveal that chimpanzees consume at least 26 plant species, many of which are used in traditional medicine to treat internal parasites and related gastrointestinal conditions (Engel 2007). Interestingly, this behaviour of eating plant to prevent parasitic infection is not unique to primates. Carnivores such as wolves and tigers have also been observed consuming plant material, likely as a strategy to expel intestinal worms.

The genus *Vernonia* includes several species with food, medicinal, and industrial applications. Ethnomedicinally significant species include *V. amygdalina*, *V. condensata*, *V. cineria*, *V. guineensis*, and *V. conferta*, all known for their pharmacological efficacy against a range of diseases (Toyang and Verpoorte 2013). Across Africa, decoctions made from *V. amygdalina* are commonly used in traditional medicine to treat malarial fever, schistosomiasis, amoebic dysentery, and various intestinal parasites. In ethnoveterinary practices, *V. amygdalina* is often used to combat parasitic infections, especially those affecting the gastrointestinal tract. For instance, Ugandan farmers feed young branches and leaves of *V. amygdalina* to pigs as a natural remedy for intestinal parasites (Huffman 2001). There are numerous other examples of animal-inspired plant medicines used in traditional medicine worldwide. A recent publication documented 14 case studies highlighting various preventative or therapeutic self-medicative behaviours observed in over 20 wild and domestic animal species, along with ethnomedicines reportedly derived from observing these behaviours in animals (Huffman 2021).

Elephants and Ethnomedicinal Knowledge: The self-medication behaviours of elephants have been documented for a long time. For example, African elephants suffering from gastrointestinal disturbances have been observed chewing the leaves of *Piliostigma thonningii* (commonly known as monkey bread or camel's foot), a leguminous plant. These elephants temporarily store the chewed leaves in their oesophageal pouch along with water. After allowing the mixture to soak, they discard the leaves and swallow the water. Notably, *P. thonningii* is widely used in traditional medicine to treat ailments such as dysentery, intestinal upsets, diarrhoea, flatulence, malaria, fever, respiratory infections, snakebites, hookworm infestations, and skin diseases, among others (Huffman 2021).

Geophagy, the deliberate ingestion of soil, is another common self-medication behaviour observed in many animal species, including mammalian herbivores including elephants. Soil-eating has been reported in all three elephant species: African savannah elephants (*Loxodonta africana*), African forest elephants (*L. cyclotis),* and Asian elephants (*Elephas maximus*). Elephant geophagy is thought to serve multiple adaptive purposes: remedying mineral deficiencies in their diet, as the soil provides essential nutrients absent in their natural habitat, and alleviating gastrointestinal issues by binding to toxins or acting as a digestive aid (Darker 2022). A further physico-chemical reason for geophagy is thought to be the detoxification of toxic secondary plant compounds. Many of the trees and shrubs consumed by elephants produce secondary compounds, such as tannins and alkaloids, which can be toxic. Geophagy may help neutralize these toxins. For example, in the rainforests of the Central African Republic, elephants are known to consume clay-rich soils from termite mounds (with a clay content exceeding 35%) or dig into the earth to access clay deposits. Their diet primarily consists of leaves, which often contain defensive secondary compounds to deter herbivores. However, ripe fruits, which are free of these harmful metabolites, are a seasonal dietary component. During September, when elephants consume large quantities of fruit, their visits to clay licks significantly decrease. This suggests a link between toxin consumption and the need for clay ingestion (Klaus 1998).

Domestic elephants (*Elephas maximus*) in Asia are traditionally managed by mahouts—a term derived from the Hindi mahaut—who devote their lives to the care and observation of these animals. Through close daily interaction, mahouts have long recognized that elephants rarely suffer from serious ailments, a trait often attributed to their instinctive self-medication behaviour. Such observations form the foundation of many ethnoveterinary and ethnomedicinal practices. A study from the Lao People's Democratic Republic highlighted that mahout observed elephants selectively consuming specific plants in response to ailments. For example, elephants with diarrhoea were noted to eat the roots of *Harrisonia perforata*, *Castanopsis indica*, and *Terminalia elliptica* Willd. Similarly, elephants with fever consumed *Tinospora crispa* and reportedly recovered quickly. Based on these observations, mahouts would guide ailing elephants to areas rich in these plants. The elephants would uproot and consume the plants (Fig. 5.1), often leading to rapid recovery. In addition, mahouts fed raw plant material directly to sick elephants or sometimes add salt to enhance its palatability, particularly for elephants suffering from diarrhoea or fever (Dubost *et al.* 2019). Although case-controlled studies on these practices are limited, these plants are widely used in traditional medicine, and pharmacological studies have identified diverse bioactive compounds with therapeutic potential. *Harrisonia perforata* contains limonoids, prenylated polyketides, and chromones, with its root extract showing significant anti-inflammatory effects. *Tinospora crispa* is rich in alkaloids, flavonoids, flavone glycosides, triterpenes, diterpenes, and diterpene glycosides exhibiting anti-inflammatory, antioxidant, immunomodulatory, cytotoxic, antimalarial, cardioprotective, and anti-diabetic properties.

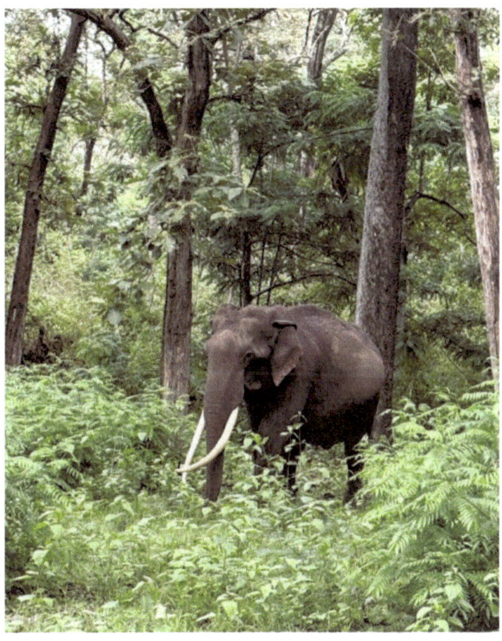

Fig. 5.1. *Elephants are known to exhibit self-medication behaviour, selectively consuming certain plants in response to specific ailments. Such observations offer valuable insights into the development of ethnomedical knowledge (Photo courtesy of Vinay Swarup).*

Complementing these findings, Wildlife SOS studies in India documented 90 plant species consumed by elephants, of which 16 are primary food sources (Wildlife SOS, pers. comm., 2025). Prominent among them are bamboo (*Bambusa arundinacea*), oleander (*Nerium oleander* L. syn. *Nerium odorum*), bidi leaf tree (*Bauhinia racemosa*), mahua (*Madhuca longifolia*), Indian coral tree (*Erythrina suberosa*), and Indian frankincense (*Boswellia serrata*). These plants contain diverse bioactive compounds—flavonoids, triterpenes, saponins, and phenolics—known for anti-inflammatory, antimicrobial, antioxidant, and tonic properties. For example, *Boswellia serrata* yields boswellic acids with potent anti-inflammatory effects; *Madhuca longifolia* provides saponins and triterpenoids with nutritive and restorative actions; and *Bambusa arundinacea* offers silica and flavonoids beneficial for joint and connective tissue health. Likewise, *Bauhinia racemosa* contains β-sitosterol, quercetin, kaempferol, and catechin, and its stem, bark, and leaves are traditionally used to treat diabetes, hepatic and gastrointestinal disorders, and malaria (Prabhu *et al.* 2021). The occurrence of such phytochemicals in key fodder species underscores the zoopharmacognostic behaviour of elephants—selectively feeding on plants that promote health maintenance and disease prevention.

Self-medication in Domestic Animals: Although domestication is believed to have influenced natural instincts—potentially reducing animals' innate ability to select diets that optimize their fitness—self-medication behaviours (Figs. 5.2-5.3) are still observed in domestic animals. Such behaviours are particularly prominent in gastrointestinal parasitic infestations. Surveys and field observations, as well as controlled studies, indicate that parasitized ruminants exhibit self-medication. In Uganda, shepherds observed that goats browsing on the anti-parasitic plant *Acacia anthelmintica* subsequently expelled worms in their faeces, leading to a noticeable reduction in the worm burden (Gradé *et al.* 2009). In Mediterranean rangelands, goats have been observed consuming significant amounts of *Pistacia lentiscus*, a shrub with known anthelmintic properties. This behaviour is most notable in the fall when the likelihood of gastrointestinal infections (GIN) is highest, despite the fact that the shrub's tannins impair protein metabolism and deter herbivory. A case-controlled study involving Mamber and Damascus breeds of domestic goats confirmed this self-medication behaviour. The study further revealed that goats of different breeds likely employ distinct self-medication strategies. Some goats consume significant amounts of anthelmintic plants regularly, irrespective of their metabolic cost, as a preventive measure, whereas others avoid consuming these plants until infection occurs, using them as a targeted treatment (Amit *et al.* 2013).

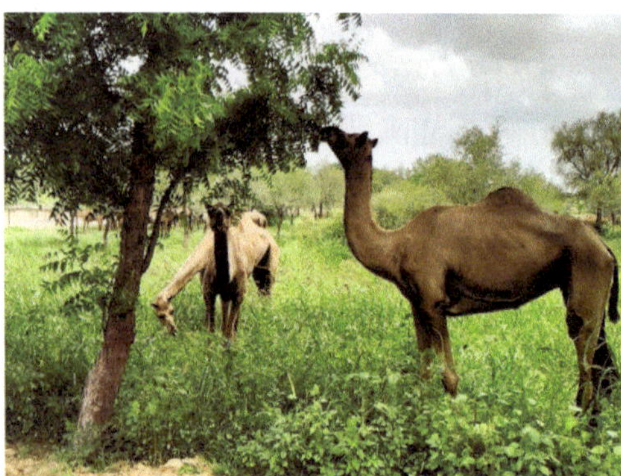

Fig. 5.2. Camels exhibit selective browsing behaviour and may even self-medicate (?). They forage on highly nutritious plants such as ber (Ziziphus mauritiana) and are among the few animals that consume Neem (Azadirachta indica), renowned for its medicinal properties (Ref: Kohler-Rollefson et al.2013). (Photo courtesy of Dr. A. Sahoo ICAR-NRC on Camel).

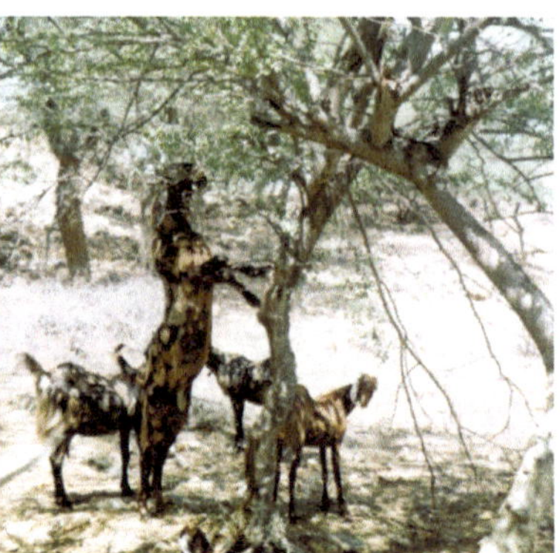

Fig. 5.3. Preference for browsing tannin-rich and antiparasitic plants such as Albizia anthelmintica is found to increase in goats following gastrointestinal parasitic infection indicating the possibility of self-medication behaviour (Photo source: ICAR-CIRG).

Similarly, sheep infected with gastrointestinal worm infections exhibit selective feeding behaviours to reduce parasite loads through self-medication. For instance, sheep infected with *Haemonchus contortus* consume more tannin-rich plants, which help decrease parasite burdens and those parasitized by larvae of the intestinal nematode *Trichostrongylus colubriformis* show a marked preference for high-protein feed, likely to meet the increased protein demands caused by parasitism (Villalba *et al.* 2014). These self-medication behaviours in domestic animals provides important indication for farmers, enabling the development of effective grazing strategies to manage parasitic burdens while maintaining animal health and welfare.

Methods and Mechanisms

The self-medication behaviours can be preventive, performed before an individual becomes infected or diseased, and/or therapeutic, performed after an individual becomes infected or diseased. It is hypothesized that animals self-medicate to compensate for increased exposure to parasites and pathogens. Additionally, animals with pathologies may self-medicate by manipulating their microbiome, such as by modifying food preferences. For example, sheep fed on acid-producing grains tend to consume bicarbonate-producing foods and solutions to mitigate acidosis (Villalba *et al.* 2007). Presently, self-medication behaviours have been classified into four basic modes: *Optimal avoidance*: Reducing likelihood of disease transmission through behaviour, such as avoiding food, water, or substrates contaminated with faeces, and substrates; *Dietary selection*: Consuming specific bioactive materials such as plants and mineral in small or limited amounts for preventative or health maintenance purposes; *Therapeutic ingestion*: Eating substances for the treatment of diseases or their symptoms, including the selective use of toxic or biologically active items at low frequency or in small quantities; and *External application:* Applying a substance to the body for the treatment or control of disease-bearing insects (e.g., fur rubbing, anting, den/nest fumigation). Sick animals also exhibit behavioural changes like lethargy, depression, anorexia, behavioural fever, or basking, which may assist in their recovery (Huffman 2021).

Despite growing interest, the precise evolutionary mechanisms behind self-medication behaviours remain inconclusive. These behaviours are often under reported in the literature, suggesting that their occurrence may be significantly more widespread across taxa than currently documented. Based on existing studies, some researchers suggest that self-medication behaviour may have evolved multiple times in mammals. In primates, it appears to be a life-history trait associated with longevity, absolute brain size, and body mass (Neco *et al.* 2019).

Previous experience and learning play a crucial role in self-medication behaviours among animals. For instance, lambs that have previously experienced the beneficial effects of condensed tannins during parasitic infestations show a stronger preference for tannin-rich feed compared to those without such experience. This suggests that individual experiences with the medicinal effects of tannins enhance both the intake and preference for tannins during subsequent parasite infections. Learning behaviours related to self-medication are often transmitted socially, either from mothers to their offspring or from pioneering individuals to followers within a group. Parasitic infestations are known to influence the ingestive responses of ruminants. Negative internal states induced by endoparasites can modify how lambs select novel foods and flavours. Parasitized animals may display increased attraction to novel foods and orosensory stimuli, which reduces neophobia and encourages a more diverse diet. This adaptive behaviour enhances the likelihood of sick herbivores consuming therapeutic doses of medicinal plants or nutritious forages that contribute to their recovery (Villalba *et al,* 2014. Egea *et al.* 2014). Chickens also have the ability to learn self-medicate to mitigate stress. With their acute colour vision, birds can quickly learn to associate specific colours with beneficial effects. For example, broiler chickens learned to recognize coloured feed supplemented with vitamin C within just three days and began self-medicating as needed. Similarly, one-month-old lame broiler chickens quickly learned to select feed containing the pain-relieving analgesic carprofen. The consumption of the painkiller increased in proportion to the severity of their lameness (Engel 2007).

In addition to ingestive changes, adaptive behavioural responses during sickness help animals fight illness, increasing their chances of recovery and survival. Lethargy conserves energy by minimizing expenditure, anorexia encourages sick animals to become more selective in their diet, favouring foods that reduce infection risks or contain anti-infective compounds, and isolation not only helps animals avoid predators but also limits the spread of contagious diseases within their group or herd. Overall, self-medication behaviours in animals illustrate the complex ways in which they adapt to health challenges, emphasizing the role of learning and experience in enhancing survival strategies. These behaviours, particularly in livestock, have far-reaching benefits: they promote healthier animals, support more sustainable farming practices, and yield economic advantages for farmers. Self-medication serves as animals' first line of defence against illness and has the potential to revolutionize sustainable grazing systems. By incorporating these natural behaviours, farmers can improve land quality, as well as the health and welfare of their livestock. Viewing foraging as a dynamic process aimed at achieving homeostasis can inspire the development of management programs that provide herbivores with access to diverse and nutritious foods, alongside an array of medicinal plants (Villalba *et al.* 2007). However, proof of self-medicative behaviour requires a clear demonstration of cause and effect that can only be achieved in controlled studies.

Ethnoveterinary Materia Medica

Ethnoveterinary Materia Medica (EVMM) refers to the collection of traditional knowledge, practices, and materials used in the treatment and management of animal health. It includes three important components application of natural products (medicinal plants, animal products, minerals, and other natural substances), manipulation and surgery and appeal to spiritual forces (rituals, incantations and prayers), which are sometimes connected with particular plants and special ingredients (Toyang *et al.* 2007).

Natural Products

Ethnoveterinary medicine uses a wide range of natural products derived from plants, minerals, and animal sources to prevent and treat livestock diseases.

Medicinal Plants and their Products: Herbs and botanicals have been widely used ingredients in the preparation of ethnoveterinary medicines for centuries, forming the foundation of traditional medicinal systems across the globe. Various plant parts, including roots, stems, leaves, bark, fruits, flowers, seeds, and plant derived oils, gums, resins and latex are utilized for their diverse pharmacological properties to treat a wide range of conditions, from minor ailments like colds to severe diseases. In ethnoveterinary practice, plants are also utilized for managing fractures and enhancing fertility, appetite, productivity, and more. Prominent examples include neem (*Azadirachta indica*), known for its insecticidal and antiparasitic properties; turmeric (*Curcuma longa*), valued for its wound-healing capabilities; and garlic (*Allium sativum*), recognized for its antibacterial and antifungal effects. *Jivanti* (Creeping milkweed, *Leptadenia reticulata*), *Shatavari* (Asparagus, *Asparagus racemosus*), *Methi* (Fenugreek, *Trigonella foenum-graecum*), *Gālikā* (Goat's rue *Galega officinalis*), and *kalonji* (Black cumin, *Nigella sativa*) are known for their galactagogue effects and their role in improving nutrient utilization. The knowledge of medicinal plants is often passed down through generations, preserving cultural heritage while contributing to the discovery of new drugs. According to the International Union for Conservation of Nature and the World Wildlife Fund, an estimated 50,000 to 80,000 flowering plant species are presently used for medicinal purposes worldwide (Chen *et al.* 2016).

Animals and Animal Products*:* For millennia, animals and their by-products have served as valuable medicinal resources, used to treat and alleviate a wide array of illnesses and diseases across diverse human cultures The healing of human ailments by using therapeutics based on medicines obtained from animals or ultimately derived from them is known as zootherapy (Costa-Neto 2005). The term also applies to the use of such animal-based medicine for the prevention, treatment, and healing of diseases in animals. Zootherapy remains an integral part of traditional medical system worldwide, including Ayurveda and Traditional Chinese medicine (TCM), where animal-derived substances are widely documented as effective ingredients in curative, protective, and preventive remedies. For example, 11 animal species were found to be used for ethnoveterinary purposes to cure diseases in livestock and pets in East Brazil (Confessor *et al.*2009). and use of 21 animal species in ethnoveterinary preparations was recorded from the state of West Bengal, India (Mandal and Rahman 2022).

Animal-based medicines are derived from various parts of animals, including their bodies, metabolic products such as secretions and excretions, and even non-animal materials like nests and cocoons. Zootherapy also involves live animals such as leeches and insects. The traditional healers and indigenous communities around the world possess vast knowledge about animal based therapeutics and using them as a vital component of both human and veterinary healthcare.

Hirudotherapy (Leech Therapy): Hirudotherapy, a branch of zootherapy, involving the use of medicinal leeches to treat various medical conditions has a rich history in both human and veterinary medicine. This ancient practice remains relevant in modern medicine for specific treatments. In Indian tradition, Dhanvantari, the God of Ayurveda, is often depicted holding a *jaluka* (leech) in one of his four hands, symbolizing the significance of leech therapy in both human and veterinary medicine in ancient India. The Sushruta Samhita, a foundational text of Ayurveda, recommends leech therapy for various ailments, including eye diseases and internal tumors (*gulmas*) characterized by pain, burning sensations, inflammation, and piercing discomfort. Chapter XIII of the Sushruta Samhita- Sutrashanam (*Jalauká-vacháraniyamadhyáyam*) provides an extensive account of leech therapy, and gives habits, habitats and morphological features of leeches (Kunja Lal 1907). The leeches are classified into 12 species, with six being non-venomous and preferred for medical use. Detailed instructions are given on the selection of patients suitable for leeching, the method of applying leeches, and the procedures for collecting and maintaining them. Non-venomous species, such as *Sarávikás*—characterized by their cold bodies, lotus-leaf-like markings, and a length of 18 finger-widths—were preferred for treating animals. The Samhita emphasizes the importance of considering the season and specific condition requirements when performing leech therapy. The Sushruta Samhita also emphasizes that leeching and cauterization should be performed with due consideration of the season and the specific requirements of the condition. If a leech refuses to detach after achieving the desired therapeutic effect, it can be removed by dusting it with *Saindhava* (rock salt). This meticulous guidance reflects the advanced understanding of leech therapy in ancient Indian medical practices.

Hirudotherapy has been successfully applied in modern veterinary medicine to treat various animal diseases, particularly in dogs, cats, and horses. It is often used when traditional treatments prove ineffective, are too slow to act, or during post-surgical recovery when tissues are at risk due to venous congestion. Common indications for leech therapy include joint disorders (hip and elbow dysplasia, acute and chronic arthritis), soft tissue inflammation (diseases involving tendons, ligaments, and fascia), vertebral disorders and wound treatment. Leech therapy is a painless procedure, typically lasting 30 to 120 minutes depending on the size of the animal. For safety and efficacy, medical leeches must be sourced exclusively from certified biofarms. Additionally, sterile conditions must be maintained during leech culture, transport, and storage to prevent microbial infections (Sobczak and Kantyka 2014).

The most commonly used medicinal leech species include *Hirudo medicinalis, Hirudo asiatica, Hirudo manellensis, Hirudo orientalis, Hirudo michaelseni, Hirudo nipponia, Hirudo granulosa* and *Macrobdella decora.* The saliva of these leeches contains a diverse range of bioactive compounds with therapeutic properties, including hirudin, hyaluronidase, calin, destabilase, apyrase, eglins, bdellins, decorsin, hirustatin, tryptase inhibitors, and histamine like substances, complement inhibitors, carboxypeptidase A- inhibitors acetylcholine. These compounds exhibit anticoagulants, vasodilator, thrombolytic, anti-inflammatories and analgesic activies, along with extracellular matrix-degradative and antimicrobial effects. They improve blood circulation, reduce swelling and pain, and promote healing in conditions such as venous congestion, arthritis, and skin graft recovery. Leech therapy is contraindicated in animals suffering from acute infections, anaemia or haemophilia, immunosuppressive disorders, skin cancer, pregnancy, or septic conditions (Sig *et al.* 2017). Although leeches have recognized therapeutic value, they may also cause *hirudiniasis*—a water-associated parasitic infestation. This condition is prevalent in domestic animals, especially cattle, during dry or hot seasons in developing regions of Africa and Asia (Abdisa 2018).

Body Parts and By-products of Animals: Various body parts and by-products of domestic and wild animals have been utilized since the inception of human-animal interactions. These include bones, nails, horns, antlers, sinew, skin, hair, urine, dung, beaks, feathers, body fat, bile, flesh and visceral organs, and milk and milk products such as curd, butter, buttermilk, clarified butter (*ghrita* or *ghee*), and honey. In West Bengal, traditional healers use zootherapeutic remedies for the purported treatment of cattle diseases like foot and mouth disease, joint problems, wounds, fever, and diarrhoea. The animal-derived materials used include: hunted blue jay (*Coracias benghalensis*), skull and beak of kingfisher (*Halcyon smyrnensis*), bones of vulture (*Gyps bengalensis*), skull and wing bone of fruit bat (*Cynopterus sphinx*), antler of spotted deer (*Axis axis*), Indian green frog (*Euphlyctis hexadactylus*), nails of fruit bat (*Cynopterus sphinx*), parietal bone of long-whiskered catfish (*Sperata aor*), umbilical cord of Bengal mongoose (*Herpestes javanicus palustris*), teeth of bear (*Melursus ursinus*), front appendage of crab (*Cancer pagurus*), body fat from Bengal monitor (*Varanus bengalensis*), Russell's viper (*Daboia russelii*), and pig (*Sus scrofa domesticus*) and honey.

These parts were used either in their raw form or combined with medicinal herbs and minerals. Furthermore, some animal species were used based on magico-religious beliefs to heal diseases in domesticated animals, which were thought to result from the influence of evil spirits (Mandal *et al.* 2022). In the semi-arid regions of Brazil, commonly used animal species for treating livestock diseases include Teju lizards (*Tupinambis merianae*), iguanas (*Iguana iguana*), pigs (*Sus scrofa domesticus*), and rattlesnakes (*Crotalus durissus* Linnaeus, 1758). The animal-derived products used in these treatments were fat, feathers, horns, eggs, bones, milk, and leather (Confessor *et al.* 2009).

Another study from Brazil reported the use of 15 animal species in folk veterinary medicine. These animals included both domestic and wild mammals like sheep (*Ovis aries*), pigs (*Sus scrofa*), cattle (*Bos taurus*), and foxes (*Cerdocyon thous*). Reptiles such as chameleons (*Iguana iguana*) and rattlesnakes (*Crotalus durissus*), along with domestic birds like chickens (*Gallus domesticus*), turkeys (*Meleagris gallopavo*), and quail (*Nothura maculosa cearensis*), were also utilized. Folk remedies were primarily applied to relatively simple conditions, such as furuncles, injuries caused by embedded thorns, or skin eruptions. However, more complex diseases, like rabies and brucellosis, were notably absent from the treatments reported. Among the resources cited, animal fat was the most frequently used, and valued for its medicinal and veterinary properties (Barboza *et al.* 2007). Animal-based products were also a significant component of the Mediterranean pharmacopeia, playing an essential role in the traditional care of livestock, particularly sheep and goats (Piluzza *et al.* 2015). Contemporary Spanish ethnoveterinary practices incorporate numerous remedies derived from domestic animals such as sheep, goats, cattle, pigs, mules, donkeys, horses, dogs, cats, and chickens (González and Vallejo 2021).

Ayurveda, one of the foremost ancient healing sciences, provides an extensive list of medicines derived from the animal kingdom. It specifically highlights the medicinal properties of milk from various domestic animals and the preparation of medicated *ghrita* (prepared by processing clarified butter or *ghee* with herbal decoctions and pastes) for treating medical conditions. Even today, farmers in many parts of India offer a draught of milk mixed with turmeric and *ghee* to revitalize their bullocks after strenuous work. Medicated milk and butter milk are also prescribed for ayurvedic treatment of many equine ailments. Honey and butter are used in ethnoveterinary medicine for their healing and preservative properties. However, despite the historical and cultural significance of such practices, case-control studies on the efficacy of zootherapies, especially in treatment of animal diseases are lacking. Additionally, the use of wild animals and their body parts poses a significant threat to wildlife conservation and raises concerns about ethical and sustainable practices. The effective use of zootherapeutic products sourced from domestic animals offers a sustainable and ethical alternative to products derived from wild animals, promoting both ecological conservation and the preservation of traditional veterinary practices.

***Entomotherapy*:** Derived from the Greek words *entomon* (insect) and *therapeia* (treatment), entomotherapy refers to the preventive or therapeutic use of insects and their by-products in medicine. While insects are often perceived as repugnant or unclean, many species and their derivatives have been used as medicinal resources since ancient times in both human and veterinary medicine, including in India (Costa-Neto 2005b). Globally, approximately 1,000 medicinal insect species have been documented, with a significant proportion (about 50%) originating from China, encompassing 70 genera, 63 families, and 14 orders. In India, over 50 insect species from 28 families and 11 orders are employed to treat as many as 50 different human diseases and health conditions (Siddiqui *et al.* 2023). Medicinal insects are integral to traditional medical preparations, primarily used for managing skin and digestive disorders, asthma and respiratory problems, kidney and urinary ailments, arthritis, and wound care.

Compared to human medicine, the application of entomotherapy in veterinary medicine is less well-documented. A study conducted in Spain reported the use of 18 invertebrate species, predominantly insects and molluscs, in contemporary ethnoveterinary medicine to treat or prevent approximately 50 animal diseases and conditions. These include skin and subcutaneous tissue diseases, eye disorders, indigestion, mastitis, intestinal parasites, colic, pneumonia, wounds, and infectious diseases such as foot-and-mouth disease (FMD), foot rot, and pasteurellosis. Among the most commonly used insect-derived products are honey and cobwebs. Honey, produced by the honey bee (*Apis mellifera* Linnaeus, 1758), is highly regarded in ethnoveterinary medicine for its effectiveness in treating wounds and eye infections (González *et al.* 2016). It is frequently used alone or combined with herbs, minerals, and other medicinal ingredients to address respiratory problems, FMD lesions, burns, canine recurrent dermatitis, canine wounds, and mastitis by traditional healers in many countries including India.

Scientific studies have revealed that insects and insect-derived products contain several natural compounds with significant biological properties, including immunological, analgesic, antibacterial, diuretic, anaesthetic, and antirheumatic effects. For example, bee venom, used to treat conditions such as arthritis, rheumatism, pain, and even cancer contains proteins and other bioactive compounds with diverse pharmacological properties. Studies have also verified antimicrobial activity in the products of bees such as honey and propolis (a resinous substance collected by honeybees from tree buds and bark, used to seal and protect their hives). The therapeutic use of bee- venom and other natural products from bees derived is known as apitherapy (Dossey 2010). Insect derivatives have been found to inhibit at least 30 species of bacteria, 13 species of fungi, 5 viruses, and 10 parasitic pathogens. These include bacteria associated with wound infections e.g., *Bacillus* sp., *Staphylococcus* sp., and *Proteus* sp., digestive system infections e.g., *Helicobacter pylori*, *Bacillus cereus*, *Citrobacter freundii*, *Escherichia coli*, and *Salmonella enterica* urinary tract infections e.g., *Enterobacter cloacae*, *Enterococcus faecalis*, *Acinetobacter baumannii*, and *Serratia marcescens*, and other infections e.g., *Listeria monocytogenes* and *Haemophilus influenzae*; dermatophytes; viruses causing Rift Valley fever v, Hepatitis A and B, and Herpes simplex infections and parasites including *Trypanosoma cruzi*, *Leishmania* sp., *Plasmodium* sp., and *Haemonchus contortus.* The mechanisms of action include reducing bacterial adherence to human keratinocytes, disrupting biofilm formation, altering membrane permeability, deforming peptides, generating reactive oxygen species (ROS), and inhibiting or damaging DNA formation. These effects are largely attributed to antimicrobial peptides (Siddiqui *et al.* 2023).

Traditional healers often use honey either alone or as a medium for plant-derived medicines. Honey possesses remarkable therapeutic properties, including antimicrobial, anti-inflammatory, antioxidant, immunomodulatory, antidiabetic, and antineoplastic effects. These benefits arise from its complex composition, which includes phenolic compounds, flavonoids, short-chain fatty acids, fermentable sugars (e.g., nigerooligosaccharides), hydrogen peroxide, acidic pH, and non-peroxide components (Nweze *et al.* 2020). Some recent innovations in entomotherapy include: *Maggot therapy* involving the use of live, disinfected blowfly larvae to selectively remove necrotic tissue from soft tissue wounds. Studies in the area of *apitherapy* have explored the use of bee products like propolis and royal jelly to treat conditions such as Parkinson's disease. Melittin, a peptide found in bee venom, has shown potential in managing inflammation associated with rheumatoid arthritis and multiple sclerosis by blocking inflammatory gene expression and reducing pain (Siddiqui *et al.* 2023). Compared to human medicine, the application of entomotherapy in veterinary medicine remains underexplored and lacks scientific validation. A systematic study involving traditional healers and modern veterinary practitioners, combined with evidence-based therapeutic assessments, could pave the way for the discovery of new, cost-effective drugs for livestock treatment, alternative materials for pharmaceutical applications to reduce emerging antimicrobial resistance problem and promotion of organic farming practices.

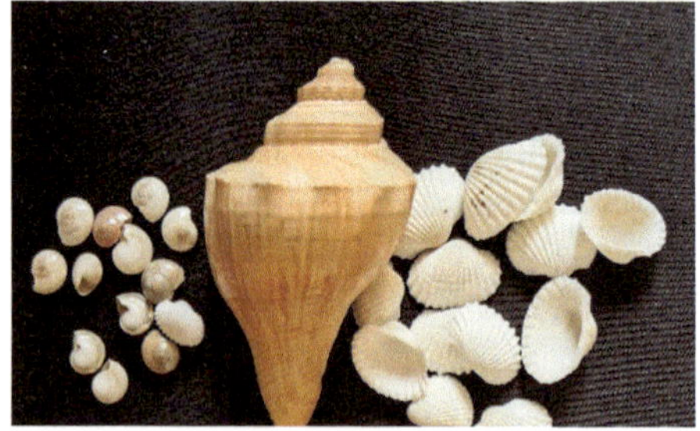

Fig. 5.4 *Marine organisms, as the richest natural sources of minerals like calcium and phosphorus, play a significant role in Ayurvedic and traditional veterinary medicine. (Photo by the Author).*

Marine Animal Products: Marine animal products (Fig. 5.4) are highly valued in Ayurveda for their medicinal properties, particularly after undergoing purification (*Shodhana*) and incineration (*Marana*). Some examples include: pearl (*Mukta*) from *Pinctada margaritifera*, red coral (*Pravāl*) from *Corallium rubrum*, conch shell (*Shankh*a) from *Turbinella rapa* or *Xancus pyrum,* cowries (*Kapard*) from *Cypraea moneta*, and cuttlefish bones (*Samudraphen*) from *Sepia officinalis*. These marine products are rich in calcium carbonate (over 80%) and also contain minerals such as phosphate, sulphate, iron, and magnesium (Saroch and Kundailia, 2014). They are traditionally used in Ayurveda to treat a range of conditions and are also incorporated into ethnoveterinary practices worldwide.

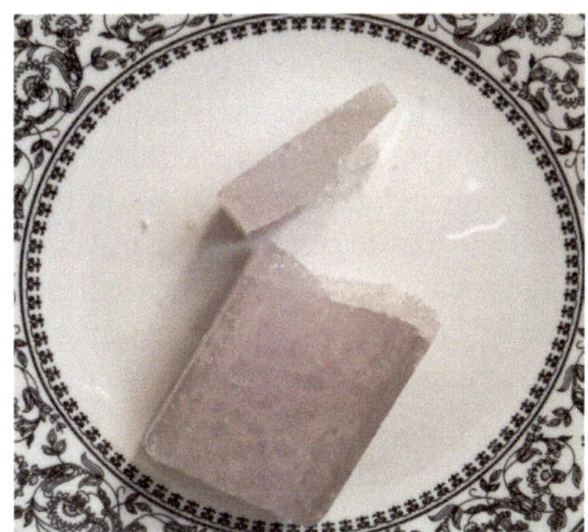

Fig. 5.5. *Alum stone: Phitkari or alum (Potassium Alum or Potassium Sulphate) is a crystalline (sphaṭika kṣāra) salt-like substance. First mentioned in ancient Ayurvedic texts for its medicinal value, alum has been widely used for its antiseptic and astringent properties. Raika pastoralists value it highly as an effective medicine for their animals (Photo by the Author).*

Minerals, Clay and Other Natural Substances: Ayurveda classifies medicinal substances into three broad categories: animal and animal products, herbs and botanicals, and minerals and other natural substances. The mineral group includes a variety of naturally occurring substances such as ores, silica, lime, gold, silver, calcium, copper, antimony, red and yellow arsenic, sulphur, lead, and zinc. Majority of these minerals and their compounds particularly copper sulphate, ammonium chloride, zinc oxide are used in ethnoveterinary practices. Additionally, various types of clays and naturally occurring substances—such as kaolin, Fuller's Earth (*Multani Mitti*), Bentonite clay, Indian red earth or Ochre (*Geru*), chalk, alum (*Phitkari*), and different salts like common salt, rock salt (Fig. 5.5, 5.6) and black salt—are utilized in ethnoveterinary practices. These natural substances are essential to ethnoveterinary medicine across cultures, utilized for preventive and curative

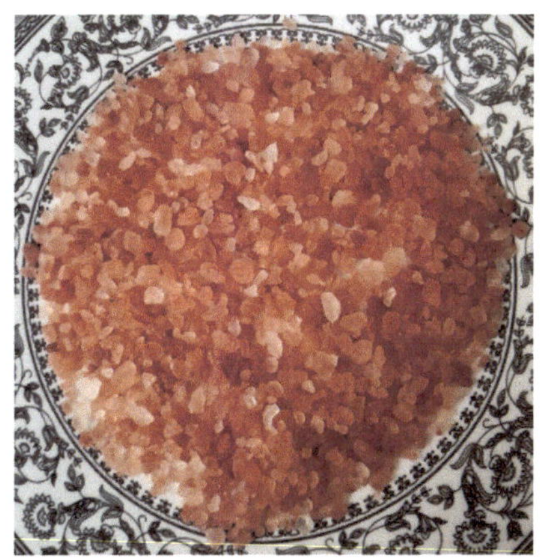

Fig.5.6. *Commonly found in the Himalayan region, rock salt consists of approximately 85% sodium chloride. The remaining 15% includes various elements and minerals such as iron, copper, zinc, iodine, manganese, magnesium, and selenium. Rock salt offers numerous health benefits and is widely used in ethnoveterinary medicine across the world (Photo by the Author).*

therapies, as well as nutritional supplements, to enhance fertility and overall animal health (Table 5.1). Salt is also used as a preservative in ethnoveterinary medicine to prevent the spoilage of herbal extracts. It creates an inhospitable environment for pathogens. Since water promotes the growth of microorganisms, salt reduces the water content in extracts and food by binding its sodium and chloride ions to water molecules (Dzoyem *et al.* 2020). Limestone is often added to decoctions to enhance their efficacy. It aids in breaking down plant materials and other ethnoveterinary substances, helping to release their active ingredients and making the medicinal preparation more effective (Toyang *et al.* 2007).

Table 5.1. Examples of non-herbal ethnoveterinary remedies documented in literature*

EVM practices	Used for	References
Fuller's Earth (*Multani Mitti*) 50g soaked in whey for three hours.	Traditional treatment of diarrhoea in livestock practiced by farmers in parts of Rajasthan	Garg *et al.* (2019)
Fuller's Earth (*Multani Mitti*) 100 g mixed with 500 g curd		
Red soil 10 kg kept overnight in 20 litres of water; filtered water given @ 2 litre for 3 days		
Powdered alum 100 g in water orally		
Paste of alum in jaggary, boiled with water for 30 minutes, kept overnight and given orally for 4-5 days	Diarrhoea in sheep and goats practiced by Raika pastoralists of Rajasthan	Meena *et al* (2020)
Paste of alum powder orally followed by water for 2-3 days	Fever in sheep and goats practiced by Raika pastoralists of Rajasthan	
Copper sulphate in water (1: 9 ratio) orally	Deworming livestock used by herders in Tamil Nadu	Balakrishnan *et al.* (2009)
Paste of common salt in butter	Mastitis in cows by herders in Tamil Nadu	
Salt (2 tablespoons) dissolved in 250 ml water	Keratoconjunctivitis in cattle in Sub-Saharan Africa	Toyang *et al.* (2007)
Paste prepared by boiling 1 kg clay soil dissolved in clean water (2 litre) applied on horn stump and bandaged	Broken horn in cattle	
Copper sulphate scrubbed on affected areas	Mange in pigs, dogs and cattle in Sardinia	Bullitta *et al.* (2018)
Lard	Mange in pigs, bloat in cattle, wound and hoof infection in horses in Sardinia	
Salt dissolved in warm water	Gastrointestinal problem and washing wounds and FMD lesions in Sardinia	

***Note:** *Mineral compounds and animal products (butter, wax, honey) are also used as preservative or medium in herbal ethnoveterinary remedies and many ethnoveterinary formulations incorporate more than one group of the medicinal substances (herbs, animal products and minerals).*

Acupuncture

A key component of Traditional Chinese Veterinary Medicine (TCVM), acupuncture is increasingly being integrated into ethnoveterinary practices worldwide to promote animal health and well-being. This ancient technique involves inserting fine needles into specific points on the body to stimulate healing and balance energy flow. In ethnoveterinary medicine, acupuncture is used to treat a variety of conditions in animals, including:

- Alleviating chronic pain associated with arthritis and musculoskeletal diseases.
- Managing neurological conditions such as paralysis and nerve injuries.
- Addressing respiratory problems like bronchitis.
- Improving gastrointestinal function and treating disorders such as colic and diarrhoea.
- Supporting fertility and addressing reproductive disorders.

Acupuncture has also been reported as effective in managing bovine mastitis. Research indicates that it reduces N-acetyl-beta-D-glucosaminidase (NAGase) activity in cows with subclinical mastitis, suggesting it may promote the healing of damaged mammary epithelial cells (Holyoak and Ma 2022). Additionally, modern veterinary acupuncturists have treated pets with metabolic diseases associated with impaired organ function— such as dogs with diabetes, kidney or liver failure, pancreatitis, Cushing's disease, and Addison's disease —resulting in reduced nausea and increase in appetite after acupuncture sessions.The use of veterinary acupuncture for pain relief is expanding, particularly among small animal practitioners. It is employed as an adjunct to conventional treatments, as an alternative when traditional methods fail to resolve pain, or as a drug-free option for pain management. In TCVM, acupuncture points are thought to represent areas of concentrated Qi (energy or life force). Stimulating these points encourages the smooth and harmonious flow of Qi along the meridians—channels that link acupuncture points throughout the body. There are 12 principal meridians named after Chinese or Zhang Fu organs. While TCVM acupuncture focuses on restoring the balance of Qi, Western medical acupuncture emphasizes restoring physiological homeostasis and leveraging the body's internal mechanisms to relieve pain. Overall, acupuncture seamlessly integrates into a multimodal approach for managing acute and chronic pain, serving as a safe and complementary modality when performed by trained practitioners in companion animal care (Huntingford and Petty 2022).

Another traditional healing technique, acupressure, involves applying pressure to acupuncture points instead of inserting needles. This less invasive method is often preferred for hard-to-reach locations or for pets that may not tolerate needles. Both acupuncture and acupressure, though rooted in traditional practices, are increasingly utilized by modern therapists. They serve as effective adjunct therapies to routine treatments, helping to alleviate symptoms and reduce suffering in patients with chronic diseases.

Surgical Practices

In ethnoveterinary medicine, routine surgical methods are often employed to treat various ailments in livestock. These methods have been developed over generations through trial and error and are deeply rooted in indigenous knowledge. Some common surgical techniques include:

Castration: Traditionally practiced to control breeding and reduce aggression in male animals, castration was often performed at a young age using sharp tools or heated instruments. Herbal remedies and other natural products with antiseptic and analgesic properties—such as turmeric, neem, and alum —are applied to reduce pain and infection. In some regions, castration methods involve bloodless methods like tight ligatures or crushing.

Dehorning (or Disbudding): Dehorning helps prevent injuries among animals and handlers. It is typically done in early life using hot irons, sharp tools, or plant-based caustics. Herbal treatments such as aloe vera, turmeric, or medicinal plant ash are applied post-procedure to promote healing and prevent infections.

Wound Treatment- Traditional practitioners often use herbal pastes and poultices to treat wounds and promote healing. They may also employ techniques like suturing with natural fibres.

Abscess Drainage- Traditional healers use sharp instruments to lance and drain the infected area, followed by the application of herbal antiseptics.

Fracture Management- Fracture management in animals often involves splinting and bandaging to immobilize fractures and promote healing. In traditional practices, natural materials such as bamboo or wood are commonly used as splints. Also, traditional healers frequently utilize herbal pastes and poultices for managing fractures. A recent study from the Eastern Ghats in Andhra Pradesh, India, identified 65 plant species from 59 genera and 42 families used by ethnoveterinary practioners and tribal communities for treating bone fractures. The procedure involves preparing poultices using a combination of herbal pastes or powders mixed with pastes made of black pepper powder (2 to 10 seeds), garlic (1 to 10 cloves), Shell lime powder (1 to 10 grams), jaggery powder (5 to 20 grams) and egg white (adequate quantity for forming a fine paste). The poultice is uniformly applied as a coat on the skin around the fractured bone. A thin, clean white or muslin cloth is tightly wrapped over the poultice as a bandage. Bamboo splints are then placed over the bandage for additional support and stability, and the bandage is wrapped again to secure the splints. The practice is used for both pet and farm animals. Depending on the animal's size, the weight of the poultice applied externally varies between 10 and 500 g. The poultice is reapplied weekly, and complete healing, including pain management, is typically achieved within 3 to 4 weeks (Babu *et al.* 2024). This traditional technique is an excellent example of integrating natural materials and indigenous knowledge for effective fracture management in animals. The other routine ethnoveterinary surgical practices include rumen trocarisation, branding, hoof trimming, shoeing, docking, nose ringing, ear-cropping or notching.

Disease Preventive Practices

Besides treatment of sick animals, traditional animal husbandry practices such as housing design, grazing strategies, supplementary feeding, and calf-rearing are not only aimed at managing livestock but also play a critical role in preventing diseases and ensuring the health and well-being of animals. These time-tested methods protect livestock from adverse weather conditions, stress, predators, and diseases caused by pests and parasites. Such practices remain highly relevant for sustainable livestock development and improving animal health and productivity. For example, the Fulani herdsmen of Northern Nigeria practice transhumance, an annual migration in search of water. Migration routes are carefully chosen to avoid tsetse fly-infested areas, thereby reducing the risk of trypanosome infections. Additionally, the Fulani employ strategic herd movements to manage foot-and-mouth disease (FMD). They sometimes move their cattle upwind of infected herds to prevent the disease from spreading. In other instances, they move cattle downwind to expose animals to mild infections, ensuring immunity against future, more severe outbreaks (Leeflang 1993). Similarly, the pastoral Maasai have, for generations, understood that wild animals are silent carriers of malignant catarrhal fever (MCF). Based on this indigenous knowledge, they take precautionary measures by keeping livestock away from wild animals, particularly during calving, to minimize disease transmission (Jacob *et al.* 2004). Interestingly, magico-religious beliefs and rituals also influence these traditional practices, often serving practical purposes. While some rituals may appear unconventional, they contribute to livestock protection by preventing the spread of pests, avoiding poisonous plants, conserving animals, or safeguarding sacred herbs and areas. For instance, specific taboos can act as unintentional but effective disease prevention measures (Minja 2004). Another notable example is the Andean livestock herders, who avoid keeping animals in cold, breezy areas believed to harbour evil winds. Modern analysis reveals that this practice is, in fact, an effective strategy to prevent respiratory illnesses such as pneumonia in livestock (McCorkle 1986).

Ethnoveterinary Pharmacy Preparations

Following are the commonly used preparations in ethnoveterinary medicine (in alphabetical order).

Decoction: Decoctions are commonly used to extract medicinal properties from the hard parts of plants, such as seeds, roots, and bark. The process involves boiling the plant material, usually for 15–30 minutes. The material is first chopped into small pieces or powdered and then boiled in water, typically using clay or steel pots. Vegetable oils or butters can be combined with powders or decoctions and then boiled with limestone. The limestone acts as an emulsifier, facilitating the mixing of fats with the liquid for improved consistency and effectiveness (Toyang *et al.* 2007). Decoctions are used for both internal and external treatments. Some commonly used herbal decoctions in ethnoveterinary medicine include those made from the bark of acacia, cinchona, *jaumn* (black plum or Indian blackberry), and neem, as well as from tobacco leaves, linseed, and barley.

Fumigation: The practice of exposing animals or their environment to smoke (fumigation), is an important traditional method used in ethnoveterinary medicine for treating and preventing various ailments in animals. This method serves multiple purposes, including disinfection of animal shelters and living area, repelling insects and parasites and treating respiratory problems. Fumigation is typically performed by burning dry or wet medicinal plants, botanicals, alone or along with animal products such as ghee, milk, or honey. Animal fat and resins help plants to burn well for fumigation. Cow dung cakes are commonly used as a fuel source to produce the smoke, which is then directed toward the animal or its surroundings. The antimicrobial effects of fumigation are attributed to the presence of antimicrobial volatile compounds in the plant materials. Common plants and substances used in fumigation practices include neem, eucalyptus, arjuna tree, long pepper, *guggul (Guggulu:* Indian bdelljium*)*, turmeric powder, *haritaki* (Indian walnut), *jaiphal* (nutmeg) and various aromatic herbs and resins known for their antimicrobial and insect-repellent properties.

Infusion: It is obtained by steeping drug materials in hot water similar to making tea without boiling. Herbal infusions are commonly used in ethnoveterinary medicine. These are prepared by adding hot boiled water to plant powder or chopped plant in a container, which is covered for 10–20 minutes until the medicinal components are extracted. The extract is filtered and given to the animal, cooled or warm water instantly or within 12 hours.

Medicinal Extracts: Extracts are typically semi-solid preparations that contain the active components of drugs, obtained through one or more extraction methods. In some cases, the juice of fresh plants is directly extracted and purified. In others, the active ingredients are dissolved in water, which is later removed through evaporation or distillation (Srinivasan 1990). Since heat can destroy active ingredients, cold-water extracts of herbs are commonly used in ethnoveterinary medicine. These extracts are not only effective but also simple to prepare. To make a cold-water extract, leaves or roots (cut into small pieces and pounded) are soaked overnight in water in a 1:1 ratio (1 ml of water to 1 g of herb). Cold-water extracts should be prepared fresh daily to ensure their efficacy.

Ointment and Cream: Ointments and creams are semisolid preparations commonly used for external applications in ethnoveterinary practices, but they differ in composition. Ointments have a higher oil content and less water compared to creams, making them thicker and more occlusive. They are typically prepared by mixing finely powdered mineral compounds, plant materials, or herbal extracts with wax, butter or cooking oil. Ointments are used for treating skin rashes, wound care, sprains, mastitis and eye conditions. Creams, in contrast, contain nearly equal proportions of oil and water or slightly more water than oil. They are lighter in consistency, absorb into the skin faster, and are suitable for covering larger areas. Creams are ideal for treating various skin conditions due to their quick absorption and ease of application.

Plaster: A plaster consists of medicinal agents with adhesive substances. In ethnoveterinary practices, plasters are used similarly to poultices but often have a firmer consistency. They are usually made by mixing medicinal herbs with a binding agent like clay, flour, or wax to form a thick paste. This paste is then spread on a cloth or directly on the skin and allowed to dry. Plasters are used to treat various ailments, including inflammation, bruises, and wounds, by providing a protective barrier and delivering the medicinal properties of the herbs directly to the affected area.

Poultice (Cataplasm): Poultices, also known as cataplasms, are widely used in ethnoveterinary medicine for their healing properties. These soft, pasty preparations made from medicinal herbs or other compounds are applied to specific areas of the body to treat inflammation, bruises, cuts, and wounds. They help reduce pain and swelling, promote the drainage of pus from abscesses, and draw out toxins or embedded particles from the skin. In ethnoveterinary practices, herbal poultices are prepared by mixing herbal powders with hot water to form a paste. This paste is then spread evenly on a piece of cloth and placed over the affected area. Poultices are cooling in nature and are popular as cost-effective and easy-to-use treatments for performance animals.

Powder: A pharmaceutical powder is a dry, solid substance composed of finely divided drugs, with or without excipients, intended for internal or external administration. It is typically prepared through mechanical processes such as crushing, grinding, and pounding the material into a finely divided form. Powders may contain one or more active ingredients mixed in precise proportions. They are categorized into two types: standardized vegetable (herbal) powders and compound powders (Srinivasan 1990). Both types are widely used in ethnoveterinary pharmacy. Herbal powders are derived from various plant parts, such as bark, stems, roots, leaves, flowers, or even entire plants. The preparation involves drying the plant material, followed by pounding it into a powder form. Coarse powders can be further sieved to achieve a finer consistency. Powder from medicinal plants can be preserved by mixing it with fat. Powders are administered to sick animals in different ways, such as: directly feeding them the powder, mixing the powder with salt, using powder in decoctions or poultices.

Tincture: Tinctures are liquid herbal preparations made by combining water (70–80%), alcohol (20–30%), and medicinal substances. They are one of the most commonly dispensed forms of herbal remedies due to their convenience and long shelf life. Alcohol acts as an effective solvent, ensuring the tinctures remain stable for extended periods unless precipitation occurs. The alcohol-to-water ratio varies based on the specific constituents to be extracted. Manufacturers adjust this ratio to achieve the ideal extract for each herb. The folk method of preparing tinctures is simple. A jar is loosely packed with fresh or dried, cut herbs. The solvent (a mixture of alcohol and water) is poured over the herbs until fully covered. The mixture is left for some days before use, either internally or externally. In standard method (weight-to-volume), the herb is weighed, and the solvent is added in a specific proportion to the herb's weight, typically 1: 2 for fresh herb and 1: 5 for dried herb. The method ensures a more precise and consistent concentration of the tincture (Fougère and Wynn 2007). Other preparations commonly used for dispensing ethnoveterinary remedies include syrups, electuaries, mixtures in water, boluses, sprays, and salt licks. Honey, milk, buttermilk, whey, curd, jaggery, and sugar are often used in their natural form. Ghee, butter, animal fat, ginger, rock salt, and honey are common preservatives used for ethnoveterinary remedies.

Conclusion

Ethnoveterinary medicine is practiced wherever humans live in close association with animals, playing a particularly significant role in societies where animal husbandry serves as a primary means of subsistence. It encompasses traditional methods used by livestock keepers to address animal health issues. Interest in documenting and validating ethnoveterinary practices gained traction in the early 1980s, resulting in numerous studies on traditional remedies. While these studies primarily focus on the use of herbal medicines for the prevention and treatment of animal diseases, they also underscore the role of non-herbal substances—such as zootherapeutics, minerals, and other natural resources—as integral components of the *ethnoveterinary materia medica.* Although traditional knowledge about animal healthcare remains invaluable for livestock management in rural societies and is increasingly relevant to organic farming systems in industrialized regions, it continues to be an understudied aspect of ethnobiology.

Zoopharmacognosy, which traditionally focused on the self-medication behaviours of primates and other wild mammals and birds, is gaining recognition in veterinary medicine. Increasing evidence suggests that domestic animals also exhibit self-medication behaviours, mirroring what has been observed in the wild. It has been hypothesized that veterinary medicine has developed, to some extent, from observing animal self-treatment. When animals experience discomfort, they engage in exploratory behaviours, trying various remedies to relieve symptoms. Reports indicate that behavioural changes, including reduced neophobia (fear of new things) and a more diverse diet with a preference for medicinal plants, often represent first way of defence adopted by animals against illness. This self-medication behaviour may or may not directly affect the underlying pathogen. For example, apes consuming specific plants to scour intestinal parasites achieve relief while simultaneously eliminating the parasite. Understanding such behaviours in domestic animals opens exciting opportunities to encourage or even harness their ability to self-regulate their health. One promising area of study involves self-administration of specific medications, both herbal and non-herbal. Self-selection of appropriate levels of veterinary medication shows potential, particularly for analgesics and carminatives, offering a novel approach to improving animal health and welfare (Engel 2007). It is also possible that remedies used by animals for self-medication are later applied for human health.

Traditional methods of treatment often apply to both humans and animals, with healers frequently treating both groups using similar techniques and materials. Many ethnoveterinary practitioners believe that remedies effective for human health are equally beneficial for animals. Among these materials, plants are the most commonly used remedies. Studies from various parts of the world indicate that the same plant species can be employed for both veterinary and human medicinal purposes, often in similar ways (Miara *et al.* 2019). However, compared to human medicine, the evaluation and use of non-herbal substances in ethnoveterinary medicine—such as zootherapeutics, entomotherapy, and by-products from domestic animals and marine organisms—are less documented. According to Ayurveda, every substance in the universe has the potential to serve as a medicinal remedy, provided it is used with a rational method and a clear objective. This profound idea is encapsulated in the words of Lord Punarvasu Atreya in the Charaka Samhita (Sutra Sthana 26.12): *Anēnōpadēśēna nānauṣadhibhūtaṁ jagati, kiñciddravyamupalabhyatē tāṁ tāṁ yuktimarthaṁ ca taṁ tamabhiprētya.* Translation: 'On this basis, there is no substance in the universe which cannot be used as a medicinal drug, provided it is employed with a rational method and a clear objective.' The Charaka Samhita further stresses that the efficacy of a drug is not determined solely by its observable properties, but also by its intrinsic nature, the manner of its application, and several contextual factors. These include the appropriate time, mechanism of action, site of action, and the therapeutic intent behind its use. This holistic understanding is elaborated in the following verse (Charaka Sutra Sthana 26.13): *Na tu kēvalaṁ guṇaprabhāvādēva dravyāṇi kārmukāṇi bhavanti; dravyāṇi hi dravyaprabhāvād guṇaprabhāvād dravyaguṇaprabhāvācca tasmiṁs tasmin kālē tattad adhikaraṇam āsādya tāṁ tāṁ ca yuktim arthaṁ ca taṁ tam abhiprētya yat kurvanti, tat karma; yēna kurvanti, tadvīryaṁ; yatra kurvanti, tadadhikaraṇaṁ; yadā kurvanti, sa kālaḥ; yathā kurvanti, sa upāyaḥ; yat sādhayanti, tat phalam.* Translation: 'The activity of a drug is not determined by its properties alone. Rather, it is the combined effect of its intrinsic nature and properties, in conjunction with the specific time, site of action, method of use, and therapeutic purpose. What the drug performs is its karma (action); the means by which it acts is its veerya (potency); the place it acts upon is the *adhikarana* (locus of action); the time it acts is *kala* (time); the way it acts is the *upaya* (mechanism); and the outcome it achieves is the *phala* (result)' (Dubey *et al.* 2020). These Ayurvedic *sutras* hold significant relevance for the field of ethnopharmacology and offer a foundational framework for understanding ethnoveterinary practices. They highlight the importance of contextual intelligence and rational methodology in the selection and application of medicinal substances in traditional animal healthcare. They provide a framework for exploring and validating novel therapeutic substances that could be incorporated into the *ethnoveterinary materia medica* for the effective treatment of animal diseases.

References

Abdisa T. 2018. Therapeutic importance of leech and impact of leech in domestic animals. *MOJ Drug Design Development & Therapy* **2**(6): 235–42. DOI: 10.15406/mojddt.2018.02.0006.

Álvaro MM, Luis RR, de Lollano S and Joaquin P. 2019. The origins of zoopharmacognosy: How humans learned about self-medication from animals. *International Journal of Applied Research* **5** (5): 73-9.

Amit M, Cohen I, Marcovics A, Muklada H, Glasser TA, Ungar ED and Landau SY. 2013. Self-medication with tannin-rich browse in goats infected with gastro-intestinal nematodes. *Veterinary Parasitology* **198** (3-4): 305-11.

Babu NJ, Sekhar BR, Rani KS and Rao GN. 2024. External application of ethno-veterinary plants to treat bone fractures in domestic and pet animals of the villages in Nallamalla forest region of Eastern Ghats of AP, India. *Scholars Journal of Agriculture and Veterinary Sciences* **11**(3): 30-37. DOI: 10.36347/sjavs. 2024.v11i03.002.

Balakrishnan V, Robinson JP, Kasamy AM and Ravindran KC.2009 Ethnoveterinary studies among farmers in Dindigul district Tamil Nadu, India. *Global Journal of Pharmacology* **3**(1): 15-23.

Barboza RR, de MS Souto W, and da S Mourão J. 2007. The use of zootherapeutics in folk veterinary medicine in the district of Cubati, Paraíba State, Brazil. *Journal of Ethnobiology and Ethnomedicine* **3**: 1-14. doi:10.1186/1746-4269-3-32.

Bullitta S, Re GA, Manunta MD and Piluzza G. 2018. Traditional knowledge about plant, animal, and mineral-based remedies to treat cattle, pigs, horses, and other domestic animals in the Mediterranean island of Sardinia. *Journal of Ethnobiology and Ethnomedicine* **14**: 1-26. https://doi.org/10.1186/s13002-018-0250-7.

Chen SL, Yu H, Luo HM, Wu Q, Li CF and Steinmetz A. 2016. Conservation and sustainable use of medicinal plants: problems, progress, and prospects. *Chinese Medicine* **11** (37): https://doi.org/10.1186/s13020-016-0108-7.

Confessor MV, Mendonça LE, Mourão JS, and Alves RR. 2009. Animals to heal animals: ethnoveterinary practices in semiarid region, Northeastern Brazil. *Journal of Ethnobiology and Ethnomedicine* **5**:37 doi:10.1186/1746-4269-5-37

Costa-Neto EM. 2005. Animal-based medicines: biological prospection and the sustainable use of zootherapeutic resources. *Anais da Academia Brasileira de Ciências (Annals of the Brazilian Academy of Sciences)* **77**(1): 33-43 https://doi.org/10.1590/S0001-37652005000100004.

Costa-Neto EM. 2005b. Entomotherapy, or the medicinal use of insects. *Journal of Ethnobiology* **25**(1):93-114.

Darker KN. 2022. *Enzootic Gophagy by Elephants (Loxodonta Africana) in Relation to Geochemical Composition of Mineral Licks in Addo Elephant National Park, South Africa.* MSc dissertation. 150p. Department of Zoology and Entomology, Faculty of Natural and Agricultural Sciences, University of the Free State, South Africa.

Dossey AT. 2010. Insects and their chemical weaponry: new potential for drug discovery. *Natural Product Reports*. **27**(12):1737-57

Dubey SD, Singh AN, Singh A, and Deole YS. 2020. *Atreyabhadrakapyiya Adhyaya*. In: *Charak Samhita New Edition*. 1st edn. pp.28. (Eds.) Sirdeshpande MK, Deole YS and Basisht G. CSRTSDC ebook, Jamnagar, India. Doi:10.47468/CSNE.2020.e01. s01.028. Available at: https://www.carakasamhitaonline.com/mediawiki-1.32.1/index.php?title=Atreyabhadrakapyiya_Adhyaya&oldid=44492.

Dubost JM, Lamxay V, Krief S, Falshaw M, Manithip C and Deharo E. 2019. From plant selection by elephants to human and veterinary pharmacopeia of mahouts in Laos. *Journal of Ehnopharmacology* **244:** https://doi.org/10.1016/j.jep.2019.112157.

Dzoyem JP, Tchuenteu RT, Mbarawa K, Keza A, Roland A, Njouendou AJ and Assob JC. 2020. Ethnoveterinary medicine and medicinal plants used in the treatment of livestock diseases in Cameroon. In. *Ethnoveterinary Medicine: Present and Future Concepts*. pp. 175-209. McGaw, LJ and Abdalla MA (Eds). Springer Nature, Switzerland AG.

Egea AV, Hall JO, Miller J, Spackman C and Villalba JJ. 2014. Reduced neophobia: A potential mechanism explaining the emergence of self-medicative behavior in sheep. *Physiology & Behavior* **135**: 189-97. https://doi.org/10.1016/j.physbeh.2014.06.019.

Engel C. 2007. Zoopharmacognosy In: *Veterinary Herbal Medicine*. pp. 7-15. (Eds) Wynn SG and Fougère B. Mosby Elsevier, St Louis, Missouri, USA.

Fougère BJ, and Wynn SG. Herb manufacture, pharmacy, and dosing. In: *Veterinary Herbal Medicine*. pp. 221-36. (Eds) Wynn SG and Fougère B. Mosby Elsevier, St Louis, Missouri. USA.

Garg SL, Sharma NK, Rajput DS, Rathore SS and Mishra P. 2019. Ethnoveterinary practices of diarrhoea with their extent of use followed by livestock owners in western zone of Rajasthan. *Veterinary Practitioner* **20**(1): 138-40.

González JA and Vallejo JR. 2021. The use of domestic animals and their derivative products in contemporary Spanish ethnoveterinary medicine. *Journal of Ethnopharmacology* **271**:113900. doi.org/10.1016/j.jep.2021.113900.

Gradé JT, Tabuti JR and Van Damme P. 2009. Four footed pharmacists: indications of self-medicating livestock in Karamoja, Uganda. *Economic Botany* **63** (1):29-42.

Holyoak GR and Ma A.2022. Evidence-based application of acupuncture in theriogenology. *Veterinary Sciences*. **9**(2): 53. https://doi.org/10.3390/vetsci9020053.

Huffman MA. 2001. Self-medicative behavior in the African great apes: An evolutionary perspective into the origins of human traditional medicine: *BioScience* **51** (8): 651-61.

Huffman MA. 2021. Folklore, animal self-medication, and phytotherapy–something old, something new, something borrowed, some things true. *Planta Medica* **88**(03/04):187-99.

Huntingford JL and Petty MC. 2022. Evidence-Based application of acupuncture for pain management in companion animal medicine. *Veterinary Sciences*. 2022; **9**(6): 252. https://doi.org/10.3390/vetsci9060252.

Jacob MO, Farah KO and Ekaya WN. 2004. Indigenous knowledge: the basis of the Maasai Ethnoveterinary Diagnostic Skills. *Journal of Human Ecology* **16**(1): 43-48.

Jones SD and Koolmees PA. 2022. *A Concise History of Veterinary Medicine*. pp 1-13. Cambridge University Press, Cambridge, UK.

Klaus G, Klaus-Hügi C and Schmid B. 1998. Geophagy by large mammals at natural licks in the rain forest of the Dzanga National Park, Central African Republic. *Journal of Tropical Ecology*. **14**(6): 829-39.

Köhler-Rollefson I, Rathore S, Rollefson A and Hardy K .2013. The Camels of Kumbhalgarh. A Biodiversity Treasure. Lokhit Pashu-Palak Sansthan, Sadri. http://www. lpps. org/wp-content/uploads/2013/10/Camels Of_ Kumbhalgarh_web. pdf. Downloaded on 17-11-2023.

Kunja Lal K. 1907. *An English Translation of the Sushruta Samhita, Vol. I. Sutrashanam*. pp 98-105. (Ed. & Publ.), Kaviraj Kunja Lal Bhishagratna. Calcutta (Kolkata), India.

Leeflang P. 1993. Some observations on ethnoveterinary medicine in Northern Nigeria. *Veterinary Quarterly* **15** (2): 72-74.

Liolios CC, Graikou K, Skaltsa E and Chinou I. 2010. Dittany of Crete: a botanical and ethnopharmacological review. *Journal of Ethnopharmacology* **131**(2): 229-41. https://doi.org/10.1016/j.jep.2010.06.005.

Mandal SK and Rahman CH. 2022. Perception and application of zootherapy for the management of cattle diseases occurred in northern laterite region of West Bengal, India. *Asian Journal of Ethnobiology* **5**(1): 12-19.

McCorkle C M. 1986. An introduction to ethnoveterinary research and development. *Journal of Ethnobiology* **6** (1): 129-49.

Meena DC, Garai S, Maiti S, Bhakat M, Meena BS and Kadian KS. 2020. Ethno-Veterinary practices used for common health ailments of sheep and goat: A participatory assessment by the Raika pastoralist of Marwar Region, Rajasthan. *Indian Journal of Animal Sciences* **90**(9): 1310-5.

Miara MD, Bendif H, Ouabed A, Rebbas K, Hammou MA, Amirat M, Greene A and Teixidor-Toneu I. Ethnoveterinary remedies used in the Algerian steppe: Exploring the relationship with traditional human herbal medicine. *Journal of Ethnopharmacology* **244**: 112164. doi.org/10.1016/j.jep.2019.112164.

Minja MM. 2005. *Towards Networking Among Institutions and Individuals Working in the Field of Ethnoveterinary Knowledge in Tanzania: Status of Ethnoveterinary Knowledge*. 34 p. FAO LinKS project Report 15. Gender and Population Division FAO, Rome, Italy. https://agris.fao.org/search/en/providers/122621/records/6472475353aa8c896304a06a.

Monteiro JP, Domingues MR, and Calado R. 2024. Marine animal co-products—how improving their use as rich sources of health-promoting lipids can foster sustainability. *Marine Drugs* **22**(2):73.https://doi.org/10.3390/md22020073.

Neco LC, Abelson ES, Brown A, Natterson-Horowitz B and Blumstein DT. 2019. The evolution of self-medication behaviour in mammals. *Biological Journal of the Linnean Society* **128**(2): 373-78.

Nweze AJ, Olovo CV, Nweze EI, John OO and Paul C. 2020. Therapeutic properties of honey. In: *Honey Analysis - New Advances and Challenges* pp. 1-22. (Eds) Alencar Arnaut de Toledo V, and Dechechi Chambó E. IntechOpen; http://dx.doi.org/10.5772/intechopen.86416, downloaded on 056-12-2024.

Piluzza G, Virdis S, Serralutzu F and Bullitta S. 2015. Uses of plants, animal and mineral substances in Mediterranean ethno-veterinary practices for the care of small ruminants. *Journal of Ethnopharmacology* **168**:87-99. doi.org/10.1016/j.jep.2015.03.056.

Rodriguez E and Wrangham R. 1993. Zoopharmacognosy: The use of medicinal plants by animals. In: *Phytochemical Potential of Tropical Plants. Recent Advances in Phytochemistry, Vol 27.* pp. 89-105. (Eds) Downum K R, Romeo J T and Stafford HA. Springer, Boston, MA, USA. https://doi.org/10.1007/978-1-4899-1783-6_4.

Saroch V and Kundailia NA 2014. review on marine originated drug tradition in *Ayurveda. Ayurpharm - International Journal of Ayurveda and Allied Sciences* **3**(9): 241-47.

Sharma TR (Trans.). 2013. *Atharva-Veda Vol. I.* Vijaykumar Govindram Hansnand, New Delhi (Digital Distributer Agniveer). https://archive.org/details/atharva-veda-vol-2-of-2, pdf downloaded on 05-06-2023.

Siddiqui SA, Li C, Aidoo OF, Fernando I, Haddad MA, Pereira JA, Blinov A, Golik A and Câmara JS.2023. Unravelling the potential of insects for medicinal purposes–a comprehensive review. *Heliyon.* **9** (5): e159385. doi: 10.1016/j.heliyon. 2023.e15938.

Sig AK, Guney M, Guclu AU, and Ozmen E. 2017. Medicinal leech therapy—an overall perspective. *Integrative Medicine Research* **6**(4):337-43.

Sobczak N and Kantyka M. 2014. Hirudotherapy in veterinary medicine. *Annals of Parasitology* **60**(2): 89-92.

Srinivasan V. 1990. *Pharmacology Materia Medica and Therapeutics for Veterinary Students.* 10th edn. 393 p. Scientific Book Company Patna, India.

Toyang NJ and Verpoorte R. 2013. A review of the medicinal potentials of plants of the genus *Vernonia* (Asteraceae). *Journal of Ethnopharmacology* **146**(3): 681-723.

Toyang NJ, Wanyama J, Nuwanyakpa M and Diango S. 2007. *Ethnoveterinary Medicine. A Practical Approach to the Treatment of Cattle Diseases in Sub-Saharan Africa.* 2nd edn. 88p. Agromisa Foundation and CTA, Wageningen, The Netherlands.

Villalba JJ, Miller J, Ungar ED, Landau SY and Glendinning J. 2014. Ruminant self-medication against gastrointestinal nematodes: evidence, mechanism, and origins. *Parasite* **21**(31): doi: 10.1051/parasite/2014032.

Villalba JJ, Provenza FD and Shaw R. 2007. Sheep self-medicate when challenged with illness-inducing foods. *Animal Behaviour* **71**(5): 1131-39.

Wanzala W, Zessin KH, Kyule NM, Baumann MPO, Mathias E and Hassanali A. 2005. Ethnoveterinary medicine: a critical review of its evolution, perception, understanding and the way forward. *Livestock Research for Rural Development* **17:** 1-31.

6

Ethnoveterinary Medicine in India: Current Status and Future Prospects

D. Swarup and R. Somvanshi

Sarvāḥ samagrā oṣadhīrbodhantu vacaso mama. Yathemam pārayāmasi puruṣam duritādadhi.
May all these herbs and medications together, without exception or exclusion or negation, know and act according to my word of healing so that we may take this patient across and out of the crisis of his life-threatening disease.

(Atharva Veda 8.7.19; translation by Sharma 2013)

1. Introduction
2. Ethnoveterinary Medicine: Curremt State of the Art
   - Pastoralists and Livestock Raisers and their Ethnoveterinary Knowledge: Bakarwals (Bakerwals) and Gujjars, Bhotias of Central Himalayas, Gaddi Pastoralists, Monpa and Chiru Tribes of Northeastern States, Rabari /Raikas of Western India, Todas of Niligiri Hills.
   - Pharmacological Relevance of Ethnoveterinary Practices used by Pastoralists
   - Field Veterinarians and Local Animal Healers
3. Role of Modern Veterinary Research and Development (R&D) and Academic Institutions in Ethnoveterinary Medicine.
4. Modern Veterinary Science in India: Evolution and Integration of Ethnoveterinary Medicine— A Brief Historical Overview
5. EVM Challenges and the Way Forward
6. Conclusion

Introduction

Ethnoveterinary medicine (EVM) in India has a rich heritage and continues to play a vital role in animal healthcare, particularly in rural areas. Over time, as diseases affected the health and welfare of humans and animals, various beliefs and concepts emerged about their causes and mitigation. This evolution led to the development of diverse healing practices for both humans and animals. Traditional knowledge-based systems such as ethnomedicine and ethnoveterinary medicine encompass the use of local knowledge, beliefs, skills, practices, and resources to diagnose, treat, and manage diseases. In India, the traditional knowledge system is broadly categorized into two distinct forms. The *Formal Codified Systems*—including Ayurveda, Siddha, and Unani-Tibb—are systematically formulated and documented, with established principles and practices for disease diagnosis and healing in both humans and animals. In contrast, the *Informal Traditional Systems* have evolved through community innovations and lived experiences, transmitted orally over generations. Despite their differences, there are notable similarities between these two forms of traditional knowledge, which is widely practiced by traditional healers across the country.

Ethnoveterinary Medicine: Current State of the Art

The animal husbandry and healthcare practices in India have evolved over several millennia, creating a vast knowledge base on traditional practices encompassing animal breeding, feeding, grazing, housing, and healthcare. Today, this knowledge can be delineated into three interrelated domains: Traditional Pastoralists, Livestock Raisers, and Traditional Animal Healers; Scientific Research and Development (R&D) Organizations; and Veterinary Professionals. These three domains collectively contribute to the preservation, evolution, and application of ethnoveterinary medicine in India, ensuring its relevance and sustainability in the face of modern challenges. Traditional pastoralists, livestock raisers, farmers, ancient Ayurvedic and veterinary Ayurvedic literature, and local animal healers are the primary sources of Ethnoveterinary Medicine (EVM) knowledge and practices. R&D organizations and veterinary professionals provide scientific and technological support to promote the application of EVM practices.

Pastoralists and Livestock Raisers and their Ethnoveterinary Knowledge

Pastoralists in India are defined as members of caste or ethnic groups with strong traditional association with livestock-keeping, where a substantial proportion of the group derive over 50% of household consumption from livestock products or their sale, and where over 90% of animal consumption is from natural pasture or browse, and where households are responsible for the full cycle of livestock breeding (Sharma *et al.* 2003). Livestock raisers, also known as livestock keepers, are individuals or communities that primarily focus on raising animals for various purposes, such as meat, milk, wool, and other animal products. Unlike traditional pastoralists, livestock raisers may not necessarily follow a nomadic lifestyle. They often have permanent or semi-permanent settlements and use a combination of grazing and supplementary feeding to maintain their animals.

Although there are no reliable figures on the current number of active pastoralists in India, a 1999 article estimated that more than 200 tribes, accounting for approximately 6% of the country's population, were engaged in pastoralism

(Khurana, 1999). Some of the well-known pastoralist groups include:

- **Northern and Central India**: *Bakarwals* (Kashmir), *Brokpas* and *Changpas* (Ladakh), *Darmi* or *Darmi Bhotiyas* (Uttarakhand), *Gaddis* (Kangra and Dharamshala regions of Himachal Pradesh, parts of Uttar Pradesh and Punjab), *Gujjars* (Jammu, Himanchal Pradesh and Uttarakhand), *Kinnauras* (Kinnaur district of Himachal Pradesh), *Tharus* (Uttarakhand and Uttar Pradesh), and *Gonds* and *Yadavas* (central and northern India).
- **Western India**: *Ahir*, *Bharwad*, *Charan* and *Maldharis* (Gujarat), *Dhangar* (Maharasthra, also in Madhya Pradesh), *Raika* and *Rebari* (Rajasthan and part of Gujarat).
- **Eastern India**: *Santhals*, *Maria* and *Muria* (West Bengal, Jharkhand, and Odisha).
- **Southern India**: *Gollas* (Karnataka and Andhra Pradesh), *Kurubas* (Karnataka), and *Toda* (Karnataka, Tamil Nadu, and Kerala).
- **Northeastern India**: *Adi*, *Monpas*, *Nyishi* (Arunachal Pradesh), *Bhutiyas* (Sikkim), and *Khasis* (Assam).

Many of these pastoral tribes trace their connection to specific livestock species through origin myths, which often depict their ancestors as divine creations, tasked by God to care for these animals (Sharma *et al.* 2003). The livestock management practices of pastoralists are deeply rooted in centuries-old traditions and rely on locally available natural resources. These include medicinal plants, animal products, minerals, earthy substances, water, medicinal smoke, fire, often combined with rituals, to treat animals and maintain their health effectively. A brief introduction of some of the pastoral groups and ethnoveterinary methods used by them for treatment of animal diseases in India is summarized here.

Bakarwals (Bakerwals) and Gujjars: The Bakarwals and Gujjars are two of the most prominent pastoral communities in Northern India, each with distinct practices and traditions. Primarily herding sheep and goats, the Bakarwals inhabit the region of Jammu and Kashmir. They are migratory pastoralists who follow a transhumant lifestyle. During the winter months, they migrate to the plains of Punjab, returning to the higher alpine valleys of the Himalayas in Kashmir during the summer. In the monsoon season, they move to lower-altitude pastures to graze their livestock. The Gujjars are found across Kashmir, parts of Himachal Pradesh, and Uttarakhand. They primarily raise buffaloes and are often referred to as *Dudh* Gujjars due to their association with milk production. In addition, they also rear sheep, goats, and maintain bullocks, horses, and ponies as pack animals. The Gujjars of Himachal Pradesh are particularly known for their skill in crafting intricately embroidered caps. Similar to the Bakarwals, the pastoral Gujjars of Northern India practice transhumance, migrating to the plains of Punjab and Uttar Pradesh (particularly the Saharanpur region) during the winter (Sharma *et al.* 2003).

The Bakarwals and Gujjars, as pastoralist communities, forage their livestock across vast stretches of pasturelands while living in close harmony with nature. They possess extensive traditional knowledge, particularly in livestock care. Limited access to modern veterinary facilities has led them to rely heavily on ethnoveterinary practices, which have been developed and refined over generations. These practices primarily involve the use of various plant parts such as inflorescences, flowers, stems, seeds, fruits, leaves, roots, and rhizomes. A study conducted in the Hirpora Wildlife Sanctuary in the Kashmir Himalaya found that the Gujjar and Bakerwal communities utilize as many as 29 plant species from 21 families to treat a wide range of livestock ailments. These include digestive issues, respiratory conditions, allergies, foot and mouth disease, ecto- and endo-parasites, dysentery, and general weakness. The plants used include 23 herbs, 3 shrubs, 2 climbers, and 1 sub-shrub, found across diverse habitats ranging from forests to sub-alpine and alpine meadows at altitudes of 2,000–4,200 masl (Dar *et al.* 2018). Some of the plants and their ethnomedicine uses reported in the study by these two communities included:

- *Achillea millefolium* L.: Paste of aerial parts administered orally for deworming.
- *Allium victorialis* L.: Whole plant used to treat cold and cough in cattle and buffaloes.
- *Artemisia scoparia* Waldst. & Kitam: Paste of aerial parts, mixed with common salt to treat intestinal worms and flatulence.
- *Euphorbia wallichii*: Latex from the green stem applied to treat fungal infections and foot and mouth disease in cattle.
- *Nepeta cataria* L.: Decoction of shoots used to treat dysentery and diarrhea in cattle.
- *Rheum webbianum* Royle: Rhizome paste applied to wounds and scabies in sheep.
- *Trifolium pratense* L.: Whole plant fed to cattle and goats as a galactagogue (to enhance milk production).

Bhotias of Central Himalayas: The Bhotia (also spelled Bhotiya) tribals are a pastoralist community primarily engaged in sheep herding. They inhabit the northern regions of Bhutan, Sikkim, and the Indo-Tibetan border areas of Uttarakhand and Himachal Pradesh. Known as the most ancient tribe in Uttarakhand, the term Bhotia originates from Bhot or *Bod*, the traditional name for the Tibetan people. A remarkable aspect of the Bhotia tribe is their close association with the *Bhotiya* dog, a robust working breed integral to their way of life. These dogs are renowned for their loyalty, strength, and courage, making them invaluable companions in the harsh Himalayan terrain. Traditionally, Bhotiya dogs are used for guarding livestock, herding, and protecting tribal homes from threats. Adapted to extreme weather and treacherous mountain conditions, these dogs play a critical role in safeguarding the tribe's herds of sheep, goats, and yaks. These dogs also provide protection from wild predators like leopards and wolves, ensuring the safety of the tribal homes and their livestock (https://www.uttarakhandi.com/bhotia/, accessed on 13-1-2025).

The Bhotias are traditionally traders, with their livelihood combines trade, terraced cultivation, pastoralism, wool production, and other services. They have dual settlements: summer settlements (May-November) for cultivating limited crops like buckwheat and winter settlements for growing wheat, rice, maize, and potatoes. Bhotia's herds primarily consist of pack animals such as sheep, goats, yaks, and ponies. The indigenous knowledge of the Bhotia community encompasses agriculture, forestry, and animal husbandry. It integrates values for subsistence (e.g., food, medicine and energy), socio-cultural practices (e.g., rituals, education, and spirituality), and economic activities (e.g., agriculture, tourism, and traditional medicine). It serves as both cultural and natural capital, rooted in their historical harmony with nature. As modern technologies often fail in their mountainous terrain due to challenges like inaccessibility, fragility, marginality, and diversity, the Bhotias rely on their indigenous knowledge to sustain their livelihoods and conserve natural resources effectively (Samal *et al.* 2010).

The Bhotias possess profound traditional knowledge in animal husbandry and veterinary practices, utilizing their natural surroundings to manage livestock health. A study on the Darmi group of Bhotias in the Darma Valley of Pithoragarh revealed their expertise in producing hybrids of yaks and local cows. Their traditional veterinary methods involve the use of plants, animals, and minerals to treat a variety of animal ailments. Research indicates that the Bhotias used more than 50 indigenous methods, utilizing over 40 plant species to manage 40–45 animal diseases and disorders (Tiwari and Pandey 2005). Below are some examples of ethnoveterinary practices documented in this study:

Dysentery

- Root of *chhipi/gonab* (Himalayan angelica-*Angelica glauca* Edgew.) roasted in 100 ml ghee, powdered, given orally twice a day.
- Fresh roots of lafu/mooli (Radish-*Raphanus sativus L.)* are crushed in 1 L of water and given orally. Alternatively, 100 g of crushed roots fried in 100 ml of ghee until they become blackish-brown and then administered orally in lukewarm ghee.
- Dried leaves of *pindalu* (*Arabi*, Taro-*Colocasia esculenta* Schott.), given orally with salt.
- Lukewarm ghee (250 ml), given orally.

- Paste of *kutki* (*Picrorhiza kurrooa*- Royle ex Benth.) roots, given orally; also effective in anorexia.

Constipation and Indigestion

- Paste of *mepar* (Hairy spurge- *Euphorbia pilosa* L.) with half litre water, given orally.
- Fresh roots (5-6) of *lafu / mooli* (Redish-*Raphanus sativus* L.) crushed in 1 litre butter-milk: Given orally.

Tympany

- Paste of *dolu* (Indian rhubarb- *Rheum australe* D. Don), given orally in tympany and by dysentery.
- Fresh roots of *saduwa* (spiked ginger lily-*Hedychium spicatum* Buch. -Ham. ex Sm.) and *chhipi/gonab* (Himalayan angelica-*Angelica glauca* Edgew.) mashed together: Given orally.

Haematuria

- Whole plant of *akaasbel* (Himalayan woodbine-*Parthenocissus semicordata* Planch.) crushed with gur (jaggery): Given orally.
- Paste of root of *peela jari* (*Thalictrum javanicum* Blume), given orally with half litre of water.
- Gruel of *masoor* (lentil- *Lens culinaris* Medik.): Given orally.

Foot and Mouth Disease (locally known as *Genu*) Foot Lesions

- Aqueous extract of roots of *kutki* (*Picrorhiza kurrooa* Royle ex Benth).
- Juice of fresh leaves of *bajrabhang* (*Chenopodium ambrosioides* L.).
- Sulphur powder spray.

Internal Injury

- Paste of *dolu* (Indian rhubarb, *Rheum australe* D. Don) roots orally twice a day.
- Paste of *chhipi/gonab* (Himalayan angelica-*Angelica glauca* Edgew.) root, given orally.

Broken Horns and Wounds

- Paste of *masoor* (lentil *Lens culinaris* Medik.) seeds applied on the wound.
- Lukewarm ghee applied on the wound.
- Paste of rose leaves applied on cuts and wounds.

Sprain

- Fresh leaves of *shikwa* (*Allium consanguineum* Kunth), roots of *dolu* (Indian rhubarb, *Rheum australe* D. Don), fresh rhizome of *haldi* (turmeric-*Curcuma domestica* Val., *Curcuma longa* L) and salt powdered together, and boiled in about 1 litre water used as fomentation.

Snakebite

- Root paste of *nirvish* (Himalayan Bog Star-*Parnassia nubicola* Wall. ex-Royle): Given orally, as well as applied on the bite site.
- *Kasturi*, obtained from the *kasturi mrig* (musk deer-*Moschus moschiferus* L.) as antivenom.

Scabies and Other Ectoparasites

- Dried *tambaku* (tobacco -*Nicotiana tabacum* L.) leaf powder mixed with mustard oil (*Brassica campestris* L.) and a pinch of salt, or dried leaves boiled in water with mustard oil (*Brassica campestris* L.) and salt applied externally in scabies.
- Powder of *timoor* or *timur* (*Zanthoxylum armatum* DC.) seeds and tobacco leaves mixed with mustard oil and a pinch of salt is rubbed on the skin to expel external parasites.
- Charcoal powder mixed with butter is applied to expel lice.

Internal Parasites

- Aqueous juice of *kutki* (*Picrorhiza kurrooa* Royle ex Benth.): Given orally.
- Roasted common salt (about 100 g) in water: Given orally.

Galactagogue

- Roasted seeds of *chuwa* (amaranth-*Amaranthus paniculatus* L.) boiled with jaggery, given orally.
- Feeding fresh leaves of *kanya* (*Ilex dipyrena* Wall.) to increase lactation.
- Extract of *ajwain* (carom seed-*Trachyspermum ammi* Sprague), given orally.

Cough and Cold

- Fresh Rhizome of *haldi* ((turmeric- *Curcuma domestica* Val., *Curcuma longa* L.) 10g, chillies (*Capsicum annuum* L.) 4-5 pods and root of *chhipi/ gonab* (Himalayan angelica-*Angelica glauca* Edgew.) are grounded and mixed with water: Given orally to cattle (also used for internal parasites).

- Cooked fruit juice of *garchuk/ritulchukh* (sea-buckthorn-*Hippophae rhamnoides* L.)) 2-3 teaspoonful: Given orally.
- Powdered bark of *angu* (*Fraxinus micrantha* Lingesh.) mixed with water: Given orally.

Fever in Cattle

- Paste of fresh roots of *kutki* (*Picrorhiza kurrooa* Royle ex Benth.): Given orally.
- Feeding leaves of *fargyo* (*Phytolacca acinosa* Roxb.).
- Dried plant powder of *chirayata* (*Swertia chiravita* Karstent) in water: Given orally.

Gaddi Pastoralists: The Gaddis are a traditional hill community residing in the states of Himachal Pradesh, Punjab, and Uttarakhand. Predominantly semi-nomadic, they maintain permanent dwellings in the Kangra Valley while practicing long-distance herding with large flocks of sheep and goats (Sharma *et al.* 2003). The term *Gaddi* in Sanskrit means seat. According to tradition, the Gaddis are devout followers of Lord Shiva, who is believed to have created them while seated on his gaddi (seat). Another significant deity for the Gaddi community is the *Gunga Devata* (the mute deity), who is worshipped annually to protect their sheep and goats from wild animals (Devi 2021). The Gaddi is also a registered indigenous breed of sheep found in the Kishtwar and Bhaderwah regions of Jammu, as well as in Ramnagar, Udhampur, Kullu, and Kangra valleys of Himachal Pradesh. Additionally, the breed is distributed across the Dehradun, Nainital, Tehri Garhwal, and Chamoli districts of Uttarakhand. An old Hindi word *gādar* (sheep) is believed to have given rise to the term *Gadariā*, referring to a herding caste in North India historically engaged in livestock breeding, particularly sheep (Ghurye 1969).

The Gaddi community has preserved its cultural heritage and continues to rely on traditional knowledge for treating various ailments of sheep and goats in migratory conditions. These practices are crucial for the Gaddi nomads, who migrate year-round with their livestock and often lack timely access to state-provided veterinary services along their routes and difficult geographical conditions. The Gaddi pastoralists of the Northwestern Himalayan region employ a variety of traditional ethnoveterinary methods to address livestock health issues. These practices involve the use of locally available plants and natural resources, reflecting their deep knowledge of animal care in challenging environments. Below is a categorized overview of some of scientifically documented ethnoveterinary medicines (Thakur *et al.* 2020).

Maggot Wounds

- *Butea monosperma*: Seed powder mixed with phenyl and applied as a paste.
- Turmeric (*Curcuma longa*): Powder or crushed immature lantana plant applied locally.

Skin Infections

- *Deodar* oil (*Cedrus deodara*): Applied topically.
- Clove oil (*Syzygium aromaticum*): Applied topically.

Ticks and Lice

- *Deodar* oil (*Cedrus deodara*): Applied topically.

Diarrhoea

- *Ajwain* seeds (*Trachyspermum ammi*): Administered orally.
- *Khair* (*Acacia catechu* Willd.): Decoction given orally.

Indigestion

- *Ajwain* (*Trachyspermum ammi*) + Salt water: Given orally.
- Fenugreek (*Trigonella foenum-graecum*) + Salt: Given orally.
- Jaggery: Administered orally.

Tympany (Bloating)

- *Ajwain* (*Trachyspermum ammi*) or Turpentine oil: Administered orally.
- *Chora* (*Angelica nuristanica*): Leaf powder drenched orally.

Lantana Poisoning

- Butter milk with mustard oil (*Brassica*) and *Aonla* (Indian gooseberry-*Emblica officinalis*): Given orally.
- Immature lantana (*Lantana camara*) flower or root decoction: Given orally.
- *Khair* (*Acacia catechu*): Decoction fed orally.
- Other remedies include feeding *Imli* (tamarind- *Tamarindus indica*), *Khatta* (*Citrus reticulata*), Lemon (*Citrus limon*), and Cucumber (*Cucumis sativus*).
- Bloodletting from the ear and housing animals under shade.

Mastitis

- *Hing* (*Ferula asafoetida*): Mixed with water and applied topically.
- Washing the udder with saline or water.

- Chanting mantras while using *Baan* (*Quercus* spp.) leaves.
- Amulets made from *Biskhapra* (*Trianthema portulacastrum* Linn.).

Foot and Mouth Disease (FMD)

- Honey or potassium permanganate: Applied to ulcers or erosions.
- Hot ghee: Applied to foot lesions.

Leech Infestation

- Salty water: Poured intranasally.

Lameness

- Bamboo sticks: Padded with hair to support the limb.
- Salt water: Used for fomentation.

Fractures

- Bamboo sticks: Used to immobilize the affected part.
- *Gumma* salt (Himalayan rock salt): Used for fomentation.
- Turmeric (*Curcuma longa*): Mixed with oil and applied locally.

Monpa and Chiru Tribes of Northeastern States: The Monpas, one of the 28 major tribes of Arunachal Pradesh, inhabit high-altitude regions ranging from 3,000 to 5,000 masl. They are the primary pastoral community in Western Arunachal Pradesh, with yak rearing serving as a crucial source of livelihood. Like many other tribal groups, the Monpas traditionally depend on nature and its resources for their sustenance and well-being. Arunachal Pradesh boasts a rich biodiversity, including nearly 5,000 species of angiosperms, with over 500 plant species actively used in traditional healthcare to treat various ailments. Beyond their use in traditional medicine, plants and plant products play a vital role in the Monpa community's daily life. They are utilized for food supplementation, dyeing clothes, veterinary healthcare, handicrafts, rituals, brewing local beverages (such as beer), and even in seasonal fishing and hunting activities (Namsa *et al.* 2011).

The Monpas have developed eco-friendly practices for yak husbandry, feeding, and healthcare, primarily using natural resources. Their ethnoveterinary practices, rooted in the early domestication of yaks, rely heavily on plant-based remedies. For example, all seven documented ethnomedicinal treatments for ephemeral fever in yaks involve plant-derived solutions. These include roots of *Thalictrum foliosum* DC, *Aralia* sp., *Phytolacca acinosa* Roxb., entire plant of *Pterocephalus hookeri* (CB Clark) E Pritz, leaves of *Nardostachys jatamansi* DC, and branches and twigs of *Rubus ellipticus* and *Rubus ideaeus* L. In addition to ephemeral fever, these plants are also used to treat a range of conditions such as fever, inflammation, cough, cold, and joint pain. Participatory assessments and validation studies have identified *Thalictrum foliosum* DC as the most effective remedy for treating ephemeral fever in yaks (Maiti *et al.* 2013). Furthermore, after calving, yaks are given a mixture of common salt and flour made from *ragi*, barley, and maize, which helps alleviate post-calving distress and boosts milk production (Pandey *et al.* 2020).

The Chirus, one of the Kuki Scheduled Tribe groups, are among the earliest inhabitants of Manipur and Assam. Predominantly found in four districts of Manipur-Tamenglong, Kangpokpi, Churachandpur, and Thoubal–they have traditionally relied on cattle farming as a primary source of livelihood. Over generations, the Chirus have developed a unique ethnoveterinary system, primarily based on plant-derived remedies, to maintain the health of their livestock. According to a study, the Chirus use 36 plant species to treat as many as 17 ailments affecting cattle, buffaloes, pigs, dogs, and other animals (Rajkumari *et al.* 2014). Some of these traditional practices as documented in the study are given here:

- ***Anorexia in cattle:*** *Terminalia citrina* (Gaertn.) Roxb. –6-7 fresh fruits are mixed with cattle fodder and fed for 2-3 days.
- ***Bloat in cattle and buffaloes:*** Juice of *Citrus lemon* L. (3 fruits) is given orally.
- ***Constipation in cattle:*** *Cassia fistula* L. –3-4 pods are fed daily until recovery.
- ***Bovine mastitis:*** *Curcuma longa* L.– Ground rhizome (10 g) is mixed with mustard oil and applied locally to the tips of affected teats 2-3 times a day.
- ***Burns:*** *Aloe* vera L. leaf pulp or *Ziziphus jujuba* leaf paste is applied locally to the burn site.
- ***Endoparasites:*** Cold water extract of *Areca catechu* L.–3 nuts soaked overnight in water and the extract is given orally; or chopped rind of pumpkin (*Cucurbita maxima* Duchesne)- 250 g is fed orally.
- ***Foot and Mouth Disease:*** About 30 whole plants of *Elsholtzia communis* (Coll. et Hemsl.) Diels- are mixed with fodder and fed to infected cattle for two weeks.
- ***Wounds and cut injuries:*** *Basella alba* L. – Leaf paste is applied locally to the affected area.
- ***Yoke gall in oxen and buffaloes:*** Mustard oil (*Brassica rapa* L. seed oil) is applied regularly to the affected part.

Rabari /Raikas of Western India: The Rabaris, also known as Raikas, Rewari, or Desai, are one of the largest and most prominent pastoral communities in western India. They are primarily found in Rajasthan and Gujarat, with smaller populations in neighboring states such as Punjab, Uttar Pradesh, and Madhya Pradesh. The term Raikas specifically refers to camel herders in Rajasthan, while Rabari is a broader term encompassing pastoral groups across Rajasthan, Haryana, and other states. Historically known as the camel people, the Raikas still retain their reputation for camel herding, although only a minority of them are now engaged in camel breeding. Today, most Raikas raise sheep, goats, cattle, or, in some regions, buffalo. While the Rabaris were traditionally nomadic, some have adopted modern lifestyles and settled in cities. However, the majority remain connected to livestock, earning their livelihoods through the sale of animals and animal products. Even those who do not own livestock often pursue professions that involve animal care. For example, many Raikas work as village cowherds, caretakers in *gaushalas* (cow sanctuaries), or labourers in organizations associated with camels (Sharma *et al.* 2003).

Box 6.1. Origin and History of the Rabari Community

Members of the Rabari community are renowned for their traditional knowledge, making them exceptional guides. The Rabari community traces its origins to the Persian word Rahbar, meaning "guide," reflecting their traditional role as expert pathfinders. This is exemplified by Ranchhod Bhai Rabari, a renowned Pagi—a tracker skilled in reading footprints—who served in the Indian Army during the 1965 and 1971 wars. His extraordinary ability to interpret tracks earned praise from Field Marshal Manekshaw. These skills were rooted in his pastoral upbringing, where Rabaris traditionally herded camels, sheep, and goats, migrating seasonally in search of fodder. Their nomadic way of life (raah-baari) is believed to have influenced the name "Rabari," also linked to "Raibari" in local genealogies.

Legend and Myth: *According to Rabari legend, they descend from Goddess Parvati and Lord Shiva. Parvati created a camel from clay, which Shiva brought to life. To protect it, Shiva fashioned the first Rabari, Chamad (later Samad), from his own ashes. Over time, the name Chamad evolved into Samad. Even today, a clan named Samad holds a special status within the Rabari community as the descendants of the first Rabari. Samad was later married to a celestial nymph, Rai, and their descendants were called Raika. Blessed with wealth and camels, the Rabaris spread across regions including Punjab, Rajasthan, Gujarat, and Sindh, with Jaisalmer regarded as their ancestral homeland.*

Titles and Regional Names: *The Rabari community comprises 133 sub-castes. In Rajasthan, they are commonly known as Raikas, split into two groups: Maru (around Jodhpur and Pali) and Godwar (in southern Pali, Jalore, and Sirohi). In Gujarat, Rabaris—believed to have migrated from Marwar—include subgroups like Kutchi-Dheberya, Vagariya, Sorathi, Bhopa, and Gujarati. Here, they are also referred to as Maldhari, meaning "cattle keeper."*

Compilation Sources: *(Sharma et al. 2003 and https://www.rabarisamaj.in/p/history-of-rabari-raika-dewasi-samaj.html#:~:text=; https://www.atlasofhumanity.com/rabari; https://iturl.in/81b81ea7?utm_source=sharetext&utm_medium=copy accessed on 17-1-2025).*

Table 6.1. Ethnoveterinary practices (EVP) followed by Rabaris/ Raikas pastoralists

Disease	Commonly used EVP (Animal species)	Mode of application
Bloat/Tympany	• Husk of isabgol mixed in water (camel) • Turpentine oil-100 ml+ back salt-100 g + asafoetida -30 g + linseed oil-500 ml (camel, (sheep & goat) • Asafoetida + Ajwain + jaggery paste (buffalo)	• Given orally • Initially, linseed oil is mixed with turpentine oil and black salt, followed by the addition of 30 g asafoetida. Animals are then not allowed to drink water for two hours • Given orally
Diarrhoea	• Alum + jaggery paste (sheep & goat) • A paste made from dry leaves or stem of *arvi* (*Colocasia esculenta*) is mixed with water and given to buffaloes.	• A paste prepared by mixing smaller amount of alum with a larger quantity of jaggery is boiled with water for 30 minutes, kept overnight. Given in the early morning for 4–5 days • The paste is given orally. A frothed solution of green leaves of *arvi* plant is also used
Fever	• Onion (*Allium cepa*), leaves + ajwain (*Trachyspermum ammi)* + maithi (*T. foenum-graecum)* + dhania (*Coriandrum sativum*)	• Paste made in jaggery is given orally
Jaundice	• Palash (*Butea monosperma*) flower tea or bark decoction (sheep and goat)	• Given orally for 7–8 days. Bark decoction is made by boiling it in water for 2–3 hours
Intestinal worms	• Pumpkin seed powder (sheep and goat)	• Mixed with fodder for 4-5 days
Mange	• Turmeric+ butter+ mustard oil • Crystalline sulphur 500 g + Copper sulphate 500 g (camel)	• Mixture in water given for 4 days • Mixed in boiled solution of ark (*Calotropis* sp) applied locally on affected part
Surra in camel	• *Khejri* (*Prosopsis cineraria*) bark • *Paneer dodi* (*Withania coagulans*) fruits • *Nirgundi* (*Vitex negundo)* + *Sahjan* (*Moringa oleifera)* + *desi ajwain* (*Trachyspermum ammi*) + salt	• Bark boiled with water, kept overnight. Given orally in the early morning • Fruits of plants mixed in water given to animals in the morning for 5-6 days • Powder of *nirgundi* leaves, *sahajan* root, *desi ajwain* and little salt is mixed with ghee and given to animals for 4 – 5 days both in evening and morning.
Camelpox	• Neem (*Azadirachta indica)* leaves • Hydrogenated vegetable oil + camel milk	• Paste applied on affected part • Paste applied on the affected part

(Ref. Ghoke *et al.* 2012, Dudi and Meena 2017, Meena *et al.* 2020, 2020b, 2023)

Despite changes in lifestyle and economic activities, the deep association of the Rabaris/Raikas with pastoral traditions continues to define their cultural identity. They possess a wealth of traditional knowledge on various aspects of animal husbandry, including the diagnosis, prevention, and treatment of animal diseases. This knowledge is accumulated over generations due to their intimate connection with animals. For instance, Raikas are well-versed in the effects of various trees and shrubs on the health of camels, as well as the quality and taste of camel milk (Köhler-Rollefson *et al.* 2013). Their diagnostic skills include their ability to identify trypanosomiasis based on the smell of urine. The method involves making a ball from sand on which the suspected animal has just urinated. If the sand sample emits a sweet and pungent odour 2 to 4 hours later, the diagnosis is considered positive (Köhler-Rollefson *et al.* 2001). Even today, Raikas have limited access to modern veterinary facilities due to the remote locations of their migratory routes. Consequently, they rely heavily on their traditional knowledge to treat diseased animals. Interestingly, many pastoral communities like Raikas have buildup a large network of traditional healers-*bhopas*, *gunis*, and *daam* to make use of local resources to treat their animals. Some of the ethnoveterinary method used by the Raikas use to treat their animals are listed in Table 6.1.

Todas of Nilgiri Hills: Indigenous to Karnataka, pastoral Todas immigrated into the Nilgiri several centuries ago with their buffaloes (Fig. 6.1). They were the first to introduce their native domestic cattle and buffaloes. It is also believed that some of the free ranging feral buffaloes in the upper Nilgiris are left by the Todas (Banumathi and Vaseeharan 2015). Living in settlements of three to seven small thatched houses scattered over the pasture slopes, Todas have a unique lifestyle centred around buffalo rearing, which serves as the cornerstone of their subsistence. They are traditionally a milk-producing community engaged in the trade of dairy products. Toda pastorals observe rituals for nearly every aspect of dairy-related activities. These include ceremonies for milking and feeding salt to the herds, churning butter, seasonally shifting pastures, ordaining dairymen-priests, rebuilding dairies and rethatching funerary temples (https://www.britannica.com/topic/Toda-people-India, accessed on 6-1-2025). The Toda faith revolves around sacred locations associated with their network of dairy temples

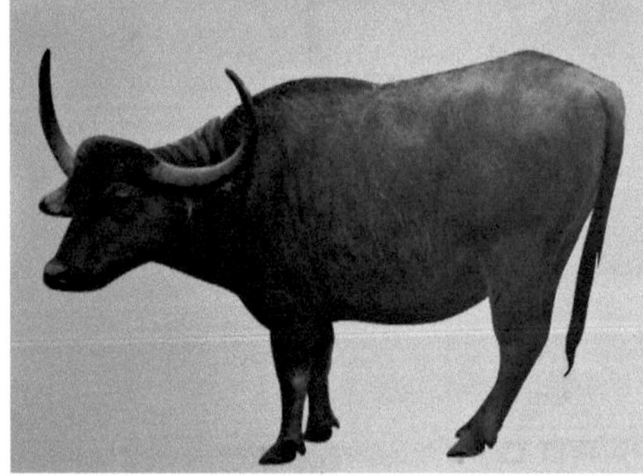

Fig. 6.1. *Maintained under semi-wild conditions by the aboriginal Toda tribals, the Toda buffalo is a registered indigenous breed. Considered more treasured than gold and worshipped for centuries, the Todas share a deep bond with their buffaloes, which they believe were created by the Goddess of the Mountains. (Photo source: ICAR-CIRB).*

and the buffalo herds linked to them. Toda temples feature a carved representation of a buffalo's horn, symbolizing its sacred significance. Access to these sacred dairy temples is restricted, preserving their sanctity. For this gentle and simple pastoral community, the buffalo holds a central place in every aspect of life. It is integral to traditional Toda rituals, including marriages, births, and deaths, and serves as a source of milk and companionship. Scholars often remark, 'A Toda is nothing without his buffalo', highlighting the profound connection between the people and their animals (Adharshana and Aishwarya 2023). The Todas exemplify how traditional pastoral communities integrate animal husbandry with cultural heritage, achieving a harmonious balance between livelihood, ecology, and tradition.

A survey of ethnoveterinary practices among the Toda people revealed their extensive use of medicinal plants for treating both human and veterinary ailments (Banumathi and Vaseeharan 2015). The study found that Toda tribes traditionally utilize various plant types, including lichens (10%), shrubs (50%), and herbs (40%), to address a wide range of conditions such as food poisoning, snake bites, indigestion, diarrhoea, bone fractures, and management of wound infections. Medicinal plants were also used as insect repellents, dewormers and galactagogue. The list of plants included sweet flag (*Acorus calamus* Linn.), ossicula (*Berberis tinctoria* Lesch.), velari (*Dodonaea viscosa* (L.) Jacq.), Crofton weed (*Euphorbia rothiana* Spreng.), wild tobacco (*Lobelia leschenaultiana* (C. Presl) Skottsb.), shield lichen (*Parmelia* sp.), bracken fern (*Pteridium aquilinum* L. Kuhn.), wild tomato (*Solanum sisymbrifolium* Lam.), and *kurinji* (*Strobilanthes foliosus* (Wight) Anders.).

Pharmacological Relevance of Ethnoveterinary Practices used by Pastoralists: Ethnoveterinary practices, followed by pastoral and tribal communities in India, hold significant pharmacological importance. These communities possess extensive knowledge of the pharmaceutical properties of numerous plants in their environment and their applications in treating both animals and humans. Many of these plants are rich in phytochemicals with therapeutic properties, offering effective remedies for various ailments. Some examples are:

- Neem (*Azadirachta indica* A. Juss) is widely used for its antifungal and antibacterial properties, while turmeric (*Curcuma longa*) is valued for its anti-inflammatory and wound-healing effects. Several pharmacological studies have reported presence of secondary metabolites in these plants with strong biological activities including antibacterial, antiviral, immunomodulatory and anti-inflammatory effects. *Ashwagandha* (*Withania somnifera* (L.) Dunal) and aloe vera (*Aloe vera* (L.) Burm.f.) are scientifically validated for their immunomodulatory and healing properties.

- The root extract of *Thalictrum javanicum* is used by the Darmi Bhotia community to treat haematuria in cattle and for its diuretic, purgative, and tonic properties in human patient by the traditional healers of high hills of Nilgiris. The roots of *Thalictrum foliosum* DC are utilized by the Monpa community as a highly effective remedy for ephemeral fever in yaks. Pharmacological studies revealed that *Thalictrum* species contain a variety of benzylisoquinoline-derived alkaloids, including berberine, a potent antimicrobial compound. Other alkaloids, such as magnoflorine, palmatine, and thalicarpine, exhibit pharmacological activities like antitumor, antimicrobial, anti-amoebic, and antiviral effects. These plants also contain unsaturated and saturated fatty acids, which enhance their medicinal value (Gurunathan and Subramaniam 2014).

- The Bhotia community uses a mixture of tobacco (*Nicotiana tabacum*) leaf powder and mustard oil to treat scabies and other ectoparasites in animals. Tobacco leaves, powder, extracts, and fumigants have been traditionally used to control agricultural pests and parasites of medical and veterinary importance. Pharmacological studies indicate that *N. tabacum* leaves contain numerous alkaloids, including nicotine, which acts as a contact insecticide. Additionally, tobacco exhibits various pharmacological effects, such as antioxidant, antimicrobial, antiparasitic, analgesic, antidiabetic, antifertility, cytotoxic, and neuropharmacological properties (Al-Snafi 2022).

- *Elsholtzia communis,* locally known as *Lomba* and *Youngpa*, is used by the Chirus tribals in Manipur to treat foot and mouth disease (FMD). This plant is also used in treating colds, headaches, fevers, dyspepsia, and for relieving exterior syndrome. Tribes in Nagaland and Arunachal Pradesh include *Elsholtzia communis* in their diet and use it for its medicinal properties. Nutritionally significant, it boasts high levels of minerals, essential fatty acids, essential oils, fibres, and proteins. This plant is a rich source of phytochemicals like flavonoids, phenolic acid, and terpenoids, contributing it antiviral, antibacterial, antioxidant, anti-inflammatory, adaptogenic, and insecticidal properties and supporting its extensive use in traditional medicine systems, underscoring its pharmacological significance (Barua *et al.* 2018).

- Raika pastoralists use the flowers of *Butea monosperma* (*palash*) to treat jaundice in sheep and goats. The flower extracts of this plant contain flavonoids such as butin, butein, butrin, isobutrin, palasitrin, coreopsin, isocoreopsin, sulphuresin, monospermoside, isomonospermoside, and 7,3,4-trihydroxyflavone. Among these, butrin and isobutrin have demonstrated antihepatotoxic activity in experimental animals. Various flower extracts also exhibit free radical scavenging activity due to their high phenolic content (Sindhia and Bairwa 2010).

- Raikas use a mixture of *Vitex negundo*, *Moringa oleifera*, and *desi Ajwain* with salt to treat trypanosomiasis in camels. *Vitex negundo* is rich in chemical compounds such as polyphenolics, terpenoids, glycosidic iridoids, and alkaloids. This shrub is one of the richest sources of stable vitamin C, making it one of the best anti-inflammatory herbs, effectively reducing temperature (Kumar *et al.* 2018). *Moringa oleifera* contains over 40 natural antioxidants and is one of the richest plant sources of vitamins A, B, C, D, E, and K. It also contains essential minerals like calcium, copper, iron, potassium, magnesium, manganese, and zinc. These compounds help to relieve mineral and vitamin deficiencies, neutralize free radicals, and support the body's anti-inflammatory mechanisms. Moringa also boosts the immune system and mitigates anaemia (Mahmood *et al.* 2010).
- Many plants used by the Toda community in their ethnoveterinary practices have been scientifically studied and found to contain phytoconstituents with diverse pharmacological properties. For example, the Toda people traditionally use *Acorus calamus* to treat snake-bites and poisoning. Scientific studies have confirmed that its rhizome extracts exhibit antioxidant, anticonvulsant, antidepressant, and neuroprotective effects in laboratory animals. The Toda community applies a paste made from the leaves of wild tobacco (*Lobelia leschenaultiana)* to wounds to serve as an insect repellent and prevent the formation of maggots. The ethanolic extracts of leaves of this plant have demonstrated insecticidal properties in scientific research. A paste prepared from the leaves of *Solanum sisymbrifolium*, garlic (*Allium sativum*), and salt is traditionally used by the Todas to deworm calves. Phytochemical analyses of *Solanum sisymbrifolium* leaf extracts have revealed the presence of carbohydrates, phenols, flavonoids, alkaloids, proteins, steroids, saponins, and terpenoids. Among these, alkaloids and terpenoids are recognized for their antimicrobial, antifungal, antiparasitic, antiallergenic, and anti-inflammatory properties (Gebrewbet and Hndeya 2023). Scores of pharmacological studies have identified garlic as a potent parasiticide, amebicide, acarifuge, vermifuge, larvicide, fungicide, and immunostimulant. Extracts of garlic leaves have shown anthelmintic activity against *Ascaris lumbricoides* larvae in rats, with effects comparable to standard allopathic drugs. This activity is attributed to allicin (diallylthiosulfinate or diallyldisulfide), one of the most abundant active compounds in garlic (Akoh *et al.* 2020).

These examples not only validate traditional knowledge but also underscore the potential of ethnoveterinary practices as valuable resources for modern pharmacological research, particularly for exploring herbs used in ethnoveterinary practices by pastoralists for reverse pharmacology and developing scientifically validated cost-effective herbal drug technology.

Field Veterinarians and Local Animal Healers

Field veterinarians play a crucial role in ensuring the health and welfare of livestock and pets. Their responsibilities encompass diagnosing, treating, and preventing animal diseases, as well as providing guidance on animal husbandry practices. These professionals work across diverse settings, including rural communities, urban clinics, and government agencies. In addition to clinical duties, field veterinarians are actively involved in research, education, and public health initiatives. They collaborate with experts such as animal scientists, epidemiologists, and policymakers to develop and implement strategies that enhance animal health and productivity. In rural and tribal areas, field veterinarians often gain significant experience in ethnoveterinary medicine. By integrating traditional knowledge with modern veterinary science, they deliver essential care to animals that might otherwise lack access to professional medical services. Moreover, they serve as a valuable resource for documenting and preserving ethnoveterinary practices in their areas of work.

Local animal healers, also known as traditional healers or ethno-veterinarians, play a vital role in providing accessible and affordable healthcare solutions for livestock in remote and underserved areas. These healers possess profound knowledge of the medicinal properties of various plants and natural substances, which they use to diagnose and treat a wide range of animal ailments. However, changing technological and environmental conditions, coupled with shifts in animal husbandry practices, have significantly impacted the survival of this traditional knowledge. Once considered invaluable for sustainable and culturally relevant livestock healthcare, this knowledge is now at risk of being lost. Its decline not only affects the availability of affordable veterinary solutions but also erodes the rich cultural heritage of rural and tribal communities in India. Preserving and integrating the wisdom of local animal healers with modern veterinary practices is essential for sustainable animal healthcare. It ensures the continuation of a culturally significant tradition while meeting the evolving needs of livestock management in diverse settings.

Role of Modern Veterinary Research and Development (R&D) and Academic Institutions in Ethnoveterinary Medicine

The combined efforts of R&D and academic institutions, Non-Government Organizations (NGOs), and pharmaceutical industry have played a pivotal role in preserving, validating, and integrating ethnoveterinary practices into modern animal healthcare. R&D and academic initiatives focus on documenting, scientific validation and preserving traditional ethnoveterinary knowledge. These can help in different ways as discussed here:

- Providing evidence based ethnoveterinary practices.
- Safeguarding indigenous practices and ensuring their transmission to future generations.
- Identifying active compounds in traditional remedies leading to the development of new veterinary drugs and treatments, thus promoting sustainable and eco-friendly practices.
- Facilitating the integration of ethnoveterinary practices with modern veterinary medicine.

Modern Veterinary Science in India: Evolution and Integration of Ethnoveterinary Medicine— A Brief Historical Overview

The development of modern veterinary science in India highlights its vital contribution to the growth of the livestock sector and the broader goals of socioeconomic progress. Over time, the integration of ethnoveterinary knowledge with contemporary scientific practices has further enriched the field.

The Beginning

Modern research and development in veterinary science, along with the introduction of a Western-style veterinary education system, began in India during the British colonial period, approximately 150 years ago (see Chapter 9 also). The last quarter of the 19th century was a transformative era, marked by significant advancements in veterinary education and research.

Formal veterinary education in India commenced in 1862 with the establishment of an army veterinary school in Pune. The first civilian veterinary school was founded in Babugarh (Hapur), Uttar Pradesh, in 1877. This was followed by the establishment of Lahore Veterinary College (now in Pakistan) in 1882, making it the first institution in the Indian subcontinent to offer a Western-style veterinary education. The college introduced a two-year Veterinary Assistant program for matriculated students. Further developments included the founding of Bombay Veterinary College in 1886, Bengal Veterinary College in 1893, Madras Veterinary College in 1903, and Bihar Veterinary College in Patna in 1927, all of which played a crucial role in advancing modern veterinary education in pre-independence India (Rahman 2004).

In 1889, India's first veterinary research facility, the Imperial Bacteriological Laboratory (IBL), was established in Pune. Its primary mission was to investigate diseases in domestic animals and provide free biological supplies to the military. In 1893, the laboratory was relocated to Mukteswar in the scenic Kumaon region (then United Provinces), nestled in the Himalayas. Lt. Col. J.H.B. Hallen, the first Inspector General of the Civil Veterinary Department, made substantial contributions to these efforts. Hallen also authored *More Deadly Forms of*

Diseases in India in 1871, a notable addition to veterinary literature. Another key figure, Major Griffith Evans (1835–1935), an army veterinarian, discovered the blood flagellate protozoan *Trypanosoma evansi*, the causative agent of surra, in camel blood. This groundbreaking discovery led to the species being named in his honour.

Pre-Independence Advancements

Significant progress was made during the pre-independence era to combat deadly cattle diseases such as rinderpest, haemorrhagic septicaemia, anthrax, highly contagious foot-and-mouth disease, east coast fever, and diseases caused by mineral deficiencies. Much of this research was conducted at the Imperial Bacteriological Laboratory, renamed the Imperial Veterinary Research Institute in 1925. A prominent figure of this period, Sir (Col) Arthur Olver, India's first Animal Husbandry Commissioner, played a crucial role in promoting indigenous cattle breeds and advancing all disciplines of veterinary science. In 1938, Olver authored *A Brief Survey of Some Important Breeds and Cattle in India*, a foundational text. Along with Vaidyanathan, he presented a research paper emphasizing the vital contributions of animal husbandry to the Indian economy. Their work highlighted the importance of livestock in rural livelihoods and economic development, influencing higher authorities to allocate increased funding for research and development programs.

The publication of India's first veterinary journal, *The Quarterly Journal of Veterinary Science in India and Army Animal Management* (1882–1892), marked the beginning of veterinary science documentation in the country. This was followed by the launch of two enduring indigenous journals: *The Indian Veterinary Journal* (1924) and *The Indian Journal of Veterinary Science and Animal Husbandry* (1930), now known as *The Indian Journal of Animal Sciences* (Somavanshi *et al.* 2017). These journals continue to play a significant role in advancing veterinary research and knowledge.

Despite significant changes over time, animal healthcare and welfare remained largely ethnomedicine-centric until the latter half of the 20th century. Traditional knowledge, which was dynamic and evolving, formed the cornerstone of animal care. The primary focus was on disease prevention. Sick animals were isolated to prevent the spread of illness, and some innovative methods were adopted to maintain animal health. For instance, records from the British colonial period highlight how camel herders in South-East Punjab and Rajasthan used a rudimentary inoculation technique to reduce the severity of camelpox in young calves. This method involved taking crusts from camelpox lesions, crushing them, and mixing them with a small amount of milk to prepare an inoculum. The lip of a young camel was then pricked multiple times with a needle, and the inoculum was applied over four consecutive days. Typically, this procedure was performed when the camel was about four months old, although in some cases, it was delayed until the camel reached 16 months. The inoculation, usually carried out in May or early June on one or two calves per herd, proved effective in mitigating the severity of camelpox (Leese 1927).

Post-Independence Developments

The livestock sector has remained a vital resource for supporting socioeconomic progress and ensuring food security in independent India. Significant emphasis has been placed on advancing scientific research and education in veterinary science and animal husbandry to improve the health and productivity of domestic animals. In 1947, the Government of Uttar Pradesh established the U.P. College of Veterinary Science and Animal Husbandry in Mathura. This veterinary college conferred a degree in Veterinary Science (BVSc & AH). It also pioneered postgraduate degree programs (MVSc) in several veterinary and animal science disciplines in 1951, followed by the introduction of PhD programs in 1953. Since then, numerous research institutes, veterinary colleges, and universities have been established across the country. Today, India boasts 19 animal science institutes under the Indian Council of Agricultural Research (ICAR), including two Deemed Universities—the Indian Veterinary Research Institute and the National Dairy Research Institute—engaged in diverse R&D programs in veterinary science. The National Dairy Development Board, established in 1965 and declared an institution of national importance by an Act of Parliament, supports dairy development in rural India through services, projects, and policies for animal breeding, nutrition, health, engineering, finance, and marketing of dairy products. As of March 2024, India has a network of 70 government and private veterinary colleges, comprising 56 recognized and 14 provisionally recognized institutions under the Veterinary Council of India (VCI)—a statutory body established in 1984 under the Indian Veterinary Council Act. These colleges, affiliated with 17 animal science and veterinary universities—including two ICAR Deemed Universities and 14 agricultural or other recognized private universities—form an integral part of the nation's veterinary education and research. In addition, several other public and private universities, research organizations and agencies, Non-Government Organizations (NGO) and veterinary pharmaceuticals are directly or indirectly associated with veterinary Education, Research and Development (ERD) programmes in India.

Role of Veterinary Herbal Pharma Industry

The ERD initiatives aimed at testing and integrating traditional knowledge into veterinary practices in India predates global recognition of EVM as legitimate branch of science. A range of herbal products were commercially available in the Indian Market in 1950s. The emergence of these initiatives can be traced back to the establishment of Veterinary Ayurvedic Pharmaceutical Companies, which introduced a range of herbal products. These companies combined ancient wisdom with modern scientific methodologies to develop plant-based and natural veterinary drugs. Beyond commercial interests, they also promoted clinical research on their products, thereby preserving indigenous animal healthcare knowledge among modern veterinarians at a time when allopathic medicine was becoming dominant in veterinary practices. For instance, Indian Herbs Pvt. Ltd., established in 1951 with the vision Nature's Way to Animal Health, pioneered the concept of herbal rumenotorics and introduced its flagship product, *Himalayan Batisa*. This polyherbal-mineral digestive stimulant and tonic for ruminants was based on traditional remedies for digestive disorders. Today, the company claims to manufacture over 200 herbal products for animals and 30 for human use. Furthermore, it has supported more than 250 Master's and PhD research programs and contributed over 1,200 research papers on herbal veterinary medicine. Another notable player in the field was Cattle Remedies Pvt. Ltd. (now Vamso), founded in 1969 by a veterinarian and an Ayurvedic doctor. The company also encouraged the scientific research and clinical trials on its products.

Alarsin Pharmaceutical Company, established in 1947 with a focus on developing research-based products combining ancient and modern medical knowledge, introduced *Leptaden*, a galactagogue for veterinary use containing *Jivanti* (*Leptadenia reticulata*) and *Kamboji* (*Breynia retusa*) in equal proportions. This was perhaps the first commercial herbal preparation to be scientifically evaluated for its efficacy in various animal species, including cows, buffaloes, sheep, and goats (Anjaria and Gupta, 1967). In 1965, Dr J.V. Anjaria submitted an MVSc thesis to Agra University on the evaluation of the galactagogue properties of *Leptaden* tablets and powdered *Jivanti* (*Leptadenia reticulata*), a plant known for its medicinal properties since the Vedic age. His work, published in a series of research papers and PhD dissertation included studies on pharmacognosy, chemical analysis, identification of lactogenic phytoingredients, and toxicity evaluation of *Leptadenia reticulata.* Using a straightforward method, the author successfully isolated phytosterols and tocopherols (with alpha-tocopherol being the major component) from *Jivanti*, thereby validating its galactagogue property (Anjaria, 1973).

Over time, contemporary veterinary herbal pharmaceutical industry has evolved into a multi-million-dollar sector. Pharma Hopers has listed 1073 Veterinary Herbal Manufacturer in India (https://www.pharmahopers.com/pharma/veterinary-herbal-manufacturer, accessed on 30-01-2025). Supported by a network of state-sponsored and private universities, research institutions, hospitals, and treatment facilities, the veterinary herbal pharma industry has facilitated the integration of traditional and modern veterinary practices. Moreover, it has played a pivotal role in promoting eco-friendly and sustainable veterinary practices, significantly reducing reliance on synthetic drugs.

Scientific Research, Validation and Value Addition to Ethnoveterinary Practices

Early scientific studies aimed at validating traditional animal healing methods primarily focused on evaluating medicinal herbs for common digestive and reproductive disorders, as well as for treating gastrointestinal worms and ectoparasites in animals. For instance, research demonstrated the curative efficacy of *Karanj* (*Pongamia pinnata*) oil, and a formulation containing equal parts of *tuvari/tara* (*Eruca stiva*) oil, tar oil (*oleum picis carbonis*), and sulphur in treating sarcoptic mange in goats and buffaloes (Kale and Panchegaonkar1969, Srivastava and Chhabra 1971). These ingredients have long been used in traditional medicine for skin disease treatment.

Interest in various aspects of ethnoveterinary medicine emerged in the 1970s and gained momentum in the early 1980s. This shift was driven by a growing recognition and appreciation of traditional animal healthcare practices, ultimately leading to the formal establishment of ethnoveterinary medicine as an academic field of study. The Food and Agriculture Organization (FAO) also advocated for the use of traditional medicine in animal treatment, similar to the World Health Organization's (WHO) efforts for human healthcare. In 1984, FAO initiated documentation and compilation of reports on traditional veterinary medicine practices used by small-scale farmers in Asia, including India (FAO, 1984). In India, the Indian Council of Agricultural Research (ICAR) and various funding agencies launched initiatives to promote scientific research, documentation, validation, and dissemination of ethnoveterinary medicine (EVM) knowledge and practices. Alongside ICAR institutes and publicly funded veterinary universities, colleges, and research institutions, several other organizations have played an active role in EVM research, development, and extension programs. These include the National Dairy Development Board (NDDB), the National Innovation Foundation (NIF), *Anthra*, the Society for Research and Initiatives for Sustainable Technologies and Institutions (SRISTI) the Honey Bee Network, the Gujarat Grassroots Innovation Augmentation Network (GIAN), and the Foundation for Revitalization of Local Health Traditions (FRLHT), Bhartiya Agro Industries Foundation (BAIF), among others.

Education, Research, Development, and Extension (ERDE) Initiatives and Advancements in Ethnoveterinary Medicine: Over the past five decades, various institutions have undertaken significant ERDE initiatives to advance ethnoveterinary medicine:

- **The Indian Veterinary Research Institute (IVRI).** The institute played a significant role in leveraging traditional knowledge to develop cost-effective and eco-friendly veterinary treatment technologies. In 1989, the institute formulated a polyherbal treatment using *Vetiveria zizanioides* (Linn.) Nash, *Annona squamosa* (Linn.), *Argemone mexicana* (Linn.), *Butea* *monosperma* (Lam.) Kuntze, and *Azadirachta indica* (A. Juss.) in specific proportions. This formulation proved highly effective in treating various skin diseases in livestock and pets, including mange, pyoderma, scabies, and fungal infections. Following rigorous clinical trials, the product was commercialized under the brand name *Olinall.*

- **Other ICAR Institutes:** Research on ethnoveterinary medicine, particularly with a focus on medicinal herbs, has also been undertaken by other ICAR institutes, including ICAR-CIRG, ICAR-NRCE, and several others. The ICAR-Central Institute for Research on Goats (ICAR-CIRG) scientifically validated the efficacy of *Devadaru* (*Cedrus deodara*) oil in treating severe mange in sheep. The study demonstrated that this herbal remedy was as effective as the chemical drug benzyl benzoate (Sharma *et al.* 1997). *Devadaru* is widely recognized for its diverse pharmacological properties. Its heartwood oil has been traditionally used as a home remedy for cough, constipation, and skin ailments. In veterinary medicine, it has shown effectiveness in treating mange across various animal species and has been used for managing ulcers and skin conditions in horses, as well as sore feet in cattle. ICAR-CIRG furthered research in this area under the NATP on *Evaluation of Medicinal Plants for Control of Parasitic Diseases in Livestock* and documented medicinal plants with antiparasitic potential for veterinary use. The institute also developed a novel herbal ectoparasiticidal drug, which was later commercialized as ALQUIT™, marking a significant advancement in natural veterinary treatments. Additionally, ICAR-CIRG has patented pharmacological properties of some novel herbal formulations.

- **NATP- Mission Mode Project on Indigenous Technical Knowledge (ITK):** The Indian Council of Agricultural Research (ICAR) launched a Mission Mode Project on the Collection, Documentation, and Validation of ITK under the National Agricultural Technology Project (NATP) between 2002 and 2004. ITK data was gathered from primary sources through voluntary disclosures and from existing literature, including books, journals, and theses.

  This resulted in an inventory of 4,033 ITKs in agriculture, published in three volumes. Among them, over 1,200 practices were related to veterinary science and animal husbandry. Scientists of the Indian Council of Agricultural Research (ICAR), in collaboration with researchers from State Agricultural and Veterinary Science Universities, validated 32 veterinary Indigenous Technical Knowledge (ITK) practices. Several of these demonstrated promising therapeutic outcomes, including the treatment of foot lesions associated with foot-and-mouth disease (FMD) using a decoction prepared from the bark of babul or Indian gum Arabic tree (*Vachellia nilotica* syn. *Acacia nilotica*) and *jamun* or Indian blackberry

(*Syzygium cumini*). Wounds and FMD lesions were effectively managed using a paste prepared from fresh leaves of peach (*Prunus persica*) (Fig. 6.2). Among other practices, diarrhoea in calves was successfully managed using shisham or Indian rosewood leaves (*Dalbergia sissoo*) and bael or Bengal quince fruit powder (*Aegle marmelos*), while joint swelling and yoke gall in cattle were managed using a herbo-mineral-based ITK. This initiative was a major milestone in systematically documenting and validating traditional knowledge agriculture and allied subjects. Under another NATP project *Identification and Evaluation of Medicinal Plants for Control of Parasitic Diseases in Livestock*, 158 medicinal plants were catalogued, of which 50 were evaluated for their antiparasitic properties (Anonymous 2003).

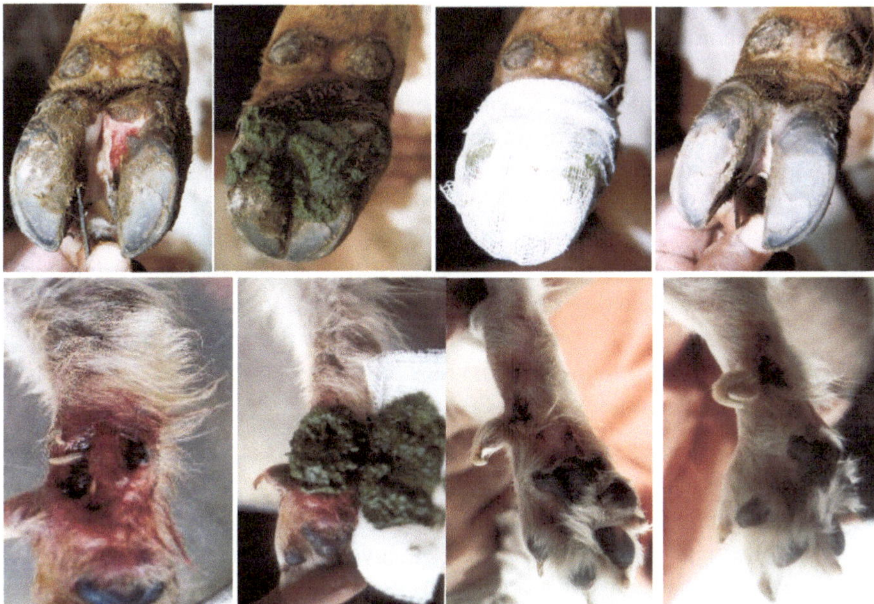

Fig. 6.2. *An Indigenous Traditional Knowledge (ITK) practice using a paste made from fresh peach leaves for treating foot-and-mouth disease (FMD) wounds was clinically validated. It was found effective in treating maggot wounds in foot lesions (FMD) in cattle, and in dogs. The wounds healed completely within 7–10 days, and the tested ITK exhibited maggoticidal effects within 24 hours. Farmers use this ITK to cure wounds both for family members and animals (Source: Swarup et al. 2004).*

- **ICAR-Ad Hoc Research Scheme on Ethnoveterinary Medicine:** To advance research in ethnoveterinary medicine (EVM), ICAR launched a transdisciplinary, multicentre mega project in 2005 as an ad-hoc scheme, coordinated by the Indian Veterinary Research Institute (IVRI) and implemented at seven centres across the country. The project evolved into an Outreach Programme in 2010 with 10 participating research centres.

Currently, it operates as a network program involving nine veterinary colleges, ICAR institutes, and two CSIR institutes—the Indian Institute of Chemical Technology, Hyderabad, and the Central Institute for Medicinal and Aromatic Plants, Lucknow. Notable outcomes include the development of herbal drug formulation for fluorosis management, herbal spray for subclinical mastitis, herbal shampoo for pet skin care, wound healing compounds from medicinal plants to cite a few.

- **National Dairy Development Board (NDDB):** Established in 1965, NDDB has been actively promoting ethnoveterinary medicine to enhance the health and productivity of dairy animals. As part of its initiatives, NDDB has developed brochures and video tutorials detailing the preparation and application of ethnoveterinary formulations for 20 common ailments in dairy animals. These resources are available in all major regional languages, ensuring widespread accessibility for farmers across India (https://www.nddb.coop/farmer/health/evm, accessed on 4-2-2025). To further popularize the concept of Ayurvedic veterinary medicine, NDDB has initiated intensive propagation drives in collaboration with the Department of AYUSH, the Department of Animal Husbandry and Dairying (DAHD), State Animal Husbandry Departments, Milk Federations, and Milk Unions to educate and encourage farmers to adopt these traditional practices. Additionally, NDDB is developing a comprehensive database to track the efficacy of each formulation, which will serve as a key tool in expanding their adoption (https://www.nddb.coop/services/animalhealth/ayurvedic-veterinary-medicine, accessed on 31-1-2025).
- **The National Innovation Foundation (NIF)-India:** Established in March 2000 as an autonomous institute of the Department of Science and Technology, Government of India, NIF has played a crucial role in documenting and validating ethnoveterinary practices used by local communities across the country. These practices include herbal remedies, healing techniques, and preventive measures for common livestock diseases such as mastitis, digestive disorders, and parasitic infestations. To promote these practices, NIF has developed training manuals and programs for veterinary doctors and farmers, integrating validated ethnoveterinary knowledge. The institute also supports grassroots innovators who have developed unique ethnoveterinary solutions, recognizing and awarding them for their contributions. This encouragement fosters greater exploration and documentation of traditional knowledge. Currently, several ethnoveterinary practices and herbal formulations used by individual traditional healers and communities are undergoing validation at the ICAR-National Dairy Research Institute (ICAR-NDRI) and Veterinary Colleges across India. To further raise awareness, NIF has also published research papers, case studies, and success stories, highlighting the effectiveness of these practices. The

institute has taken a big step to protect Intellectual Property Right (IPR). As many as 59 veterinary patents have been granted to individual innovators and communities for their traditional knowledge, with the support of NIF-India. (Source: VARD Human Health & Veterinary - National Innovation Foundation-India, accessed on 31-01-2025).

- **Centre for Development of Education, Science and Technology (C-DEST) Rajiv Gandhi Centre for Biotechnology (BRIC-RGCB):** An autonomous institute of government of India, BRIC-RGCB, has developed a Community Knowledge Register on ethnoveterinary practices and scientifically validated herbal formulations. The institute also launched *Gau Mitra*, a mobile app under the DST-funded Tribal Heritage Programme, helping farmers to diagnose and treat primary cattle health issues using ethnoveterinary methods (Source: https://rgcb.res.in/thp/portfolio-details.php, accessed on 29-01-2025).
- **The Rajasthan University of Veterinary and Animal Sciences (RAJUVAS):** Established the Centre for Ethno-Veterinary Practice and Alternative Medicine. This centre focuses on documenting traditional knowledge, scientific validation, and developing protocols to integrate ethnoveterinary practices into mainstream veterinary medicine.
- **Foundation for Revitalisation of Local Health Tradition (FRLHT)**: A public trust since 1991, FRLHT has worked extensively on human and animal healthcare. In collaboration with the National Dairy Development Board (NDDB) and NGOs in Southern India, it documented and validated plant-based ethnoveterinary treatments for gastrointestinal disorders (constipation, indigestion, bloat, and diarrhoea), infectious diseases (mastitis, FMD, and ephemeral fever), reproductive and metabolic conditions (repeat breeding, hypogalactia, and helminthiasis). FRLHT has also developed an extensive database on Indian medicinal plants, incorporating 7,263 botanical names representing Indian medicinal plant taxa. These botanical names have been correlated with more than 150,000 vernacular names in ten different Indian languages. Additionally, the database includes over 5,000 authentic images of Indian medicinal plants, each duly linked to the specific botanical entities. (https://envis.frlht.org/frlht, accessed on 31-01-2025).
- **Anthra:** Founded in 1992 by women veterinarians, Anthra documented ethnoveterinary healing practices among farmers in Andhra Pradesh and Maharashtra. The organization has made significant contributions to the field of ethnoveterinary practices, including clinical validation of 165 traditional treatments for ruminants and poultry with reported cure rates of 92% and 100%, respectively, publication of *Plants Used in Animal Care* (2008), cataloguing 375 medicinal and fodder plants used for therapeutic and nutritional purposes and release of *Annotated Bibliography* on

Ethnoveterinary Research in India (2004) and *Indigenous Knowledge Applications for Livestock Care* (2016).

- **Society for Research and Initiatives for Sustainable Technologies and Institutions (SRISTI):** Established in 1992, SRISTI is a developmental voluntary organization. Evolved and expanded through the Honey Bee Network, SRISTI has undertaken various projects focused on documenting, experimenting with, adding value to, and disseminating local innovations. SRISTI has played a crucial role in validating and enhancing traditional knowledge-based practices including veterinary medicine by value addition, as well as the development and commercialization of veterinary formulations based on indigenous innovations for treating animal diseases. The organization aims to build a comprehensive database of indigenous and herbal medicines while employing state-of-the-art laboratory facilities for quantitative analysis of active ingredients (Source: Validation & Value Addition – SRISTI, accessed on 02-02-2025). Notably, SRISTI has published *A Glossary of Selected Indigenous Medicinal Plants of India*, which documents medicinal plants used in both human and animal healthcare practices (Anjaria *et al.* 2002).

Training, Education, and Policy Integration: Since the 1997 International Conference on Ethnoveterinary Medicine in Pune and the 1998 ICAR Summer Short Course on Techniques for Scientific Validation and Evaluation of Ethnoveterinary Practice at ICAR-IVRI, numerous academic activities — including conferences, workshops, and training programmes — have been held across India to promote ethnoveterinary research. In 2017, Tamil Nadu Veterinary and Animal Sciences University (TANUVAS) launched a Postgraduate Diploma in Ethnoveterinary Practice at the Veterinary College and Research Institute, Orathanadu. (tanuvas.ac.in). The University of Trans-disciplinary Health Sciences and Technology, along with TANUVAS, trained 1,750 veterinarians from organizations like the National Dairy Development Board (NDDB) and Karnataka Milk Federation(downtoearth.org.in). Additionally, university reported potential role of ethnoveterinary practices (EVP) in management of mastitis. The university also reported the potential role of EVP in the management of mastitis. A clinical intervention using EVM preparations on 181,252 cows in a multicentric field study over a period of five years assessed the efficacy of EVP for subclinical, clinical, and chronic mastitis with multifactorial aetiology. The study resulted in a clinical recovery rate of 84.9% of cases (Nair and Natesan 2024). In 2018, ICAR-IVRI organized a summer school on the practicability, scope, and future prospects of ethnobotanicals in minimizing antibiotic resistance, emphasizing the significance of ethnoveterinary medicine (EVM) in mitigating antimicrobial resistance (AMR). More recently, in 2023, the ICAR-National Meat Research Institute organized a workshop on the role of EVM in organic livestock production, highlighting the global demand for natural and organic foods (icar.org.in). Furthermore, the Deen

Dayal Kamdhenu Gaushala Samiti in Farah, Mathura, is working to introduce a six-month Postgraduate Diploma in Animal Ayurveda at its upcoming Shalihotra Institute of Veterinary Ayurveda, in alignment with the Veterinary Council of India's Continuing Veterinary Education objectives.

Ethnoveterinary practices are now endorsed as a treatment option in the *Standard Veterinary Treatment Guidelines for Livestock and Poultry*, released by the Ministry of Fisheries, Animal Husbandry & Dairying, Government of India, in collaboration with FAO. This is a comprehensive document that outlines best practices for veterinary care, aimed at improving the overall health and productivity of livestock and supporting to the national action plan for anti-microbial resistance. *The Handbook for Pashu Sakhi*, a Women Empowerment Module under the National Livelihood Mission, recommends ethnoveterinary practices for a wide range of livestock diseases (Source: https://www.pashudhanpraharee.com/wp-content/uploads/2019/08/Pashu-Sakhi-Hand-book.pdf, accessed on 24-1-2025). The Ministry of AYUSH and the Department of Animal Husbandry have signed an MoU to develop guidelines for Ayurvedic treatments in animal healthcare.

These are just a few representative examples of initiatives and advancements in ethnoveterinary research, development, and education over the past 50 years. Notably, there has been remarkable progress in scientific research and education in this field across the country, reflected in a growing number of publications, including books, monographs, conference proceedings, and research articles. In the last decade alone, over 150 research papers and reviews have been published on ethnoveterinary practices and the scientific validation of traditional healing methods, particularly plant-based therapeutics (Source: Google Scholar; keyword *"ethnoveterinary practices in India"*, searched on 31-01-2025). Additionally, several patents have been filed or granted for the novel medicinal properties of indigenous herbs (Fig. 6.3) traditionally used in ethnoveterinary medicine. Some

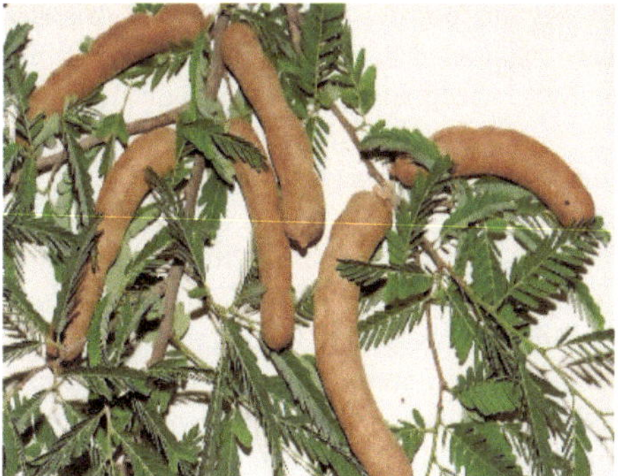

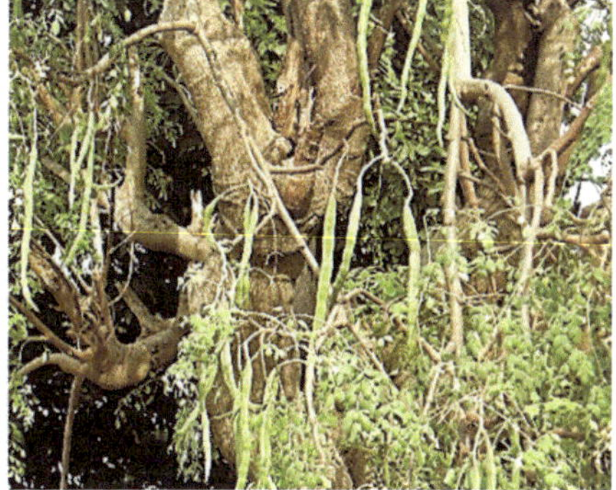

Fig. 6.3. *From Traditional Use to Patented Ethnoveterinary Innovation: Drawing on the traditional digestive, detoxifying, and nutritive uses of Tamarindus indica L. and Moringa oleifera Lam., a patented herbal product* ***(Patent No.*** *416413, Government of India) containing tamarind fruit pulp and immature drumstick pods has been developed to ameliorate fluorosis in animals (Source: Dr. S. Dey, ICAR–IVRI).*

scientifically validated EVM practices for treatment of common ailments of animals are presented in Table 6.2.

Table 6.2. Scientifically documented/ validated ethnoveterinary remedies for animal diseases

Condition	EVM practices/formulations used
Anorexia	• Mixture of powdered *Saunph* (Fennel seed, *Foeniculum vulgare*) + Jaggery 60 g each + Black salt 20 g applied as electuary. • Mixture of powdered seed of *Ajwain* (Wild celery, *Trachyspermum ammi,* or *Carum copticum)* + Salt 20 g each in 20 g Molasses given twice daily orally.
Rumen indigestion	• Magnesium sulphate 500 g + Common salt 200 g + *Adrak* (Ginger, *Zinger officinale)* powder 10 g in 500 ml lukewarm water given orally for adult cattle.
Constipation/ purgation	• Vegetable oil 500 ml orally for adult cattle or decoction of 100 g *Haldi* (Turmeric, *Curcuma longa*) powder in a litre water given daily for 2-3 day. • Powered *Isvarmul* (Indian Birthwort, *Aristolochia indica)* leaves 250 g + Molasses 50 g three time at ½ hourly interval.
Bloat	• Vegetable oil 500 ml given orally to cattle. • *Hing (*Asafoetida, *Ferula assa-foetida*) - 5g+ black salt- 100 g+ *Soowa dana* (*Garden* dill, *Anethum sowa*) seed- 50g + *Adrak (*Ginger, *Z officinale)* powder 25 g + *Ajwain* (Wild celery, *T ammi (L), C. copticum* L.) + Jaggery. Boil the ingredients in 1000 ml of water until the volume is reduced by half. Administer orally.
	• *Pyaaz* (Onion, *A cepa L.)* - 100 g+ *Lahsun (* Garlic, *Allium sativum)-* 10 pearls + Dry chilies *(Capsicum annuum)-* 2+ *Jeera (* Cumin, *Cuminum cyminum)* seeds - 10 g+ *Haldi* (Turmeric, *C. longa*) powder -10 g+ Jaggery-100 g+ *Kaali Mirch (*Pepper, *Piper nigrum*)- 10 g + *Paan (*Betel, *Piper betel*) leaves - 10+ *Adrak (*Ginger, *Z. officinale)* powder - 100 g. Soak pepper and cumin seeds for 30 minutes, then blend with the other ingredients to form a paste. Administer orally in small portions with salt, 3–4 times a day for 3 days.
Diarrhoea	• *Bartundi* (Indian mulberry, *Morinda citrifolia)* flower buds- 50g + *Pipali* (Long pepper, *Piper nigrum*) powder-1tsp + *Dhania* (Coriander, *Coriandrum sativum*) powder- 1tsp boiled in 200-300 ml of water for 1-2 minutes; decoction given orally to sheep and goats twice daily for 10-12 days in dysentery. • Powder of half ripe *Bael (*Stone fruit, *Aegle marmelos)* given @15-25 g per kg body weight orally for calves. • Kaolin- 5 g + chalk- 5 g + catechu- 0.8 g + *Bael (*Stone fruit, *A marmelos)* -1 g + alum 0.8 g + *Motha* (*Cyperus rotundus)-* 2g + *Kutja* (*Holarrhena antidysenterica)-* 3g, given as a drench twice daily for 5 days. • Fenugreek (*Trigonella foenum-graecum*) seeds - 10 g+ *Pyaaz* (Onion, *A cepa L.)* - 1 + *Lahsun (* Garlic, *A. sativum)-* 1 pearl + *Jeera (* Cumin, *C cyminum)* seeds- 10 g+ Turmeric (*C longa*) powder - 10 g+ Curry (*Murraya koenjii)* leaves - 1 handful + *Khus khus* (Poppy, *Papaver somniferum)* seeds - 5 g+ *Kaali Mirch (*Pepper, *P. nigrum*)- 10 g+ Jaggery - 100 g+ Hing (Asafoetida *F. assa-foetida*) - 5 g. Fry cumin seeds, asafoetida, poppy seeds, and fenugreek seeds until they emit smoke. Allow to cool, then grind into a fine powder. Blend with the remaining ingredients to form a paste. Given orally in small portions with salt, 3–4 times a day for 3 days.

Condition	EVM practices/formulations used
Ectoparasites (ticks)	• *Lahsun (Garlic, A sativum)* – 10 pearls + *Neem* (*Azadirachta indica*) leaves – 1 handful + *Neem* (*A. indica*) fruit – 1 handful + Acorus (*Acorus calamus*) rhizome – 10 g+ Turmeric (*C. longa*) powder – 20 g+ Lantana (*Lantana camara*) leaves – 1 handful +*Tulsi* (*Ocimum sanctum*) leaves. Blend all the ingredients thoroughly. Add 1 litre of clean water and mix well. Strain the mixture using a fine sieve or muslin cloth. Transfer the liquid into a bottle fitted with a sprayer. Spray evenly over the entire body of the animal. Apply to cracks and crevices in the cattle shed. Alternatively, soak a clean cloth in the solution and apply manually. Repeat once a week until the condition resolves. Apply only during sunny hours for best results. • *Gulvel/ Giloe* (*Tinospora cordifolia*) stem-150 g + 500 g *Chibad* (*Cucumis sativus* var. *hardwickii*) fruit- 500 g+ *Kadunimb/ Neem* (*A indica*) bark-100 g. + *Nirgundi* (*Vitex negundo*) leaves 130 g + 25 g *Vekhand* / acarus (*Acorus calamus*) rhizome. Crush all the plants to get the fine paste and keep it in 10 litres of water overnight. Filter and use as spray once (Nimbalkar *et al.* 2020).
Fever	• *Lahsun (* Garlic, *A sativum)*- 2 pearls+ Coriander (*C. sativum*) - 10 g+ Cumin seeds (*Cuminum cyminum*) -10 g; *Tulsi* (*Ocimum sanctum*)- 1 handful + Dry cinnamon (*Cinnamomum zeylanicum*) leaves - 10 g + *Kaali Mirch (*Pepper, *P nigrum*) - 10 g + Betel leaves (*Piper betel*) - 5 count + *Shallots*/onion (*A. cepa, var aggregatum*) - 2 bulbs+ Turmeric (*C. longa*) powder - 10 g + *Chiraita* (*Andrographis paniculata)* leaf powder - 20 g; Sweet basil (*Ocimum basilicum)* - 1 handful +Neem (*A. indica*) leaves - 1 handful +Jaggery - 100 g. Soak cumin, pepper and coriander seeds in water for 15 minutes. Blend and mix all ingredients to form a paste. Given orally in small portions in the morning and evening.
FMD lesions	• Decoction made of bark of *babul;* Indian gum Arabic tree (*Acacia nilotica* ssp *indica*) + *jamun;* java plum (*Syzygium cumini*) in equal parts; wash foot lesions thrice daily for 3-5 days. • Apply paste of finger millet flour in honey (50% v/v) after washing with 1% potassium permanganate solution on foot and mouth lesion. Give gruel prepared by cooking equal proportion of whole rice, wheat flour and finger millet flour in adequate quantity of water, jaggery (10%) and mineral mixture @ 2 kg/day for 20 days (Ranjan *et al.* 2016). • *Harita Manjari*-Indian Acalypha *(Acalypha indica)* leaves - 1 handful + Garlic *Lahsun (Garlic, A sativum)*- 10 pearls + *Neem (A. indica*) leaves 1 handful+ Coconut or Sesame oil - 500 ml +Turmeric (*C. longa*) powder - 20 g+ *Mehandi* (*Lawsonia innermis*) leaves - 1 handful+ *Tulsi* (*O. sanctum*) leaves - 1 handful. Blend all the ingredients thoroughly. Mix with 500 ml coconut or sesame oil and boil and bring to cool. Clean the foot lesions/ wound and apply directly or bandage with a medicated cloth. Apply Anona (*Anona squamosa)* leaf paste or camphorated coconut oil for the first day only if maggots are present.

Condition	EVM practices/formulations used
	• Cumin seeds (*Cuminum cyminum*)- 10 g+ Fenugreek (*Trigonella foenum-graecum*) seeds - 10 g+ *Kaali Mirch (*Pepper, *P nigrum*)- 10 g + Turmeric (*C.* longa) powder - 10 g+ *Lahsun (*Garlic, *A sativum)*- 4 pearls+ Coconut – 1+ Jaggery- 120 g. Soak cumin, fenugreek, and black pepper seeds in water for 20–30 minutes. Blend all ingredients into a fine paste. Add one fully grated coconut to the paste and mix thoroughly by hand only. Prepare a fresh dose for each application. Apply gently inside the mouth, on the tongue, and across the palate. Repeat three times daily for 3–5 days.
Intestinal parasites	• Powder of *Kutja (H antidysenterica*) bark + *Kala jeera, Somraj* (Black cumin/ Black Caraway, *Vernonia anthelmintica)* + *Baberang/ Vidagna (*Embelia, *Embelia ribes)* + *Neem (*Margosa/ Chinaberyy, *A indica)* + *Motha;* cyperus *(Cyperus rotundus)* + *Karanj* (Fever nut, *Caesalpinia bonduc* (L.) Roxb) in equal part and ¼ part of *Dakamali* (Gummy gardenia, (*Gardenia gummifer).* Given as electuary or as drench preferably empty stomach @ 10-100 g.
	• *Pyaaz* (Onion, *A cepa L.)* - 1 + *Lahsun (*Garlic, *A. sativum)*- 5 pearls +Mustard (*Brassica nigra)* seeds - 10 g+ *Neem* (*A. indica*) leaves - 1 handful+ Cumin seeds (*Cuminum cyminum*)- 10 g+ Bitter gourd (*Momordica charantia)* - 50 g+ Turmeric (C. longa) powder - 5 g+ *Kaali Mirch (*Pepper, *P. nigrum*) - 5 g+ Banana (*Musa paradisiaca)* stem - 100 g+ Common leucas *(Lucas aspera)* -1 handful+ Jaggery - 100 g. Soak pepper, cumin and mustard seeds for 30 minutes and blend them with remaining ingredients to form a paste. Roll the paste into small balls. Give small portions with salt once daily for 3 days.
Mastitis	• **Water-based Preparation**. *Aloe vera* - 250 g+ Turmeric (*C. longa*) powder-50 g+ Calcium Hydroxide (lime)-15 g+ Lemon - 6 (for one day). Remove thorns from Aloe vera leaves and cut them into small pieces. Blend with turmeric powder and lime to form a reddish paste. Wash, clean, and completely milk out all quarters, including unaffected ones. Take a handful of the paste and mix with 200 ml of water to create a thin solution. Apply the diluted paste ten times a day for 5 days. The final application of the day should be an oil-based preparation. Feed two lemons (cut into halves) orally, three times a day for 3 days. • **Oil-based Preparation.** Remove thorns from *Ghrit Kumari (Aloe vera)* leaves and cut them into small pieces. Blend with turmeric powder and lime to form a reddish paste. Wash, clean, and completely milk out all quarters, including unaffected ones. Dry the udder thoroughly. Take a handful of the paste and mix with 200 ml of mustard or gingelly oil to create a thin solution. Apply the diluted paste three times a day for 5 days. Feed two lemons (cut into halves) orally, three times a day for 3 days.
Pneumonia	• Inhalation of steam of mixture of *Chai patti* (tea leaves, *Camellia sinesis*) + *Neem (*margosa/ chinaberry *A. indica)* leaves with eucalyptus (*Eucalyptus globules*) or turpentine oil.
	• Massage of liniment of camphorated oil (250 ml vegetable oil + 50 g camphor) or turpentine oil on either side of chest.

Condition	EVM practices/formulations used
Retained placenta and Infertility	• White radish (*Raphanus sativus*) -1 full tuber+ *Bhindee* (Okra, *Abelmoschus esculentus*) - 1.5 kg+ Jaggery - as required+ Salt - as required. *For Initial Treatment*: Cut fresh okra into two pieces. Feed 1.5 kg of okra mixed with jaggery and salt if ROP persists 8 hours after calving. If *Retention Persists Beyond 12 Hours*: Tie a tight knot close to the base of the retained placenta. Cut 2 inches below the knot and leave it—do not attempt manual removal. The knot will retract naturally. *White Radish Supplementation:* Feed one full tuber of radish within two hours of calving. Repeat the radish feeding weekly for four weeks. • Administer ripened fruits of brinjal (eggplant) — 1 kg — followed by horse gram (Kulthi) — 250 g, soaked and ground. Give brinjal first, then horse gram, daily for one week in cases of infertility.
Wound	• Apply a paste made from fresh *Adhu* (Peach, *Prunus persica*) leaves on the wound and bandage it. • Crush the leaves of *Tulsi* (Holy Basil, *O sanctum*) or *Neem* (Chinaberry, *A. indica*), apply the paste to the wound, and bandage. • After cleaning the wound, apply a powder mixture of *Neem* (Chinaberry, *A. indica*), *Sitaphal* (Custard Apple, *Annona squamosa*) in a 2:1 ratio, and *Katahal* (Jackfruit, *Artocarpus heterophyllus*) leaves mixed with oil. • Prepare a poultice using a paste of *Sahajan* (Drumstick, *Moringa oleifera*) leaves and apply to the affected area. • Apply a powder made from *Nirgundi* (Chaste Tree, *Vitex negundo*) leaves in a paraffin base.
Yoke gall and Joint swelling	• *Snail shell* powder10 g + *Alua (*Dried Aloe *Aloe vera)* gel10 g+ *Sahajan* (Drum stick*, Moringa oleifera*)-10g + *Geru,* red earth- 30 g. Mix all the powdered ingredients thoroughly. Add the mixture to 150 ml of castor oil and heat gently. Allow it to cool slightly, ensuring it remains warm but not too hot. Apply the warm preparation to the affected area *two to three times a day.*
Respiratory signs in poultry	• Whole plant of *Kalmegh* (Green Chiraitta, *Andrographis paniculata*) boiled in 2 litre waters, reduced to half + 2 handful of uncooked, milled rice. Let the preparation sit overnight to enhance its potency. Feed the mixture to the flock to reduce mortality caused by respiratory infections.
Roundworm in poultry	• Give juice obtained from unripe fruit of *Papita*; (Papaya, *Carica papaya*) 10-15 ml in 50 ml water to 10 birds for 5 days for Ascarids. • Give juice from 250 g fresh rhizome of *Haldi* (Turmeric, *C longa*) in drinking water of 10 birds at monthly intervals.

(*Sources:* Anjaria *et al.* 2000; Anonymous 2002-04; Swarup *et al.* 2013; Ethnoveterinary Formulations - English | Dairy Knowledge Portal :Accessed on 4-2-2025)

Box 6.2. Ethnoveterinary Remedy for Lumpy Skin Disease

Lumpy Skin Disease (LSD), is a highly contagious viral disease affecting ruminants. It is caused by the Lumpy Skin Disease Virus (LSDV), a member of the Capripoxvirus genus. The disease is characterized by fever, nodules on the skin, mucous membranes, and other parts of the body. LSD is a non-zoonotic transboundary disease transmitted by arthropod vectors, including biting flies, mosquitoes, and ticks. LSD first emerged in India in 2019 in Odisha, subsequently spreading to multiple states, causing significant economic losses. Control and preventive measures include: movement control of bovines and quarantining, implementing biosecurity measures, vector control by sanitising sheds and spraying insecticides, and mass awareness campaigns. ICAR-NRCE, in collaboration with ICAR-IVRI, has developed a 100% effective vaccine named Lumpi-ProVacInd. However, there is no specific treatment for LSD. Symptomatic treatment involves the use of anti-inflammatory drugs and antibiotics. The National Dairy Development Board (NDDB) has scientifically validated the following ethnoveterinary formulations as a first-line management approach for LSD:

Oral preparation I (one dose): *Betel (P. betel) leaves -10 + Kaali Mirch (Pepper, P. nigrum)- 10 g + salt - 10g. Prepare a paste by blending betel leaves, black pepper, and salt. Mix the paste with jaggery and administer as follows: Day 1: Every 3 hours. Day 2 onwards: 3 times daily for 2 weeks.*

Oral preparation II: *Garlic (Allium sativum) - 2 pearls + Coriander (C sativum) seeds - 10 g + Cumin (C cyminum) - 10 g + dry Cinnamon leaves- Indian bay (Connamomum tamala) leaves - 10 g + Black pepper (P nigrum)- 10 g + Betel (P betel) leaves - 5 + Shallots (A cepa, var aggregatum) - 2 bulbs + Turmeric (C. longa) - 10g + Chirata ((S chirata) leaf powder - 30 g + Sweet basil (Ocimum basillicum)*

1 handful + Neem (A indica) leaves - 1 handful + Stone fruit (A marmalos) 1 handful + Jaggery - 100 g. Blend all ingredients into a paste and mix with jaggery. Divide into two portions and administer as follows: Day 1: Feed small portions every 3 hours. Day 2 onwards: Feed twice daily until recovery

External application: *Indian nettle (Acalypha indica) leaves - 1 handful + Garlic (A sativum) - 2 pearls + Neem (A indica) leaves - 1 handful + Coconut or Sesame oil - 500 ml + Turmeric (C longa) powder - 20 g + Henna leaves - 1 handful + Tulsi leaves - 1 handful. Blend all ingredients and mix with coconut or sesame oil. Boil the mixture, let it cool, and apply gently as a fomentation on lumps and swollen areas. If wounds are present- clean with a soft cloth and apply gently, avoiding excessive rubbing. For maggot-infested wounds, apply Custard apple (A squamosa) leaf paste or camphorated coconut oil only on the first day.*

(Source: Ethnoveterinary formulations at www.nddb.coop ; Punniamurthy, 2022)

EVM Challenges and the Way Forward

Despite growing scientific interest in EVM, several challenges hinder its widespread adoption:

- **Lack of Formal Education and Training:** Veterinary professionals receive little to no formal training in ethnomedicine or herbal veterinary care. There is an urgent need to integrate EVM into veterinary education and establish structured training programs.
- **Limited Scientific Validation:** Although interest in ethnomedicine is rising, few controlled studies have been conducted to assess the safety, efficacy, and quality of traditional remedies.
- **Standardization and Knowledge Transmission:** Efforts should focus on standardizing EVM practices and disseminating knowledge to similar agro-climatic regions through an efficient extension system.
- **Access to Medicinal Plants:** Promoting herbal gardens and local cultivation of medicinal plants would ensure their availability and sustainability.
- **Data Collection and Networking:** Developing a comprehensive database on livestock populations, veterinary infrastructure, and ethno-veterinarians, including those in the NGO and private sectors, would facilitate collaboration and policy-making.

Conclusion

Folk medicine forms the bedrock of India's healing traditions. Charaka, often hailed as the Father of Ayurveda, emphasized the importance of indigenous knowledge by consulting shepherds and forest dwellers to identify medicinal plants. This ancient wisdom thrives among tribal communities across the Indian subcontinent. The written tradition began with the Atharva Veda, marking advancements in healing practices for both humans and animals, deeply rooted in faith. Today, this traditional knowledge, recognized as Ethnoveterinary Medicine (EVM), remains integral to animal husbandry and healthcare in India. Prior to the introduction of Western veterinary education in the 19th century under British rule, traditional knowledge guided livestock care. However, the rise of modern veterinary infrastructure, including fast-acting synthetic drugs, led to a decline in these traditional practices. Despite this, many animal owners, particularly pastoral and tribal communities, continue to rely on EVM for maintaining livestock health and treating diseases. These communities possess a rich repository of practical knowledge, gained through experience and a deep understanding of animal behaviour, nutrition, and health. They can accurately identify disease symptoms, determine seasonal disease patterns, and diagnose and treat illnesses using natural remedies. Their expertise extends to recognizing the pharmaceutical properties of medicinal plants in their environment. In resource-limited and ecologically diverse regions, pastoralists not only excel in animal healthcare but also contribute to biodiversity conservation, including indigenous livestock genetic diversity and medicinal plants. Over time, many traditional practices have been documented and scientifically validated, leading to their increasing integration into modern veterinary treatment protocols. This fusion of traditional wisdom and scientific research enhances the credibility and acceptance of EVM in contemporary veterinary medicine.

Given the global trade landscape and the limitations of single-molecule drug technologies, there is renewed interest in traditional practices. Efforts to document, validate, and integrate EVM with modern veterinary science are gaining momentum, ensuring its preservation and wider acceptance. Today the EVM is projected as a sustainable alternative for animal healthcare and disease management. High cost and inaccessibility of modern veterinary drugs, along with concerns such as antibiotic resistance, ecotoxicity, and drug residues in animal products, pose significant challenges. In contrast, EVM is cost-effective, eco-friendly, and often safer, making it a viable alternative to synthetic drugs. Several countries have already banned or restricted synthetic chemicals in animal healthcare, favouring ethnoveterinary practices, particularly herbal treatments, as safer options for disease management and antibiotic resistance (AMR) control. EVM is also gaining attention as a key component of organic farming in both developing and developed nations. Medicinal plants used in EVM have been found to boost immunity, reduce infection severity, and promote faster recovery. Many herbs, such as barberry, have shown effectiveness against drug-resistant bacterial strains due to their natural phytochemical composition. Research highlights the potential of herbs and botanicals as alternatives to chemotherapy and as supportive therapies for enhancing immunity and reducing antibiotic dependence.

To sum up, ethnoveterinary medicine remains a valuable resource for animal healthcare in India. As scientific validation progresses, its integration with modern veterinary practices is becoming more feasible. With continued research, policy support, and educational reforms, EVM has the potential to be a mainstream, sustainable, and effective approach to livestock healthcare in the future.

References

Adharshana S and Aishwarya K . 2023. Belief system and oral tradition of Toda tribal religion. In: *Proceedings of ICSSR Sponsored National Seminar on Actions@75 -ek Bharat Shrestha Bharat: Culture, Skills, Beliefs and Rituals of Janajatis of India with Special Reference to the Scheduled tribes of the Nilgiris District.* 12-13 October 2023, Sri Ramkrishna College of Art and Science, Coimbatore. pp.11-13. Coimbatore Institute of Information Technology, Coimbatore, Tamil Nadu, India.

Akoh OU, Mac-Kalunta OM and Amadi OK. 2020. Phytochemical screening and *in-vivo* anthelmintic activity of *Allium sativum* leaf extract. *Communication in Physical Sciences* **7**(1): 18-23.

Al-Snafi AE. 2022. Pharmacological and toxicological effects of *Nicotiana tabacum*. *World Journal of Advanced Pharmaceutical and Medical Research* **3**(1): 6-18.

Anjaria J V, Dwivedi S K, Desai P, Thaker A and Parabia M. 2000. *Animal Friends*. Shri Jivdaya Kendra, Luni-Mumbai, India

Anjaria JV. 1973. *Some Pharmacological Studies on the Isolated Principles of Leptadenia reticulata.* PhD thesis. 172 p. Department of Pharmacology. Gujarat College of Veterinary Science and Animal Husbandry, Anand, Gujarat, India.

Anjaria JV and Gupta, I. 1967. Studies on lactogenic property of *Leptadenia reticulata* (*Jivanti*) and leptaden tablets in goats, sheep, cows and buffaloes. *Indian Veterinary Journal* **44**: 967-74.

Anonymous. 2002-2004. *Mission mode Project on Collection, Documentation and Validation of Indigenous Technical Knowledge. Document 1, 2.1, 2.3 and 3.* Directorate of Information and Publications of Agriculture (DIPA), Indian Council of Agricultural Research, New Delhi, India.

Anonymous. 2003. *Identification and Evaluation of Medicinal Plants for Control of Parasitic Diseases of Livestock.* Technical Report. CIRG, Makhdoom, Mathura, Uttar Pradesh, India.

Banumathi B and Vaseeharan B. 2015. A report on medicinal plants used in ethnoveterinary practices of Toda tribe in the Nilgiri hills. *Journal of Veterinary Science & Technology* **6** (5): 245. doi:10.4172/2157-7579.1000245.

Barua CC, Yasmin N and Buragohain L. 2018. *Elsholtzia communis*: A review of its traditional uses, pharmacological activity and phytochemical compounds. *EC Pharmacology and Toxicology* **6**(9): 806-13.

Dar MS, Khuroo AA, Malik AH and Dar GH. 2018. Ethnoveterinary uses of some plants by Gujjar and Bakerwal community in Hirpora Wildlife Sanctuary, Kashmir Himalaya. *SKUAST Journal of Research* **20** (2): 181-86.

Devi Shivani. 2021. The Gaddi schedule tribe of Jammu and Kashmir (Historical, socio-cultural, religious, economic over view). *Ilkogretim Online - Elementary Education Online* **20** (3): 4933-40. doi: 10.17051/ilkonline.2021.03.506.4933 http://ilkogretim-online.org.

FAO. 1984. Traditional (indigenous) systems of veterinary medicine for small farmers in India (based on the work of Anjaria JV). FAO Regional Office for Asia and the Pacific, Bangkok, Thailand.

Gebrewbet GH and Hndeya AG.2023. Phytochemical screening and antibacterial activity studies on the crude leaf extract of *Solanum sisymbriifolium*: Traditional Ethiopian medicinal plant. *Advanced Gut & Microbiome Research* **2023** (1): 5525606. https://doi.org/10.1155/2023/5525606.

Ghoke SS, Jadhav KM and Thorat KS. 2012. Ethnoveterinary practices in camels of north Gujarat. *Journal of Camel Practice and Research* **19** (1): 79-80.

Ghurye GS. 1969. Features of caste system. In: *Caste and Race in India.* 5th edn. pp. 1-30. Popular Prakashan, Mumbai, India

Gurunathan A and Subramaniam P. 2014. Preliminary phytochemical studies in the leaf, stem and root extracts of the traditional medicinal plant species, *Thalictrum javanicum* Blume. *Ruhuna Journal of Science* **5**: 7-15.

Kale SM and Panchegaonkar MR. 1969. Treatment of sarcoptic mange in goats with oil of Karanj. *Indian Veterinary Journal* **46**: 622-25.

Khurana I. 1999. The milk that ate the grass. *Down to Earth* **April 15, 1999.** 24-31.

Köhler-Rollefson I, Mundy P and Mathias E. 2001. *A Field Manual of Camel Diseases: Traditional and Modern Healthcare for the Dromedary*. ITDG Publishing, London, UK.

Köhler-Rollefson I, Rathore S, Rollefson A and Hardy K. 2013. The Camels of Kumbhalgarh. A Biodiversity Treasure. Lokhit Pashu-Palak Sansthan, Sadri. http://www. lpps. org/wp-content/uploads/2013/10/Camels Of_ Kumbhalgarh_web. pdf. downloaded on 17-11-2023.

Kumar D, Kumar R and Sharda K. 2018. Medicinal property of *Nirgundi. Journal of Pharmacognosy and Phytochemistry* **7**(1S): 2147-51.

Leese AS. 1927. A *Treatise on the One-Humped Camel in Health and in Diseases*. pp.264-65. Haynes & Sons, Maiden Lane, Stampford, Lincolnshire, UK. https://archive.org/details/treatiseonehumpedcamel/ pdf downloaded on 20-01-2025.

Mahmood KT, Mugal T and Haq IU. 2010. *Moringa oleifera*: a natural gift-A review. *Journal of Pharmaceutical Sciences and Research* **2**(11): 775-81.

Maiti S, Chakravarty P, Garai S, Bandyopadhyay S and Chouhan VS. 2013. Ethno-veterinary practices for ephemeral fever of Yak: A participatory assessment by the Monpa tribe of Arunachal Pradesh. *Indian Journal of Traditional Knowledge* **12** (1): 36-39.

Meena DC, Garai S, Maiti S and Mandi K. 2019. Pastoralists in modern India: Current status and future prospectus. In: *Research Trends in Multidisciplinary Research.* 1st edn. pp. 21-33. (Ed) Jayakumar R. Akinik Publications, New Delhi, India.

Meena DC, Garai S, Maiti S, Bhakat M, Meena BS and Kadian KS. 2020. Ethno-Veterinary practices used for common health ailments of sheep and goat: A participatory assessment by the Raika pastoralist of Marwar Region, Rajasthan. *Indian Journal of Animal Sciences* **90** (9): 1310-15.

Meena DC, Garai S, Maiti S, Bhakat M, Meena BS and Kadian KS. 2023. Ethno-veterinary practices for camel diseases: A participatory assessment by the Raika pastoralist of Rajasthan. *Indian Journal of Animal Sciences* **93**(1): 45-50.

Meena DC, Garai S, Maiti S, Bhatt N, Meena BS. 2020b. Ethno-veterinary practices followed by Raika pastoralists of Rajasthan: A descriptive study. Journal of Pharmacognosy and Phytochemistry **9** (2S): 63-66.

Nair BM and Natesan P. 2024. Management of mastitis using trans-disciplinarily validated ethno-veterinary practices. *IntechOpen*. doi: 10.5772/intechopen.112976.

Namsa ND, Mandal M, Tangjang S and Mandal SC. 2011. Ethnobotany of the Monpa ethnic group at Arunachal Pradesh, India. *Journal of Ethnobiology and Ethnomedicine* **7**:1-15. http://www.ethnobiomed.com/content/7/1/31.

Nimbalkar SD, Patil DS and Deo AD. 2020. Ethnoveterinary practices (EVP) for control of ectoparasite in livestock. *Indian Journal of Traditional Knowledge* **19**(2): 401-05.

Pandey NK, Somvanshi SP, Prakash O and Kumar S. 2020. Indigenous knowledge of agriculture and animal husbandry practiced by Monpa tribes of Tawang Arunachal Pradesh. *The Pharma Innovation Journal* **9**(4): 1012-16.

Punniamurthy N. 2022. *Down to Earth*, November 21, 2022. https://www.downtoearth.org.in/health/antimicrobial-resistance-use-these-ethnoveterinary-medicines-for-lumpy-skin-disease-86096, accessed on 3-02-2025.

Rahman SA. 2004.The history of veterinary education in India. *Journal of Veterinary Medical Education* **31**(1): 55-61.

Rajkumari R, Nirmala RK, Singh PK, Das AK, Dutta BK and Pinokiyo A. 2014. Ethnoveterinary plants used by the Chiru tribes of Manipur, Northeast India. *Indian Journal of Traditional Knowledge* **13** (2): 368-76.

Ranjan R, Biswal JK, Sharma AK, Kumar M and Pattnaik B. 2016. Managements of Foot and Mouth Disease in a dairy farm: By Ethnoveterinary practice. *Indian Journal of Animal Sciences* **86** (3): 256-59.

Samal PK, Dhyani PP and Dollo M. 2010. Indigenous medicinal practices of Bhotia tribal community in Indian Central Himalaya. *Indian Journal of Traditional Knowledge* **9** (2): 256-60.

Santhanakrishnan R, Hafeel A, Hariramamurthi BA and Unnikrishnan PM. 2008. Documentation and participatory rapid assessment of ethnoveterinary practices. *Indian Journal of Traditional Knowledge* **7**(2): 360-64.

Sharma DK, Saxena VK, Sanil NK and Singh N. 1998. Evaluation of oil of *Cedrus deodara* and benzyl benzoate in sarcoptic mange in sheep. *Small Ruminant Research* **26**(1-2): 81-85.

Sharma VP, Köhler-Rollefson I and Morton J. 2003. *Pastoralism in India: a scoping study.* Indian Institute of Management and League of Pastoral Peoples, Ahmedabad, India.

Sindhia VR and Bairwa R. 2010. Plant review: *Butea monosperma. International Journal of Pharmaceutical and Clinical Research* **2**(2): 90-94.

Somavanshi R, Saminathan M and Singh RK. 2017. *Veterinary Science and Animal Husbandry in Medieval and Modern India.* 88 p. ICAR- Indian Veterinary Research Institute, Izatnagar, Uttar Pradesh, India.

Srivastava GC and Chhabra RC. 1971. Treatment of sarcoptic mange in buffaloes with indigenous remedies. *Indian Veterinary Journal* **48**: 196-99.

Swarup D, Dey S and Dwivedi HP. 2013. Indigenous technical knowledge in animal husbandry and ethnoveterinary medicine. *Handbook of Animal Husbandry*. pp 953-79. Directorate of Knowledge Management in Agriculture, Indian Council of Agricultural Research, New Delhi, India.

Swarup D, Kumar N, Sharma AK, Chander M and Naresh R. 2004. Evaluation of peach (*Prunus persica*) leaves with fresh milk in the treatment of FMD lesions/wounds. In: *Validation of Indigenous Technical Knowledge in Agriculture Mission mode Project on Collection. Documentation and Validation of Indigenous Technical Knowledge Document 3.* pp. 254-57. Indian Council of Agricultural Research, New Delhi, India.

Thakur A, Sharma M, Thakur R, Sharma A, Suman M, Verma N and Vanita B. 2020. Ethnoveterinary practices among Gaddi pastoralists of North-Western Himalayan region, Himachal Pradesh. *Indian Journal of Animal Production and Management* **36** (3-4): 97-100.

Tiwari L and Pande PC. Indigenous veterinary practices of *Darma* valley of Pithoragarh district, Uttaranchal. *Indian Journal of Traditional Knowledge* **5** (2): 201-06.

7

Evidence-Based Ethnoveterinary Medicine

S. Dey

Śāstraṁ jyōtiḥ prakāśārthaṁ darśanaṁ buddhirātmanaḥ| tābhyāṁ bhiṣak suyuktābhyāṁ cikitsannāparādhyati||ncikitsitē trayaḥ pādā yasmādvaidyavyapāśrayaḥ| tasmāt prayatnamātiṣṭhēdbhiṣak svaguṇasampadi|

Scientific scriptures provide light for illumination (to remove darkness of ignorance or to know things) and one's own intellect is like eyes. The physician who uses both (scientific knowledge and own intellect) properly, does not commit mistakes during treatment because in treatment, the other three components are dependent on the physician. Hence the physician should make all efforts to enrich his qualities.

(Charaka Saṁhitā, Su. Sth. 9.17.24–25; translation by Tomar and Kumar 2020)

Introduction

All living beings face the disease related challenges. Since the beginning of civilizations, humans have sought ways to keep themselves and their socio-economically important animals healthy. Ethnoveterinary medicine (EVM), acquired through practical experience over millennia, encompasses people's knowledge, skills, methods, tools, technologies, practices, and beliefs about caring for and alleviating health constraints in domestic animals. In addition to healing practices, EVM includes healthful animal husbandry practices such as breeding, feeding, housing, and human resource management. Traditionally passed down orally from generation to generation, EVM was the cornerstone of animal husbandry and healthcare, contributing to human well-being through sustainable and healthy livestock raising. The advent of modern therapeutic practices in the veterinary profession and the global promotion of Western knowledge-based veterinary education systems endangered these age-old, experience-based traditional knowledge systems. This shift made it difficult for younger generations to appreciate and use the beliefs and practices of their forefathers. It was during the last quarter of the 20th century that EVM received global recognition as a legitimate field of scientific research. It was acknowledged as a potential resource that could play a pivotal role in grassroots development and poverty alleviation, empowering people by enhancing the use of their own knowledge and resources, especially in developing countries (Iqbal *et al.* 2005). Studies revealed that despite modern scientific and technological advancements, a significant number of animal owners worldwide still use EVM, particularly ethnoveterinary botanical medicine for their animals (Souto *et al.* 2012). However, in the modern era of evidence-based veterinary medicine, many professionals question the usefulness, applicability, and adaptability of EVM. Critics argue that traditional practices lack scientific evidence and may not be as effective as claimed. Some practices are also considered harmful or may not be readily available (Swarup *et al.* 2013).

Evidence-Based Veterinary Medicine (EBVM)

Evidence-based medicine (EBM) is defined as the conscientious, explicit and judicious use of current best evidence from research for the care of an individual patient. It integrates individual clinical expertise with the most reliable clinical evidence derived from systematic research. Individual clinical expertise refers to the proficiency and judgment that clinicians develop through their experience and practice. The best available external clinical evidence encompasses research that is clinically relevant, often originating from basic medical sciences, and particularly from patient-centred clinical research. This type of research focuses on evaluating the accuracy and precision of diagnostic tests (including clinical examinations), the predictive value of prognostic markers, and the effectiveness and safety of therapeutic, rehabilitative, and preventive strategies. External clinical evidence plays a crucial role in refining medical practices. It challenges and updates previously accepted diagnostic tests and treatments, and also introduces newer, more effective, accurate, and safer alternatives (Sackett *et al.* 1996).

The concept of EBM was first described in human medicine in the early 1990s and was introduced to veterinary medicine a decade later. However, it is not clear whether the EBM approach used in human medicine can be applied to the same extent as to veterinary medicine (Vandeweerd *et al.* 2012). The EBVM is broadly defined as the use of the current best evidence in making clinical decisions (Cockcroft and Holmes 2003). According to the Evidence-Based Veterinary

Medicine Association (EBVMA), EBVM is a formal approach that integrates the best research evidence, clinical expertise, and the specific needs or preferences of each client in clinical practice. This approach heavily relies on findings from research studies that were critically designed and statistically evaluated (https://ebvma.org/, accessed on 24.10.24).

Evidence-based veterinary medicine has the potential to help clinicians to make more informed decisions, but many veterinarians have various reasons for not fully adopting this approach. Some argue that since veterinarians have always used evidence to guide their clinical decisions, they are inherently practicing EBVM. However, the evidence they often rely on tends to be informal, unsystematic, and sometimes haphazard. The core principle of EBVM is that, for any clinical decision, all relevant research evidence should be systematically searched for, rigorously evaluated for its quality, and assessed for its applicability to that specific decision. This process aims to provide the best available evidence and offers a clear grading of its quality or reliability, making the decision-making process transparent and repeatable. Further, veterinary practitioners, compared to those in human medicine, often face a shortage of high-quality evidence, such as systematic reviews, meta-analyses, and resources akin to the Cochrane Reviews. There is also a lack of high-quality patient-centred research, the basic understanding of clinical epidemiology by veterinary practitioners and the inadequacy of EBVM tools that can be applied to the busy daily practice of veterinarians. Moreover, private practitioners frequently have to pay for access to full-text articles, creating further barriers. Many veterinarian express concerns that EBVM's emphasis on clinical trials may not always reflect the realities of their local populations, and they feel that it can undervalue their clinical experience and expertise. Moreover, a lack of time and training is commonly cited as a significant obstacle to adopting EBVM (Vandeweerd *et al.* 2012, Turner and Royle 2015, Gibbons *et al.* 2021).

One of the most significant advances in veterinary medicine has been the collective expansion of knowledge. This growth includes a deeper understanding of animal diseases and health, as well as insights into the efficacy of diagnostic and therapeutic techniques. While the ease of accessing such information through online databases and search engines is beneficial, it also presents challenges. Practitioners must navigate the task of assessing the quality of the information and organizing it into a form that is practical and usable for clinical decision-making (Constable *et al.* 2017). Evidence synthesis is a crucial component of EBVM. It involves identifying relevant evidence, critically appraising it, and ultimately combining it into a format that can guide clinical decision-making. Effective evidence synthesis requires several key steps: finding the most efficient ways to search for existing veterinary evidence, assessing the quality of that evidence, improving reporting standards within the scientific literature, organizing the evidence into a practical and usable format, and developing methods for effectively delivering high-quality evidence to practitioners (https://www.nottingham.ac.uk/cevm/evidence-synthesis/evidence-synthesis. aspx., accessed on 23-10-2024). The most crucial aspect of evidence synthesis is the assessment of the quality of evidence provided by scientific articles. This assessment depends on the type of study and the authors' ability to clearly report what they did and how they did it. High-quality evidence is essential for the adoption of a particular treatment, diagnostic test, or prophylactic measure. The systematic reviews being designated a *priori* as the highest level of evidence and observational studies providing a lower quality of evidence. A poorly documented report usually provides unreliable evidence regarding the efficacy and safety of treatments (Constable *et al.* 2017). Toolkits have been developed for various aspects of evidence-based veterinary medicine, including evidence synthesis and critical appraisal. These toolkits contain standardized questions that can be applied to different types of research, such as systematic reviews and meta-analyses, randomized controlled trials, prognosis studies, diagnostic testing studies, cohort studies, case-control studies, as well as narrative texts and websites (https://www.nottingham.ac.uk/cevm/index.aspx., accessed on 23-10-2024).

Evidence- Based Ethnoveterinary Medicine (EBEVM)

Evidence-Based Ethnoveterinary Medicine (EBEVM) combines traditional animal health practices with modern evidence-based principles to improve veterinary care, especially in rural or resource-limited settings. It involves systematically researching and validating traditional knowledge and practices used by local communities to treat and manage animal health issues. The goal of EBEVM is to assess the effectiveness, safety, and applicability of these traditional remedies through rigorous scientific methods. The process includes field studies, laboratory tests, and clinical trials to determine the efficacy and safety of traditional treatments. By applying evidence-based approaches, EBEVM aims to create a more inclusive and culturally appropriate framework for veterinary care. It respects and preserves indigenous knowledge while ensuring that traditional practices are validated through modern scientific methods. This integration can result in more accessible, sustainable, and effective solutions for animal health, particularly in areas where conventional veterinary services may be limited.

Why EBEVM?

EVM encompasses traditional animal healthcare practices rooted in indigenous knowledge and cultural beliefs. While these practices have been utilized for generations, many remain undocumented and lack scientific validation through rigorous methods like randomized controlled trials. Without the application of rigorous evidence-based standards, anecdotes can easily evolve into widely accepted dogmas over time–even, if those beliefs are inaccurate (Chicoine 2024). Many experts and critics have raised concerns that while the popularity of traditional and complementary medicine is growing, the field continues to struggle with establishing appropriate models and providing sufficient scientific evidence. In philosophy, evidence is closely linked to epistemology, which examines the nature of knowledge and the processes through which it is acquired. Proponents of traditional and complementary medicine argue that the inability to measure certain phenomena using current scientific methods does not prove their non-existence. However, the inability to measure something is also not proof of its existence (Patwardhan 2014). The impact of ethnoveterinary medicine on the target-animal and its utility in local ecosystem must be considered before discarding it as pure myth.

Approaches to EBEVM

The approaches to EBVM involve five steps: formulating a clinical question, searching the literature for relevant evidence, critically appraising that evidence, applying the findings, and evaluating performance. Essential professional skills, such as patient advocacy, safeguarding animal welfare, and effective communication, are also academically important for EBVM (Dean *et al.* 2017). These EBVM approaches can be adapted with minor adjustments to support Evidence-Based Ethnoveterinary Medicine (EVEVM). For example, in EVM, knowledge is often passed down orally, meaning that peer-reviewed journals and scientific publications may not be the sole sources of the best evidence. As such systemic documentation and critical analysis of EVM practices are the necessary initial steps. Steps for research on traditional herbal medicine and folklore medicine suggested by the Central Council for Research in Ayurvedic Sciences (CCRAS) are shown in Figs 7.1. and 7.2 (Anonymous 2018).

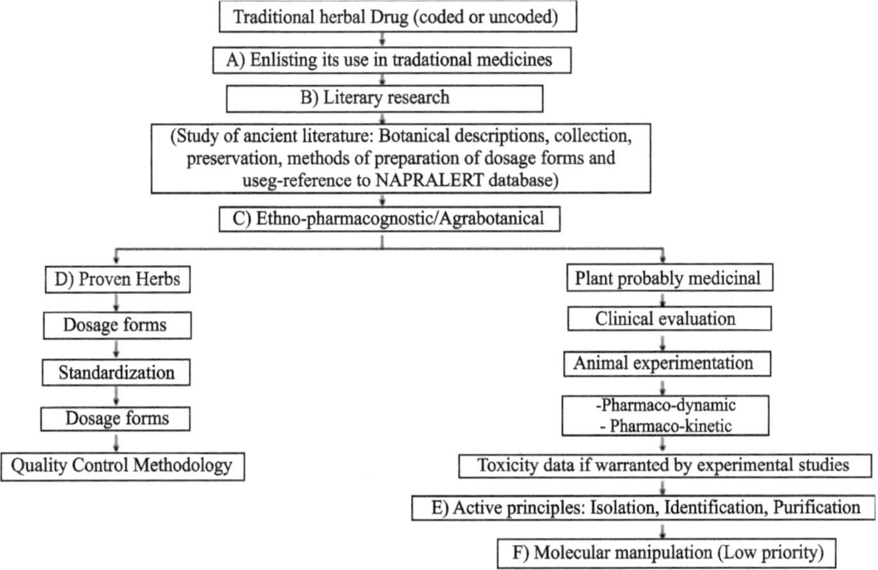

Fig. 7.1. *Approaches to validate traditional herbs (Source: Anonymous 2018).*

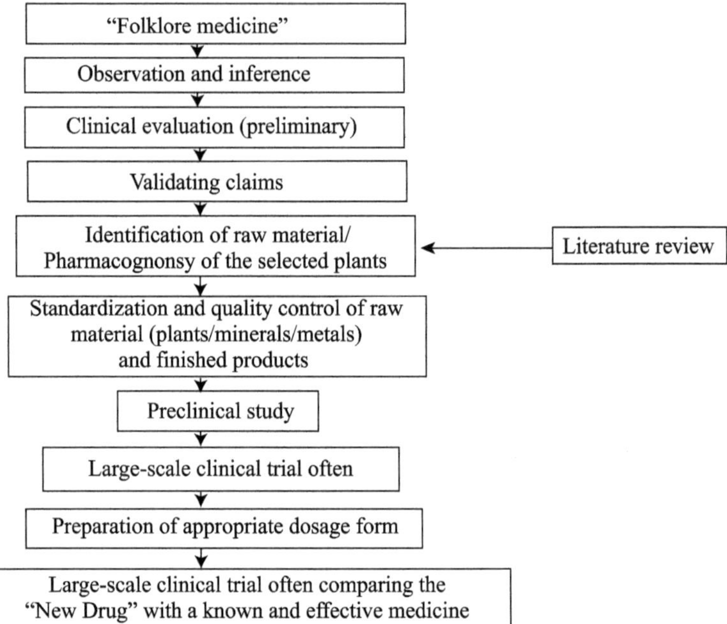

Fig. 7.2. *Approaches to validate ethnomedicines (Source: Anonymous 2018).*

Documentation and Scientific Validation of EVM

Documenting and validating traditional knowledge are crucial for developing an evidence-based healthcare system that effectively integrates Indigenous Technical Knowledge (ITK) with modern technologies. This integration aims to provide cost-effective, eco-friendly, and safe solutions for managing livestock health. Proper documentation allows for the evaluation of traditional practices, quantification of their effectiveness, preservation for future generations, and understanding of their scientific basis. It also addresses Intellectual Property Rights (IPR) issues related to indigenous knowledge. The absence of scientific validation and proper documentation limits the clinical and raises concerns about efficacy and safety, leading to hesitancy among veterinarians and farmers in adopting EVM treatments. A study among state-employed veterinarians and animal health technicians in South Africa's North West province found that while 77.4% were aware of EVM practices, 65.9% questioned their effectiveness. They perceived EVM as lacking a scientific foundation compared to Western veterinary medicine, which is grounded in science. Additionally, they noted that EVM lacks standardized dosages, information on side effects, and withdrawal periods (Ndou *et al.* 2024). The scientific validation increases the acceptability among modern clinicians and other stakeholders as part of standard treatment. For example, a substantial body of scientific evidence has been developed over time for various forms of Traditional Chinese Medicine (TCM). The clinical efficacy of acupuncture in humans has been evaluated through several hundred controlled clinical trials, with numerous systematic reviews available. Based on meta-analyses demonstrating its efficacy for specific conditions, acupuncture is gaining acceptance in academic medicine. In veterinary medicine, different forms of acupuncture are now used to treat small animals, horses, and livestock (Arlt and Heuwieser 2010).

Step 1–Documentation: The initial phase involves collecting and identifying potential ethnoveterinary technologies. In India, many pastoralist and tribal communities have a rich tradition of livestock rearing, utilizing locally available natural resources such as plants, animals, and minerals for animal treatment (See Chapter 6). Gathering information about these practices requires personal interactions with elderly community members, beneficiary farmers, local veterinary officers, and organizing workshops or group meetings with community representatives. However, traditional healers may sometimes be reluctant to share their knowledge. To encourage the sharing of Indigenous Technical Knowledge (ITKs), initiatives like the Mission Mode National Agricultural Technology Project (NATP) have introduced incentives.

Documentation of EVM should include details such as the practitioner's name, socio-cultural and geographical background, ingredients of the remedy, treatment methods, and the claimed effectiveness by traditional healers. Additional sources of information encompass scientific survey reports, books, ancient literature, and reports from various organizations. Reviewing published literature is essential to determine if there is existing information on the properties of the ingredients used or if validation studies have already been conducted on similar EVM practices. Traditional healers often recommend medicinal herbs or procedure-based therapies accompanied by specific dietary and lifestyle guidelines to promote health. Quantifying Indigenous Knowledge (QuIK) using Participatory Rural Appraisal (PRA) is a field method for assessing the extent and acceptance of ITK among farmers for managing farming systems. This approach identifies whether farmers are using traditional practices and captures their perceptions of these practices (Das *et al.* 2002). In PRA for veterinary remedies, a minimum of 20-25 respondents (animal owners) who use the technology are asked to score various aspects of EVM on a 1–10 scale. Parameters include effectiveness, treatment duration, cost, safety, accessibility, and comparison with standard allopathic treatments. If a technology is no longer in use or is ineffective, it may be deemed unsuitable for further validation. The literature review further aids in assessing which technologies warrant additional validation (Swarup *et al.* 2013).

Step 2–Identification, Collection and Processing of Medicinal Herbs: Medicinal plants are a key component in many ethnomedicinal practices, used either in whole or in parts (leaves, stem, roots, bark, flowers, fruits, and seeds). As such, proper identification and authentication of medicinal plants and raw materials is a vital step to EBEVM approaches. In traditional pharmacology (*Dravyagunasastra*), the entire plant or its specific parts are studied holistically, focusing on their *in vivo* effects on parameters such as the six *Rasa* (tastes), which indicate composition, properties, and biological activity. Other essential factors include *Guna* (inherent qualities of a substance), *Vīrya* (the substance's potency upon ingestion), *Vipaka* (the substance's properties post-digestion), and *Prabhava* (unique biological activity, utilized therapeutically). The active ingredients and pharmacological properties of medicinal herbs can vary significantly depending on plant species and variety, soil type, geoclimatic conditions, and harvesting and post-harvesting methods. Recognizing the influence of these factors on a plant's medicinal value, Ayurveda provides specific guidelines on identifying, collecting, processing, and storing plant materials. The Suśruta Saṃhitā describes the habitats and foliage characteristics of various plants to distinguish them from closely related species. In Chapter XXXVII, Suśruta recommends that medicinal plants be identified with the assistance of cowherds, hermits, hunters, forest dwellers, and gatherers of wild fruits and edible roots (Kunja Lal 1907). Similarly, Charaka emphasizes the importance of consulting such local experts for identifying medicinal herbs, stating: *Ōṣadhīr nāmarūpābhyāṁ jānatē hy ajapā vane, avipāś caiva gopāś ca ye cānye vanavāsinaḥ* (Charaka Saṃhitā, Sūtra Sthāna 1.120), which indicates that, goat-herds, shepherds, cowherds, and forest dwellers are well acquainted with the names and forms—that is, the identification—of various medicinal herbs and plants (Singh *et al.* 2020). A medical practitioner was also expected to be proficient in ten arts, including horticulture and the analysis and separation of metabolic compounds. (Anonymous 1949). According to Ayurveda, medicinal herbs and plants should be collected at specific seasons and stages of maturation to achieve optimal medicinal properties. Research indicates, for example, that the tender leaves of *Mangifera indica* (mango) collected in the spring exhibit the highest anti-neoplastic activity (Bhutia 2009). It is also recommended that medicinal plants be cultivated in clean, pollution-free environments to prevent contamination from toxic metals and other pollutants (Dey *et al.* 2009). Chapter 12 in this book summarizes guidelines for the cultivation, harvesting, collection, post-harvest processing, and storage of medicinal plants and botanicals, as well as methods for their authentication.

Ethnobotany — an interdisciplinary field of modern science — plays a crucial role in evidence-based traditional medicine. It examines the relationships between humans- and plants, exploring how people use them while integrating knowledge from botany, anthropology, and linguistics. Researchers in this field require botanical expertise to accurately identify and preserve plant specimens, anthropological insight to understand cultural perceptions and uses of plants, and linguistic skills to accurately transcribe local terms and comprehend native language structures. A thorough understanding of ethnobotany is crucial for the proper identification and authentication of plants. In modern pharmacology, active chemical components of plants are isolated and studied for their effects on microorganisms and body tissues, both *in vitro* and *in vivo.* While indigenous knowledge systems evaluate the systemic effects of plants, Western medicine often focuses on analysis at the atomic or cellular level (Shankar 2010).

Step 3–Evidence for Clinical Efficacy: Research and development on ethnic practices and traditional medicine, particularly on medicinal herbs, began in the late 19th and early 20th centuries. This led to significant progress in understanding plant pharmacognosy, discovering phytomolecules, and identifying their pharmacokinetic and pharmacodynamic mechanisms. Systematic reviews, meta-analyses, and clinical trials have validated the efficacy and, in many cases, have indicated the superiority of these molecules over synthetic counterparts (Leaviss *et al.* 2014). Clinical research in EVM aims to evaluate efficacy, ensure safety, and minimize bias. While randomized clinical trials (RCTs) remain the gold standard, evidence-based medicine also considers cross-sectional studies for diagnostic accuracy and basic sciences for understanding therapeutic questions (Sackett *et al.* 1996). The hierarchy of quality of clinical evidence is depicted in Fig. 7.3. In principle, evidence-based medicine should emphasize consistency in clinical practice quality and the reliability of scientific evidence to develop robust, evidence-based practices (Fig. 7.4).

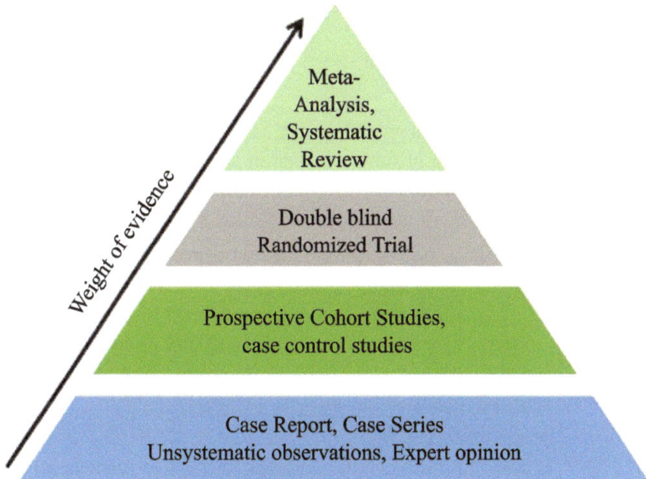

Fig. 7.3. *The hierarchy of clinical evidence (Source: Izzo et al.2016).*

Step 4–Translation of Evidence Based Phytotherapy into Clinical Practice: Documenting safety profiles and adverse reactions of herbal formulations is a prerequisite for clinical translation, and progress in this area has been observed in India over the past decade (Chaudhary *et al.* 2010). According to *AYUSH* guidelines, the initial steps involve demonstrating consistent, precise, and reproducible outcomes, with proven efficacy and minimal toxicity in preclinical studies. Despite the extensive traditional knowledge in herbal medicine, systematic studies yielding reproducible data are limited. Conducting double-blind, randomized controlled trials with standardized treatment protocols is crucial for this integration (Table 7.1). Quality guidelines for clinical evaluation of herbal medicines, as recommended by The Italian Pharmacological Society, are summarized in Table 7.2.

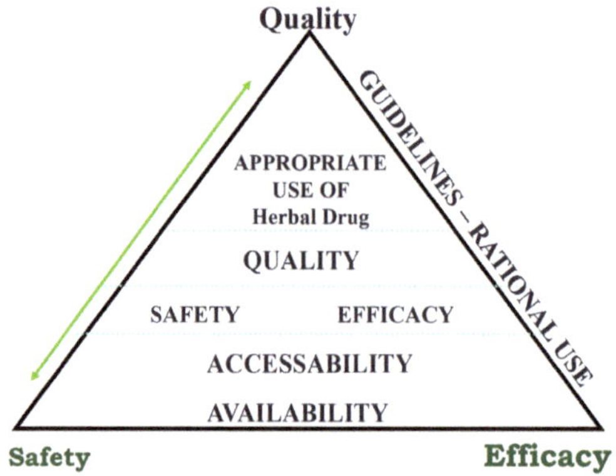

Fig. 7.4. Essential parameters for assessment of quality in evidence based ethnoveterinary medicine into a clinical practice.

Table 7.1. Criteria for quality clinical trial

Criteria	Description
Study design	• Must focus to a specific question • Randomized, in subject selection and grouping • Subject as well as investigator blind about treatment allocation • Application of appropriate statistical method
Enrolment and treatment	• Must define size of sample method of recruitment and details of follow-up • There should be parity among control and treatment groups • Additional treatment to any patient of any group should be avoided strictly
Outcome	• Must be measured in standard, valid reliable method of recruitment and details of follow-up • Primary and secondary outcomes must be estimated and reported with precision • Number dropout patient should be less than 20 % of the total subject in any particular group • In multicentre study difference among centres should be within certain limit
Bias	• Multiple analysis of results • Possible bias should be reported
Overall	• Interpretation should be on balancing benefit and adverse effect of the treatment

Table 7.2. Guidelines for preclinical and clinical evaluation of herbal medicine

Criteria	Description
Description of plant material	• Name of medicinal plant should be described in Latin binomial system (genus, species) variety, family and part of the plant used • Authentication of plant, method of reparation (such as fresh/dried/ powdered), drying and storage conditions • Details of geographical origin, harvest time method of storage, name and details of person /institution for authentication, and batch number • If test material is an extract detail method of extraction type of solvent used, time, temperature and yield must be recorded • Chemical profile of the extract (fingerprint) through chromatographic analysis
Description of plant extract	• Extract must be titrated; description of their content must be given. Pharmacological markers (if known) must be provided • Molecular formula, relative molecular mass, structural formula along with analytical procedure must be provided • For extract where active constituents are unknown pharmaceutical markers used/correlate to identify the provable compounds present must be justified
Specific criteria	• If the product is a mixture of plant materials, the composition and percentage of each individual component must be clearly specified • For plant materials that have been processed or enriched, details of the manipulation—including the type of processing, the procedure used, the manufacturer's name, lot number, chemical profile, and content of constituents with known therapeutic activity—must be provided • For products sold under a trade name, the manufacturers or supplier's name, source of materials, and therapeutic markers must also be specified

Ethnoveterinary medicine, particularly herbal products, has a longstanding tradition of efficacy, and is generally perceived as safe and non-toxic due to its natural components. However, despite extensive traditional use, evidence of safety — especially regarding subtle, long-term toxicities with delayed onset — is often lacking (DeSmet 2004). Use of indigenous drugs from plant origin forms a major part of ethnoveterinary medicine. Alongside traditional applications, the herbal products are marketed both as prescribed drugs and nutraceuticals (phytonutrients). The toxicity of herbal products can arise not only from adulteration, contamination, or misidentification of plant species but also from the inherent toxicity of the plants themselves (intrinsic factors). Proper toxicological assessment is essential to identify and mitigate potential safety concerns (Jordan *et al.* 2010). An increasing number of case reports since the late 1990s have documented both acute and chronic toxic effects from herbal product use. These effects vary, ranging from mild gastrointestinal distress and allergic reactions to serious renal and hepatic toxicity, haematological, cardiovascular, and neurological complications, and, in some cases, carcinogenic effects and even death, depending on the amount consumed and the duration of use (Bhowmik *et al.* 2009, Schilter *et al.* 2003).

The risk of adverse reactions from herbal remedies is influenced not only by the remedy itself and its dosage but also by consumer-specific factors such as age, genetic makeup, existing health conditions, and concurrent drug use. The quality of herbal remedies is also a crucial factor in determining their potential toxicity. Information on the known risks associated with herbal remedies should be systematically gathered, shared, and addressed. Unknown risks must be identified through rigorous post-marketing surveillance and experimental research (DeSmet 1995). Without targeted investigations, only acute and severe adverse effects are likely to be observed, and the absence of obvious toxic effects should not be interpreted as complete safety. Furthermore, the mechanisms underlying these toxicities need to be thoroughly understood to ensure the safe use of herbal products.

Intrinsic Toxicity Evaluation

The toxicity of medicinal plants and herbal products is often linked to the presence of bioactive compounds with known toxic potential (Woo *et al.* 2012). This issue becomes even more complex with heterogeneous and complex herbal mixtures, which can lead to unpredictable effects (Efferth and Greten 2012). Numerous examples of toxic endogenous compounds exist in the plant kingdom, including pyrrolizidine alkaloids (hepatotoxic, genotoxic, cytotoxic, and phototoxic), furan derivatives (hepatotoxic, possibly carcinogenic), epoxy-diterpenoids (hepatotoxic), anthraquinones (hepatotoxic), bis- benzylisoquinoline alkaloids (pulmonary toxicity), alkenyl benzenes (genotoxic, and carcinogenic), and ginkgolic acids (embryotoxic, cytotoxic, and neurotoxic) (Wang *et al.* 2021). For phytometabolites with confirmed toxic potential, regulatory authorities impose concentration limits to ensure the quality and safety of herbal medicines. Medicinal herbs are generally classified into three safety categories:

1. *High-risk herbs:* These contain high levels of potentially harmful substances, including *Atropa belladonna*, *Arnica* spp., *Aconitum* spp., and *Digitalis* spp.
2. *Potent-effect herbs*: Herbs with strong effects that may cause symptoms such as nausea or vomiting but are safe when used correctly, like *Lobelia* spp. and *Euonymus* spp.
3. *Specific-toxicity herbs:* Herbs known to have specific types of toxicity, such as *Comfrey* (*Symphytum* spp.), which is hepatotoxic due to pyrrolizidine alkaloids. Other examples include *Dryopteris* (male fern), *Viscum* (mistletoe), and *Corynanthe* (yohimbe)

***Acute/Sub-acute/Chronic Toxicity Evaluation*:** The preclinical toxicological assessment of herbal medicines utilizes both *in vitro* and *in vivo* models. Animal models are commonly used to evaluate acute and chronic toxicity levels. Guidelines for toxicity testing of chemical compounds were established by the Organization for Economic Cooperation and Development (OECD), providing standardized protocols for such evaluations (Fig. 7.5).

Acute toxicity assessment involves administering a single dose of the test product to each animal, with toxicity signs and mortality monitored over 14 days. This process determines parameters such as the maximum tolerated dose (MTD) and the median lethal dose (LD_{50}). For sub-acute and chronic toxicity evaluations, the test product is administered daily to the animals over extended periods, typically 28 days (OECD 407), 90 days (OECD 408), or 12 months (OECD 452). Key toxicity metrics such as NOAEL (no observed adverse effect level), NOEL (no observed effect level), LOAEL (lowest observed adverse effect level), and LOEL (lowest observed effect level) are determined. For medicinal plants and herbal products, oral administration is most common, though other routes like dermal, intraperitoneal, and inhalation are also employed. Inhalation exposure is mainly used for essential oils, while dermal toxicity is assessed for products intended for skin applications. Rodents (mice or rats) are the preferred animal models, though rabbits are also used for dermal exposure studies (Mekonnen *et al.* 2019, Liyanagamage *et al.* 2020).

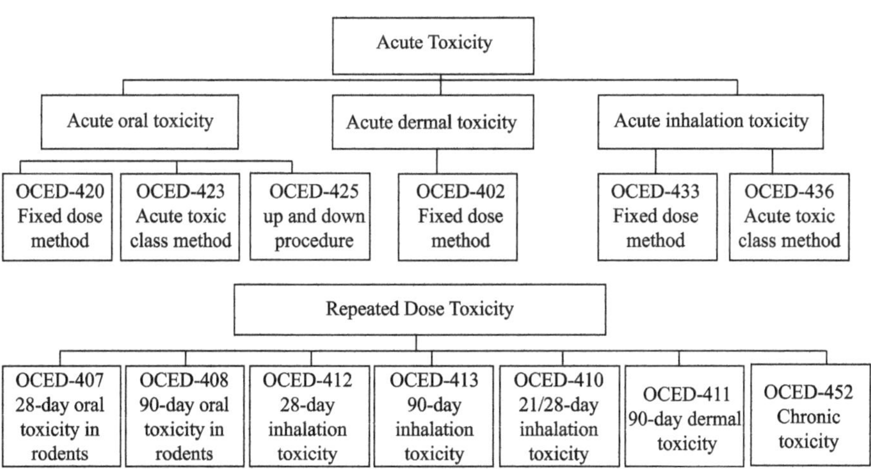

Fig. 7.5. *Guidelines for toxicological studies (Source: OECD 2018).*

***In vitro* Model for Toxicity Study:** Conducting *in vivo* studies with experimental animals presents significant ethical concerns. To address these issues and reduce the reliance on animal testing, *in vitro* models were developed to simulate *in vivo* conditions for toxicity testing, particularly through cell culture systems. However, cell culture systems have limitations, such as altered cell morphology, limited cell-to-cell interactions, and potential transformations of test materials. These factors can impact the accuracy of bioactivity predictions (Badr-Eldin *et al.* 2022).

Carcinogenic and Genotoxic Studies: Carcinogenesis is a complex process that can arise through various mechanisms. The induction of cancer involves the accumulation of genomic alterations, which can be induced directly or indirectly. Carcinogens are substances capable of inducing tumours (benign or malignant), increasing tumour incidence, or reducing the latency period for tumour development upon entry into the body via inhalation, injection, dermal contact, or ingestion. Carcinogens have conventionally been divided into two categories according to their presumed mode of action, genotoxic carcinogens and non-genotoxic carcinogens. Genotoxic carcinogens initiate carcinogenesis by directly interacting with DNA and/or the cellular apparatus involved in the preservation of the integrity of the genome. A non-genotoxic carcinogen has the potential to induce cancer without interacting directly with either DNA or the cellular apparatus involved in the preservation of the integrity of the genome. The genotoxicity assays are typically used to distinguish those chemicals with the potential to directly affect the integrity of DNA from those that do not (Jacobs *et al.* 2020).

Although often perceived as innocuous by the general public, many herbs harbour phytochemicals that are either directly reactive towards DNA or likely to disturb cellular homeostasis, cell-cycle, and/or genome maintenance mechanisms; this may translate into genotoxicity, carcinogenicity, or co-carcinogenicity (Poivre *et al.* 2017). Studies on certain herbs highlighted genotoxic and carcinogenic risks associated with herbal medicines. This area requires careful investigation to ensure consumer safety. Certain plant-derived alkylating agents, considered pro-carcinogenic, interact with DNA bases, leading affected cells toward apoptosis or carcinogenesis (Kristanc and Kreft 2016). For instance, aristolochic acids (AAs), naturally occurring in many Aristolochiaceae plants, pose a severe risk for nephropathy, urological, hepatobiliary cancers, and more, often carrying a distinctive mutational signature. Despite these risks, herbal products containing AA are still manufactured and marketed worldwide with limited regulation, and potential environmental exposure receives minimal attention (Das *et al.* 2022). Case-control studies in Scandinavia, France, and Switzerland have linked Digoxin-a common medication derived from the digitalis plant-to an increased cancer risk. Besides digitalis, extracts from *Aloe vera* (whole leaf), *Ginkgo biloba*, Goldenseal root powder, and Kava are classified as possibly carcinogenic to humans (Group 2B) based on sufficient evidence from animal studies (Grosse *et al.* 2013). Since no specific guidelines for testing carcinogenicity of herbal medicinal products are available, OECD guidelines (OECD 451 & OECD 453) for pharmaceutical compounds are used for carcinogenicity studies for herbal products (Poivre *et al.* 2017). Animal models can also be used for carcinogenicity testing of herbal products used as medicine or nutraceutical. Long-term animal studies have also raised concerns about the carcinogenic potential of essential oils and herbal medicines derived from *Panax ginseng*, *Hydrastis canadensis*, *Piper methysticum*, and *Silybum marianum* (https://monographs.iarc.who.int/, accessed on 28.08.2024).

Genotoxicity refers to the ability of a substance to damage genetic material (DNA) within a cell, which can lead to mutations, disruptions of normal cell function, or cell death. Genotoxic substances can cause structural changes in chromosomes (chromosome aberrations) or impact the replication process, potentially leading to cancer and other genetic diseases if the damage is not properly repaired. Mutagenicity, a subset of genotoxicity, specifically involves the ability of a substance to cause genetic mutations—permanent alterations in the DNA sequence of a cell. These mutations can affect a single gene or larger regions of the chromosome and can be inherited if they occur in germ cells (sperm or egg cells), or can lead to cancer and other health issues if they occur in somatic (body) cells. It should be noted that not all genotoxic events lead to mutagenicity. A systematic review of 239 articles published between 1975 and 2020 showed that 18% of 478 medicinal plant species, spanning 111 botanical families, contain secondary metabolites with mutagenic potential, such as pyrrolizidine alkaloids (da Silva Dantas *et al.* 2020). These findings underscore the need for more stringent safety assessments of herbal medicines. Different *in vitro* and *in vivo* methods are available to assess genotoxicity, and they cover the different mechanisms of genotoxicity (such as gene mutations, primary DNA damage, and numerical and structural chromosomal damage). For more reliable evaluation, more than one assay is required; the bacterial reverse mutation assay, which covers gene mutations, and the *in vitro* micronucleus test, which covers chromosome aberrations. In case *in vitro* test identifies positive genotoxic endpoints, then further *in vivo* testing is required.

Evidence of Toxic Interaction: The increasing demand for the toxicological evaluation of herbal medicinal products has led to the development of various methods for toxicity testing (Woo *et al.* 2012). The Omics approach provides reliable information at the cellular level about the interactions between toxic xenobiotics and biological systems. The ultimate goal is to uncover the mechanisms behind the effects of specific compounds. Omics-based approaches in toxicology evaluate the interactions between xenobiotics and living cells at different levels. Sometimes medicinal plants can initiate the metabolic activation of phytometabolites. In these situations, omics technologies can identify reactive metabolites of natural molecules and the targeted peptides modified by these interactions. Toxico-transcriptomics detects effects on gene transcription, Toxico-proteomics identifies protein alterations, and Toxico-metabonomics analyses physiological changes, such as perturbations in the metabolic profile.

The purpose of this approach is to assess protein alterations as a consequence of exposure to xenobiotics. The changes can consist of modified protein levels, increased/decreased activation of key proteins (for example, apoptosis-related proteins), structural modifications, and post-translational protein modifications (e.g., phosphorylation, glycosylation, acetylation, and proteolysis). The proteomics research has different areas of interest: protein profiling proteomics (quantitative evaluation), structural proteomics, functional proteomics, and protein-protein interactions. The identification of biomarkers that are closely connected to the toxicity signature of xenobiotic compounds (Fig. 7.6) represents an important issue for the use of proteomics in toxicology (Jităreanu *et al.* 2023).

Toxico-metabonomics: It is a subset of metabolomics, which involves the quantitative analysis of all metabolites, focusing on the metabolic response of organisms to toxic agents over time. This approach has several applications-evaluating the levels of endogenous biochemicals potentially affected by interaction with toxic agents, identifying metabolites of toxic compounds to reveal their molecular mechanisms of action and discovering novel biomarkers of toxicity. Toxico-metabonomics can also be used in herbal medicinal products to evaluate herb-host interactions. Most studies use experimental animal models to evaluate the metabolic response to these interactions.

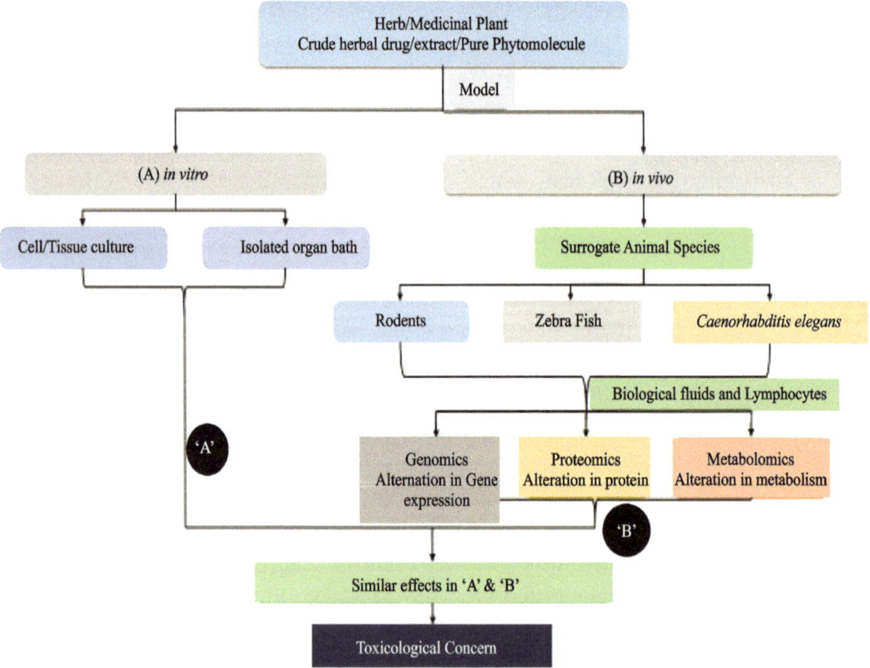

Fig. 7.6. *Crucial steps in assessing evidence of toxicity (Source: Ouedraogo et al. 2012).*

Toxicity due to Extrinsic Factors

Over recent decades, the increasing demand for natural products has propelled significant growth in the phyto-industry, resulting in a diverse array of herbal products used as medicines, cosmetics, and phytonutrients. However, this expansion has also led to fraudulent practices, including the adulteration and substitution of herbal materials and the addition of synthetic compounds. Common contaminants in herbal medicinal products include dust, pollen, insects, rodents, parasites, microbes, fungi, mold, toxins, pesticides, toxic heavy metals, and/or prescription drugs (Posadzki *et al.* 2013). Misidentification of medicinal plants and/ or substitution of medicinal plants with unknown harmful botanicals also contribute to the possibilities of the adverse effects. Traditionally, medicinal plants were cultivated on quality land or harvested by experienced collectors from pristine forests with minimal human interference. Today, many medicinal plants are commercially grown across varied environments, potentially compromising their purity and quality. To reduce costs, some manufacturers substitute authentic medicinal plants with others that may have similar properties but lack the same efficacy. Additionally, many producers fail to adhere to Good Manufacturing Practices (GMP) throughout the entire process, from herb collection to final product delivery. Poor quality control of herbal products can pose health hazards, as some products may contain unusually high concentrations of potent and poisonous ingredients, leading to serious adverse effects if consumed (WHO 2007). Implementing stringent GMP guidelines is essential to ensure the quality, safety, and consistency of herbal medicines. These guidelines encompass appropriate personal hygienic practices, design and maintenance of production facilities, and rigorous production and process controls. Adherence to these standards helps prevent contamination and adulteration, safeguarding consumer health.

Contaminants in Medicinal Herbs and Products: The risk of toxicity in medicinal herbs and herbal products is significantly increased by extrinsic contaminants, which primarily include chemical contaminants like mycotoxins, toxic heavy metals (e.g., lead, mercury, cadmium, thallium, and arsenic), polycyclic aromatic hydrocarbons, fumigants, pesticide residues and residual solvents. These contaminants are introduced during cultivation, processing, or storage and may have adverse health effects on consumers. Environmental pollution, as well as the use of fertilizers and pesticides, contributes to contamination of soil, irrigation water, and air, leading to the uptake and accumulation of heavy metals in medicinal plants (Dey *et al.* 2009).

Studies reported the presence of both biological and chemical contaminants in traditional herbs and herbal products at concentrations exceeding permissible limits. A systematic review and meta-analysis of 91 scientific articles, published in peer-reviewed journals from 1982 to 2021, examined studies from 28 countries across Asia, Africa, Europe, and South America. Conducted in accordance with the

Preferred Reporting Items for Systematic Reviews and Meta-Analyses (PRISMA) guidelines, the review identified metals (56.0%), microbial contaminants (27.5 %), and mycotoxins (18.7 %, 17/91) as the most prevalent contaminants. Approximately 16.4 % (1236 out of 7518) of the analysed samples had contaminant levels exceeding regulatory limits (Opuni *et al.* 2023). The World Health Organization (WHO) issued guidelines for monitoring heavy metals in medicinal plants and herbal products, establishing maximum permissible limits for toxic metals such as lead, arsenic, and cadmium to ensure consumer safety (WHO 1998).

Mycotoxins are produced as secondary metabolites by wide range of fungi usually found in hot and humid climatic conditions. Increasing evidence of microbial toxins in herbal products is reported due to both field and post-harvest contamination by various toxic fungi and bacteria. In addition to environmental conditions, plant genotype and fungus strain also affect mycotoxin occurrence. Mycotoxin contamination is more prevalent in developing countries, largely due to inadequate storage practices and limited adoption of Good Agricultural Practices (GAP) and Good Harvesting Practices (GHP). Numerous reports from India highlight cases of mycotoxin contamination in aromatic medicinal plants and herbal products (Tripathy *et al.* 2015). Major mycotoxins in herbal medicines include aflatoxin, ochratoxin A, trichothecenes and fumonisin B, mainly produced by *Aspegillus, Penicillium* and *Fusarium* (Yu *et al.* 2022). Mycotoxin contamination in food and feed poses significant health risks to both humans and animals. For instance, ochratoxin A is linked to nephropathy across animal species, and the International Agency for Research on Cancer has classified it as a possible human carcinogen (Category 2B). Mycotoxins can also lead to hepatotoxicity, nephrotoxicity, immunotoxicity, neurotoxicity, and teratogenicity, underscoring their global health importance (da Rocha *et al.* 2014). The presence of mycotoxins in herbal medicines may also lead to drug interactions, influence therapeutic effects, and potentiate adverse effects.

Pesticides are a class of substances or mixtures of substances designed to prevent, destroy, repel, or control pests, including insects, weeds, fungi, rodents, bacteria, and other organisms that can harm crops, animals, and human health. They are widely used in agriculture to protect crops from damage, increase yields, and prevent the spread of disease. However, direct or indirect exposure to pesticides may pose potential health risks to man and animals. Health hazards associated with pesticide exposure include hepatotoxicity, nephrotoxicity, neurotoxicity, diabetes, cancer, and endocrine disruption. Pesticide residues are reported in medicinal herbs from several countries, including India. Analysis of 75 samples of 33 different dried herbs from Brazil demonstrated that 26 samples (34.6 %) contained at least one pesticide. While many of the reported levels were within regulatory limits, some pesticides degrade slowly and can bioaccumulate, posing potential health risks over time (Mello *et al.* 2024).

Residual solvents are volatile organic chemicals used or produced during the manufacturing of drug substances, excipients, and medicinal products, including herbal drug substances and herbal medicines. These solvents, on the basis of their potential health risks are classified into three categories: Class 1, Class 2, and Class 3. Class 1 solvents, such as 1,1,1-trichloroethane, 1,1-dichloroethene, 1,2-dichloroethane, benzene, and carbon tetrachloride, are known or strongly suspected human carcinogens. Residual solvents are indeed a significant concern in the manufacturing of herbal products. The presence of Class 1 solvents in herbal products, as reported in studies from Africa and Asia, highlights the need for stringent quality control to ensue consumer safety (Opuni *et al.* 2023).

Adulteration: Adulteration in herbal products refers to the presence of chemical substances or other botanicals that are not labelled or prescribed as part of the intended use in herbal medicine. It involves intentionally or unintentionally substituting or adding other substances that compromise the quality, purity, and therapeutic effectiveness of the products. Adulteration of medicinal herbs and products can also lead to the possibility of overdose, interactions, and serious health complications. Additionally, it reduces consumer's trust in herbal products, affecting the market and livelihoods of genuine producers, underscoring the need for stringent quality control, authentication methods, and regulatory oversight in the herbal product industry to ensure safety and efficacy. Adulterants can be intentional or unintentional and can occur in following forms:

Substitution with Similar-looking Plants: The growing international demand for herbal medicines has led to widespread adulteration and species substitution in the raw herbal product trade. Such practices can reduce therapeutic efficacy and may introduce toxic compounds if the substituted plant has harmful properties. Often, less expensive or more readily available plant species are used in place of valuable ones owing to their similar appearance. For instance, bark preparations of *Saraca asoca*, traditionally used in India to treat uterine bleeding and in various Ayurvedic formulations, are frequently adulterated with bark from *Polyalthia longifolia* (Indian fir or mast tree), *Shorea robusta* (sal tree), *Mallotus nudiflorus* (false white teak), and *Humboldtia vahliana* (Srirama *et al.* 2017). Ayurveda recognizes the issue of species substitution through the concept of *Abhava Pratinidhi Dravya*, which focuses on the rational substitution of crude drugs when the desired plant species or other drugs is unavailable. This concept is documented in Bhavaprakasha, one of the Laghutrayi texts written in the 16th century AD. The *Abhava Pratinidhi Dravya* compilation includes 47 plant-based drugs (*Sthavara Dravya*), 2 animal-based drugs (*Jangama Dravya*), 7 mineral- and metal-based drugs (*Bhoumya Dravya*), and 5 food substances (*Ahariya Dravya*) pairs. The substitution is based on Ayurveda principles, that both the drugs *Abhava Pratinidhi* should possess similar *Guna* and proven pharmacological and therapeutic activities (Giri 2013).

***Use of Exhausted or Depleted Plant Material*:** After the active compounds have been extracted from medicinal plants, the leftover material (often of low therapeutic value) is sometimes reused as adulterated raw material. Products made from depleted material have little to no therapeutic benefit, misleading consumers and potentially delaying effective treatment.

Adulteration with Non-medicinal Plant Parts: Parts of a plant that lack the required active compounds, such as stems or leaves when the root is needed, are sometimes added to increase bulk. This reduces the therapeutic value of the preparation, and depending on the plant, the substituted parts may have undesired or harmful effects.

Intentional Substitution with Hazardous Plants: In some cases, plants with similar appearance but toxic properties are added intentionally, either for cost savings or due to unavailability of the genuine plant. This can result in severe health effects, including poisoning, organ failure, or even death in extreme cases.

Addition of Artificial Colouring Agents or Chemical Substances: Artificial dyes and synthetic chemicals are sometimes added to enhance the colour or perceived potency of herbal products. Some of these additives may cause allergic reactions, toxicity, or other health issues, especially if they include hazardous chemicals not intended for human consumption.

Mixing with Inorganic Substances: Weight enhancers, such as sand, soil, or stones, are sometimes mixed with powdered herbs to increase product weight and volume. This type of adulteration dilutes the potency of the herb and poses health risks from ingestion of non-medicinal substances, which can cause digestive and kidney issues.

Substitution with Synthetic Drugs: Certain synthetic drugs are sometimes added to herbal products to mimic therapeutic effects. The most common chemical drug adulterants in herbal medicinal products reported during 2004-2015 included sildenafil, famotidine, ibuprofen, promethazine, diazepam, nifedipine, captopril, amoxicillin and dexamethasone (Calahan *et al.* 2015). The adulteration with these synthetic prescription drugs can have serious side effects and may interact dangerously with other medications, posing significant health risks.

In summary, assessing the safety of scientifically-backed ethnoveterinary practices is essential, especially for herbal or herbo-mineral drugs and nutraceuticals used in animal healthcare and productivity enhancement. Adherence to Good Agricultural Practices (GAP), Good Manufacturing Practices (GMP), Good Laboratory Practices (GLP), and other guidelines established by national and international agencies is crucial for producing quality herbs and herbal products. Several guidelines are available online, including: *FAO-Good Agricultural and Collection Practices for Medicinal Plants* (https://dmapr.icar.gov.in/Downloads/ Illustratedbooklet.

pdf#:), *WHO-Guidelines on Good Agricultural and Collection Practices (GACP) for Medicinal Plants* (https://www.who.int/publications/i/item/9241546271), *FDA- Current Good Manufacturing Practices (CGMPs) for Food and Dietary Supplements | FDA-National Medicinal Plant Board-Good Agricultural Practices Standard for Medicinal Plants-Requirements* (https://www.nmpb.nic.in/sites/default/files/STANDARD_FOR_GAPMP.pdf), *National Medicinal Plant Board-Standard for Good Field Collection Practices of Medicinal Plants* (https://nmpb.nic.in/sites/default/files/STANDARD_FOR_GFCP2.pdf), *WHO Guidelines for Selecting Marker Substances of Herbal Origin for Quality Control of Herbal Medicines Anex-1*(iris.who.int/bitstream/handle/10665/258720/9789241210034-eng.pdf?sequence=1), *CCRAS-General Guidelines for Safety/Toxicity Evaluation of Ayurvedic Formulations* (https://ccras.nic.in/wp-content/uploads/2024/07/CCRAS_Guideline-of-Safety_Toxicity.pdf) and *CCRAS-General Guidelines for Drug Development of Ayurvedic Formulations* (CCRS-Guidline of Drug_Book-7_CD MATTER.pdf). These guidelines support the development and use of safe, high-quality herbal products in animal care.

Conclusion

For centuries, ethnoveterinary medicine (EVM) was central to animal husbandry and healthcare. In the mid-1800s, a scientific approach to healthcare began to emerge in medical schools, soon influencing veterinary medicine. The discovery of causative agents—such as bacteria, viruses, protozoa, and metazoans-and the development of antitoxins and vaccines marked a shift from traditional practices to a modern healthcare system (Dossey and Swyers 1991). A pivotal moment occurred in 1910 with the adoption of the Flexner Report, which emphasized the need to update medical curricula and enforce scientific methods in medical education. This shift led to substantial funding for modern medical practices, while support for other healthcare systems waned (Wynn and Schoen 1998). The introduction of modern therapeutic practices and the spread of a Western knowledge-based veterinary education system significantly undermined traditional knowledge systems, making it challenging for younger generations to appreciate and utilize the practices of their ancestors. It was not until the last quarter of the 20th century that EVM gained global recognition as a potential alternative for mitigating the negative socioeconomic and environmental impacts of contemporary treatment and management approaches for domestic animals. This sparked widespread interest in documenting and validating EVM practices, beginning in the early 1980s. Since then, numerous studies have been conducted, many reports published, and various conferences and workshops held. Although these efforts have helped to preserve EVM knowledge from extinction, scepticism and concerns about effectiveness of ethnoveterinary practices have persisted, especially in the context of modern evidence-based therapeutic practices.

Evidence-Based Medicine (EBM) relies on quantitative evidence on healthcare practices and the effects of interventions on diagnosis, treatment, and prevention of health issues. It helps to minimize reliance on anecdote, personal experience, and opinion. For any healthcare practice to be accepted or rejected, there must be sufficient evidence demonstrating that the intervention has a beneficial, harmful, or negligible effect, typically through randomized controlled trials. EBM, therefore, offers a more systematic, reliable, and reproducible method of documenting outcomes than unverified personal experiences or anecdotal reports. While the philosophy of EBM also encompasses skills and experience in patient management, critical appraisal, and causal reasoning (Bonnett and Reid-Smith 1996), the randomized controlled trials (RCT) and high-quality clinical trials remain a gold standard. However, RCT based studies remain relatively scarce in ethnoveterinary practices. Instead, many traditional practices are accepted as proven-to-work without rigorous testing. In many cases, efficacy studies rely on descriptions of clinical cases, often conducted retrospectively without a robust study design. Additionally, evidence derived from *in vitro* or experimental studies may not accurately reflect real-world clinical outcomes for specific populations. Since the World Health Organization (WHO) recognized the value of traditional medicine in 1976, efforts have grown to integrate EVM with mainstream practices. Research into EVM has, though gained considerable attention, a substantial proportion of the available studies remain field reports, anecdotal or poorly documented. Poor data quality and inadequate documentation have hindered the full integration of EVM practices into mainstream veterinary medicine. Additionally, the erosion of traditional knowledge and resources—including authentic ethnolects (language varieties associated with specific ethnic or cultural groups) —has led to the rise of quackery and unethical practices under the guise of ethnoveterinary medicine. Many formulations used by so-called traditional practitioners contain spurious ingredients or are adulterated with synthetic drugs. Reports on adverse effects, sale of adulterated plant products and misleading health claims of herbal products demand proper regulations and legislation to ensure acceptable quality, safety and efficacy of medicinal plant preparations. These issues highlight an urgent need for rigorous scientific research to validate the efficacy, safety, and mechanisms of action of traditional remedies. High-quality research—including clinical trials, pharmacological studies, safety evaluation and systematic reviews—can help to validate EVM remedies. Collaborative initiatives between scientists, healthcare professionals, traditional healers and policy makers could bridge EVM and modern science. Integrating Indigenous Technical Knowledge with contemporary methods may provide cost-effective, sustainable solutions for global livestock health management.

References

Anonymous. 1949. The method of theoretical and practical study. In: *The Caraka Samhita pp. 187-217.* Shree Gulabkunverba Ayurvedic Society, Jamnagar. (2015.63710.The-Caraka-Samhita1.pdf (archive.org), downloaded on 21-08-2024.

Anonymous. 1992. Evidenced based working group: Evidenced based medicine, A new approach to teach in the practice of medicine. *American Medical Association* **268:** 2420-25.

Anonymous. 2018. *General Guidelines for Clinical Evaluation of Ayurvedic Interventions.* Vol III, 123p. Central Council for Research in Ayurvedic Sciences, Ministry of Ayush, Government of India, New Delhi, India. pdf down loaded on 23-10-2024.

Arlt S and Heuwieser W. 2010. Evidence-based complementary and alternative veterinary medicine-A contradiction in terms. *Berl Munch Tierarztl Wochenschr* **123**(9-10): 377-84.

Badr-Eldin SM, Aldawsari HM, Kotta S, Deb PK and Venugopala KN. 2022. Three-dimensional *in vitro* cell culture models for efficient drug discovery: Progress so far and future. *Prospects in Pharmaceuticals* **15** (8): 926-27. https://doi.org/10.3390/ph15080926.

Bhowmik D, Chiranjib Dubey P, Chandira M and Kumar KPS. 2009. Herbal drug toxicity and safety evaluation of traditional medicines. *Archives of Applied Science Research* **1:** 32-56.

Bhutia Doma. 2009. *Evaluation of Antineoplastic Activity of Medicinal Plants.* 128p. MVSc thesis, Division of Medicine, Indian Veterinary Research Institute, Izatnagar, Uttar Pradesh, India.

Bonnett B and Reid-Smith R.1996. Critical appraisal meets clinical reality: evaluating evidence in the literature using canine hemangiosarcoma as an example *Veterinary Clinics: Small Animal Practice* **26:** 29-63.

Calahan J, Howard D, Almalki AJ, Gupta MP and Calderón AI. 2015. Chemical adulterants in herbal medicinal products: a review. *Planta Medica* **82**(6): 505-15.

Chaudhary A, Singh N and Kumar N. 2010. Pharmacovigilance boon for the safety and efficacy of Ayurvedic formulation. *Ayurveda and Integrated Medicine* **1:** 251-56.

Chicoine A. 2024. Evidence-based veterinary pharmacology: How to critically assess therapeutic efficacy. https://www.mmhimages.com/production/Creative/1OldBackup/fetch_Backup/CVC_SD_2013_proceedings_proof/data/PDFs/, pdf downloaded on 26-10-2024.

Cockcroft PD and Holmes MA. 2003. Introduction. In*: Handbook of Evidence-Based Veterinary Medicine*. pp. 1-22. Blackwell Publishing, Oxford, UK.

Constable PD, Hinchcliff KW, Done SH and Grünberg W. 2017. *Veterinary Medicine: A Textbook of the Diseases of Cattle, Horses, Sheep, Pigs and Goats*. 11th edn. pp. xiii-xv. Elsevier, St Louis Missouri, USA.

da Rocha ME, Freire FD, Maia FE, Guedes MI and Rondina D. 2014. Mycotoxins and their effects on human and animal health. *Food control* **36**(1): 159-65.

da Silva Dantas FG, de Castilho PF, de Almeida-Apolonio AA, de Araújo RP and de Oliveira KM. 2020. Mutagenic potential of medicinal plants evaluated by the Ames Salmonella/microsome assay: A systematic review. *Mutation Research Review* **786:** 108338.

Das S, Thakur S, Korenjak M, Sidorenko VS, Chung FF and Zavadil J. 2022. Aristolochic acid-associated cancers: A public health risk in need of global action. *Nature Reviews Cancer* **22** (10): 576–91. https://doi.org/10.1038/s41568-022-00494-x.

Das SK, Arya HPS, Subba Reddy G and Mishra A. 2002. *Inventory of Indigenous Technical Knowledge in Agriculture Document 1.* 411p. Mission Unit, Division of Agriculture Extension, Indian Council of Agricultural Research, New Delhi, India

Dean R, Brennan M, Baillie S, Brearley J, Cripps P, Eisler MC, Ewers R, Handel I, Holmes M, Hudson C and Jones P. 2017. The challenge of teaching undergraduates evidence-based veterinary medicine. *Veterinary Record* **181**(11): 298–99.

DeSmet PAGM. 1995. Health risks of herbal remedies. *Drug-Safety* **13**: 81–93.https://doi.org/10.2165/00002018-199513020-00003.

DeSmet PAGM. 2004. Health risks of herbal remedies: An update. *Clinical Pharmacology and Therapeutics* **76:** 1–17. doi 10.1016/jelpt2004.03.005.

Dey S, Saxena Anju, Dan Ananya and Swarup D. 2009. Indian medicinal herb a source of lead and cadmium for man and animals *Archives of Environmental and Occupational Health* **64** (3): 164-67.

Dossey L and Swyers JP. 1991. *Introduction in Alternative Medicine: Expanding Medical Horizons*. 763 p. US Government Printing Office, Washington, USA.

Efferth T and Greten HJ. 2012. Potential of 'Omics' technologies for implementation in research on phytotherapeutical toxicology. In: *Advances in Botanical Research.* Vol 62. pp. 343–63. (Eds) Shyur L.-F and Lau, Allen SY. Elsevier Academic Press: Cambridge, MA, USA.

Gibbons PM, Anderson SL, Robertson S, Thurman FK and Hunt JA. 2021. Evaluation of an evidence-based veterinary medicine exercise for instruction in clinical year of veterinary medicine program. *Veterinary Record Open* **8** (1): e3. https://doi.org/10.1002/vro2.3.

Giri CM. 2013. Concept of *Abhava pratinidhi dravyas*, a rational substitution of drugs-a review. *International Journal of Advanced Ayurveda, Yoga, Unani, Siddha and Homeopathy* **2**(1): 148-61.

Grosse Y, Loomis D, Lauby-Secretan B, El Ghissassi F, Bouvard V, Benbrahim-Tallaa L, Guha N, Baan R, Mattock H and Straif K. 2013. Carcinogenicity of some drugs and herbal products. *Lancet Oncology* **14**(9): 807-08.

Iqbal Z, Jabbar A, Akhtar MS, Muhammad G and Lateef M. 2005. Possible role of ethnoveterinary medicine in poverty reduction in Pakistan: Use of botanical anthelmintics as an example. *Journal of Agriculture and Social Sciences* **1:** 187-95.

Izzo AA, Hun-Kim S, Radhakrishnan R and Williamson EM. 2016. A critical approach to evaluating adverse events and drug interactions of herbal remedies. *Phytotherapy Research* **30:** 691-700.

Jacobs MN, Colacci A, Corvi R, Vaccari M, Aguila MC, Corvaro M, Delrue N, Desaulniers D, Ertych N, Jacobs A and Luijten M. 2020. Chemical carcinogen safety testing: OECD expert group international consensus on the development of an integrated approach for the testing and assessment of chemical non-genotoxic carcinogens. *Archives of Toxicology* **94**: 2899-923. https://doi.org/10.1007/s00204-020-02784-5.

Jităreanu A, Trifan A, Vieriu M, Ioana-Cezara Caba, Mârt I and Agoroaei L. 2023. Current trends in toxicity assessment of herbal medicines: A narrative review. *Processes* **11**: 83 https://doi.org/10.3390/pr11010083.

Jordan SA, Cunningham DG, and Marles RJ. 2010. Assessment of herbal medicinal products: Challenges, and opportunities to increase the knowledge base for safety assessment. *Toxicology and Applied Pharmacology* **243:** 198–216.

Kristanc L and Kreft S. 2016. European medicinal and edible plants associated with subacute and chronic toxicity part I: Plants with carcinogenic, teratogenic and endocrine-disrupting effects. *Food and Chemical Toxicology* **92:** 150–64. https://doi.org/10.1016/j.fct.2016.04.007.

Kunja Lal K.1907. *An English Translation of the Sushruta Samhita, Vol. I Sutrashanam.* (Ed. & Publ.), Kaviraj Kunja Lal Bhishagratna., 10, Kashi Ghose's Lane, Calcutta (Kolkata), India.

Leaviss J, Sullivan W, Ren S, Everson-Hock, E, Stevenson M, Stevens J W and Cantrell A. 2014. What is clinical effectiveness of cytosine compared with varenicline for smoking cessation? A systematic review and economic evaluation. *Health Technology Assessment* **18:** 120-24.

Liyanagamage DSNK, Jayasinghe S, Attanayake A P and Karunaratne V. 2020. Acute and subchronic toxicity profile of a polyherbal drug used in Sri Lankan traditional medicine. *Evidence Based Complementary and Alternative Medicine* **2020:** 1-12. 2189189, https://doi.org/10.1155/2020/2189189.

Mekonnen A, Tesfaye S, Christos SG, Dires K, Zenebe T, Zegeye N, Shiferaw Y and Lulekal E. 2019. Evaluation of skin irritation and acute and subacute oral toxicity of *Lavandula angustifolia* essential oils in rabbit and mice. *Journal Toxicology* **2019**: 1-8.5979546, https://doi.org/10.1155/2019/5979546.

Mello DC, Pires NL, Evangelista CS and Caldas ED. 2024. Pesticide residues in dry herbs used for tea preparation by UHPLC-MS/MS: Method validation and analysis. *Journal of Food Composition and Analysis* **125**: 105817. https://doi.org/10.1016/j.jfca.2023.105817.

Ndou RV, Materechera SA, Mwanza M and Otang-Mbeng W. 2024. Perceptions of ethnoveterinary medicine among animal healthcare practitioners in South Africa. *Onderstepoort Journal of Veterinary Research* **91**(1): a2138. https://doi.org/ 10.4102/ojvr. v91i1.2138.

OECD 2007. Detailed review paper on cell transformation assays for detection of chemical carcinogens. In: *OECD Series on Testing and Assessment, No. 31.* OECD Publishing, Paris, France. https://doi.org/10.1787/8b8ef5ba-en, accessed on 10-12- 2024.

OECD.2018. *Guidelines for the Testing of Chemicals, Section 4.* Organization for Economic Cooperation and Development (OECD) Publishing, Paris, France. DOI: 10.1787/20745788.

Opuni KF, Kretchy JP, Agyabeng K, Boadu JA, Adanu T, Ankamah S, Appiah A, Amoah GB, Baidoo M and Kretchy IA. 2023. Contamination of herbal medicinal products in low-and-middle-income countries: A systematic review. *Heliyon:* **e19370**. https://doi.org/10.1016/j.heliyon.2023.e19370.

Ouedraogo M, Baudoux T, Stévigny C, Nortier J, Colet JM, Efferth T, Qu F, Zhou J, Chan K, Shaw D and Pelkonen O. 2012. Review of current and "omics" methods for assessing the toxicity (genotoxicity, teratogenicity and nephrotoxicity) of herbal medicines and mushrooms. *Journal of Ethnopharmacology* **140**(3): 492-512.

Patwardhan B. 2014. Bridging Ayurveda with evidence-based scientific approaches in medicine. *EPMA Journal* **5**: 19 http://www.epmajournal.com/content/5/1/19.

Poivre M, Nachtergael A, Bunel V, Philippe ON and Duez P. 2017. Genotoxicity and carcinogenicity of herbal products. In: *Toxicology of Herbal Products.* pp. 179-215. (Eds) Pelkonen O, Duez P, Vuorela P and Vuorela H. Springer International Publishing, Switzerland. DOI 10.1007/978-3-319-43806-1_9, accessed on 06-11-2024.

Posadzki P, Watson L and Ernst E. 2013. Contamination and adulteration of herbal medicinal products (HMPs): an overview of systematic reviews. *European Journal of Clinical Pharmacology* **69** (3): 295-307. DOI: 10.1007/s00228-012-1353-z

Sackett DL, Rosenberg WM, Gray JM, Haynes RB and Richardson WS. 1996. Evidence based medicine: What it is and what it isn't. *BMJ* **312**(7023): 71-72. doi: https://doi.org/10.1136/bmj.312.7023.71.

Schilter B, Andersson C, Anton V, Constable A, Kleiner J, O'Brien J, Renwick AG, Korver O, Smit F and Walker R. 2003. Guidance for the safety assessment of botanicals and botanical preparations for use in food and food supplements. *Food and Chemical Toxicology* **41:** 1625-49.

Shankar D. 2010. Conceptual framework for new models of integrative medicine. *Journal of Ayurveda and Integrative Medicine* **1**(1): 3-5. doi: 10.4103/0975-9476.59817. PMID: 21829291; PMCID: PMC3149389.

Singh RH, Singh G, Sodhi JS and Dixit U.2020. *Deerghanjiviteeya Adhyaya.* In: *Charak Samhita New Edition.* 1st edn. pp.3. (Eds) Dixit U, Deole YS and Basisht G. Jamnagar,

India CSRTSDC ebook. Available at: https://www.carakasamhitaonline.com/index.php?title=Deerghanjiviteeya_Adhyaya&oldid=45351.

Souto WM, Pinto LC, Mendonça LE, Mourão JS, Vieira WL, Montenegro PF and Alves RR.21012. Medicinal animals in ethnoveterinary practices: A World Overview. In: *Animals in Traditional Folk Medicine*. pp.43-66. (Eds) Alves R and RosaI I. Springer, Berlin, Germany. https://doi.org/10.1007/978-3-642-29026-8_4.

Srirama R, Santhosh Kumar JU, Seethapathy GS, Newmaster SG, Ragupathy S, Ganeshaiah KN, Uma Shaanker R and Ravikanth G. 2017. Species adulteration in the herbal trade: causes, consequences and mitigation. *Drug Safety* **40:** 651-61. https://doi.org/10.1007/s40264-017-0527-0.

Swarup D, Dey S and Dwivedi HP. 2013. Indigenous Technical Knowledge in animal husbandry and ethnoveterinary medicine. In: *Handbook of Animal Husbandry*. pp. 953-79. Directorate of Knowledge Management in Agriculture, Indian Council of Agricultural Research, New Delhi.

Tomar GS and Kumar N. 2020. *Khuddakachatushpada Adhyaya.* In: *Charak Samhita New Edition.* 1st edn. pp.11. (Eds) Dixit U, Deole YS and Basisht G. CSRTSDC ebook, Jamnagar, India. Available at: https://www.carakasamhitaonline.com/mediawiki1.32.1/index.php?title=Khuddakachatushpada_Adhyaya&oldid=44475.

Tripathy V, Basak BB, Varghese TS and Saha A. 2015. Residues and contaminants in medicinal herbs-A review. *Phytochemistry Letters* **14**: 67-78. https://doi.org/10.1016/j.phytol.2015.09.003.

Turner SW and Royle N. 2015. Evidence-based veterinary medicine. *Veterinary Record* **177**(11): 293-94.

Vandeweerd JM, Kirschvink N, Clegg P, Vandenput S, Gustin P and Saegerman C. 2012. Is evidence-based medicine so evident in veterinary research and practice? History, obstacles and perspectives. *Veterinary Journal* **191**(1): 28-34.

Wang Y-K, Li WQ, Xia S, Guo L, Miao Y, and Zhang B-K. 2021. Metabolic activation of the toxic natural products from herbal and dietary supplements leading to toxicities. *Frontiers in Pharmacology* **12**: 758468. doi: 10.3389/fphar.2021.758468.

WHO. 1998. *Quality Control Methods for Medicinal Plant Materials*. 154 p. World Health Organization, Geneva, Switzerland.

WHO. 2007. *WHO Guidelines on Good Manufacturing Practices (GMP) for Herbal Medicines*. 72 p. World Health Organization, Geneva, Switzerland. https://www.who.int/publications/i/item/9789241547161.

Woo CSJ, Lau JSH and El-Nezami H. 2012. Herbal medicine: Toxicity and recent trends in assessing their potential toxic effects. In: *Advances in Botanical Research.* Vol 62. pp. 365–84. (Eds) Shyur LF and Lau Allen SY. Elsevier Academic Press, Cambridge, MA, USA.

Wynn SG and Schoen AM. 1998. Fundamentals of complementary and alternative veterinary medicine In: *Complementary and Alternative Veterinary Medicine: Principles and Practices*. pp. 3-15. (Eds). Schoen AM and Wynn SG. Mosby, St. Louis, USA.

Yu J, Yang M, Han J and Pang X. 2022. Fungal and mycotoxin occurrence, affecting factors, and prevention in herbal medicines: A review. *Toxin Reviews* **41**(3): 976-94.

8

Overview of Ayurvedic System of Human and Animal Healthcare and Well-being

S.K. Kumar

āyuḥ-kāmayamānena dharmārtha-sukha-sādhanam; āyur-vedopadeśeṣu vidheyaḥ param ādaraḥ.

Life is the implementation of our desires (kāma). Dharma, artha, and sukha are part of it, as are the sādhanas—the means, the method, the practices of that implementation. One who is interested in how life works should pay humble attention to Ayurveda.

(Aṣṭāṅga Hṛdaya, Sūtra Sthāna 1.2; ayurveda-online.net)

1. Introduction
2. Evolution of Early Healing Practices and Brief History of Ayurveda:
   - Vedic Origin of Ayurveda: From God to Humans
   - Ayurveda in Buddhist Literature
   - Golden Age of Ayurveda: Samhita Period
   - Universal Education and Medical Institutions in Ancient India
   - Stagnation Phase
   - Modern Period and Resurgence of Ayurveda
3. Classical Texts in Ayurveda: Caraka Saṃhitā (Charaka Samhita); Suśruta Saṃhitā (Sushruta Samhita); Aṣṭāṅga Saṃgraha (Ashtanga Samgraha) and Aṣṭāṅga Hṛdaya (Ashtanga Hridaya); Laghu-trayī (Laghutrayee / the Lesser Triad)
4. Philosophy and Fundamental Principles of Ayurveda
5. Pramāṇa in Ayurveda: A Fundamental Concept of Knowledge Acquisition
6. Ayurveda and One Health
7. Conclusion

Introduction

Ayurveda, often referred to as the *Science of Life* and *Mother of All Healing* is among the oldest holistic healing systems, originating in India over 5,000 years ago. Its name derives from the Sanskrit words *āyus, Āyu* (Ayu-life) and Veda (knowledge). Unlike conventional medical approaches that primarily address disease symptoms, Ayurveda emphasizes maintaining a harmonious balance between the body, mind, spirit, and environment to promote overall well-being. According to Cāraka (Charaka), Ayurveda is that which deals with good, bad, blissful and sorrowful life, and with what is wholesome or unwholesome for it, as well as principle of longevity. Ayu itself is defined as 'the conjunction of the physical body, senses, mind, and soul, and is known by the synonyms dhāri (that which preserves vitality), *jīvita* (that which is alive), *nityaga* (that which is continuous), and *anubandha* (that which is interdependent, or a link between past and future lives)' (Singh et al. 2020):

hitāhitaṁ sukhaṁ duḥkhamāyustasya hitāhitam;
mānaṁ ca tacca yatrōktamāyurvēdaḥ sa ucyatē (Ch. Su. 1. 41).

śarīrēndriyasattvātmasaṁyōgō dhāri jīvitam;
nityagaścānubandhaśca paryāyairāyurucyatē (Ch. Su. 1.42).

The Charaka Samhita further emphasizes:

tasyāyuṣaḥ puṇyatamō vēdō vēdavidāṁ mataḥ; vakṣyatē yanmanuṣyāṇāṁ lōkayōrubhayōrhitam (Ch Su 1.43).

Translated as: 'Among the Vedas, Ayurveda is considered the most sacred, as it promotes the well-being of humans in both' (Singh *et al.* 2020).

Evolution of Early Healing Practices and Brief History of Ayurveda

The origins of both human and animal healing practices in India trace back to the Indus Valley Civilization (IVC). Archaeological evidence indicates that, alongside magico-religious rituals, the inhabitants utilized medicinal plants, minerals, and animal-derived substances—practices characteristic of early Ayurvedic medicine. Notably, depictions of flora such as neem (*Azadirachta indica*), pipal (*Ficus religiosa*), and acacia (*Acacia catechu*) have been found in Indus Valley artifacts (Arnott 2024). These plants are esteemed in Ayurveda for their therapeutic properties. The Pashupati seal from Mohenjo-Daro, portraying a figure seated in a cross-legged posture, suggests the existence of yogic practices during this era. The excavations of Neolithic archaeological sites in south central Asia, including the pre-Harappa phase in the Baluchistan region along with Vedic references also point to a connection between the Indus Valley sites and Vedic culture (Kizhakkeveettil 2024). Most likely, early healing practices of the IVC influenced the development of Ayurveda during the Vedic period, which evolved further as Vedic civilization transitioned from the Indus to the Gangetic Valley over more than two millennia.

Vedic Origin of Ayurveda: From God to Humans

Ayurveda, often regarded as an extension of the Atharva Veda, traces its earliest concepts to this ancient text from the 2nd millennium BCE. The Vedic medical tradition, spanning until approximately 800 BCE, addressed ailments such as fever (*takman*), cough, constipation, diarrhoea, dropsy (generalized oedema), abscesses, seizures, tumours, and skin conditions, including leprosy. Treatment methods prominently featured various herbs (Anonymous 2025). Herbs were often administered alongside hymns and rituals detailed in the *Kauśika Sūtra* of the Atharva Veda (Valiathan 2006). Traditionally attributed to the *Atharvans*, a group of sacred sages, the Atharva Veda details various treatment modalities, elaborates on the origins and pathogenesis of numerous diseases, and enumerates corresponding remedies. It serves as a compendium of medicine in its various stages of evolution, containing both primitive and highly advanced stages of therapy. The Atharva Veda combines psychosomatic techniques of healing—such as charms, incantations, prayers, and amulets—with the use of various herbal medicines. The following hymn from the Atharva Veda recounts four types of remedies or therapies to protect life:

Atharvanīrāngirasīrdaivīrmanuṣyajā uta. Osadhayaḥ pra jāyante yadā tvaṁ prāṣa jinvasi (Atharva Veda11.4.16); Translated as: 'O, life! You are propitious, the drug of *Atharvans* (charm), the drugs of *Angirasis* (juices of plants and animal parts), the divine drugs (prayers to the sun, water, and other natural elements), and drugs of human artifice, all bear fruition' (Anonymous 1949). Sharma (2013) interpreted these remedies as follows: *Atharvani* intended for psychic cures; *Angirasis* used as energizing tonics and tranquilizers; *Daivi* meant for sensuous purposes and *Human artifice remedies* included those prepared by people in laboratories. The esteemed 12th -century commentator on the Charaka Samhita, Chakrapani Datta, observed that the Atharva Veda itself evolved into Ayurveda, as its content primarily focuses on therapeutics. It also portrays Ayurveda as a system that harmonizes individuals with their inherent nature to maintain health (Kizhakkeveettil 2024).

The historical evidence for Ayurvedic texts, terminology and concepts appears from the middle of the first millennium BCE onwards. The main classical Ayurveda texts begin with accounts of the transmission of medical knowledge from the gods to sages, and then to human physicians. The Charaka Samhita offers a compelling narrative on the divine descent of Ayurveda to earth, marking a significant epoch in medical history. The introductory part of the Samhita mentions that knowledge was first recited by Brahma, to Daksha Prajapati. It was then transmitted to the Ashwin twins, the divine healers, and subsequently to Indra. Sage Bharadwaja, eager to acquire this wisdom, to find out way to overcome the diseases that assailed lives of righteous people, learned it directly from Indra, becoming the first human custodian of Ayurvedic knowledge (in that age of epoch). He shared this profound understanding with Atreya, who passed it to Punarnavasu, and ultimately to Acharya Agnivesha (Singh *et al.* 2020).

dīrghaṁ jīvitamanvicchanbharadvāja upāgamat;
indramugratapā buddhvā śaraṇyamamarēśvaram (Ch. Su.1.3).

Translated as: 'Bharadwaja, a great scholar, went to the King of Gods and the saviour Indra in quest of longevity' (Singh *et al.* 2020).

brahmaṇā hi yathāprōktamāyurvēdaṁ prajāpatiḥ;
jagrāha nikhilēnādāvaśvinau tu punastataḥ (Cha. Su. 1.4).

aśvibhyāṁ bhagavāñchakraḥ pratipēdē ha kēvalam;

ṛṣiprōktō bharadvājastasmācchakramupāgamat (Ch. Su. 1. 5).

Translated as: 'Ayurveda in its entirety as recited by Brahma was received by Prajapati at first. Then the Ashwins received the knowledge. From Ashwins, lord Indra received it fully. That is why Bharadvāja (Bharadwaj), as beseeched by the sages, came to Indra' (Singh *et al.* 2020).

The key highlights of the divine descent of Ayurveda to Earth include:

- **Eternal existence of Ayurveda:** Charaka posits that Ayurveda, the science of life, is without beginning, having eternally existed. This suggests that humanity has periodically received divine guidance in the art of healing.
- **Divine Bestowal to Bharadwaj:** In response to a profound health crisis afflicting humanity, a congregation of wise sages from India and neighbouring regions convened in the sacred Himalayas. They elected Bharadwaj to seek a remedy. He approached the deity Indra, who imparted to him the wisdom of Ayurveda in the following words: 'Ayurveda provides knowledge of *hetu* (etiology), *linga* (symptomatology), and *auṣadha* (therapeutics), and lays down the best ways for both the healthy and the sick. This tri-aphoristic, virtuous knowledge, continuing from time immemorial, was first revealed to Brahma.' (Singh *et al.* 2020).
- **Systematic Compilation:** Satisfied with the results, the sages commissioned six eminent scholars to compile and categorize the amassed data on diseases and remedies from various regions. After rigorous evaluation, Agnivesha's compilation, under the mentorship of the esteemed teacher Atreya, was deemed the most authoritative and was proclaimed as the definitive medical text.
- **Earliest Recorded Instance of a Medical Conference:** This account is notable as it may represent the earliest recorded instance of a medical conference convened to systematize knowledge derived from divine revelation, deep meditation, empirical observation, and generational experience. The assembly comprised numerous eminent sages, including Aṅgiras, Jamadagni, Vasiṣṭha, Kaśyapa, Bhṛgu, Ātreya, Gautama, Pulastya, Nārada, Asita, Agastya, Vāmadeva, Mārkaṇḍeya, Aśvalāyana, Parīkṣit, Bhikṣu Ātreya, Bharadvāja, Viśvāmitra, Cyavana, Dhaumya, Marīci, Śaunaka, and Maitreya among others, along with sages of the Vaikhānasa and Vālakhilya orders and several other revered seers (Ch. Su. 1. 5-15).

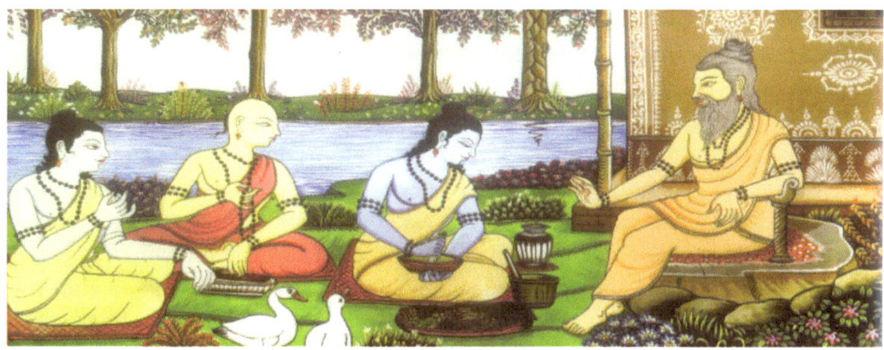

Fig. 8.1. *An artistic depiction of transfer of knowledge of Ayurveda*

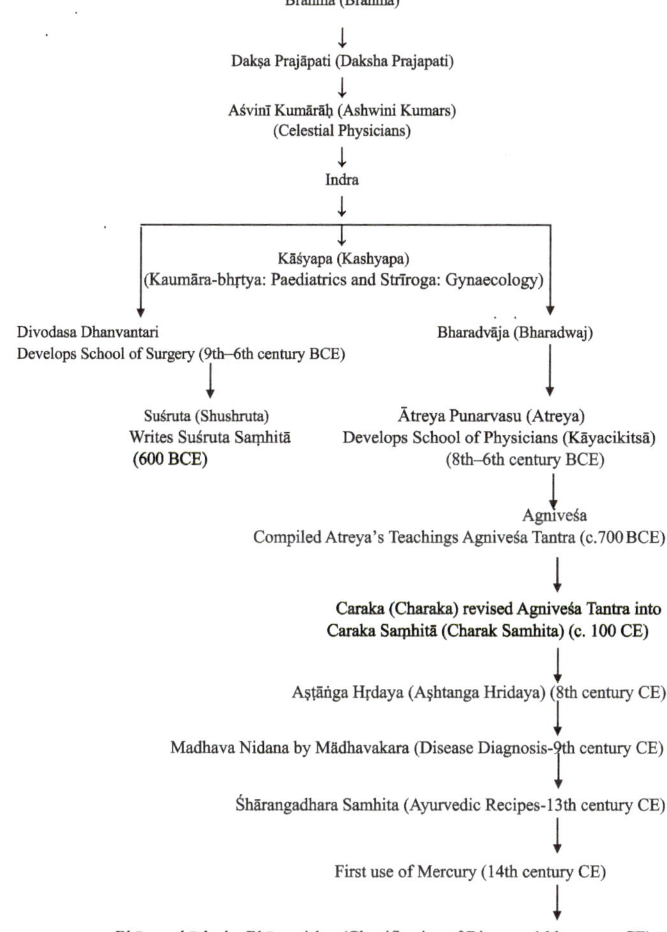

Fig. 8.2. *Chronology of Ayurveda knowledge transmission (Āyurveda Āvatarana): From divine revelation to founders of schools and classical texts (Flowchart by the Author).*

Alternative version describing the transmission of Ayurvedic knowledge are also found (Fig. 8.2). The Sushruta Saṃhitā (Sushrut Samhita) recounts that Divodāsa Dhanvantari (Dhanvantari, or Divodasa), received this wisdom from Indra. The Kashyapa tradition mentions that sages like Kāśyapa (Kashyapa), Vasiṣṭha (Vasishta), Ātreya (Atreya, Atri), and Bhṛgu (Bhrigu) directly learned from Indra. The Charaka Samhita offers another perspective, stating that sages such as Bhrigu and Aṅgiras (Angira) approached Indra to acquire specific knowledge, particularly related to *Rasayana* (rejuvenation therapies). These contradictions have been explained plausibly by some learned commentators (Anonymous 1949). However, undisputedly all these narratives underscore the profound reverence and divine origin attributed to Ayurveda in ancient Indian tradition.

Ayurveda in Buddhist Literature

While Ayurveda is not explicitly mentioned in Buddhist texts, its foundational concepts and practices were prevalent during the Buddhist era. Lord Buddha was revered as both a physician *(bhisakka)* and a surgeon (*sallakatto*). He provided detailed guidance on various medical treatments, including dietary recommendations; preparation of plant-based remedies using roots, leaves, gums, and salts; application of lime for treating ulcers with scabs; use of ointments for eye ailments; administration of oil for nasal cleansing; consumption of oil decoctions and fermented beverages; therapeutic use of hot baths; application of salves and bandages; induction of emesis for poisoning and other conditions; and the intake of sour gruel with salt to alleviate flatulence. Vāgbhata (Vagbhata) honoured him as the supreme healer, capable of alleviating the suffering (*dukkha*) arising from birth, aging, and disease. Concepts from the Buddhist period, such as codes for longevity (*āyussa dhamma*) and notions of timely and untimely death (*kāla maraṇa* and *akāla maraṇa*), resonate within the teachings of the Charaka Samhita (Valiathan 2006). Buddhist monks played a significant role in propagating Ayurveda to countries like Malaysia, Cambodia, Thailand, Myanmar, Japan, Singapore, Korea, and Tibet (Potbhare 2019). Additionally, Acharya Vagbhata, author of the Ashtanga Samgraha and Ashtanga Hrudaya, is believed to have been a disciple of Avalokita, a chief monk of Mahayana Buddhism (Acharya Vagbhata: Work, Text Books, Legacy, Amazing Facts, accessed on 22-02-2025).

Golden Age of Ayurveda: Samhita Period

The period from about 800 BCE to 1000 AD is celebrated as the golden age of Indian medicine. This period was marked by production of medical treatise (Anonymous 2025). In the early days of Ayurveda, its principles were transmitted orally by sages who shared the knowledge they had intuited while deep in meditation with their disciples. During the Samhita period, this knowledge was codified in the classic works of Ayurvedic literature, and the main therapeutic branches emerged as full- fledged schools of medicine, such as Atreya (internal medicine), Dhanvantari (surgery), and Kashyapa (paediatrics). This era witnessed the systematic development of foundational medical treatises, notably the Charaka Samhita, the Sushruta Samhita, and the Ashtanga Samgraha. These foundational texts of Ayurveda, attributed to ancient sages like Charaka, Sushruta, and Vāgbhata, respectively provide comprehensive insights into disease prevention, health maintenance, and longevity. This Greater Trio of Ayurveda (*Brahatrayee*) has profoundly influenced various traditional medicine systems worldwide, including Traditional Chinese Medicine and Unani. The Charaka Samhita, in its current form, is believed to date back to the 1st century CE, though earlier versions likely existed. The Sushruta Samhita possibly originated in the final centuries BCE, achieving its present form by the 7th century CE. These seminal works analyse the human body in terms of five elements—earth, water, fire, air, and ether—and discuss the three bodily humors.

Ayurveda gained global prominence, with Sushruta—revered as the Father of Surgery—pioneering complex surgical techniques such as rhinoplasty and cataract surgery. These methods influenced surgeons across the ancient world, including in Europe. Ancient Ayurvedic physicians were highly regarded for their medical expertise and were often invited to treat complex ailments. In *The Golden Road* (2024), British historian William Dalrymple highlights Ayurveda's influence on the Arab world. He recounts how an Indian delegation from Sindh to Baghdad in 733CE included Ayurvedic doctors. Citing the 9th century historian Al-Tabari, Dalrymple describes an instance where an Indian physician successfully treated Caliph Al-Mansur's digestive ailment after his court doctors had failed. The physician prepared an Ayurvedic digestive powder with hot spices, providing the Caliph with relief and earning praise for Indian medicine. Ayurvedic practices, based on the works of Charaka—known as the Father of Ayurveda—were followed in hospitals in Baghdad, established by the influential Barmakid family. Several Indian physicians worked there, and two translators were tasked with rendering Charaka's Sanskrit medical texts into Arabic, including his renowned treatise on poisons and antidotes. Dalrymple also notes that Barmark, father of the Abbasid vizier, travelled to Kashmir—a centre of Indian learning—to study astrology, medicine, and philosophy.

Universal Education and Medical Institutions in Ancient India

In ancient India, Vedic sages, or *Rishis*, were renowned for their intellectual prowess and multifaceted virtues. During the early Vedic period, these sages not only composed hymns but also engaged in warfare and various life-sustaining activities. A distinct group among them dedicated themselves to profound psychological and scientific inquiries, delving into thought, imagination, reasoning, and generalization. Resembling modern scientific scholars, these sages resided in forest retreats known as *Ashrams*, which evolved into esteemed centres of learning for the Vedic people. Many sages earned reputations as great teachers, ascending to the esteemed ranks of Maharishis and Brahma Rishis. Notably, the Saptarishi—

Agastya, Atri, Bhardwaja, Gautama, Jamadagni, Vashistha, and Vishvamitra—are revered as the seven great sages. In ancient Indian astronomy, the constellation Ursa Major, or the Big Dipper, is referred to as Saptarishi, with its seven stars symbolizing these illustrious sages.

Each *Ṛṣi* (Rishi, Sage) family functioned as an autonomous university, fostering an atmosphere of learning, scholarship, sacrifice, worship, and self-realization. These unitary *Ṛṣi-kulas*, or educational settlements, evolved into more complex forms—initially as *āśrama-kulas* in forest settings and later as Gurukulas in urban areas. Both types served as early universities, with āśrama-kulas resembling residential universities and Gurukulas akin to affiliating and partly residential universities. Renowned sages such as Vyāsa, Dhaumya, Agastya, Vaśiṣṭha, Viśvāmitra, Jābāli, Vālmiki, and Kanva were honoured with the title *Kulapati*, denoting those who imparted knowledge of all four Vedas to ten thousand students, providing free lodging and boarding in their Ashrams or Gurukuls. These institutions were typically situated in serene, natural settings and are immortalized in revered texts like the Purāṇas, the Rāmāyaṇa, and the Mahābhārata (https://www.hindupedia.com/en/Medical_Institutions_and_Universities_in_Ancient_India, accessed on 21-02-2025). Ayurveda was an important part of the curriculum at these teaching institutions across the country. The students were bound to study compulsory five fundamental subjects such as *Śabdavidyā* (Grammar or lexicography) *Śilpasthānavidyā* (art), *Chikitsavidyā* (medicine), *Hetuvidyā* (logic) and *Adyatmavidyā* (science of spiritual philosophy). On completing these courses, students were considered fit to opt a subject of their choice for higher studies. This education system continued to thrive at least until the 7th century AD (Anonymous 1949).

In post-Vedic India, especially during Buddhist period, the tradition of forest-dwelling Ṛṣi-kulas evolved into Gurukuls and Buddhist monasteries (*Viharas*) that flourished in urban settings. The merchant class played a pivotal role in disseminating diverse philosophical and religious ideas, leading to the emergence of approximately sixty-two new schools of thought, including Jainism (Lowe and Yasuhara 2017). Prominent centres of learning in ancient India—such as Takṣaśilā (Takshashila, Taxila, near present-day Rawalpindi, Pakistan), Kāśi (modern Varanasi, Uttar Pradesh), Ujjain (Madhya Pradesh), Mithilā (in present-day Bihar), Vikramaśīlā (Vikramashila, Bhagalpur, Bihar), Nālandā (Bihar), Kanchipuram (Tamil Nadu), and Valabhi (present-day Vala in Gujarat)—gained renown for their comprehensive curricula. These institutions offered advanced studies in philosophy, theology, literature, history, political and military science, marine science, geography, geometry, astronomy, mathematics, and medicine (Ayurveda). Other eminent centres of Ayurvedic education included: Śrughna (near Yamunanagar, Haryana), known for its surgical training and botanical gardens; Pātaliputra (modern Patna, Bihar), a major intellectual hub during the Mauryan period; Pushkar (Rajasthan), associated with early healing practices and medicinal plant traditions; Kāñcī (Kanchipuram), which hosted scholars of both Buddhist and Brahmanical traditions; Madurai (Tamil Nadu), a southern centre of Siddha and Ayurvedic integration and Sharada Peeth (Kashmir), a renowned seat of learning and Junnar and Nasik (Maharashtra), known for their Buddhist monastic universities and Ayurvedic propagation. These centres not only preserved and transmitted Ayurvedic knowledge but also fostered interdisciplinary scholarship, attracting students and physicians from across South Asia and beyond.

The medical teaching also became more systematized with emergence of major institutions of higher learning. Takshashila, one of the oldest known higher education institutes and medical school, was esteemed for its medical faculty. It is considered to be first medical school. The university emphasized the study of medicinal plants and offered instruction in both medicine and surgery. Jīvaka (Jīvaka or Jivaka) Kaumārabhartya, the personal physician to Gautama Buddha, was among its distinguished alumni. Atreya, a renowned medical teacher at Takshashila, is credited with laying the foundational principles of Ayurveda. Archaeological findings, including copper medical instruments, suggest that surgical practices were part of the curriculum (Paul 2022).

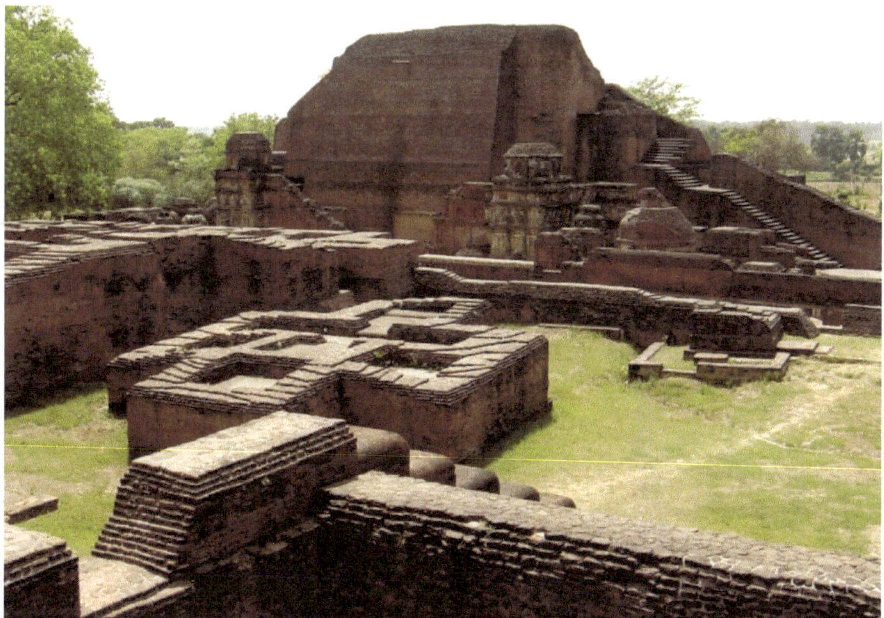

Fig. 8.3: *Remains of the ancient Nalanda Mahāvihāra, regarded as the world's first residential university (427 CE to circa 1400 CE). This eminent centre of learning offered instruction in a wide range of disciplines, including medicine, logic, grammar, and Sāṃkhya philosophy. (Source: File: Temple No. 3, Nalanda Archaeological Site.jpg – Wikimedia Commons).*

The University of Nalanda (Fig. 8.3), flourishing from the 5th to the 12th century CE, was another eminent institution. It combined monastic and educational functions, housing numerous lecture halls and a vast library to support its scholars and students. The library complex (*Dharma-gañja,* the mart of knowledge) was located in three splendid buildings – Ratnāsagara, Ratnodadhi and Ratnarañjaka. While primarily a *Mahāyāna* Buddhist establishment, Nalanda's curriculum encompassed a wide array of subjects beyond religious studies, including the Vedas, *Hetuvidyā* (logic), the *Sabda-vidyā* (grammar), *Chikitsāvidyā* and *Samkhya* philosophy. This diverse academic environment attracted scholars from various regions, contributing to its reputation as a premier centre of learning (Altekar 2009). According to the memoirs of a contemporary Chinese student, medicine at Nalanda was taught by highly competent teachers to students not only from India but also from countries such as Nepal, China, Java, Sri Lanka, Sumatra, Cambodia, and even distant Korea. Acharya Shilbhadra, the legendary master of *Yogācāra* (the Practice of Yoga), was a distinguished faculty member in Ayurveda at Nalanda. In the sixth century, the Chinese monk Xuanzang enrolled at the renowned monastery and university of *Nalanda*, where he studied Buddhist scriptures alongside the Vedas, Sanskrit grammar, logic, philosophy, divination, mathematics, astronomy, literature, and medicine for over five years. Upon returning to China, Xuanzang carried a small library of Buddhist medical and astronomical texts, along with a precious sapling of the Bodhi tree, sent as a gift by Emperor Harsha to Emperor Taizong of China (Dalrymple 2024).

Stagnation Phase

Following the era of Vagbhata, Ayurveda entered a prolonged period of stagnation lasting approximately a millennium. This era was characterized by a notable decline in creativity and innovation within the field. While some advancements occurred, they did not match the intellectual vigor of earlier centuries. During this time, significant texts such as Mādhavanidāna, Śārṅgadhara Saṃhitā, and Bhāvaprakāśa were composed, alongside numerous dictionaries and commentaries on ancient works. A notable development in this period was the rapid growth of alchemy, especially in centres like Nalanda, Vikramaśīla, and Udāntapura (Odantapuri, identified with present-day Bihar Shariff in Nalanda district in Bihar). Indian alchemy focused on achieving self-realization, transmuting base metals into gold, and rejuvenating the body. This tradition drew heavily from the Tantric cult and evolved over time to include practical applications in medicine, particularly through the development of various mercury and metal-based preparations (Ali 1993). Despite these advancements, the preference of Muslim rulers for Unani medicine accelerated the decline of Ayurveda. Surgical techniques detailed by Sushruta and Jīvaka had largely vanished from mainstream practice by Vagbhata's time. The discontinuation of cadaveric dissection and hands-on surgical training led to a significant loss of anatomical and surgical knowledge. Social and cultural factors further exacerbated this decline, including the relegation of certain medical practices to lower castes and the discouragement of manual work among the intellectual elite (Valiathan 2006). Additionally, the absence of standardized education and training systems allowed quackery to flourish, making it challenging to distinguish qualified practitioners from impostors. This period of stagnation persisted until a renewed interest in Ayurveda emerged in more recent times.

Modern Period and Resurgence of Ayurveda

The modern resurgence of Ayurveda began in the early 19th century, driven by the efforts of renowned Ayurvedic scholars and some western enthusiasts. As European medicine gradually gained prominence in India, notable figures like H.H. Wilson (1786–1860), an English orientalist, introduced ancient Indic medicine to Western academia through his 1823 essay, *The Medical and Surgical Sciences of the Hindus*. In 1836, Madhusudan printed and published the Sushruta Samhita, followed by other significant publications of ancient Ayurvedic texts. A major shift from traditional practice occurred with the contributions of Gananathji Sen, an eminent scholar in both Ayurveda and modern medicine. He authored *Pratyaksha Shariram*, marking a new phase in Ayurvedic scholarship. The first institution to offer education in both Ayurveda and Western medicine (Allopathy) was the Gurukula Vidyalaya, established in 1918 at (Kangri), with Hindi as the medium of instruction. Many of the Sanskrit Ayurvedic texts available today with Hindi translations were contributed by scholars from this institution. Other prominent centres of Ayurvedic education at the time included Banaras Hindu University (BHU) and the Rishikul Brahmacharya Ashram in Haridwar (https://indicportal.org/classical-indic-medicine-ii-history-of-ayurveda-3/, accessed on 05-02-2025).

Following India's independence in 1947, the government took several initiatives to promote Ayurveda, including the establishment of Ayurvedic colleges and research institutions. The Ministry of AYUSH (Ayurveda, Yoga & Naturopathy, Unani, Siddha, and Homoeopathy) and the Central Council for Research in Ayurveda and Siddha (CCRAS) were founded in 1978. The latter was renamed the Central Council for Research in Ayurvedic Sciences (CCRAS) in 2011 and operates as an autonomous body under the Ministry of AYUSH to promote and regulate traditional medicine. The research activities of the Council include medicinal plant research, drug standardization, pharmacological and clinical research, and documentation of traditional healthcare practices. The activities are carried out through its 30 Institutes/Centres/Units located all over the country. Efforts by CCRAS have facilitated the collaboration of Ayurveda with modern medicine through joint research, the establishment of integrated healthcare facilities, and the inclusion of Ayurvedic treatments in hospitals and clinics.

As of 14-03-2023, there are 495 Ayurveda colleges in India (Source: https://ncismindia.org/A, accessed on 02-03-2025), along with over 500,000 registered Ayurveda practitioners. Ayurvedic formulations are documented in official Ayurvedic formularies and pharmacopeia of India. *The Ayurveda Formulary of India* provides details on 985 formulations, including 50 Ayurvedic veterinary formulations, while the *Ayurveda Pharmacopoeia of India* includes over 100 monographs on herbs, extracts, and products, along with more than 650 pharmacopeial monographs. The Drugs & Cosmetics Act of 1940 and its associated rules provide exclusive provisions for the regulation and quality control of Ayurvedic medicines. The First Schedule of the Act recognizes 57 Ayurvedic texts as classical and authoritative references, detailing ingredient compositions, usage levels, manufacturing processes, dosages, and therapeutic indications (Source:https://ccras.nic.in/wp-content/uploads/2024/07/CCRAS-AGNI-1.pdf, accessed on 05-02-2025).

Recently National Commission for Indian System of Medicine (NCISM), a statutory body constituted under the NCISM Act of 2020 via a gazette notification on 21.09.2020, came into force on 11th June 2021. NCISM aims to enhance medical education, ensure the availability of high-quality professionals in the Indian System of Medicine across the country, and promote equitable and universal healthcare. It also encourages a community health perspective, facilitates the integration of modern medical research into Ayurvedic practice, maintains a medical register for the Indian System of Medicine, enforces high ethical standards, and establishes a responsive grievance redressal mechanism. These advancements have significantly contributed to the growth and integration of Ayurveda into mainstream healthcare.

Classical Texts in Ayurveda

Ayurveda, is founded upon a rich tradition of classical texts that have shaped its principles and practices. These texts are primarily categorized into two groups: the *Brihatrayee (Bṛhat-Trayī,* The Great Triad) and the *Laghutrayee* (Lesser Triad). Among the available Samhitas, Charaka Samhita focuses on medicine, Sushruta Samhita emphasizes surgery, and Kashyapa Samhita specializes in paediatrics. Together with Ashtanga Hridaya, these are considered the Brihatrayee. Laghutrayee comprise three treatises- Sarangadhara Samhita, Bhavaprakasha and Madhava Nidana covering Ayurvedic basics and description of diseases, formulations and treatments in a simplified way.

Caraka Saṃhitā (Charaka Samhita)

Origin and Compilation: Charaka Samhita originated from the teachings of Punarvasu Atreya, compiled by Agnivesa, and later redacted by Charaka. The name "Charaka" is traditionally understood to derive from the Sanskrit root chara, meaning "to wanderer," and has been mentioned in various works. While some believe Charaka and Patanjali are the same, others assert they were distinct individuals. Despite covering all branches of Ayurveda, Charaka Samhita is particularly renowned for its contributions to general medicine (*Kayachikitsa*).

Structure: The text is divided into 8 sections and 120 chapters.

Time Period: Estimated between the 1st and 2nd century BCE, with final revisions by Dridhabala around the 4th century CE. Vagbhata's references to Charaka's work confirm its existence before his time.

Special Features- *Triskandha* Ayurveda: Key features of Charaka Samhita include:

- Advanced diagnostic methods, including pathogenesis and examination techniques.
- Emphasis on importance of both theoretical knowledge and clinical practice for physicians.
- Highlighting rejuvenation therapies aimed at enhancing immunity and promoting longevity.

Initially, Ayurveda was categorized into aetiology, symptoms, and treatment. Charaka advanced diagnostic methods by introducing concepts like pathogenesis and techniques such as palpation and percussion. Emphasis was placed on examining the patient's digestion, psychological state, and constitution.

Seminars and Conferences: Charaka introduced the tradition of arranging seminars and symposiums for knowledge exchange and clarification of doubts, with participation from renowned Ayurvedic physicians.

Advances in Principles: Explained bioenergetics and foundational theories like *pañcamahābhūta* (Panchamahabhutas) and *Rasaguna Veerya Vipaka.*

Highlighted rejuvenation treatments to strengthen immunity as a priority in therapy.

Emphasized the dual importance of theoretical and clinical knowledge for physicians.

Medicines and Homeostasis: Acharya Charaka introduced the concept that medicines not only treat diseases but also restore homeostasis.

Commentaries: Several Sanskrit commentaries have been written on Charaka Samhita, prominent being:

- Charaka Nyasa by Bhattara Harischandra (4th century CE).
- Ayurveda Deepika by Chakrapani (11th century CE).
- Charaka Pradipika by Jyotischandra Saraswathi (20th century CE)

Suśruta Saṃhitā (Sushruta Samhita)

Origin and Overview: The Sushruta Samhita is a seminal text in Ayurveda, primarily focusing on surgery and associated disciplines. Attributed to the sage Sushruta, a disciple of King Divodasa Dhanvantari of Kashi, this compendium is a cornerstone of ancient Indian medical literature. Historically, Sushruta and his mentor, Divodasa Dhanvantari, are esteemed figures in the annals of Ayurveda. Traditional accounts sometimes place them as early as 1500–1000 BCE, but most modern scholars suggest that Sushruta lived around the 6th century BCE.

Time Period: The dating of the Sushruta Samhita has been a subject of scholarly debate due to the lack of definitive historical evidence. Some scholars suggest that the original composition occurred between the time of Gautama Buddha (6th century BCE) and that of Kātyāyana, based on references within the text. For instance, the Sushruta Samhita mentions Subhūti Gautama, a direct disciple of Buddha, participating in discussions on embryological development, implying that Sushruta, a disciple of Dhanvantari, lived around the late 6th or early 5th century BCE. The text underwent significant redaction by Nāgārjuna, a renowned alchemist and medical scholar. The Chronology Committee of the National Institute of Sciences of India posits that this recession occurred between the 3rd and 4th centuries CE, forming the basis for subsequent commentaries, such as that by Dalhana (Ray 1980). This layered composition suggests that the Sushruta Samhita evolved over several centuries, integrating surgical knowledge from various periods.

Structure and Content: The Sushruta Samhita is originally divided into five sections and 120 chapters (*Purvatantra*): *Sutrasthana* (46 chapters), *Nidanasthana* (16 chapters), *Sharirasthana* (10 chapters), *Chikitsasthana* (40 chapters), and *Kalpasthana* (8 chapters). Additionally, when the 66 chapters of the *Uttaratantra*, composed by Nagarjuna, are included, the total number of chapters in this Samhita reaches 186. The extant form contains descriptions of 1,120 illnesses, 700 medicinal plants, 64 preparations from mineral sources and 57 preparations based on animal sources. Broad aspects covered in different chapters include:

- *Sutrasthana:* Fundamental principles, surgical instruments, and general guidelines.
- *Nidanasthana*: Aetiology and pathogenesis of surgical diseases.
- *Sharirasthana*: Anatomy, embryology, and physiology.
- *Chikitsasthana*: Therapeutic approaches and management of diseases.
- *Kalpasthana*: Toxicology and management of poisons.
- *Uttaratantra*: Specialized areas such as: *Shalakya*-Ophthalmology and ENT disorders; *Kaumarabhritya*- Paediatrics; *Kayachikitsa*- General medicine and *Bhutavidya*: Psychiatry and demonic afflictions.

Key features and Notable Contributions: Some of the notable features of Sushruta Samhita are:

- **Cosmic Evolution and Creation of Life:** Fertilization, according to Sushruta, occurs through the union of sperm and ova, but the involvement of a superior agency is necessary for life.
- **Tridosha (Tridosha) Theory:** Detailed discussions on physiological, pathological, and therapeutic aspects of the Tridoshas (*Vāta, Pitta, Kapha*).
- **Surgical procedures:** The Sushruta Samhita is the oldest known surgical text, offering a comprehensive account of medical practices from its time. It provides detailed descriptions of various complex surgical procedures, including rhinoplasty (nasal reconstruction), otoplasty (ear surgery), cataract removal, prostate surgery, hernia repair, and caesarean section, among others.
- **Training and Ethics:** Comprehensive guidelines for training, duties of physicians, surgeons, and nurses.

***Commentaries*:** Key commentators include Jejjata, Gayadasa (Nyaya Chandrika), Dalhana (Nibandha Sangraha), and Chakrapani (Bhanumati).

Aṣṭāṅga Saṃgraha (Ashtanga Samgraha) and Aṣṭāṅga Hṛdaya (Ashtanga Hridaya)

These classical Ayurveda texts were authored by two different scholars. Ashtanga Samgraha leans more toward the teachings of Sushruta, while Ashtanga Hridaya is influenced by Charaka. Both Samhitas contain descriptions of Sharira Rachana in Sutra Sthana, Sharira Sthana, and Uttar Sthana (Sewada *et al.* 2023).

Ashtanga Samgraha: Composed by Vridha Vagbhata (500 CE), Ashtanga Samgraha synthesizes essential topics on human illness and therapy from the Charaka Samhita and Sushruta Samhita while introducing new subjects systematically. This compendium is organized into six sections and 150 chapters:

- *Sutrasthana* - 40 chapters
- *Nidanasthana* - 16 chapters
- *Sharirasthana* - 12 chapters
- *Cikitsasthana* - 24 chapters
- *Kalpasthana* - 8 chapters
- *Uttarastana* - 50 chapters

The eight branches, known as *Ashtanga* in Sanskrit, include:

- Internal Medicine- *Kaya Chikitsa*
- Paediatrics- *Koumarabhrithya*
- Psychiatry - *Griha Chikitsa*
- E.N.T.- *Shalakya*
- Toxicology- *Agada Tantra*
- Basic Surgery- *Shalya*
- Geriatrics- *Jarachikitsa*
- Science of Aphrodisiacs- *Vrushya Chikitsa*

(Source: e-Vagbhata - Institute of Ayurveda and Integrative Medicine (I-AIM). Notable features of the Samhita include:

- Inclusion of new medicinal plants
- Elaboration on the relationship between diseases and Tridoshas
- Introduction of the innovative use of processed toxins in treatment

Commentary: Shashilekha by Indu is the only surviving commentary.

Aṣṭāṅga Hṛdaya (Ashtanga Hridaya, Ashtanga Hrudaya): Written by Laghu Vagbhatta (6th century), the Ashtanga Hridaya, is better organized and more concise than Ashtanga Samgraha. This poetic text is widely used, especially in South India. The Ashtanga Hridaya encapsulates the essence of the Charaka and Sushruta Samhitas. While Acharya Charaka prioritized *Kayachikitsa* (Internal Medicine) and Sushruta focused on *Shalya* (Surgery), Vagbhata emphasized all eight branches of Ayurveda. The Ashtanga Hridaya can be considered a *Prakaran Grantha*, meaning it references other texts and is neither too abridged nor too elaborate. Topics are systematically arranged, with principles and their applications in treatment clearly explained. It is divided into six sections and 120 chapters (Gore *et al.* 2023). The special features of Ashtanga Hridaya include:

- A comprehensive guide combining principles of medicine and surgery
- Details on specific plants for diseases (e.g. *Musta* for fever, *Haritaki* for Vata and Kapha disorders)
- Introduction of rejuvenators and aphrodisiacs
- Description of diseases under headings like *Nidhana*, *Purvaroopa*, *Roopa*, *Samprapti*, and *Chikitsa*

Commentaries: Important commentaries include Sarvanga Sundara by Arunadatta and Ayurveda Rasayanam by Hemadri (Paradakar 2005).

Laghu-trayī (Laghutrayee / the Lesser Triad)

The trio of significant texts—Sharangadhara Samhita, Madhava Nidana and Bhava Prakasha—serves as foundational references for Ayurvedic practitioners and scholars. Some of their features are highlighted here:

Sharangadhara Samhita: Written by Acharya Sharangadhara, this text is known for its practical approach to Ayurveda. It provides extensive information on pharmacology, preparation of medicines, and therapeutic techniques. Sharangadhara Samhita contains three sections, 32 chapters, and 2600 verses covering topics such as diagnosis, treatment, medicinal formulations, and *Panchakarma* procedures. It also introduces the concept of pulse diagnosis (*Nadi Pariksha*), which remains an important diagnostic tool in Ayurveda.

***Bhava Prakasha*:** Composed by Acharya Bhava Mishra in the 16th century CE, this text is a comprehensive compilation of Ayurvedic knowledge, including the principles of Ayurveda, medicinal plants, and therapeutic procedures. Bhava Prakasha is known for its detailed descriptions of herbs, including new herbs and formulations not mentioned in earlier texts, along with their uses, making it an invaluable resource for practitioners and students of Ayurveda. The text is divided into three sections *Purva Khanda* (first part), *Madhya Khanda* (middle part) and *Uttara Khanda* (later part), covering Ayurveda's principles, and various aspects of disease management, and treatment including rejuvenation therapies.

***Madhava Nidana*:** Authored by Acharya Madhava in 7th century CE, this text focuses on the diagnosis of diseases (Nidana). It is highly valued for its detailed descriptions of various diseases and their symptoms, offering comprehensive insight into the cause and nature of ailments. The Madhava Nidana is particularly noted for introducing classifications for colic pain (*Sula*) and vesicles (*Vispotta*), and for its systematic approach to diagnosing diseases, making it a crucial tool for practitioners.

Significance of Laghutrayee: These texts hold considerable historical importance in Ayurveda. The following points highlight their relevance and contribution to the development of Ayurvedic knowledge:

- **Simplification and Accessibility**: The Laghutrayee was created to simplify and make accessible the vast and detailed knowledge contained in the Brihatrayee. By condensing and organizing the information, the Laghutrayee made it easier for practitioners to understand and apply Ayurvedic principles in clinical practice.
- **Comprehensive Coverage**: These texts cover a wide range of topics, including disease diagnosis, treatment methodologies, medicinal formulations, and the use of specific plants for various ailments. They provide a holistic approach to understanding and practicing Ayurveda.

- **Influence on Later Works**: The Laghutrayee has influenced numerous subsequent Ayurvedic texts and practices. The systematic approach and practical insights offered by these texts have been incorporated into later works, ensuring the continuity and evolution of Ayurvedic knowledge.
- **Educational Value**: The Laghutrayee is widely used in Ayurvedic education and training. Its concise and organized presentation of Ayurvedic concepts makes it an essential resource for students and practitioners alike.
- **Cultural and Historical Context**: These texts reflect the cultural and historical context of their time, providing insights into the medical practices, societal norms, and philosophical underpinnings of ancient India. As such they remain valuable historical documents that contribute to our understanding of the development of Ayurveda.

Collectively, the Brihatrayee and Laghutrayee form the cornerstone of Ayurvedic knowledge, offering a holistic and systematic approach to health and wellness. They continue to guide practitioners and scholars in understanding the complexities of human health and disease management.

Philosophy and Fundamental Principles of Ayurveda

The Ayurvedic healing system is rooted in the philosophy that health results from the harmonious integration of an individual's constitution with nature and the universe. Central to Ayurvedic philosophy is the concept of Ayu, which signifies the union of the physical body, senses, mind, and soul. This holistic perspective underscores the importance of aligning one's lifestyle with natural laws to achieve optimal health. Ayurveda offers personalized guidance, recognizing that each individual has a unique constitution, or *prakrti* (Prakriti), which influences their health and response to various treatments. The fundamental principles of Ayurveda that form the basis for understanding creation, health, disease, and treatment include Panchamahabhutas (the five great elements), Tridosha (the three bodily humors), Prakriti (individual constitution), *Ojas* (vital energy), *Dhatu* (tissues), *Mala* (waste products), *Agni* (digestive fire), *Manas* (mind), and *Atma* (soul). This unique and original approach to material creation allows for the integration of modern developments in elemental physics (Meena *et al.* 2015).

Aimes and Goals

The ultimate aim of Ayurveda is to guide every human being to maintain and promote health, and prevent ailments:

prayōjanaṁ cāsya svasthasya svāsthyarakṣaṇamāturasya vikārapraśamanaṁ ca.

Translated as: 'The purpose of this science (Ayurveda) is to preserve the health of the healthy and cure the disease of the unhealthy' (Patwardhan and Upadhyaya 2020).

Need of Health? A long healthy life is the wish of every being from antiquity. Ayurveda emphasises that Health is important to attain the four-goals of human life -*Dharma (*virtue*), Artha (*wealth*), Kama* (pleasure) and *Moksha* (liberation). According to Charka:

*dharmārthakāmamōkṣāṇāmārōgyaṁ mūlamuttamam (*Ch. Su. 1. 15).

rōgāstasyāpahartāraḥ śrēyasō jīvitasya ca;

prādurbhūtō manuṣyāṇāmantarāyō mahānayam (Ch. Su. 1. 16).

Translated as- 'Health is the best source of virtue, wealth, gratification and emancipation; while diseases are destroyers of this (source), welfare and life itself. Now this has appeared as a great obstacle for human well-being and life' (Singh *et al.* 2020).

Definition of Health

The World Health Organization (WHO) defines health as 'a state of complete physical, mental, and social well-being and not merely the absence of disease or infirmity.' However, many scholars contest this definition, arguing that the notion of *"complete"* well-being may inadvertently contribute to the over-medicalization of society. Callahan (1973) critiques this absolutist perspective, stating, 'Complete entails setting the stage for the worst false consciousness of all—the demand that life deliver perfection. Practically speaking, this demand has led, in the field of health, to a constant escalation of expectation and requirement, never-ending, never satisfied.' In contrast, health (*Swasthya--* self free from any limitation) in Ayurveda is not merely the absence of disease but a state of holistic well-being — a healthy mind and body.

The classical texts describe specific indicators that define an individual's health. These indicators encompass physical, mental, and spiritual balance — balance/ equilibrium/homeostasis of three physiological functions, metabolism, body tissues, excretory functions, senses, mind and soul (self). Sushruta defines health and healthy person as:

समदोषः समाग्निश्च समधातुमलक्रियिः | प्रसन्नात्मेन्द्रयिमनाः स्वस्थ इत्यभिधीयते ||
(Sushruta Sutrashanam, 15.41. Source: e-Samhita - National Institute of Indian Medical Heritage).

- 'One whose *Doṣas* (bodily humors) are balanced (*Sama*), Agni of digestion and so forth are balanced, dhatus (seven bodily elements) are balanced, Mala kriya (function of excretions) are balanced, and whose soul (*Atma*), and *Indriyas* (five sense organs, five organs of action), and mind (*Mana*) remain in a state of harmony and contentment (*prasanna*).'

Balance of *Doṣa* (*Doshas*) (*Sama Dosha*)

- The three Doshas—Vata, Pitta, and Kapha—should remain in a balanced state according to an individual's constitution (*Prakriti*).
- Imbalance (*Vikriti*) leads to disease and discomfort.

Proper Functioning of *Agni* (Sama Agni)

- *Agni* (digestive fire) governs digestion, metabolism, and transformation in the body.
- Balanced Agni ensures proper digestion, absorption of nutrients and elimination of waste materials.

Equilibrium of *Dhatus* (*Sama Dhatu*)

- The seven *Dhatus* (body tissues) should be nourished and function optimally:
    1. *Rasa* (plasma)
    2. *Rakta* (blood)
    3. *Mamsa* (muscle)
    4. *Meda* (fat)
    5. *Asthi* (bone)
    6. *Majja* (Bone marrow)
    7. *Shukra/Artava* (Reproductive tissues)

Efficient Elimination of Waste (*Sama Mala Kriya*)

- *Mutra* (Urine) – Clear, adequate quantity, and frequency
- *Purisha* (Faeces) – Well-formed, easy elimination, and regularity
- *Sweda* (Sweat) – Balanced perspiration without excessive or insufficient sweating

Mental and Emotional Well-being (*Prasanna Atma-Indriya-Mana*)

- *Atma* (Soul) – A sense of inner peace and spiritual well-being
- *Indriyas* (Senses and organs of action) – Clear perception and proper sensory function
- *Mana* (Mind) – Emotional stability, clarity of thought, and absence of excessive stress or anxiety
- *Ahara* (Food),

- *Vihara* (Lifestyle),
- *Vichara* (The mental thoughts), and
- *Vyavahara* are the pillars of health and wellness.

The Tridosha (Three Humoral Factors) Theory

The Tridosha theory in Ayurveda describes three fundamental energies—Vata, Pitta, and Kapha—that govern physiological functions in the body. Unlike biomedicine's organ-centric approach, Ayurveda views the human body as an interconnected system where balance is key to health. The term Dosha means 'that which can become vitiated,' emphasizing their potential for imbalance. According to Ashtanga Hridaya, these Doshas pervade the body but have specific areas of dominance:

te vyāpino'pi hṛnnābhyoradhomadhyordhva samśrayā: vayo 'horātribhuktānām te'ntamadhyādigā: kramāt. (As. Hr. Su.1.2.5-6)

The Tridosha are present all over the body, but their presence is especially seen in particular parts:

- Kapha – Predominantly in the upper body (head to chest)
- Pitta – Central body region (chest to umbilicus)
- Vata – Lower body (below the umbilicus)

Ayurveda focuses on maintaining the balance of these Doshas to ensure health and prevent disease.

Functions of Tridosa: In Ayurveda, the three doṣas— vāta, Pitta, and Kapha—govern all physiological and psychological functions of the body.

1. Kapha Dosha (Water Energy / Stabilizer)

- Elements: Earth and Water
- Functions: Provides structure, cohesion, and lubrication, ensuring tissue hydration, joint flexibility, and immune strength.
- Balanced Kapha: Stability, compassion, and endurance.
- Imbalanced Kapha: Lethargy, congestion, attachment, and insecurity.

2. Vata Dosha (Wind Energy / Neurological)

- Elements: Space and Air
- Functions: Governs movement, including circulation, respiration, nerve impulses, and cellular activity.
- Balanced Vata: Creativity, flexibility, and enthusiasm.

- Imbalanced Vata: Anxiety, restlessness, dryness, and joint pain.

3. Pitta Dosha (Fire Energy / Metabolizer)

- Elements: Fire and Water
- Functions: Regulates metabolism, digestion, nutrient assimilation, and body temperature.
- Balanced Pitta: Intelligence, focus, and digestion.
- Imbalanced Pitta: Irritability, inflammation, ulcers, and excessive heat.

Panchamahabhutas – The Five Supreme Powers or Fundamental Elements: Ayurveda posits that all matter consists of five fundamental elements (Panchamahabhutas):

- *Prithvi* (Earth) – Provides stability and structure.
- *Jal* (Water) – Facilitates cohesion and fluidity.
- *Agni* (Fire) – Governs transformation and metabolism.
- *Vayu* (Air) – Controls movement and circulation.
- *Akash* (Space/Ether) – Creates expansiveness and potential.

These elements form the foundation of all beings and substances, influencing both the cosmos and human physiology. Any imbalance in them can lead to disease. For instance, disruptions in Prithvi (Earth element)—predominant in bones—can cause osteoporosis or arthritis. Ayurvedic treatments aim to restore balance among these elements for overall well-being.

Body Tissues and Waste Products (Dushyas)

Maintaining a balance in tissues and efficient elimination of waste is crucial for health, as imbalances can lead to various diseases. Dushyas refer to body tissues and waste products: *Rasa asrk māmsa medo asthi majja śukrāni dhātava: sapta dūṣyā: malā: mūtra śakrt svedādavo pi ca.* (Astang Hr. Su.1.13). These are influenced by Doshas. The seven body tissues (Sapta Dhatus) include:

- *Rasa* – The first product of digestion, comparable to lymph or plasma.
- *Rakta* – Blood, essential for oxygenation and vitality.
- *Mamsa* – Muscle tissue, responsible for movement and strength.
- *Meda* – Fat tissue, providing lubrication and energy storage.
- *Asthi* – Bones and cartilage, offering structural support.
- *Majja* – Bone marrow, contributing to nervous and immune function.
- *Shukra / Artava* – Reproductive tissues, essential for fertility and vitality.

The body also produces three essential waste products *(Mala)*

- *Purisha (Feces)* – Regulates elimination and gut health.
- *Sweda (Sweat)* – Maintains temperature and detoxification.
- *Mootra (Urine)* – Balances fluid levels and removes toxins.

Maintaining a balance in tissues and efficient elimination of waste is crucial for health, as imbalances can lead to various diseases.

Ayurveda for Daily Life

Ayurveda provides a timeless framework for harmonizing with nature's rhythms, offering a holistic approach to health and well-being. Rooted in ancient Indian wisdom, it emphasizes preventive care, healing, and longevity through balanced living. Ayurvedic principles highlight the importance of *pathya*—a lifestyle aligned with individual constitution and environmental influences. Prevention is prioritized, as maintaining health is easier than restoring it once compromised. Integrating Ayurveda into daily life doesnt require drastic changes; simple shifts—such as choosing fresh, seasonal, and organic foods over processed alternatives—can significantly enhance well-being. Transitioning from a sedentary lifestyle to an active one, including activities like walking, supports overall vitality. Hydration is also crucial; drinking ample water helps detoxify the body, while a warm glass of water before bedtime aids digestion and promotes restful sleep. Ayurveda also offers gentle, natural remedies for common ailments, reinforcing its holistic and sustainable approach to health.

The Six Tastes in Ayurveda (Aahara - Shadrasa Pradhanata)

Let food be thy medicine and medicine be thy food. – Hippocrates

Ayurveda classifies food based on six fundamental tastes (*Shadrasa*):

रसाः स्वाद्वम्ललवणतिक्तोषणकषायकाः षड् द्रव्यमाश्रतिास्ते च यथापूर्व बलावहाः || (अस्.हृ.सू 1.13.5).

(Madhura, Amla, Lavana, Tikta, Ushna - Katu, Kashaya are the six types of *Rasas*).

तत्राद्या मारुतं घनन्ति त्रयस्तष्ठिादाय: कफं |कशायतक्तिमधुरा: पत्तिमन्ये तु कुर्वते || (अस्.हृ.सू 1.14).

tatrādyā mārutaṃ ghnanti traya: tiktādaya: kapham; kaṣāya tikta madhurā: pittamanye (Astang Hr. Su.1.14).

Each taste affects the body's Tridosha (Vata, Pitta, Kapha) differently and provides varying degrees of energy, with **sweet** imparting the most nourishment and **astringent** the least:

- *Madhura* (Sweet) – Nourishing, builds strength (↑ Kapha, ↓ Vata and Pitta)
- *Amla* (Sour) – Stimulates digestion (↑ Pitta and Kapha, ↓ Vata)
- *Lavana* (Salty) – Retains moisture, enhances metabolism (↑ Pitta and Kapha, ↓ Vata)
- *Tikta* (Bitter) – Detoxifies, supports digestion (↑ Vata, ↓ Pitta and Kapha)
- *Katu* (Pungent) – Stimulates circulation and metabolism (↑ Pitta and Vata, ↓ Kapha)
- *Kashaya* (Astringent) – Absorptive, drying effect (↑ Vata, ↓ Pitta and Kapha).

Diet and Individuals' Growth and Development and Causation of Diseases

Ayurveda emphasises crucial role of diet in growth, development, and disease prevention

na rāgānnāpyavijñānādāhārānupayōjayēt; parīkṣya hitamaśnīyāddēhō hyāhāRasambhavaḥ (Ch. Su. 28.41).

'One should not take food with greed and ignorance. One should consume wholesome food after evaluation as the body is formed from food' (Rao 2020).

āhārasya vidhāvaṣṭau viśēṣā hētusañjñakāḥ; śubhāśubhasamutpattau tān parīkṣya prayōjayēt. (Ch. Su 28.42).

'Eight special factors are to be considered while consuming food. These factors should be evaluated before consuming food, as they are responsible for good and bad effects on the body' (Rao 2020).

Growth and Development: Assessing the influence of dietary intake on growth and development involves evaluating nutritional adequacy, including macronutrients (proteins, carbohydrates, fats) and micronutrients (vitamins, minerals). Monitoring parameters like height, weight, and developmental milestones offers valuable insights into the sufficiency of nutrition and its impact on both physical and cognitive development.

Disease Causation: Exploring the connection between nutrition and disease (Fig. 8.4) requires an analysis of dietary patterns, nutrient composition, and lifestyle factors. Epidemiological studies investigate links between diet and disease occurrence, while clinical trials provide insights into causal relationships. Additional factors like biomarkers, genetic predispositions, and environmental influences contribute to understanding the complex interplay between diet and disease pathogenesis. Such research aids in identifying dietary factors crucial for promoting growth and minimizing disease risk.

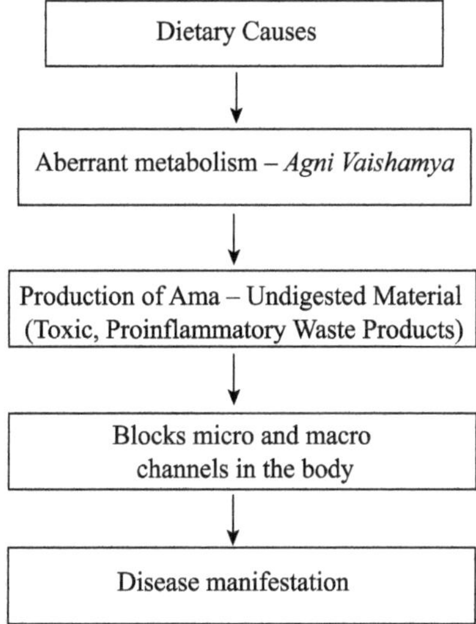

Fig. 8.4. *Graphic representation of diet and disease manifestation.*

Ayurvedic Understanding of Causes and Pathophysiology of Illness

Ayurveda offers a unique perspective on the underlying causes of disease pathogenesis, delineating three fundamental factors:

- *Asatmyendriyartha Samyoga* – Improper engagement of senses (overuse, underuse, or misuse).
- *Prajnaparadha* – Actions taken without discernment, leading to harm.
- *Parinama (Kala)* – Environmental or seasonal changes disrupting the body's balance.

These causes collectively contribute to the manifestation of various ailments through *Trividha Hetu—Atiyoga, Ayoga*, and *Mithyayoga*. *Prajnaparadha* arises from actions undertaken without discernment, whether they are beneficial or detrimental to the body and mind. *Asatmyendriyartha Samyoga* involves improper engagement of the senses with their respective objects, leading to either excessive stimulation or deficiency in sensory activity. Excessive or *Atiyoga* of *Parinama* encompasses extraordinary or unexpected climatic conditions, such as extreme heat during summer or cold during winter. These climatic fluctuations disrupt the body's equilibrium, predisposing it to illness and imbalance.

Theory of Pathogenesis (*Shat Kriya Kala*)- *Vyadhi Kriyakala:* In Ayurveda, sequential progression of a disease is explained in following 6 stages.

- *Sanchaya*- Stage of accumulation
- *Prakopa*- Stage of vitiation

- *Prasara*- Stage of dissemination
- *Sthanasamsraya*- Stage of localisation
- *Vyakti*- Stage of clinical symptoms
- *Bheda*-Stage of complication

It can be otherwise classified based on the criteria for treatment as

- *Dosha kriyakala* including *Sanchaya, Prakopa* and *Prasara.*
- *Vyadhi kriyakala,* including *Sthana samsraya*, *Vyakti* and *Bheda.*

Examination of a Patient

Examination of a Patient in Ayurveda: Patient examination in Ayurveda is a comprehensive and holistic process that evaluates both the disease (*roga*) and the patient (*rogi*). It employs three primary methods: *Trividha Pareeksha* (threefold examination), *Ashtavidha Pareeksha* (eightfold examination), and *Dashavidha Pareeksha* (tenfold examination). These methodologies aim to gain a thorough understanding of the patient's physical, mental, and emotional well-being, enabling personalized and effective treatment.

***Trividha Pareeksha* (Threefold Examination):** According to *Ashtanga Hridaya,* threefold examination (*Trividha Pareeksha*) to assess a patient include दर्शनस्पर्शनप्रश्नैःपरीक्षेत च रोगिणम् (अस्.हृ. सू. 1.22).

- ***Darshana (Inspection):*** Observing the patient's physical attributes, including appearance, posture, skin condition, and other visible signs.
- ***Sparshana (Palpation):*** Touch-based examination to assess body temperature, texture, tenderness, and other tactile characteristics.
- ***Prashna (Interrogation):*** Questioning the patient to gather information about their medical history, symptoms, habits, and lifestyle.

Ashtavidha Pareeksha (Eightfold Examination): Includes examination of pulse (*nadi*), urine (*mutra*), stool (*mala*), tongue (*jihva*), voice (*shabda*), skin (*sparsha*), eyes (*drik*), and overall appearance (*akriti*).

Dashavidha Pareeksha (Tenfold Examination): The tenfold examination focuses on factors like constitution (*prakriti*), pathological state (*vikriti*), tissue quality (*sara*), compactness (*samhanana*), body measurements (*pramana*), adaptability (*satmya*), mental health (*sattva*), digestive capacity (*ahara shakti*), physical strength (*vyayama shakti*), and age (*vaya*).

***Dravyaguna*–The Science of Medicinal Substances:** Derived from two Sanskrit terms—*Dravya* (substance) and *Guna* (qualities)—*Dravyaguna* is a fundamental branch of Ayurveda and serves as its counterpart to modern pharmacology. It involves the pharmacological and therapeutic study of medicinal substances, including herbs, minerals, and other natural materials, with a focus on their properties, actions, and clinical applications (Acharya 2000, Acharya and Acharya 2003).

Key Factors Influencing Drug Action: Following key factors can influence the action of a drug

- ***Dravya*** **(Substance)** – The physical entity with inherent properties.
- ***Guna*** **(Properties)** – Forty-one qualities affecting the body, classified into somatic, psychic, physical, and applicative.
- ***Rasa*** **(Taste)** – Six primary tastes (*Madhura*, *Amla*, *Lavana*, *Katu*, *Tikta*, *Kashaya*) influence doshas and digestion.
- ***Vipaka*** **(Final Transformation)** – The post-digestive effect of a substance, categorized as *Madhura*, *Amla*, or *Katu*.
- ***Virya*** **(Potency)** – The active principle that determines the drug's strength, generally classified as *Ushna* (hot) or *Shita* (cold).
- ***Prabhava*** **(Specific Power)** – An inexplicable unique action beyond *Rasa*, *Vipaka*, and *Virya*.
- ***Karma*** **(Action)** – The effect of a drug in the body, including its impact on *doshas*, *dhatus*, and *malas*.

Interrelation and Drug Action in Ayurveda: In Ayurveda, the action of a drug is determined by the interplay of several key factors

- ***Rasa*** (taste) influences *Vipaka* (post-digestive effect), which is further modified by *Virya* (potency or energy).
- **Prabhava** (specific or unique action), being the most dominant factor, can override the effects of the other properties.
- The body's response to a substance is guided by its inherent affinity with external elements, based on the principle of *Loka-Purusha Samya* (the correspondence between the universe and the individual).

Classification: Medicinal substances are classified based on their origin:

- **Herbal**: Plants and plant-based products.
- **Mineral**: Metals, minerals, and naturally occurring inorganic substances.
- **Animal**: Substances derived from animals.

Therapeutic Applications: *Dravyaguna* provides guidelines for using medicinal substances to:

- Prevent and treat diseases.
- Promote health and well-being.
- Balance the body's doshas (Vata, Pitta, Kapha).

Dravyaguna forms the foundation for the effective practice of Ayurveda, guiding practitioners in the selection and application of medicinal substances to promote health and treat diseases. A deep understanding of these principles is crucial for effective Ayurvedic treatment.

Pramāṇa in Ayurveda – A Fundamental Concept of Knowledge Acquisition

Pramāṇa, a foundational concept in Ayurveda, serves as the means of acquiring valid knowledge, ensuring accurate understanding, and guiding both research and clinical practice. It encompasses methods for knowledge acquisition, data analysis, and interpretation, thereby aiding in navigating the complexities of health and disease, as well as supporting diagnostic processes. In research, *Pramāṇa* provides a structured, scientific approach within the discipline of Ayurveda.

Synonyms of *Pramāṇa:* The term *Pramāṇa* is derived from the Sanskrit root '*ma*' (to measure), prefixed by *pra* and suffixed with *lyuṭ*, collectively meaning a source or means of knowledge. According to Chakrapani, Pramāṇa is instrumental in examining entities to attain true knowledge. *Uplabdhi* (availability), *Sādhana* (source, tool), *Jñāna* (knowledge), *Parīkṣā* (examination, evaluation), are used in allied or overlapping senses with Pramana in Ayurvedic literature. Ayurveda recognizes four Pramanas, namely *Aptopadesha*, *Pratyaksha, Anumana*, and *Yukti* (Ankita 2021).

Types of Pramāṇa and their Modern Correlations

Acharya Charaka identifies four primary *Pramāṇas* for investigating existent (*Sat/ Bhava*) and non-existent (*Asat/Abhava*) entities: *Āptopadeśa*, *Pratyakṣa, Anumāna*, and *Yukti Āptopadeśa* is the primary method of information acquisition, *Pratyakṣa* is direct knowledge perception, *Anumāna* deals with inferential understanding, and Yukti emphasizes rational thought (Choudhary *et al.* 2024)

Āptopadeśa **Pramāṇa (Authoritative Testimony):** This refers to knowledge acquired from authoritative scriptures and the teachings of enlightened individuals (*Āptas*) who possess pure, unobstructed, and unquestionable knowledge, free from *Rajas* (passion) and *Tamas* (ignorance). Their words and actions serve as valid sources of knowledge, aligning with modern concepts of expert testimony and historical evidence in scientific research.

***Pratyakṣa* Pramāṇa (Direct Perception):** Knowledge gained through direct interaction between the senses and external objects. Acharya Sushruta emphasizes integrating *Āptopadeśa* with *Pratyakṣa* for comprehensive learning. *Pratyakṣa* is further classified into:

- ***Laukika Pratyakṣa (Ordinary Perception):*** Knowledge obtained through regular sensory experiences.
- ***Alaukika Pratyakṣa (Extraordinary Perception):*** Knowledge acquired beyond ordinary sensory perception, akin to intuition or higher cognitive faculties. In modern reasoning, *Pratyakṣa Pramāṇa* corresponds to empirical evidence and sensory observation used in scientific research.

***Anumāna* Pramāṇa (Inference):** The process of deriving unknown knowledge from known facts through logical inference. It serves as an indirect means of acquiring knowledge and follows *Pratyakṣa* and *Āptopadeśa. Anumāna* is categorized into:

- ***Svārthānumāna:*** Individual inference driven by personal curiosity.
- ***Parārthānumāna***: Inference used for demonstrating knowledge to others, employing *Panchāvayava Vākya* (five-part logical reasoning). This aligns with deductive and inductive reasoning in modern scientific methodology.

***Yukti* Pramāṇa (Logical Reasoning):** Involves acquiring knowledge through the rational and logical integration of multiple causative factors. It is essential for understanding complex interactions and achieving objectives. *Yukti* emphasizes a structured and effective combination of various elements, similar to systematic analysis and experimental design in modern science.

Additional Pramāṇa Concepts: Other factors contributing to Ayurvedic knowledge acquisition include:

- ***Upamāna*:** Knowledge gained through comparison, akin to analogy-based reasoning.
- ***Arthāpatti*:** Understanding implied meaning through relevant references, similar to presumption or postulation.
- ***Sambhava*:** Inferring knowledge based on related references.
- ***Abhāva*:** Understanding the absence of something, comparable to negative evidence or falsification in scientific inquiry.
- ***Ceṣṭā*:** Observing expressions or behavioural cues to derive meaning.
- ***Pariśeṣa*:** Eliminating alternatives to determine the correct conclusion, similar to the process of elimination in logical deduction.

Ayurveda and One Health

The One Health approach emphasizes the interconnectedness of human, animal, and environmental health, advocating for a collaborative, multidisciplinary effort to achieve optimal well-being for all. Ayurveda, with its holistic principles, naturally aligns with this concept by promoting a balanced and integrated approach to health. Beyond individual well-being, Ayurveda extends its focus to encompass environmental and animal health, recognizing the deep interdependence between these elements. This perspective resonates with the One Health approach, which addresses the intricate relationship between human, animal, and environmental health. The AYUSH system has the potential to contribute significantly to several priority areas within the One Health framework. Some of these include (Kumar *et al.* 2023):

- **Management of Zoonotic and Tropical Diseases:** AYUSH systems offer a range of preventive measures, dietary guidelines, immunomodulatory herbs and drugs, and therapeutic interventions for disease prevention and management.
- **Prevention and Management of Noncommunicable Diseases (NCDs):** Ayurveda can play a vital role in managing NCDs such as diabetes, cardiovascular diseases, cancer, and stroke, which are often influenced by lifestyle, dietary habits, and environmental factors.
- **Mitigating the Global Emergence of Antimicrobial Resistance:** Many Ayurvedic formulations are known for their immunomodulatory, antiseptic, and antimicrobial properties. Integrating Ayurveda and other traditional medicine systems, including ethnoveterinary medicine, with modern medical and veterinary practices can significantly contribute to reducing antimicrobial resistance.
- **Plant, Food Safety and Environmental Health:** Vrikshayurveda, the ancient science of plant health, provides detailed protocols and methods to ensure the healthy growth and productivity of various tree and plant species. Many of these traditional practices are supported by modern scientific validation. The integration of Vrikshayurveda's eco-friendly principles with contemporary science and technology can offer sustainable solutions for plant production systems. Additionally, promoting safe agricultural practices can enhance food safety and environmental health. The indiscriminate use of agrochemicals, such as pesticides and insecticides, contributes to soil, water, and air pollution, biodiversity loss, and chemical residues in food. Ayurveda-based approaches can help mitigate these risks and support ecological balance.

Conclusion

Ayurveda, meaning 'Science of Life' in Sanskrit, is a holistic system of medicine that originated in India over five millennia ago. It emphasizes maintaining health through a balanced lifestyle, addressing physical, mental, and spiritual well-being. The structural, functional, and pharmacological branches of Ayurveda are conceptualized on the metaphysical doctrine of Panchamahabhutas (the five foundational elements of the universe and life) and the *Trigunas* (the three properties of nature-super power). The Panchamahabhutas are the evolved forms of *Trigunatmaka Prakriti* (supernatural power/constitution). Ayurveda emphasizes optimal health and well-being through a multifaceted strategy that harmonizes the mind, body, behaviour, and environment through dietary adjustments, lifestyle recommendations, and therapeutic interventions like Panchakarma—comprising biodetoxification and bio-purification procedures and use of natural substance for treatment of diseases. Historically, Ayurveda has significantly influenced global medicine. Pioneers like Sushruta and Charaka made notable contributions; for instance, Sushruta's surgical techniques, including early forms of rhinoplasty, laid the groundwork for modern plastic surgery. However, after the golden age of Ayurveda, marked by the contributions of great scholars like Charaka, Sushruta, and Vagbhata, Ayurveda experienced a prolonged phase of stagnation. This period, spanning roughly from the 8th century to the 18th century, was marked by several factors such as decline in scholarly activity, foreign invasions and colonial rule, rise of Unani Medicine, social and cultural changes, and lack of institutional support to cite a few.

In recent decades, the Government of India has undertaken sustained initiatives to institutionalize and mainstream Ayurveda within national healthcare systems. The establishment of the Ministry of AYUSH and research bodies such as the Central Council for Research in Ayurvedic Sciences (CCRAS) has strengthened education, research, documentation, and regulatory oversight of traditional medical knowledge. A nationwide network of Ayurvedic colleges, research institutes, and registered practitioners supports both human and animal healthcare. Authoritative compilations, including the *Ayurveda Formulary of India and the Ayurveda Pharmacopoeia of India*, document standardized formulations and authenticated medicinal plant monographs, notably including veterinary preparations. These formal systems draw substantially upon India's long-standing ethnoveterinary traditions, which preserve community-based knowledge of herbal therapies, animal management, and disease prevention. Regulatory frameworks under the Drugs and Cosmetics Act, together with the recognition of classical Ayurvedic texts, ensure quality, safety, and therapeutic consistency. Collectively, these developments reflect the potential for integrating classical Ayurveda with ethnoveterinary practices into contemporary healthcare frameworks, reinforcing their relevance for holistic, sustainable, and culturally rooted approaches to human and animal health and well-being.

Globally, Ayurveda is gaining recognition as a natural and holistic healthcare system. Its focus on individualized treatment and preventive care aligns with the growing demand for sustainable health solutions. Modern scientific research continues to validate many Ayurvedic principles, fostering a renewed interest in its practices. Additionally, Ayurveda's comprehensive approach to health, emphasizing prevention, personalized care, and environmental harmony, aligns closely with the One Health concept. Integrating Ayurvedic principles into modern healthcare can promote a more holistic and sustainable approach, benefiting humans, animals, and the environment alike. Remember Ayurveda teaches us healthy lifestyle with healthy mind and environment. It is a prototype of ecopsychology, which holds that humans need to rediscover their ties to the natural world in order to experience full mental health:

Sarve bhavantu sukhinah, Sarve santu nirāmayāḥ; Sarve bhadrāṇi paśyantu, Mā kaścid-duḥkha-bhāg-bhavet (Brihadaranyaka Upanishad).

'Let all be happy, let all be free from debilitation, let all see goodness, let there be no victims of sorrow.'

References

Acharya JT and Acharya NR. 2003. *Sushuruta Samhita of Sushruta with 'Nibandhasangraha' commentary by Dalhana.* Chaukhamba Surbharati Prakashan, Varanasi, Uttar Pradesh, India.

Acharya JT. 2000. *Charaka Samhita of Agnivesha with Ayurveda Dipika Commentary of Chakrapani.* Chaukhamba Surbharati Prakashan, Varanasi, Uttar Pradesh, India.

Ali M. 1993. A brief history of Indian alchemy covering pre-Vedic to Vedic and Ayurvedic period (circa 400 BC-800 AD). *Bulletin of the Indian Institute of History of Medicine (Hyderabad)* **23**(2): 151–66.

Altekar AS. 2009. Some educational centres and institutions. In: *Education in Ancient India.* 6th edn. pp. 245-98. Gyan Publishing House, Reprinted by Isha Books, Delhi, India.

Ankita. 2021. A review on role of *Pramanas* in Ayurvedic research methodology. *International Ayurvedic Medical Journal* **9**(2): 423-29. doi:10.46607/iamj1609022021.

Anonymous. 1949. The history of medicine in India. In: *Caraka Samhita.* pp. 9-25. Shree Gulabkunverba Ayurvedic Society, Jamnagar. Available at: https://dn790006.ca. archive. org /0/items /in. ernet.dli.2015.63710/2015.63710.The-Caraka-Samhita1_text.pdf. downloaded on 21-08-2024.

Arnott R. 2024. Healing and medicine. In: *Disease and Healing in the Indus Civilisation.* pp. 134-61. Archaeopress Publishing Ltd Summertown, Oxford, UK.

Astanga Hridaya Sutra Sthan. https://www.planetayurveda.com/ayurveda-ebooks/astanga-hridaya-sutrasthan-handbook.pdf, downloaded on 24-09-2024.

Callahan D. 1973. The WHO definition of' health. Hastings Centre Studies **1**(3): 77-87. http://www.jstor.org/stable/352746.

Choudhary R, Pathak R and Upadhyay K. 2024. A summary of *Pramanas'* part in Ayurvedic research methods. *World Journal of Pharmaceutical Research* **14** (1): 703-13.

Dalrymple W. 2024. *The Golden Road: How Ancient India Transformed the World.* pp. 105-32, 237-53, Bloomsbury Publishing, New Delhi, India

Gore V, Bhatkar A, Nimbalkar M, Bagde A and Fulkar S. 2023. A bird eye view on *Ashtanga Hridaya. World Journal of Pharmacy and Pharmaceutical Sciences* **12** (8): 784-92.

Kizhakkeveettil A, Parla J, Patwardhan K, Sharma A, Sharma S. 2024. History, present and prospect of Ayurveda. In: *History, Present and Prospect of World Traditional Medicine.* pp. 1-72. World Scientific Publishing Company https://doi.org/10.1142/9789811282171_0001.

Kumar S, Gopal KM, Choudhary A, Soman A and Namburi URS. 2023. Advancing the one health approach through integration of Ayush systems: Opportunities and way forward. *Journal of Family Medicine and Primary Care* **12**(9): 1764-70. doi: 10.4103/jfmpc.jfmpc_192_23

Lowe R and Yasuhara Y. 2016. From the Indus to the Ganges. In: *The Origins of Higher Learning: Knowledge Networks and the Early Development of Universities.* pp 31-56. Routledge. Taylor and Francis Group, London, New York, USA.

Meena DK, Upadhyay D, Singh R and Dwibedy BK. 2015. A critical review of fundamental principles of Ayurveda. A critical review of fundamental principles of Ayurveda *International Ayurvedic Medical Journal* **3** (7): 2075-8.

Paradakar HS(Ed). 2005. *Astanga Hrdayam of Vagbhata with The Commentaries of Sarvangasundara of Arunadatta and Ayurvedarasyana of Hemadri.* Chaukhamba Orientalia, Varanasi, Uttar Pradesh, India.

Patwardhan K and Upadhyaya W. 2020. *Arthedashmahamooliya Adhyaya.* In: *Charak Samhita New Edition.* 1st edn. pp.32. (Eds) Dwivedi RB, Deole YS and Basisht G. CSRTSDC ebook, Jamnagar, India. Doi:10.47468/CSNE.2020.e01.s01.032. Available at: https://www.carakasamhitaonline.com/mediawiki-1.32.1/index.php?.

Paul R. 2022. Medicine history. *Journal* of *Indian Medical Association* **120**(4): 89.

Potbhare BM, Reddy RG, Thakre PA and Sangvikar S. 2019. Samrat Ashoka's inscriptions and Ayurveda: A review. *International Journal of Ayurveda and Pharma Research* **7**(9): 69-72.

Rao M. 2020. *Vividhashitapitiya Adhyaya.* In: *Charak Samhita New Edition.* 1st edn. pp.30. (Eds.) Patwardhan K, Deole YS and Basisht G. CSRTSDC ebook, Jamnagar, India. Doi: 10.47468/ CSNE.2020.e01.s01.030. Available at: https://doi.org/10.47468/CSNE.2020.e01.s01.030.

Ray P, Gupta HN and Roy M. 1980. *Suśruta saṃhitā: (a scientific synopsis).* New Delhi: Indian National Science Academy. p. 4. OCLC 985517620. https://archive.org/details/englishtranslati00susruoft/page/n15/mode/2up.pdf, downloaded 28-02-2025.

Sewada D, Sharma M, Mishra TN and Pooja Arora P. 2023. A comparative study of *Astanga Hridaya* and *Astanga Samgraha-* A Review Article. *International Research Journal of Ayurveda & Yoga* **6** (6):78-85. DOI: 10.47223/IRJAY.2023.6612.

Sharma SP. 2006. *Ashtanga Samgraha of Vrddha Vagbhata with Sasilekha' Commentary by Indu.* Chowkhanmba Sanskrit Series Office, Varanasi, India.

Singh RH, Singh G, Sodhi JS and Dixit U .2020. *Deerghanjiviteeya Adhyaya.* In: *Charak Samhita New Edition.* 1st edn. pp.3. (Eds) Dixit U, Deole YS and Basisht G. CSRTSDC ebook, Jamnagar, India. Available at: https://doi.org/10.47468/CSNE.2020.e01.s01.003.

Valiathan MS. 2006. Evolution of Healing Art in India. In: *Towards Ayurvedic Biology: A Decadal Vision Document – 2006.* pp. 8-18. Indian Academy of Sciences, Bangalore, India.

9

Origin, Principles, and Practices of Veterinary Ayurveda (*Pashu Ayurveda*): Historical Overview and Scientific Relevance

R. Somvanshi, D. Swarup and Aruna T. Kumar

Audumbareṇa maṇinā pustikāmāya vedhasā. Paśūnām sarveṣām sphātim gosthe me savitā karat.
May Savita, creative genius, with Vedha, the expert of specialised knowledge, with Audumbara mani, a prize preparation of Ficus glomerata, develop in my cow stall plenty of all breeds of healthy animals for me as I am keen for the health, growth and development of animals.

(Atharva Veda 19.31.1. translation by Sharma 2013)

1. Introduction
2. Specialized Branches of Pashu Ayurveda
3. Origins of Veterinary Ayurvedic Medicine (Pashu Ayurveda)
4. Historical Background and Advances in Veterinary Ayurveda
5. Principal Medical Ayurveda *Āchāryas* and their Contributions to Pashu Ayurveda
6. Veterinary Ayurveda Scholars and their Work
7. Veterinary Ayurveda: Way Forward
8. Veterinary Ayurveda—Future Directions and Market Expansion
9. Conclusion

Introduction

Veterinary Ayurveda, known as *Pashu Ayurveda* or *Mrig Ayurveda*, is one of the oldest and most structured systems of veterinary medicine in the world. It reflects the deep-rooted, holistic man-animal relationship that has existed in Indian civilization for centuries. Animals have played an integral role in various socio-economic, agricultural, and cultural aspects of life in ancient India, necessitating a well-developed system of healthcare for their well-being. Ancient Indian literature is replete with references to the rearing, treatment, and management of animal health. Texts such as the Vedas, Brahmanas, Puranas, Epics (Ramayana and Mahabharata), Buddhist scriptures, and the Arthashastra of Kautilya, along with the linguistic treatises of Pāṇini and other scholarly works of ancient *Āchāryas*, provide valuable insights into the practices of animal care. These texts mention specialized physicians dedicated to the treatment of animals, referred to as *'Pashu Vaidyas'* (Veterinary physicians) or '*Shalihotriyas* (Veterinarians; Equine experts).' Not only physicians but also kings, princes, and warriors were well-versed in the knowledge of animal healthcare, as the welfare of livestock was crucial to the prosperity of kingdoms.

The principles of Veterinary Ayurveda evolved parallel to those of human medicine, applying the same fundamental doctrines of Ayurveda to animal health. Ancient Indian texts on Ayurveda provide extensive information on diagnosing and treating diseases in animals using herbs, minerals, and holistic healing methods. The Panchamahabhuta doctrine, a foundational concept in Ayurveda, emphasizes that all living beings—including humans, animals, and plants—are composed of five fundamental elements:

- *Prithvi* (Earth): Represents solidity and stability; associated with bones, muscles, and tissues.
- *Jala* (Water): Represents fluidity and cohesion; corresponds to bodily fluids such as blood, lymph, and secretions.
- *Agni* (Fire): Represents transformation and metabolism; linked to digestion and body temperature regulation.
- *Vayu* (Air): Represents movement and dynamism; governs respiration, circulation, and nervous system functions.
- *Akasha* (Ether/Space): Represents expansiveness and emptiness; associated with bodily cavities and cellular spaces.

Recognizing that all living beings share this elemental composition, Vedic sages extended the knowledge of Ayurveda beyond human healthcare to develop specialized branches for animals and plants. This led to the evolution of distinct disciplines, such as:

- ***Mṛg Āyurveda:*** Also known in later texts as *Paśu Āyurveda* (Pashu Ayurveda), this branch of Ayurveda focuses on the health and welfare of animals, particularly domesticated species.
- ***Matsya Ayurveda*:** Dedicated to the health and well-being of aquatic animals, including fish and amphibians.
- ***Vriksha Ayurveda*:** Concerned with the health, conservation, and medicinal applications of plants.

Specialized Branches of Pashu Ayurveda

Pashu Ayurveda has been further evolved into specialized branches to cater to the unique needs of various animals. These specialized branches underscore the significance of animals in Vedic society and reflect a profound understanding of their care and management.

- ***Aśvāyurveda (Ashva Ayurveda, Ashva-ayurveda,* Equine Science*):*** Horses held immense importance in ancient India, serving roles in transportation, agriculture, and warfare. Ashva Ayurveda, also known as Haya Ayurveda, is one of the earliest branches of veterinary science, focusing on the comprehensive care of horses. It encompasses the study of different horse breeds, their behaviours, physiological aspects, and medical treatments. This branch provides remedies for common equine ailments, strategies to maintain stamina and strength, and dietary guidelines to ensure optimal health. The foundational text, Shalihotra Samhita, authored by the sage physician Shalihotra, is a seminal work in this field. Relatively speaking, the medical care of the horses was in a much more advanced stage in ancient India than it is nowadays.

- ***Gajāyurveda (Gaja Ayurveda, Gaja-ayurveda,* Elephant Science*):*** In ancient India, elephants—revered as royal and sacred symbols of strength and sovereignty—played a pivotal role in the politico-economic structure of kingdoms. Their significance extended beyond ceremonial display to military strategy, diplomatic exchange, and royal prestige. Gaja Ayurveda, also known as Hastyāyurveda (Hastyā Ayurveda), is the specialized branch of Ayurvedic science devoted to the health and ethical management of elephants. It addresses both physical and psychological well-being, offering treatments for skin disorders, joint ailments, and stress induced by captivity or overwork. This branch also offers guidelines on proper diet, training, and ethical care, emphasizing the importance of suitable habitats, known as *Gajavana*, for these majestic creatures.

- ***Go-Āyurveda* (Bovine Science):** Cows have been deeply revered in Vedic society, symbolizing prosperity and benevolence. *Go-ayurveda* centres on the health and well-being of cattle, particularly cows. It includes treatments for issues affecting milk production, fertility problems, injuries, and common infections. Preventive care strategies are emphasized to maintain optimal health. Additionally, this branch highlights the role of cows in producing *Panchgavya*, a combination of five cow-derived products used for its medicinal properties.

- ***Śyen-Āyurveda* (Syen Ayurveda, Avian Science):** This specialized branch focuses on the care of birds, including falcons and other species trained for specific purposes such as retrieving medicinal plants or serving as messengers. *Syen-Āyurveda* involves diagnosing and treating various avian ailments, providing dietary recommendations, and offering preventive care to ensure the overall well-being of birds. It also addresses the rehabilitation of injured or sick birds, guiding their recovery and reintegration into their natural habitats or human care.

- ***Pet-Āyurveda* (*Pet-Ayurveda*, Ayurvedic Care for Companion Animals):** A modern extension of Pashu Ayurveda, Pet Ayurveda applies traditional Ayurvedic principles to the care of domesticated companion animals—primarily dogs, cats, and pet birds. It emphasizes natural, constitution-based, and ecologically attuned methods to promote physical health, emotional balance, and preventive wellness. Unlike the classical sub-branches of Pashu Ayurveda such as Ashva Ayurveda and Gaja Ayurveda, this category reflects contemporary adaptations of Ayurvedic principles suited to modern urban and household settings, offering holistic care tailored to the unique temperaments and lifestyles of companion animals.

Origins of Veterinary Ayurvedic Medicine (*Pashu Ayurveda*)

The roots of Veterinary Ayurveda can be traced back to the Vedas, the oldest documented records of Indian literature. The Vedas contain numerous Ayurvedic references, including those related to herbal medicine and surgical treatments for animal well-being. Among them, the Atharva Veda—a repository of ancient ethnomedical knowledge—features several hymns dedicated to animal health and protection. One significant example is found in *Kanda 6, Sukta 59*, which is devoted to the divine herb *Arundhati*. In this hymn, the Atharva Rishi prays:

Anadudbhyastvam prathamam dhenubhya-stvamarundhati. Adhenave vayase śarma yaccha catuspade (Atharva Veda 6.59.1).

Translated as:

'O Arundhati, give peace and comfort of good health first to the cow and the bullock, and give health and peace for life to all the quadrupeds other than the cow' (Sharma 2013).

Divine Transmission of Veterinary Ayurveda Knowledge

Similar to human Ayurveda, Veterinary Ayurveda is believed to have a divine origin in Hindu mythology. The knowledge of Pashu Ayurveda is said to have been bestowed upon humanity by celestial beings, including Brahma, Rudra, Indra, the Moon and Sun Gods, and twin Ashvins-the divine physicians. Raivata, the revered master of horses, and Dhanvantari, the legendary physician of the *Devas*, are also associated with the transmission of this sacred wisdom. According to mythology, the Gods revealed this knowledge to ancient sages (*Rishis*) who were deeply connected with nature and dedicated to the welfare of all living beings. This divine wisdom was then passed down through generations, forming the foundation of veterinary science in India. One of the most prominent figures in Pashu Ayurveda is Sage Shalihotra, often regarded as the father of veterinary science in India. He is believed to have received divine knowledge about animal health and welfare directly from the Gods. His teachings significantly influenced later scholars, including Nakula, the renowned equine specialist from the Mahabharata, who is said to have acquired the knowledge of Hayayurveda (equine medicine) from Shalihotra. Key exponents of veterinary ayurveda are: Surya (Sun God), Chandra (Moon God), Sage Shalihotra, Sushruta (also called Dinapat), and Garga and other sages. The significance of these sages is also reflected in Sanskrit scriptures, such as the following verses from the *Aśvaśāstram* (*Vajiprasna, Adhyaya* 6-8, Gopalan 1952):

प्रणपित्य धवलतनुं तमिरिहरं गोपतर्शिशाङ्गं च । अश्वायुर्वेदनधिर्मिहामुनर्शिालहोित्रं च ॥
ये शालहोित्रसुश्रुतगर्गादमिहर्षभिःपुरा गदताः। स्वे स्वे तुरङ्गशास्त्रे योगाःशान्त्यै वकिाराणाम् ॥
तेषां मध्यादराजन् सारतरं हयाहतार्थमुदधृत्य । रचतिःस्वयं समासेन सङ्ग्रहःसदि्धयोिगानाम् ॥ '

A rough Translation:

'The Moon, whose body is white and dispels darkness, is the lord of the cowherds. I also revere the great sage Śālihotra, the treasure house of Vedic wisdom. The names of great sages such as Śālihotra, Suśruta, and Garga are mentioned in ancient texts. The knowledge of *Ashva Shashtra* (equine medicine) is described in scriptures as a means of calming disturbances in horses.'

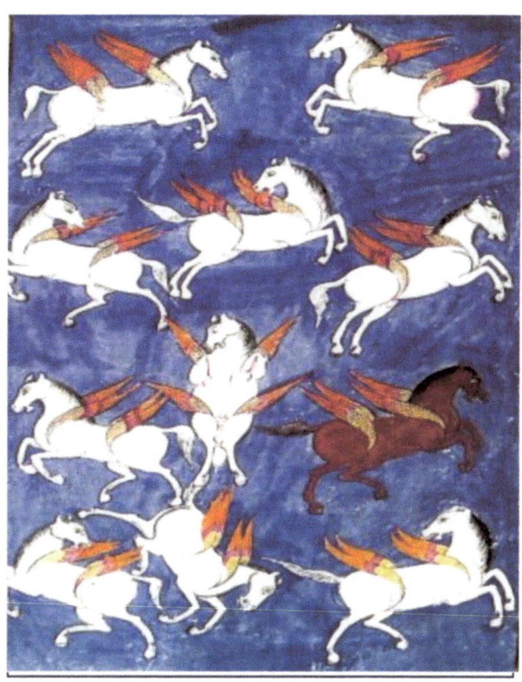

Fig. 9.1. Winged celestial progenitors of horses lose their wings at the hands of Śālihotra—the fountainhead of equine knowledge—to become chariot-pullers for Indra, thereby serving mankind more effectively (Source: Aśvaśāstram, Sri Venkateswara University Oriental Research Institute, Tirupati. Courtesy of Dr. V. V. Rao, SVVU Tirupati).

A legend about transfer of knowledge of equine medicine is given in Nakula's *Aśvaśāstram*. According to it horses were celestial creatures born with wings and could freely fly across the sky with Gandharvas (Fig. 9.1). Seeing their strength and suitability as vehicles, Indra addressed the sage Śālihotra (Shalihotra), the master of horse and knowledge holder of equinology, requesting his help in making the horses more useful for the world. Obeying Indra's command, Shalihotra removed their wings through a ritual, causing them great sorrow. Grieving and drenched in blood, they questioned the sage, arguing that the virtuous do not harm the innocent. Moved by compassion, Shalihotra reassured them that they would still hold an honoured place in the world. He foretold that horses would become the esteemed mounts of deities such as Surya and Indra, as well as revered companions of earthly rulers and assured them that he would teach men all the rare secrete of horse lore to enable to look after them properly. Shalihotra then imparted knowledge of horse care, emphasizing nourishment, healing, and well-being to earthy world and sent the horses to roam the earth and the underworld, ensuring they would continue to play a vital role in human civilization. The Vedic people admired horses for their swiftness and brilliance, with sacred texts referencing the winged steeds of deities like Surya and the Maruts. The legend portrayal symbolizes the vital energy and dynamic force that horses represented in Vedic culture and a representation of an important biological stage in animal life. Additionally, this act can be interpreted as a symbolic representation of taming wild horses by Shalihotra for human use, marking a significant advancement in domestication practices (Gopalan 1952).

Historical Background and Advances in Veterinary Ayurveda

Death and disease have troubled humanity since the dawn of civilization. Observing the instinctive healing behaviours of animals, early humans likely discovered—by chance—the medicinal properties of various herbs and natural substances (See Chapter 5). This rudimentary knowledge laid the foundation for healing practices in early societies, which evolved and expanded over time. Spanning over five millennia, the history of Indian medicine-encompassing both human and veterinary traditions—can be traced through different socio-cultural and political periods. The integration of medicinal practices with religious and philosophical thought played a crucial role in shaping India's medical heritage, influencing both practical treatments and the broader understanding of health and disease.

Vedic Period

The Vedic culture, which emerged during the 3rd and 2nd millennia BCE, was one of the world's oldest and most significant civilizations. This period saw the composition of the Vedas and the establishment of major urban centres such as Mohenjo-daro and Harappa, marking the beginning of the first urban society in South Asia (Jones 2021). The four Vedas—Rig Veda, Yajur Veda, Sama Veda, and Atharva Veda—form the foundation of Vedic knowledge. Each Veda is further divided into four sections:

- *Samhitas* – Collections of Vedic hymns,
- *Brahmanas* – Theological and ritualistic interpretations,

- *Aranyakas* – texts discussing rituals, ceremonies, sacrifices, and symbolic offerings, and
- *Upanishads* – philosophical discourses on spiritual knowledge.

Vedic literature, particularly the Samhitas, contains a wealth of information that directly or indirectly contributed to the development of ancient medical traditions.

Ayurveda Origins from Vedas: Although Ayurveda is classified as an *Upaveda* (a subsidiary Veda) of the Atharva Veda, its primary roots can be traced back to the Rig Veda, which contains numerous references to rituals, hygiene, medicinal herbs, surgery, and the duties of physicians. These elements form the foundational principles of Ayurveda for both human and animal health. The fundamental Panchamahabhuta (five-element theory) in Ayurveda has its root in the Rig Veda, where the five elements—Agni (Fire), Vayu (Air/Wind), Apas (Water), Prithvi (Earth) and Akasha (Ether/Space)—are praised for their interconnected roles in sustaining life and maintaining cosmic harmony. The Rig Veda describes *Agni* as a divine force that benefits all creatures:

saṃ-sam id yuvase vṛṣann agne viśvāny arya ā; iḻas pade sam idhyase sa no vasūny ā bhara (Rig Veda 10.191.1).

English Translation

'Agni, showerer of benefits, you who are the lord, you verily combine with all creatures. You are kindled upon the altar; bring unto us riches' (Wilson 1946).

The Rig Veda also extols the curative properties of water, the sun, and medicinal herbs. It mentions toxic germs and their eradication, noting that-sun rays eliminate diseases such as parasitic worms, cardiac ailments, and jaundice, water maintains bodily vitality and possesses medicinal properties, and fire destroys bacteria and viruses. Vayu is described as *Bhiṣak* (physician) and the reliever of disease (मयोभु): *vāta ā vātu bheṣajaṃ śambhu mayobhu no hṛade; pra ṇa āyūṃṣi tāriṣat-* (Rig Veda 10.186.1) translated as: 'May Vata breathe into our hearts a haling balm, bringing happiness; may prolong our life' (Wilson 1928). Also, divine beings are credited with medical prowess. Indra, Marut, and Rudra are invoked as celestial healers both for human and animals, with Rudra being the earliest and most accomplished among them. He is hailed as *prathamo daivyo bhiṣak* (the first divine physician), and sixty-two medical decoctions are attributed to him. Aśvinī Kumāras, twin deities, are also invoked for their healing abilities (Maji 2021). A solemn ritual of Vedic period, linked to medicinal practice, was the consumption of *Soma*, a sacred drink extracted from plant (s) to grant immortality, strength, and disease resistance:

apāma somam amṛtā abhūmāganma jyotir avidāma devān; kiṃ nūnam asmān kṛṇavad arātiḥ kim u dhūrtir amṛta martyasya (Rig Veda 8.48.3).

Translated as:

'We have drunk the Soma and become immortal; we have attained the divine light and come to know the gods. What now can our enemy do to us, or what harm can the mortal inflict upon the immortal' (Wilson 1928).

apa tyā asthur anirā amīvā nir atrasan tamiṣīcīr abhaiṣuḥ; ā somo asmām̐ aruhad vihāyā aganma yatra pratiranta āyuḥ (Rig Veda 8.48.11).

Translated as:

'May those irremovable ailments depart; let those strong pains that made us tremble be dispelled. The mighty Soma has entered us, granting the life-prolonging elixir' (Wilson 1928).

The identity of the plant used to prepare Soma remains a subject of debate among scholars, with proposed candidates including *Amanita muscaria*, psilocybin mushrooms (often called magic mushrooms), *Peganum harmala*, and *Ephedra sinica*. In South India, the flowers of *Illuppai* (*Madhuca indica*) have been identified as Soma, while *Ceropegia juncea* is used as Soma by Ayurvedic practitioners in Kerala. The history of the *Soma* plant is closely linked to the migration of Vedic *Āryans* across different regions and time periods, with the choice of plants varying based on local availability. The Soma tradition also highlights the ethnobotanical knowledge of the Vedic period and its applications in medicine (Shah 2015).

Role of Domestic Animals in Vedic Society: Domestic animals such as cattle, horses, donkeys, sheep, and goats played a pivotal role in Vedic society, shaping its socioeconomic, cultural, and religious structures. Horses and elephants, in particular, were indispensable for transportation and warfare. Cattle, buffaloes, sheep, goats, camels, asses, mules, swine, and dogs were domesticated for various purposes, many of which were directly or indirectly linked to agriculture. Cattle tending was considered a solemn religious vow (*vrata*) and was entrusted to a specific group of people who possessed extensive knowledge and expertise in the practice. Cattle rearing formed the backbone of economic management, making cattle the primary symbol of wealth. Vedic people relied on cattle for milk, food, and leather for daily use. Agricultural activities, such as tilling, were possible only with the help of bullocks, and cattle also served as a medium of exchange. Sheep provided invaluable wool for clothing, while goats supplied both milk and hide. These two small ruminants were also offered as sacrificial oblations to the gods. Milk of sheep was used for sacred rituals as indicated in Yajur Veda- *'Let the man of yajna perform the yajna in honour of Sarasvati, divine voice and mother power of enlightenment, with the holy food of sheep's milk and ghee'* (21. 44, Sharma 2013b). Dogs were trained to guard homes and livestock and possibly played a role in battles. Camels were highly valued as prestigious gifts and were also used in warfare (Kansara 2008). Though presence of poultry during Vedic period remains unattested, birds were maintained as pet and trained for specific purposes. A fascinating aspect of bird-keeping during the Rigvedic period is its association with the Soma ritual. According to the Rig Veda, *Śyena* (a falcon) or Suparna delivered the Soma plant to Indra. Based on interpretations of these hymns, Shah (2015) posited that around 3700 BCE, Vedic Aryans possibly used the fly-agaric mushroom (*Amanita muscaria*) to prepare the Soma drink. As the mushroom became scarce and was primarily found in remote mountainous regions, trained falcons—Śyena, Suparna, or Gayatri (likely *Falco columbarius*) —were employed to retrieve it:

ānyaṃ divo mātariśvā jabhārāmathnād anyam pari śyeno adreḥ; agnīṣomā brahmaṇā vāvṛdhānoruṃ yajñāya cakrathur u lokam (Rig Veda 1.93.6).

atas tvā rayim abhi rājānaṃ sukrato divaḥ; suparṇo avyathir bharat (Rig Veda 9.48.3).

viśvasmā it svar dṛśe sādhāraṇaṃ rajasturam; gopām ṛtasya vir bharat (Rig Veda 9.48.4).

Translated as:

'Agni and Soma, the wind brought one of you from heaven, a hawk carried off the other by force from the summit of the mountain; growing vast by praise, you have made the worldwide for (the performance of) sacrifice'.

'O (Soma), doer of good deeds, the unwearied hawk brought you, king over riches, from this heaven'.

'The bird brought you, the showerer of water, the protector of the sacrifice, the common property of every god' (Wilson 1866).

Animal Welfare: The Veda*s*, particularly the Rig Veda, Atharva Veda, and Yajur Veda, emphasize the interconnectedness of all living beings, reflecting a deep respect for animal welfare. This philosophy is rooted in the principle of *Ahimsa* (non-violence), advocating for compassion and care towards animals. Animals were admired in Vedic society, not just for their utility but also as sacred beings. Cows, for example, were revered and often referred to as Kamadhenu, the wish-fulfilling divine cow. The Rig Veda refers to the cow as *aghnya* (not to be killed or injured) at least 17 times. Similarly, horses, breeding bulls, and working bullocks were also protected from harm. Vedic texts prescribe severe punishments, including death or banishment, for those who kill horses or other animals or harm cows. One such verse from the Rig Veda (10.87.16) states:

yaḥ pauruṣeyeṇa kraviṣā samaṅkte yo aśvyena paśunā yātudhānaḥ; yo aghnyāyā bharati kṣīram agne teṣāṃ śīrṣāṇi harasāpi vṛśca. (Rig Veda 10.87.16).

Translated as:

'The *Yātudhāna*, who fills himself with the flesh of man, and he who fills himself with the flesh of horses or of other animals, and he who steals the milk of the cow-- cut off their heads with your flame' (Wilson 1946).

The Yajur Veda and Atharva Veda echo similar sentiments. The Yajur Veda begins with an invocation to Savita, praying for the prosperity of cows, emphasizing that they should neither be stolen nor slaughtered:

Iṣe tvorje tvā vāyava stha devo vaḥ savitā prā-rpayatu śresthatamāya karmaṇa āpyāyadhva-maghnya›indrāya bhāgam prajāvatiranamīvā ayakṣmā mā va stena'īśata māghaśamso dhruvā asmin gopatau syāta bahvīryajamānasya paśun pāhi (Yajur Veda 1.1).

Translated as:

'Lord Creator, Savita, for the gifts of food and energy, light and life, for the body, mind and soul. Pray that you dedicate yourself to the noblest action, *yajna*, and play your part in the service of the Lord. Be blest with the best of health and wealth in plenty, cows, healthy, strong and fertile, sacred, not to be killed. No thief to rule over you, no sinner to boss over you! Growing in power and prosperity, be firm and loyal to this Lord of the Nation and protect the wealth and honour of the *yajamana*' (Sharma 2013b).

Chapter 13 (Verses 42, 43, 47–51) of the Yajur Veda further emphasizes the welfare of domestic animals. The sage Virupa prays to Lord Agni, requesting protection for horses, cows, bulls, sheep, goats, birds, and aquatic creatures essential to human life; rather direct attention to forest and harmful wild animals:

Imam mā himsīrekaśapham paśum kanikradam vājinaṁ vājinesu. Gauramāranyamanu te diśāmi tena cinvänastanvo niṣīda. Gauram te śugṛcchatu yam dviṣmastam te sugrcchatu (Yajur Veda 13.48).

Translated as:

'Do not kill this one-hoofed animal, fastest among the fast, roaring in the battles. I advise you, turn your attention to the white, yellow and brown animals, the wild ones, and growing by this animal wealth, sit at peace with yourself. Let your concern address the wild animals. Let it be directed to those who hurt us' (Sharma 2013b).

Subsequent verses extend this sentiment to sheep and other animals:

Imam sahasram śatadhāramutsam vyacya-manam sarirasya madhye. Ghṛtam duhānām-aditim janāyāgne mã himsīḥ parame vyoman. Gavayamāraṇyamanu te diśāmi tena cinvana-stanvo niṣīda. Gavayam te sugṛcchatu yam dviṣmastam te śugṛcchatu (Yajur Veda 13. 49).

Translated as:

'Agni, enlightened ruler, in the world even in the best of places, do not kill the cow and the bull, infinitely useful, and spring of a hundred streams and showers of milk and ghee for the people. It is holy and worthy of protection and development. I advise you, turn your attention to the wild cow and the bull and other animals. Growing and developing the economy with animal and forest wealth, feel settled with yourself and your land. Let your attention be directed to the wild cow and the forest wealth. Let your concern take on those who hurt us' (Sharma 2013b).

Imamurṇāyum varuṇasya nābhim tvacam paśunām dvipadām catuspadām. Tvastuh prajānām prathamam janitramagne mā himsih parame vyoman. Ustramāranyamanu te diśāmi tena cinvänastanvo niṣīda. Uṣtram te sugṛcchatu yam dviṣmastam te śugṛcchatu (Yajur Veda 13.50).

Translated as:

'Agni, noble ruler, in the wonderful world of the Supreme Lord, do not hurt, do not kill the sheep and other such animals, one of the first creations of Twashta, the maker of the world, and source of comfort and providers of woollen cover to the human beings and the animals. I point out to the wild camel and other wild animals. Growing and developing the economy with that animal wealth, be at peace with yourself in your land. Let your concern turn to the camel. Let it be directed to those who hurt us' (Sharma 2013b).

Vedic scholar Saraswati suggests that the wild animals mentioned in these verses may symbolize the ancestors of domesticated species—*gaura* as the precursor to the horse, *gavaya* as the precursor to the cow, *wild ustra* as the precursor to the sheep, and *śarabha* as the precursor to the goat (Saraswati 2011). These references may reflect the symbolic nature of the verses rather than literal prohibitions. The early Vedic society was predominantly pastoral, constantly seeking new grazing lands. Fire was often used to clear forests, facilitating migration and settlement. It is possible that the ancient Aryans encountered wild ancestors or feral populations of domestic animals, which may have posed threats to their survival. Thus, these verses could represent an attempt to balance human needs with ecological awareness, encouraging the protection of valuable domestic species while managing wild populations. Protection of other animals such as birds is also appreciated in Vedic culture as reflected in Rig Veda:

āsno vṛkasya vartikām abhīke yuvaṃ narā nāsatyāmumuktam; uto kavim purubhujā yuvaṃ ha kṛpamāṇam akṛṇutaṃ vicakṣe (Rig Veda 1.116.14).

Translated as:

'Nāsatyas, leaders, you liberated the quail from the mouth of the dog that had seized her, and you, who are the benefactors of many, have granted to the sage who praises you, to behold (true wisdom)' (Wilson 1946).

Animal Healthcare: Vedic scriptures provide ample evidence of healthcare practices for domestic animals. One of the main objectives of *Yajnas* was to invoke divine blessings for abundant and healthy livestock. Many hymns highlight this aspect, including prayers to Lord Rudra, regarded as the supreme physician. The Atharva Veda invokes the sacred herb Arundhati endowed with manifold curative powers, in accordance with Rudra's injunctions, to ward off disease from both cattle and humankind:

Viśvarūpām subhagāmacchāvadāmi jīvalām. Sā no rudrasyāstām hetim dūram nayatu gobhyaḥ (Atharva Veda 6.59.3).

Translated as:

'I value and welcome Arundhati, the auspicious, rejuvenating herb of versatile efficacy, curative of all forms of ailments, and pray that the herb helps us keep away the attack of diseases caused by neglect of precautions prescribed by the physician, Rudra, and may the herb help us keep off disease from cows as well' (Sharma 2013).

Barren cows and those prone to abortion were feared and avoided, while the restoration of barren cows to fertility and lactation, possibly through the use of herbs, was highly valued (Kansara 2008). In the Rig Veda, Sage Kakṣīvān praises the Ashvins—the divine physicians—for rejuvenating a barren and emaciated cow with milk:

adhenuṃ dasrā staryaṃ viṣaktām apinvataṃ śayave aśvinā gām | yuvaṃ śacībhir vimadāya jāyāṃ ny ūhathuḥ purumitrasya yoṣām (Rig Veda 1.117.20).

Translated as:

'Dasras you filled the milk-less, barren, and emaciated cow of Śayu with milk; you brought, by your powers, the daughter of *Purumitra*, as a wife, of *Vimada*' (Wilson 1946).

The Rishi also invokes the Ashvins to bless for:

trivandhureṇa trivṛtā rathena tricakreṇa suvṛtā yātam arvāk; pinvataṃ gā jinvatam arvato no vardhayatam aśvinā vīram asme (Rig Veda 1.118.2)

Translated as:

'Come to us with your tri-columnar, triangular, three-wheeled, and well-constructed car; replenish our cows (with milk), give spirit to our horses, and augment, Aśvins, our posterity' (Wilson 1946).

The Atharva Veda also emphasizes the significance of veterinary care, invoking *Arundhati* and other divine herbs to bestow health and peace (welfare) upon livestock:

Śarma yacchatvoṣadhiḥ saha devīrarundhati. Karatpayasvantam gosthamayakṣmān uta puruṣān (Atharva Veda 6.59.2).

Translated as:

'Let divine Arundhati along with other divine herbs give health and peace to the animals and thus make the stall overflow with milk, and let it make humanity also free from consumptive diseases such as tuberculosis' (Sharma 2013).

Other Vedic scriptures also refer to animal welfare and healthcare. During the later *Sutra* period, livestock breeding remained a vital occupation, with people maintaining large herds of cattle, horses, goats, and sheep. Rituals were performed for the well-being of animals, and diseased livestock were treated appropriately. The *Srauta Sutras* describe numerous ceremonies dedicated to cattle welfare. One such ritual, *Vṛṣotsarga*, was a significant Vedic practice aimed at ensuring livestock well-being, promoting land fertility, and invoking divine favour for the prosperity of the community. The ritual involved the ceremonial release of a bull—symbolizing strength and fertility—as an offering to the gods, signifying the community's reliance on nature and divine blessings for agricultural and economic prosperity. The *Grhya Sutras* mention additional ceremonies for cattle welfare. These include rituals for restoring affection between a cow and her calf, protecting cows from harm, and ensuring the prosperity of young calves. Specific treatments for diseased cattle are also prescribed, such as administering saline water to ailing cows (Kansara 2008).

Evolution of Veterinary Surgery: The origins of veterinary surgery can be traced back to the Rig Veda, one of the oldest known texts in human history. In particular, Rig Veda (1.116.15) references the surgical intervention performed by the Ashvins, the divine twin physicians, in restoring the mobility of *Viśpalā,* a mare who had lost her leg in battle:

caritraṁ hi ver ivācchedi parṇam ājā khelasya paritakmyāyām; sadyo jaṁghām āyasīṁ viśpalāyai dhane hite sartave praty adhattam (Rig Veda 1.116.15).

Translated as:

'The foot of Vispalā, the wife of Khela, was cut off, like the wing of a bird, in an engagement by night; immediately you gave her a metallic leg, that she might walk, the hidden treasure (of the enemy being the object of the conflict)' (Wilson 1946).

The Rig Veda defines a physician as 'a scholar who possesses extensive knowledge of herbs, eradicates disease-causing germs, and safeguards both the universe and human beings' (Maji 2021). Early physicians, known as *Bhishaks*, likely treated both humans and animals, primarily using herbal medicine. However, as social and economic structures evolved, different classes of medical practitioners emerged, including veterinary surgeons. According to Kunja Lal (1907), the development of veterinary surgery was closely linked to the growth and prosperity of Aryan settlements. As the Aryan communities expanded, wealthy nobles travelled in elaborate chariots, increasing the incidence of accidents and injuries among horses and cattle. This necessitated the rise of a specialized class of surgeons devoted to the treatment of injured animals. Moreover, cattle were often maintained in large herds, making them vulnerable to injuries and requiring dedicated veterinary care. In summary, the evolution of veterinary surgery during Vedic era can be seen as a response to the increasing reliance on animals for transportation, agriculture, and warfare. Some key factors that contributed to the development of veterinary surgery include:

- **Warfare and Animal Injuries**: Horses played a critical role in battles, necessitating the treatment of wounds and fractures.
- **Agricultural Advancements**: The domestication of cattle for ploughing and milk production led to the need for medical intervention in cases of injury or disease.
- **Economic Prosperity and Animal Trade**: The expansion of trade routes required robust veterinary services to maintain the health of transport animals.

Epic Period

The Epic Period holds significant importance in the history of veterinary Ayurveda, as it laid the foundation for the development of veterinary science in India. This era (ca. 1000–600 BCE) witnessed the integration of practical knowledge with ethical principles, particularly in the treatment and welfare of animals. As in the Vedic period, domestic animals played a vital role in society, and their welfare was not only a responsibility of common people but also a duty of kings.

Role of Animals in the Epic Period: Domestic animals continued to be central to the socioeconomic and cultural fabric of the Epic Period. Cattle, buffalo, sheep, goats, and horses were essential for agriculture, transportation, and trade. Cows, in particular, were revered as symbols of wealth and prosperity, while elephants held a sacred status and were indispensable in civil and military affairs. Animals held symbolic significance in the epics. The bull was associated with supreme might, and virtuous individuals were often metaphorically referred to as 'a bull among men.' The Valmiki Ramayana and Mahabharata document the extensive use of elephants in both civil and military operations. Along with horses, elephants were crucial in warfare, serving in cavalry units and as war elephants. These majestic creatures were carefully trained, with emphasis on their lineage, strength, and appearance. Other animals such as camels, mules, and donkeys were also employed in military campaigns. The Valmiki Ramayana highlights their role: 'Many generals of the army went accompanied by elephants, horses, camels, and donkeys with chariots decorated with banners and pennons' (Valmiki Ramayana

6.53.5). Interestingly, the magnificent golden chariot of Ravana is said to have been drawn by donkeys (Valmiki Ramayana 3.49.19). Camels were also used for charioteering, transportation, and pleasure rides. The period saw advancements in breeding and training, particularly of horses for charioteering, cattle breeding, castration of bulls, and the use of nose rings to control bullocks for agricultural purposes.

Cattle wealth was considered a measure of prosperity for kingdoms. Kings maintained vast herds under their direct supervision and promoted livestock breeding. The Mahabharata explicitly references the importance of royal cattle stations: 'Listen to it, O lord of men! Our herds are now waiting in the woods of *Dvaitavana* in expectation of you! Without doubt, we may all go there under the pretext of supervising our cattle stations, for, O monarch, it is proper that kings should frequently repair to their cattle stations' (Mahabharata, 3.236; Ganguly 1886). The Valmiki Ramayana (2.50. 8–10) describes the prosperity of the Kosala kingdom, including its well-maintained cattle herds: 'Full of temples and sacrificial stakes, adorned with gardens and mango-orchards, intersected by ponds full of water, populated by contented and well-nourished people, abounded in herds of cows which deserved to be seen by all kings' (Valmiki Ramayana 2.50. 9). Similarly, the Mahabharata's *Goharana Parva* describes the immense livestock wealth of the Matsya kingdom, which Duryodhana sought to seize: 'Let us carry off by thousands his excellent kine of various species… let us lift his cattle in droves... ' (Mahabharata, Book 4.30; Ganguly 1886).

Rishi Ashramas (hermitages) and Gurukuls (traditional learning centres) served as sanctuaries not only for scholars and sages but also for animals, particularly cows. These sacred spaces emphasized harmonious coexistence with nature, where animals were cared for with reverence. Cows, in particular, played a vital role in sustaining the inhabitants of these hermitages. They provided milk, butter, and *ghee*, which were essential for the nutritional needs of students and sages. Cow dung was used as an organic fertilizer to enrich the soil, while cow urine held medicinal value and was an integral component of *Panchgavya*, a mixture used in Ayurvedic medicine and purification rituals. The significance of cows extended beyond their practical utility, as they were revered in Vedic and Epic traditions. Some of the most famous divine cows included:

- *Kamadhenu (Surabhi):* A miraculous, wish-fulfilling cow believed to grant her owner any desire. She is often regarded as the mother of all cattle and symbolizes abundance, prosperity, and dharma.
- *Nandini:* The sacred cow of Maharshi Vasishtha, known for her ability to grant wishes and bestow prosperity. She played a pivotal role in the transformation of Vishvamitra, who initially sought to take her by force but later became a great sage.

- *Shabala (Kamadhenu of Sage Jamadagni):* Another divine cow owned by Sage Jamadagni, renowned for her ability to provide unlimited resources (Fig. 9.2). She is also central to the legend of Parashurama, who avenged the unjust killing of his father after King Kartavirya Arjuna attempted to seize the cow by force.

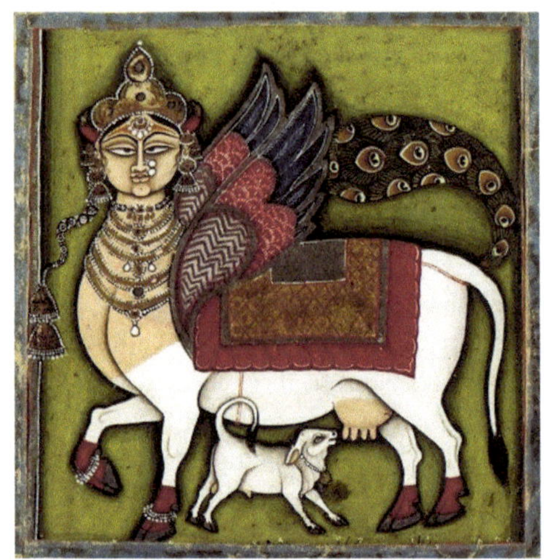

Fig. 9.2. *An artistic representation of Kamdhenu with her calf. Unknown artist Jodhpur 1825-55 (Source: https://upload.wikimedia.org/wikipedia/commons/8/81/Kamadhenu.jpg).*

These sacred cows were not just symbols of prosperity but also played crucial roles in various mythological narratives, reinforcing the deep connection between animals, *dharma*, and the spiritual traditions of ancient India.

Animal Welfare and Healthcare: The Epic Period marked the emergence of specialized knowledge in animal healthcare. The principle of Ahimsa advocating humane treatment of animals gained prominence during this era. The Ramayana and Mahabharata emphasized the interconnectedness of all living beings and promoted compassion toward animals. Lord Rama, during his exile, demonstrated compassion toward animals, reflecting the Vedic principle of Ahimsa. Lord Krishna, depicted as a caretaker of cows, underscored their spiritual significance. Nakula and Sahadeva, from the Mahabharata, were experts in horse and cattle care, respectively. Advanced procedures for treating injuries and diseases were carried out by trained physicians (Vaidhyas), who used medicinal herbs, minerals, and surgical techniques. Illustrious veterinary physicians and scholars - Palkapya, Rajputra, Jayadutta Suri, Mrgasarma, Garga, Gana, and Malladeva Pandita belong to the epic period (Garg 1987). Their work had long lasting effect on veterinary Ayurveda.

There are references of divine herbs, obtained from sacred plants. These were recognized for their spiritual and medicinal properties. These herbs were equally effective in curing man and animals. A notable reference to divine herbs is found in the *Yuddha Kanda* of the Ramayana. Upon Jambavan's advice, Hanuman retrieved four medicinal herbs from the Himalayas:

- *Mrtasanjivani* - Restores life to the dead.
- *Visalyakarani* - Extracts weapons from wounds and heals them.

- *Suvarnakarani*- Restores the body to its original complexion.
- *Sandhani*- Capable of joining severed limbs or fractured bones.

The healing properties of these herbs revived Rama's army: 'The two sons of the ruler of men inhaling the fragrance of the herbs became free from wounds. Other Vanara heroes also got restored' (Valmiki Ramayana*:* 6.74.73).

The legendary herb *Mṛtasañjīvanī* (Sanjeevani) continues to intrigue modern researchers. Numerous scientific expeditions, particularly in Uttarakhand, have sought to identify its botanical equivalent. Among the 17 species initially considered as potential candidates, the most promising are *Selaginella bryopteris*, *Dendrobium plicatile* (syn. *Desmotrichum fimbriatum*), and *Cressa cretica* (Ganeshaiah *et al.* 2009). Of these, *Selaginella bryopteris* is a particularly strong candidate for *Sanjeevani*, as it has been traditionally used to treat wounds, bleeding (including menstruation and uterine disorders), and other internal injuries. It contains a variety of secondary metabolites, including alkaloids, phenols, and terpenoids, which contribute to its antioxidant, anti-inflammatory, anticancer, antiallergic, antimicrobial, antifungal, antibacterial, and antiviral properties. Additionally, it is used as a tonic to enhance physical fitness and promote longevity (Antony and Thomas 2011). The Valley of Flowers in Uttarakhand, nestled in the Himalayan slopes, is often believed to be the legendary "mountain of herbs." However, further research is necessary to authenticate the ethnobotanical characteristics and medicinal efficacy of these plants.

In summary, the Epic Period played a foundational role in shaping veterinary science in India. The significance of livestock, the emergence of specialized veterinary knowledge, and the emphasis on ethical treatment of animals all contributed to the development of veterinary Ayurveda. The reverence for animals, coupled with practical advancements in their healthcare, highlights the profound relationship between human civilization and animal welfare during this period.

Buddhist Period to 13th Century CE

India witnessed significant socio-political and cultural developments. Majority of population was agriculturists and engaged in animal husbandry. The animal wealth was one of the most important state assets with domestic animals such as cattle, buffalo, sheep, goat, horses, donkeys, elephants and camel playing vital roles in society. Livestock was a valuable

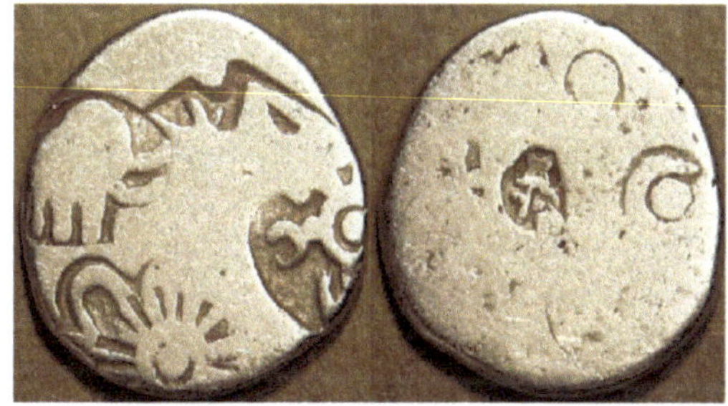

Fig. 9.3. *Mauryan Silver Karshapana (ca. 4th-2nd Century BCE depicting elephant (Photo Source https://coinindia.com/galleries-maurya.html).*

commodity in trade and diplomatic exchanges. Like Vedic and epic periods, cows continued to be adored and highly protected class of animal. The period witnessed the birth of the Great reformers, Mahaveera and Buddha propagating philosophy of Ahimsa and compassion to all. Rulers from 600 BCE used to inscribe pictures of bulls (rarely cows) on coins, which show their importance and utility. Round coins (occasionally rectangular or square) weighing 5-7 g made up of copper, silver, lead, or gold were used as currency. The earliest known coinage (Mankas) in Nepal was introduced by King Anshu Verma (also known as Amshuverma), who ruled from approximately 605 to 621 CE. These coins often featured inscriptions in the Lichchhavi script and Sanskrit, with some depicting a bull on the reverse side, signifying the importance of cattle in the region. Also, punch-marked coins, known as '*karshapana*,' were prevalent in ancient India and continued to be used in various regions during the post-Mauryan period. These coins were typically made of silver (Fig. 9.3) and bore symbols such as humped bulls, which were associated with several ancient Indian kingdoms, including: Airan, Audumbar, Ayodhya, Kaushambi, Sātavāhana, Ujjayini, Yaudheya, Krishnaraja (Kalachuri) (Somvanshi 2002). During this period, several classical texts were composed on various subjects, including Ayurveda and Veterinary Ayurveda. These texts reflect the intellectual and cultural richness of the period, with a strong emphasis on holistic knowledge and ethical practices.

Animal Welfare and Healthcare: The period from the time of Buddha (6th–5th century BCE) to 1250 CE was marked by a deep integration of ethical principles, scientific knowledge, and socio-political policies that emphasized animal welfare and healthcare. Ancient Indian texts, including Buddhist scriptures like the Jataka Tales, Vinaya Pitaka, and Suttanipata, alongside Hindu and Jain works such as Panini's Ashtadhyayi, Kautilya's Arthashastra, and the Puranas, provide extensive references to animal husbandry, ethical treatment, and welfare. The teachings of Mahaveera and Buddha, institutional frameworks, and Ayurvedic medical traditions significantly contributed to animal care and welfare during this era.

Jainism and Ahimsa: Mahaveera's Influence on Animal Welfare: While the phrase *Ahimsa Paramo Dharma* occurs in the Mahabharata, the post-epic period saw the principle of ahimsa elevated to the highest virtue within the śramaṇic traditions. In Jainism, Lord Mahāvīra (Mahaveer, 599–527 BCE), the 24th Tīrthaṅkara (supreme preacher), placed non-violence at the very core of his teachings, extending its scope universally to humans, animals, plants, and even micro-organisms. Several animal species, including domestic animals, are associated with Tirthankaras as their symbols. For example:

- **Bull or Ox** – Lord Rishabhanatha (Adinath, 1st Tirthankara)
- **Elephant** – Lord Ajitnatha (2nd Tirthankara)
- **Horse** – Lord Sambhavanatha (3rd Tirthankara)

- **Buffalo** – Lord Vasupujya (12th Tirthankara)
- **Pig** – Lord Vimalanatha (13th Tirthankara)
- **Male Goat** – Lord Kunthunatha (17th Tirthankara)
- **Lion**- Lord Mahaveera (24th Tirthankara)

(Source: https://jainsquare.wordpress.com/2011/05/01/24-tirthankars-symbols/, accessed on 21-03-2025)

The common Jain practice of *jīvadayā*, or compassion (*dayā*) towards sentient beings (*jīva*), emphasizes providing animals with food, water, shelter, and medical care, especially in situations where they would otherwise suffer neglect. Jain scriptures outline five major transgressions of ahimsa (non-violence): tying animals too tightly, beating them mercilessly, cutting their limbs, overloading them, and depriving them of adequate nourishment. This strict ethical code not only shaped the compassionate treatment of animals in Jain communities but also influenced broader societal attitudes toward animal welfare. Although historical documentation is scarce, some scholars speculate that Jain communities may have established animal sanctuaries akin to modern *pinjrapoles*—shelters for sick, injured, or abandoned animals—long before Emperor Ashoka's reign (Dickstein 2024). Such institutions would have reflected the Jain commitment to non-violence and care for all living beings, predating the formalized state-supported animal welfare measures seen in Mauryan times.

Buddhism and Animal Ethics: Siddhartha Gautama (Buddha) viewed animals as sentient beings, emphasizing their interconnectedness with humans through the doctrine of rebirth. Buddhist texts like the Jatakas highlight compassion towards animals, illustrated by stories of the Buddha's past lives where he sacrificed himself to save creatures, such as the tale of Prince Sattva offering himself to a starving tigress. Monastic codes forbade monks from killing animals or consuming meat derived from slaughter. The Mahayana *Laṅkāvatāra* and *Aṅgulimāla sutras* explicitly prohibited the consumption of meat, reinforcing the doctrine of non-violence (Somvanshi 2024 b).

***Animal Symbolism in Buddhism*:** Buddhist iconography extensively employs animal symbolism to convey spiritual ideals:

- **Lions:** Represent the power and wisdom of the Buddha; depicted as *dharma* protectors in temples and supporting Buddha's throne.
- **Elephants**: Symbolize strength, wisdom, and mental discipline; linked to the Buddha's conception in Queen Maya's dream and venerated in Buddhist mythology.
- **Horses:** Embody diligence and effort in spiritual practice; *Kanthaka*, the horse of Siddhartha, symbolizes loyalty and devotion.

- **Peacocks**: Represent wisdom and transformation; their ability to ingest poison without harm symbolizes the enlightened being's capacity to transform suffering.
- **Garuda:** The king of birds, associated with protection and healing; serves as the vehicle of Vishnu in Hinduism and A*moghasiddhi* in Buddhism.

Ashoka's Contribution to Animal Welfare: Emperor Ashoka (269–232 BCE) played a crucial role in institutionalizing animal welfare. His edicts prohibited animal slaughter for royal consumption, advocated for the establishment of veterinary hospitals (possibly the world's first), and promoted the conservation of forests and wildlife. His famous Lion Capital at Sarnath, now India's national emblem, features symbolic animals:

- **Elephant**: Represents the Buddha's conception.
- **Bull:** Symbolizes worldly desires before renunciation.
- **Horse:** Signifies the Buddha's departure from palace life.
- **Lion:** Represents the Buddha's enlightenment and spiritual sovereignty.

Asokan Rampurva Zebu Bull and its Message of Kindness to Animals: The Zebu Bull, an emblematic pillar capital from Emperor Ashoka's period, was excavated from Rampurva in Bihar and is now housed at Rashtrapati Bhavan in New Delhi. In ancient India, the bull symbolized not only prosperity but also vigour and fertility. To align with this symbolism, the Veterinary Council of India (VCI) adopted a phrase from Ashoka's IX Rock Edict (Girnar), inscribed in Pali as *'Panesu Saymo.'* This phrase, prominently featured in the VCI logo, translates closely to the Sanskrit *'Sarveshu Praneshu Samyamah,'* meaning 'The two sons of the ruler of men inhaling the fragrance of the herbs became free from wounds. Other Vanara heroes also got restored' (Pashu Sandesh, 22nd July 2020).

Ashoka's Edicts: A New Meaning to Animal Care: Emperor Ashoka revolutionized the perception of animals, advocating for their coexistence with humans. His edicts, inscribed in Prakrit (Brāhmī or Kharoṣṭhī script), as well as in, Greek, and Aramaic, were scattered across his vast empire, covering present-day India, Bangladesh, Nepal, Afghanistan, and Pakistan. These inscriptions serve as the first tangible evidence of his policy of *dhamma* (morality) and the influence of Buddhism. Ashoka's inscriptions are categorized into:

- Major Rock Edicts (14 edicts)
- Minor Rock Edicts (7 edicts)
- Major Pillar Edicts (7 edicts)
- Minor Pillar Edicts (5 edicts)

Ashoka took extensive measures for animal welfare, establishing hospitals for their treatment, ensuring the availability of medicinal herbs, and constructing wells along roads for both humans and animals. His policies extended beyond his empire to regions such as the Cholas, Pandyas, Satiyaputas, Keralaputas, and even Tamraparni (Sri Lanka) Major Rock Edict II (Girnar). One of Ashoka's most significant contributions was his prohibition of animal sacrifices, as outlined in Major Rock Edict I (Girnar) (Fig. 9.4). He actively advocated non-violence and kindness towards all living beings, embedding these values into his concept of dhamma. Non-violence became one of the four key tenets of dhamma, which he urged future generations to uphold. These principles are echoed in several of Ashoka's inscriptions, notably translated by Hultzsch (1925):

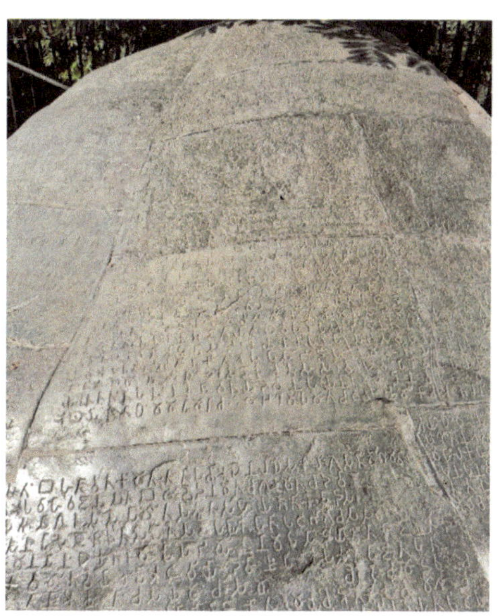

Fig. 9.4. *Replica of the Girnar Rock Edicts on display at the National Museum, New Delhi (Photo by Dr. D. Swarup).*

'King Devanampriya Priyadarśin speaks thus. (When I had been) anointed twelve years, the following was ordered by me. Everywhere in my dominions the Yuktas, Rajukas, and Pradesikas shall set out on a complete tour (throughout their charges) every five years for this very purpose, (viz.) for the following instruction in morality as well as for other business. Meritorious is obedience to mother and father. Liberality to friends, acquaintances, and relatives, to Brahmanas and Śramanas is meritorious. Abstention from killing animals is meritorious. Moderation in expenditure (and) moderation in possessions are meritorious. The council (of Makamdtras), also shall order the Yuktas to register (these rules) both with (the addition of) reasons and according to the letter' – Major Rock Edict III (Girnar).

This moral duty has to be continued for generations:

'……. through the instruction in morality on the part of king Devanampriya Piyadarśin, abstention from killing animals, abstention from hurting living beings, courtesy to relatives, courtesy to Brahmanas and Sramanas, obedience to mother (and) father, (and) obedience to the aged. In this and many other ways is the practice of morality promoted. And king Devanampriya Priyadarśin will ever promote this practice of morality. And the sons, grandsons, and great-grandsons of king Devanampriya Piyadarśin will promote this practice of morality until the aeon of destruction (of the world), (and) will instruct (people) in morality, abiding by morality (and) by good conduct' – Major Rock Edicts IV (Girnar).

'This rescript on morality has been caused to be written by king Devanampriya Priyadarśin. Here no living being must be killed and sacrificed. And no festival meeting must be held. For long Devanampriya Priyadarśin sees much evil in festival meetings. But there are also some festival meetings which are considered meritorious by king Devanampriya Priyadarśin. Formerly in the kitchen of king Devanampriya Priyadarśin many hundred thousand of animals were killed daily for the sake of curry. But now, when this rescript on morality is written, only three animals are being killed (daily) for the sake of curry, (viz.) two peacocks (and) one deer, (but) even this deer not regularly. Even these three animals shall not be killed in future' – Major Rock Edict I (Girnar).

The second pillar-edict gives prominence to various benefits conferred on animals. This statement is explained by the Fifth pillar- edict, which contains a detailed list of animals that were declared inviolable either permanently or on certain days, among them the well-known fast-days.

'King Devanampriya Priyadarśin speaks thus. (When I had been) anointed twenty-six years, the following animals were declared by me inviolable, viz.1 parrot, mainas, the aruna, ruddy geese, wild geese, --- bulls-- the rhinoceros, white doves, domestic doves, (and) all the quadrupeds which are neither useful nor edible. Those [she-goats], ewes, and sows (which are) either with young or in milk, are inviolable, and also those (of their) young ones (which are) less than six months old. Cocks must not be caponed. Husks containing living animals must not be burnt. Forests must not be burnt either uselessly or in order to destroy (living beings)' – Pillar Edict V (Delhi-Topra).

These inscriptions highlight Ashoka's deep concern for animal welfare and his condemnation of violence against them. He was arguably the first ruler in history to implement conservation policies for wildlife and animal protection. Ashoka's inscriptions share commonalities with Ayurveda, emphasizing good conduct and moral discipline. His teachings warn against jealousy, heedlessness, ruthlessness, impatience, and laziness—values echoed in Ayurveda's concept of *Sadvritta* (ethical living), which outlines proper mental, social, religious, personal, and moral conduct. Ashoka's philosophy was deeply influenced by Buddhism, specifically. *Bauddha Darshan*, a philosophical school classified under *Nastika Darshanas* (heterodox systems). The influence of *Aastika* (orthodox) and *Nastika Darshan Shastras* on Ayurveda is well known (Potbhare *et al.* 2019). The interconnectedness of these traditions underscores Ashoka's commitment to moral and ethical living, extending beyond human society to include the welfare of all living beings. He directly and indirectly promoted veterinary Ayurveda with lasting influence.

Shunga and Satavahana Period (ca. 200 BCE–300 CE): Veterinary practices continued to be influenced by earlier traditions, particularly those from the Atharva Veda and Sushruta Samhita. The importance of horses, elephants, and cattle in agriculture, transport, and warfare led to systematic breeding and healthcare practices. The Shalihotra Samhita, an early Sanskrit text on veterinary science, is believed to have originated around this time. It covered equine behaviour, diseases, treatments, and general care.

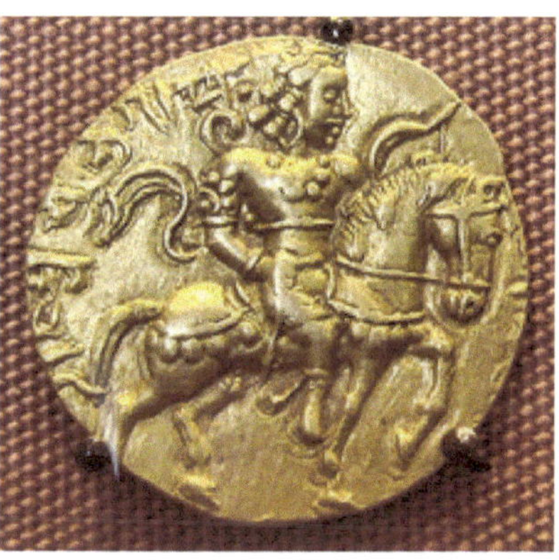

Fig. 9.5. A Gupta Coin depicting Chandragupta II astride horse holding bow signifies the military significance of horse in Gupta period (Photo source: https://www.touristlink.com/india/udayagiri-caves/photos.html).

Gupta Period (ca. 320–550 CE): The Golden Age of Veterinary Science: The Gupta period is often regarded as a 'golden age' of Indian civilization, marked by remarkable achievements in art, literature, mathematics, astronomy, science, and medicine. The Chinese pilgrim Faxian (Fa Hsien) (ca. 337–422 CE) provided firsthand accounts of the advanced healthcare system in the Gupta Empire, describing its institutional approach to medicine. The medical texts of Charaka and Sushruta set high ethical standards for physicians, advocating that they should be selfless, compassionate, and impartial toward all patients, irrespective of their social or economic status. Significant medical advancements included the discovery of distillation processes, the use of disinfectants (attributed to Nagarjuna), and even early forms of smallpox vaccination. The field of surgery also progressed, with successful procedures for amputations and reconstructive surgeries for ears and noses. Numerous surgical instruments were developed, showcasing the refinement of medical knowledge during this era. The practice of veterinary Ayurveda flourished during the Gupta period, with the use of herbal and herbo-mineral medicines, as well as zootherapeutic approaches to treat animal diseases. Horses gained prominence as key military assets due to their speed and agility, forming the core of Emperor Samudragupta's (ca. 335–380 CE) army (Fig. 9.5). The Gupta period witnessed the consolidation of veterinary knowledge into specialized treatises such as:

Shalihotra Samhita: Attributed to Shalihotra, this text became a foundational work on veterinary medicine, particularly focusing on horse care, disease management, and treatment methodologies.

Hastyayurveda: Attributed to Palakapya Muni, this text detailed the diagnosis, treatment, and management of elephants, covering aspects such as diet, disease prevention, and surgical interventions.

Veterinary hospitals, akin to those established during Emperor Ashoka's reign, continued under the Gupta rulers, providing care for elephants and horses, vital for both warfare and transportation. Advancements in animal care included improved techniques for wound healing, fracture repair, and herbal treatments.

Veterinary Ayurveda in the Purāṇas (Puranas): The Puranas, composed and compiled primarily between 300 CE and 1000 CE (drawing on earlier oral traditions), contain numerous references to veterinary medicine. Several texts, including the Skanda Purana, Devi Purana, Matsya Purana, Agni Purana, Garuda Purana, Vishnudharmottara Purana (a continuation of the Viṣhṇu Purana), and Linga Purana, discuss treatments for animal diseases. Notable authors contributing to veterinary content include Vaisampayana and Vyasa. The Vishnudharmottara Purana describes treatments for common ailments affecting cattle, including diseases of the horns, ears, eyes, teeth, and throat. Salt was administered to cattle every fifteen days to prevent constipation, colic, and appetite loss. Oilcake was considered highly beneficial for overall cattle health (Kansara 2008). The Agni Purana prescribes fumigation of cattle sheds using a mixture of *Devadāru* (Himalayan Cedar, *Pinus deodara*), *Vaca* (Sweet Flag, *Acorus calamus*), *Māṃsī / Jatāmāṃsī* (Spikenard, *Nardostachys jatamansi*), *Guggulu* (Indian Bdellium, *Commiphora wightii*), *Hiṅgu* (Asafoetida, *Ferula asafoetida*), and mustard seeds (*Brassica spp.*) to prevent disease outbreaks. A bolus prepared from black gram (*Vigna mungo*), sesame seeds (*Sesamum indicum*), wheat (*Triticum aestivum*), cow's milk, and ghee, seasoned with salt, was administered to calves to promote nourishment and the growth of strong, healthy young bulls (Agni Purana 292.32–35). Barley without the husk (*Hordeum vulgare*), Bengal gram (*Cicer arietinum*), *Vṛhī* (a kind of rice/paddy), and *Durvā* grass (*Bermuda grass, Cynodon dactylon*) were considered the preferred food for horses. *Durvā* was also recommended as a remedy for excess bile, while Arjuna (*Terminalia arjuna*) was prescribed for respiratory problems (Agni Purana 289. 49-52). Specific herbal formulations mentioned in the Puranas for veterinary conditions include:

- **Diseases of Horns (in cows):** Application of oil infused with *Śṛṅgavera / Śuṇṭhī* (Dry Ginger, *Zingiber officinale*), *Balā* (*Sida cordifolia*), and Māṃsī / Jatāmāṃsī (*Spikenard, Nardostachys jatamansi*), mixed with honey and rock salt.

- **Wounds:** Application of oil or ghee mixed with *Haritāla* (Orpiment, Yellow Arsenic Trisulfide) on bleeding wounds.

- **Ear pain:** Application of oil prepared with *Mañjiṣṭhā* (*Indian Madder, Rubia cordifolia*), asafoetida (*Ferula asafoetida*), and rock salt—or garlic (*Allium sativum*) alone—for all kinds of ear pain.

- **Stiff-neck:** Treatment included dry ginger (*Zingiber officinale*), two varieties of turmeric (*Haridrā, Curcuma longa*; *Daruharidrā, Berberis aristata*), and the *Triphala* group of three myrobalans: *Āmalakī* (Indian Gooseberry, *Emblica officinalis*), *Bibhitaka* (*Baheda, Terminalia bellirica*), and *Harītakī* (Chebulic Myrobalan, *Terminalia chebula*).

- **Dental Issues:** A paste of *Bilva* (Wood-apple, *Aegle marmelos*), *Apāmārga* (Prickly Chaff Flower, *Achyranthes aspera*), *Dhātakī* (Fire Flame Bush, *Woodfordia fruticosa*), *Pāṭalā* (Trumpet Flower Tree, *Stereospermum suaveolens*), and *Kuṭaja* (Kurchi Tree, *Holarrhena antidysenterica*) applied at the base of the teeth.
- **Sore Throat:** Formulation with *Śṛṅgavera / Śuṇṭhī* (Dry Ginger, *Zingiber officinale*), *Haridrā* (Turmeric, *Curcuma longa*), and *Triphala* (*Terminalia chebula, Terminalia bellirica, Emblica officinalis*).
- **Fractures:** Application of a mixture of *Priyaṅgu* (*Callicarpa macrophylla*) and rock salt.
- **Digestive Disorders:** Administration of cow's ghee infused with *Yaṣṭimadhu* (Liquorice, *Glycyrrhiza glabra*) or buttermilk mixed with *Pāṭhā* (*Cissampelos pareira*).

The Agni Purana also provides detailed descriptions of elephant treatment and *Gajaśānti* (propitiatory rites) for curing ailments of elephants, including information on auspicious characteristics, bodily marks, methods of capturing elephants, and their role in the army. Therapeutic practices mentioned include enemas, anointments, oil applications, and drinks prepared from *Yaṣṭikā* (Liquorice, *Glycyrrhiza glabra*) with *Śārada* (Paddy/rice harvested in autumn, *Oryza sativa*), together with soup made from *Mudga* (Green Gram, *Vigna radiata*), recommended as remedies for various ailments. Staple foods for elephants included *Śāṣṭika* (a quick-maturing rice variety, *Oryza sativa*), *Vṛhī* (Rice, *Oryza sativa*), and *Śālī* (a superior variety of rice, *Oryza sativa*). In contrast, feed consisting of *Godhūma* (Wheat, *Triticum aestivum*) and *Yava* (Barley, *Hordeum vulgare*) was considered mediocre. However, *Barley* (*Hordeum vulgare*) and *Ikṣu* (Sugarcane, *Saccharum officinarum*) were regarded as beneficial for improving the strength and vigour of elephants (Agni Purana 287, 291).

It may be noted that newly captured elephants require special care as they often undergo stress and health risks. The traditional Ayurvedic regimen followed in Kerala to ensure healthy, and strong elephant with gentle temperament include provisions for frequent baths, proper bedding, exercise, and a balanced diet. Their daily regimen includes inspections, massages, suitable medicinal treatments, and food enriched with ghee, jaggery, sesame oil, and medicinal herbs. Elephants require a substantial diet consisting of lotus stalks, plantains, sugarcane, banyan leaves, and rice grits mixed with grass, totalling approximately 160-180 kg of green fodder, 6.8 kg of groceries, and 80 kg of additional food, alongside 190 litres of water per day. Bathing is crucial for preventing skin diseases, strengthening limbs, and maintaining overall health. Their eyes are regularly anointed with ghee to preserve vision, while tusks are treated to maintain strength and durability (Geetha 2012).

In summary, The Gupta period was instrumental in advancing veterinary medicine, integrating Ayurveda into animal healthcare. The development of foundational texts like Shalihotra Samhita and Hastyayurveda, along with references in the Puranas and classical Ayurvedic texts, highlights the importance of Pashu Ayurveda in ancient India. These practices laid the groundwork for subsequent developments in veterinary science.

Post-Gupta and Early Medieval Period (ca. 550–1250 CE): The decline of centralized empires led to regional kingdoms nurturing veterinary medicine, especially for war animals. The Rashtrakutas (8th–10th century CE) and Cholas (9th–13th century CE) maintained elephant stables (*hastishalas*) and horse breeding centres, leading to the refinement of veterinary care. In Chola Dynasty, members of the royal family often held leadership positions within the cavalry forces. The kings and the royal family members were gifted with the training in horse riding. Horses were treated using traditional methods. The great Chola dynasty extensively used elephants in war and as a power house for their ambitious construction projects to move granite stones from the nearby quarry. Apart from carrying warriors and generals, the elephants themselves fought in the battles. The victorious elephants were granted honorary names to signalize their merit. The kingdom owned sixty thousand war elephants, every one seven or eight feet high. The elephants were imported mainly from Sri Lanka, and trained were highly valued in medieval trade, commanding substantial sums that reflected their strategic importance. Some were bred in South India itself. They were all carefully trained and taken care by the mahout, kept in the elephant stables, and fed with *Borassus* (palmyra palm) leaves, rice, and jaggery. Elephants were bathed in tanks or rivers and their face was painted with vermillion and armoured with face plates (Arasu 2019). There are no documentary evidences how sick elephants were treated in Chola period. Texts like Gaja Ayurveda, which predate the Chola period, were likely referenced for dietary requirement and treating ailments in elephants. In addition to war animals, livestock including cattle, buffaloes, sheep and goats contributed to rural economy. There are references of well-established medical care and hospitals in Chola empire. However, no documentary evidence is available for such veterinary facilities. Perhaps people used their traditional knowledge for treatment of animals.

Veterinary Ayurveda from Early Islamic (13th Century) to Mughul Period (18th Century)

During this period, animals continued to serve vital roles in food production, religion, transportation, agriculture, and warfare. Mughal art frequently depicted oxen for transport and draught work, cows and buffaloes for milk, camels and donkeys as pack animals, and sheep and goats for meat. Horses and elephants were particularly crucial for military purposes, with Mughal warfare relying on cavalry supported by war elephants. Each army unit maintained trained war elephants and high-quality horses, including Arabian, Persian, Turki, and Tazi breeds. Bullocks, camels, and donkeys were maintained for transporting artillery and supplies.

Animal Welfare and Healthcare Under Islamic Rule: The evolution of veterinary-medical culture in Islamic India was driven by military and civil necessities. Earlier Indian treatises appear to have provided the technical background for medieval practitioners. Horses and elephants were vital military and state assets, and the breeding of superior lineages was actively patronized by the court. Armour was also employed to protect animals on the battlefield; a distinctive example is the burqustawan, a special type of horse armour (Ahmed 2024). His administration supported the breeding of superior horse and elephant lineages, recognizing their strategic importance in warfare and governance.

Animal husbandry held strategic importance during the Mughal era, contributing to the Empire's needs in conservation, protection, and selective breeding of domestic animals. Emperor Akbar issued royal *firmans* assigning nobles the responsibility for specific animal species: Abdul Raheem Khan-e-Khana oversaw horses, Mirza Yusuf Khan camels, Raja Birbal cattle and buffaloes, Raja Todar Mal elephants and grains, and Shareef Khan sheep and goats. Branding (*dag* and *hulia*) of animals like horses, mules, elephants, and bullocks was practiced for identification of animals to prevent fraud. The elite breeding tracts for horses, mules, bovines, camels, and elephants were documented in Abul Fazl's *Ain-i-Akbari*. Akbar also banned cow slaughter across his empire and emphasized the importance of cow milk and bullocks in agriculture (Somvanshi *et al.* 2017). Contemporary historian Mulla Abdu'l Qadir Badayuni (1540–1615 CE) observed that Akbar's reverence for cows stemmed from his close association with Hindus, who regarded the cow as vital for the preservation of the world (Elliot 1867). Although Emperor Jehangir did not explicitly ban cow slaughter, he upheld Akbar's ethos of religious inclusivity. A naturalist and animal lover, Jehangir introduced turkeys via Portuguese traders, maintained extensive wildlife collections, and patronized animal paintings by artists like Ustad Mansur. His zodiac coins depicted animals such as Taurus, Capricorn, and Leo. His reign also included observations on rabies in elephants, plague outbreaks, elephant gestation, and characteristics of camel milk (Somvanshi *et al.* 2017).

Veterinary Science During the Mughal Period*:* Veterinary knowledge further advanced under the patronage of Moghul emperors. While earlier Sanskrit texts remained influential in royal stables, Persian and Central Asian practices shaped Mughal veterinary traditions. Indian veterinary texts were translated into Persian and Arabic, fostering cross-cultural knowledge exchange. Mughals actively traded animals and engaged in territorial conflicts with the Persians, particularly under Shah Abbas (1571–1629 CE), whose court was a multicultural hub where Armenians, Georgians, and Circassians contributed to veterinary knowledge. The health of war animals was critical to Mughal military success, leading to specialized care and breeding practices. Horses, being symbols of power and authority, were meticulously reared and maintained, with the Mughal state employing inspectors and veterinarians (*salutri/salotri*) to oversee their health (Chaudhary 2017). Literature from the Mughal era indicates a growing awareness of optimal breeding and feed management.

Veterinary Texts Under the Mughals: During the Mughal period, veterinary science became a formalized discipline, with animal healers compiling and documenting their knowledge. This veterinary tradition emerged from the synthesis of Indian, Persian, and Central Asian medical practices. Notable works from this period include *Tarjamah-i-Saloter-i-Asban* and *Faras-Nama-i-Rangin*, both of which reflect this cross-cultural exchange in equine care. Sayed Abdullah Khan Firoze Jung, the author of *Tarjamah-i-Saloter-i-Asban*, recorded that several chests of Indian manuscripts were seized during an expedition against Rana Amer Singh of Rajasthan. Among these texts was the *Saloter*, a Sanskrit treatise on horse care containing 19,000 *shlokas* (verses). Recognizing its significance, Mughal Emperor Shah Jahan later commissioned its translation into Persian, further integrating Indian veterinary knowledge with Islamic equine medical traditions. The *Faras-Nama* (Treatise on Horses) provided a comprehensive study of horse anatomy, diseases, and treatments, serving as a vital resource for Mughal veterinarians and equestrian experts (Choudhary 2017).

Veterinarians and Healing Methods During the Mughal Era: Mughal veterinary practices consisted of two primary groups: private veterinarians and those serving in royal institutions, particularly within the military. Veterinary professionals, known as *baytars* or *salotris*, operated under the supervision of the *atbegi*, an official responsible for overseeing government-owned horses. The Mughals, along with successive states in the 18th century, actively supported these veterinarians as well as other medical professionals, such as *hakims* (physicians), *tabibs* (general doctors), and *jarrahs* (surgeons), by providing them administrative posts and granting free endowments. Some veterinarians achieved administrative ranks (*mansabs*), reflecting their high status and importance within the empire. One notable figure was Muqarrab Khan, a prominent veterinarian during Emperor Jahangir's reign. Veterinary practices included minor surgeries and treatments performed by animal caretakers. The *Faras-Namas* provided detailed diagnostic methods, such as examining dung and eyes, and outlined the use of herbal and biomedical formulations (Choudhary 2017), many of which drew from earlier Ayurvedic traditions.

Lameness in horses was treated with poultices or hot irons (cautery), while drenching was employed for both horses and cattle to administer medications and alleviate colic. In war elephant healthcare, wounds often progressed to abscesses requiring careful draining and cleaning. Mahouts (elephant caretakers) used innovative techniques such as packing fresh wounds with sugar and employing maggots to remove gangrenous tissue. Herbal remedies, administered in substantial doses, were a prevalent method for treating elephants. Preventive care was emphasized across all species, with an understanding that proper feeding was paramount for maintaining digestion and overall health. For elephants, this involved sourcing approximately 600 pounds of digestible fodder daily—a monumental task in certain conditions. For animals traveling long distances or working in challenging environments, access to high-quality food was critical for maintaining their well-being. Preventive measures were prioritized to ensure sustained health and optimal performance (Jones and Koolmees 2022).

British Period (18th Century to 1947 CE)

The British period in India (18th century to 1947) was a significant transitional phase in veterinary medicine, characterized by the introduction of Western-based veterinary education, research, and infrastructure development (See Chapter 6).

Westernization of Veterinary Medicine: According to Jones (2021), the institutionalization of European veterinary medicine in India began in the late 18th century, driven by the East India Company's growing need for horses in transport, military, and personal use. This demand extended to improving the quality of cattle, elephants, and camels used in transportation. In 1791, the Military Auditor-General proposed establishing a Board of Agriculture, inspired by Tipu Sultan's breeding regulations, but the British Board ultimately rejected the plan. In 1793, Lieutenant William Frazer recommended creating a stud farm in the Ganges Valley and emphasized the lack of veterinary knowledge, requesting a skilled veterinarian to train local breeders. By 1799, British veterinary surgeons from the London Veterinary College arrived in India, including James Grellier, who authored *The Elements of Veterinary Science* or *The Veterinary Art in India* (1802), the first English-language Indian veterinary text. In 1808, the Company employed William Moorcroft, an English veterinarian and explorer, to improve equine breeding at the Equine Breeding Stud in Pusa, Bihar. Moorcroft introduced large-scale cultivation of horse feed oats and travelled across Central India, the Himalayas, Tibet, and Central Asia, reaching Bukhara in search of superior horses—though without success. During this period, veterinary research grew steadily, with studies published in British veterinary journals and Calcutta medical periodicals. Common topics included equine diseases like *Kumri* (cerebral nematodiasis), *Bursati* (cutaneous habronemiasis), eye-worm, and canine distemper among hunting dogs imported from England. By the late 19th century, Veterinary Colleges in India began producing graduates who served in both government and private sectors. As affluence grew, two distinct groups of practitioners emerged: Western-trained veterinarians and traditional healers known as *Salutris*. Many graduates adopted the title *Salutri* to make their role more relatable to the public. In 1934, an Ayurvedic veterinary college—*Andhra Jatiya Ayurveda Pashu Vaidya Kalashala*—was established in Andhra Pradesh. Its graduates went on to found

Ayurvedic veterinary hospitals and served their communities (Prasad and Swamy 2015)

Pinjrapoles and Gaushalas: Pinjrapoles and Gaushalas provided refuge for animals, aligning with cultural and religious values. These institutions, supported by philanthropic efforts, played a crucial role in breeding, rearing, and caring for animals in British India.

Pinjrapoles: The term *Pinjrapole* (or *Panjarapole*) originates from the Sanskrit word *pāñjara*, meaning cage or enclosure. These shelters provide refuge for elderly, infirm, and needy animals of various types. Their roots lie in ancient Jain traditions, which emphasize compassion and nonviolence (ahiṃsā). Over time, Pinjrapoles became formalized institutions of animal welfare, particularly flourishing in Gujarat with support from Jain communities. By the British era, they had become prominent centers for animal care. Today, hundreds of Pinjrapoles operate across India, varying in size, scope, and services. A study identified 284 Jain animal sanctuaries in Gujarat alone (Dickstein, 2024). Many Pinjrapoles today are equipped with state-of-the-art facilities for housing and animal welfare. For instance, the Madras Pinjrapole, established in 1906 in Chennai, Tamil Nadu, shelters over 2,000 cows. It features temperature-controlled sheds and dedicated caretakers to ensure the well-being of the animals (Madras Musings, accessed 27-03-2025).

Gaushalas: The term *Gaushala* comes from Sanskrit (*Gau* meaning cow and *Shala* meaning shelter), signifying a home for cows. While Pinjrapoles care for various animals, Gaushalas focus exclusively on cattle, particularly cows. The movement to establish Gaushalas gained momentum in the late 19th century, influenced by reformist Dayanand Saraswati, who campaigned against cow slaughter. The first organized Gaushala was founded in Punjab in 1882 during British rule, and within a few decades, hundreds of such shelters had spread across the country. These Gaushalas operated as charitable trusts or societies, sustained by donations from individuals and organizations. Today, India has over 4,000 Gaushalas, including approximately 200 model Gaushalas, which promote self-reliant cattle care while continuing their mission of animal welfare. They are becoming economically sustainable through innovative practices (https://www.pashudhanpraharee.com/avenues-for-self-reliance-for-gaushala/) such as:

- *Bio-energy Production:* Using cow dung for fuel, biogas, and organic manure.
- *Medicinal Applications*: Processing cow urine into bio-pesticides and raw materials for *Panchgavya* medicines.
- *Dairy Advancements:* Promoting indigenous cow breeds for A2 milk production, which is valued for its nutritional and therapeutic benefits.

- *Breed Conservation:* Preserving native cattle breeds, particularly male germplasm, to address the growing issue of stray cattle and support traditional Ayurvedic practices.

Several Gaushalas have gained recognition for their outstanding contributions to animal welfare and sustainability. Some exemplary Gaushalas include:

- *Pathmeda Godham, Rajasthan* – The largest Gaushala in India, housing over 85,000 cows.
- *Shri Vraj Kamad Surabhi Van Avam Shodh Sansthan, Rajasthan* – Home to over 10,000 Indian breed cows, including thousands of abandoned male , this Gaushala focuses on the conservation and improvement of indigenous breeds such as Gir, Sahiwal, Tharparkar, Rathi, Kankrej, and Haryanvi. It also operates a small biogas plant, dairy unit for A2 milk production, and an Ayurvedic medicine centre based on Panchgavya therapies (Gaushala Report,2025, accessed on 27-03-2025).
- *Shri Mataji Gaushala, Barsana, Uttar Pradesh*–Shelters over 50,000 cows, mostly abandoned males. It pioneers A2 milk production, indigenous breed improvement, and an Ayurvedic hospital/pharmacy. Additionally, it runs a biogas turbine, utilizing biogas from its organic fertilizer plant (Gaushala Report, 2025, accessed on 27-03-2025).
- *Kanpur Gaushala Society, Uttar Pradesh* – Known for harnessing bulls for rural activities and developing electricity-generation projects.
- *Sri Gobind Gaushala, Gorakhpur, Uttar Pradesh*–Specializes in bio-pesticide production, organic manure, and Panchgavya-based medicines.

In summary, both Gaushalas and Pinjrapoles stand as remarkable examples of India's commitment to animal welfare, sustainability, and cultural heritage. Their innovative approaches continue to set benchmarks in cattle care, breed conservation, and eco-friendly practices, ensuring that these ancient institutions remain relevant in modern times.

Translation and Reworking of Ancient Veterinary Ayurvedic Manuscripts: The British period in India was marked by a "printing revolution." While printing technology was introduced to India in the 16th century by Portuguese traders, who brought it to Goa, it was during British rule that multilingual printing facilities expanded, making publications more accessible. This led to the widespread printing of various manuscripts, including original texts and translations on diverse subjects such as human and animal Ayurveda, the Mahabharata, Ramayana, and Puranas. One notable example is Kautilya's Arthashastra (ca. 350–283 BCE), a text that disappeared in the 12th century but was rediscovered in 1904 by R. Shamasastry, who translated it into English and published it in 1909. The Arthashastra extends beyond statecraft, outlining a comprehensive legal and bureaucratic framework for governance, including insights into mineralogy, agriculture, animal husbandry, medicine, and wildlife management. Similarly, Kaviraj Kunja Lal published an English translation with commentary on the Sushruta Samhita in 1907.

Several manuscripts on *Hasti* Ayurveda (elephant medicine) were also published during this period. Palakapya's Hastyayurveda was printed in 1894 by Anandashrama Mudranalaya, while the Telugu manuscript of Gajashastram was transcribed into Devanagari by Pandit V. Vijayaraghavacharya in 1926. The Government Press in Trivandrum later published Nilakantha's Matangalila in 1942 (Geetha 2012). Numerous manuscripts on equine medicine, originally written in Sanskrit, were translated and adapted into various regional languages. Among these were Jayadatta's Asvavaidhyakam and Nakula's Asvhachikitsam, in Sanskrit by Vidhyasagar Bhattacharya in 1891. Asvasastram, attributed to Nakula, was translated into English and multiple Indian languages by S. Gopalan in 1942. Gopalan, who served as the Honorary Secretary of the TMSSM Library in Tanjore, worked from a rare Sanskrit manuscript preserved at the library. A significant contributor to Veterinary Ayurveda was Yejella Shri Ramulu Chaudari, a renowned Ayurvedic veterinarian from Andhra Pradesh. Between 1928 and 1947, he authored and published 23 books in Telugu, making Veterinary Ayurveda more accessible to the local population. His works covered various aspects of cattle and horse care, including disease aetiology, treatments using Ayurvedic medicine, and preventive measures. Some of his notable publications include *Pashuvaidyacintamani*, *Pashuchikitsasaramu*, *Vishanivarini*, *Pashunetrachikitsa*, *Shastravaidyamu*, *Ashvapariksha*, and *Ashvashastramu*. His publications emphasized hygienic practices, balanced diets, exercise, proper cattle housing, seasonal care, and eye disease treatment. Additionally, he launched an Ayurvedic veterinary journal (Prasad and Swamy 2015). However, not all published manuscripts maintained high standards. Many texts on equine and bovine medicine were printed in vernacular languages and sold in livestock fairs. These works often lacked adherence to standard veterinary Ayurvedic practices, limiting their credibility and effectiveness.

Principal Medical Ayurveda *Āchāryas* and their Contributions to Pashu Ayurveda

The foundational knowledge of Ayurveda was shaped by legendary scholars and divine figures whose contributions laid the groundwork for holistic healing. From the celestial healers—the Ashvin Kumars—to eminent Ayurvedic *Āchāryas* (Acharya, revered teachers and preceptors) such as Jīvaka, Charaka, Suśruta, and Vāgbhaṭa, these pioneers advanced medical science in India, influencing both human and animal healthcare. Their texts not only addressed human ailments but also contained references to veterinary treatments, highlighting the deep interconnection between Ayurveda and animal welfare.

Ashvins: The Physicians of Gods: The Ashvin Kumars (*Dasra* and *Nāsatya*) are twin gods in Vedic mythology, revered as divine physicians who bring healing and prevent diseases. Described in the Rig Veda as youthful horsemen riding a golden chariot, they are credited with remarkable medical feats, such as restoring eyesight and reviving individuals from apparent death. They are also mentioned in the Mahabharata as the fathers of Nakula and Sahadeva, two of the Pandavas. Some Vedic scholars interpret the Ashvins as a blend of cosmic and human elements—their luminous nature symbolizing celestial forces, while their legendary cures reflect their role as healers in human society(https://www.wisdomlib.org/hinduism/book/shiva-purana-english/d/doc225561.html, accessed on 17.02.2025). Certain theories suggest they may have been historical figures, renowned horsemen or warriors, whose medical knowledge inspired awe among their contemporaries.

A significant reference in Rig Veda (1.117.22) states that the Ashvins acquired medical knowledge from a horse's head, which was implanted on Dadhyañc, son of Atharvan, after he had learned the secrets of medicine from Prajapati Tvasta. Interestingly, a parallel can be found in Greek mythology—Chiron, the wise centaur, was known for his profound knowledge of medicine, which he passed on to Greek heroes like Heracles, Achilles, Jason, and Asclepius (https://www.britannica.com/topic/Chiron-Greek-mythology). This similarity in knowledge transfer between equine-related figures suggests a fascinating possibility of cross-cultural interactions between ancient civilizations.

Dhanvantari: God of Medicine: In Vedic and Puranic traditions, Dhanvantari is one of the most revered figures in Indian medical history, regarded as the divine physician and the god of Ayurveda. Alongside the twin Ashvins, he holds a pre-eminent place in the healing traditions of ancient India. Considered an *avatar* (incarnation) of Lord Vishnu, Dhanvantari is often depicted holding a pot of *amrita* (the elixir of immortality) and medicinal herbs, symbolizing his role as the harbinger of health and longevity. According to the Puranas, Dhanvantari emerged during the *Samudra Manthana* (Churning of the Ocean of Milk), carrying the amrita, which granted immortality to the gods. His divine association with Ayurveda is emphasized in texts such as the Śivapurāṇa (1.16), which states: 'The worship of Dhanvantari and the twin deities—Aśvins—alleviates ailments, prevents foul death, and suppresses all sickness instantaneously.' (https://www.wisdomlib.org/definition/dhanvantari#hinduism-general, accessed on 17.02.2025). Dhanvantari is also linked to the ancient city of Kashi (Varanasi), where he is believed to have ruled as a king and taught Ayurveda to his disciples. He is sometimes referred to as Divodāsa Dhanvantari, a semi-historical figure who is said to have systematized medical knowledge into a structured discipline.

From a historical perspective, Dhanvantari is considered the founder of the Dhanvantari School of Ayurveda, which laid the groundwork for surgical techniques and medical treatment. His disciples included Shusruta, the legendary physician and surgeon. Some scholars suggest that Dhanvantari may have been a title used for multiple eminent physicians rather than a single individual. Dhanvantari is said to have expounded the principles of equine medicine and management to Sushruta (Agni Purana 288). Furthermore, Nakula, one of the brothers and a renowned equine specialist, is believed to have composed a treatise on horse medicine under the guidance of Dhanvantari, reinforcing his influence on veterinary Ayurveda. Dhanvantari also narrated Go-Ayurveda comprising propitiation and welfare of cows (Agni Purana 292). While myth and history intertwine in the accounts of Dhanvantari, his contributions remain foundational to the evolution of Ayurveda, influencing both human and animal medical traditions in India.

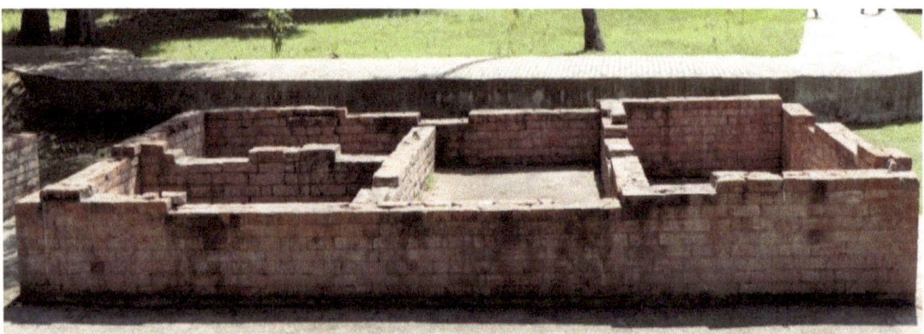

Fig. 9.6. *A 4th–5th century brick structure at Kumrahar (Patna), identified as Arogya-Vihar (hospital-cum-monastery). A potsherd inscribed with Dhanvantareh suggests its association with Dhanvantari, the renowned Gupta-era physician. Scholars also propose the existence of an ancient veterinary hospital nearby. The finding reinforces Dhanvantari's historical significance in Ayurveda. (Photo courtesy of Dr. D. Swarup).*

Jīvaka (Jivaka, Komārabhacca / Kaumārabhṛtya): The Thrice-Crowned Physician (5th Century BCE): Jīvaka, the personal physician of the Buddha, King Bimbisāra, and King Ajātaśatru, is celebrated as the 'Medicine King' and 'Thrice-Crowned Physician.' Trained in Takṣaśilā, he gained prominence for his medical skills, including complex surgeries, and remains revered in Indian and Thai traditional medicine. Jīvaka demonstrated remarkable observational abilities, distinguishing a pregnant female elephant and its rider's characteristics through subtle clues—an example of his deep understanding of both human and animal physiology (Singh *et al.* 2011).

Carak (Charaka): The Physician and Philosopher of Ayurveda (1st Century BCE – 2nd Century CE): Charaka, one of the most influential figures in Ayurveda, is credited with editing and expanding the Agnivesha Samhitā (Figs. 9.7-9.8) into what became known as the Charaka Saṃhitā, a foundational text of Ayurveda. His contributions revolutionized medical theory and practice, emphasizing holistic healing, preventive care, and the balance of bodily humors (doshas). The exact dates of Charaka's life remain uncertain. Some scholars, such as Meulenbeld (1999), suggest that Charaka lived between 100 BCE and 200 CE, while other traditions place him in the 4th century BCE. He is believed to have been a native of Kashmir and was associated with the University of Takshashila, a renowned centre of learning in ancient India. Some historical sources also identify Charaka as the court physician of King Kanishka (127–150 CE) of the Kushan Empire. However, this identification remains debated due to chronological inconsistencies. Charaka's teachings resonate with modern public health principles, particularly the emphasis on disease prevention over reactive treatment. According to the Charaka Samhita, the physician who possesses comprehensive knowledge of aetiology (*nidāna*), symptomatology (*puruṣa-vicaya*), therapeutics (*cikitsā*), and preventive strategies (*rasāyana, vṛṣya*) is considered the foremost among healers and deemed worthy of royal appointment (Sutra Sthana 919) (Sutra Sthana 9.19). Moreover, Charaka cautions that mere familiarity with the names and external forms of herbs does not constitute mastery; true understanding lies in discerning their properties, applications, and contextual efficacy (Sutra Sthana 1. 121).

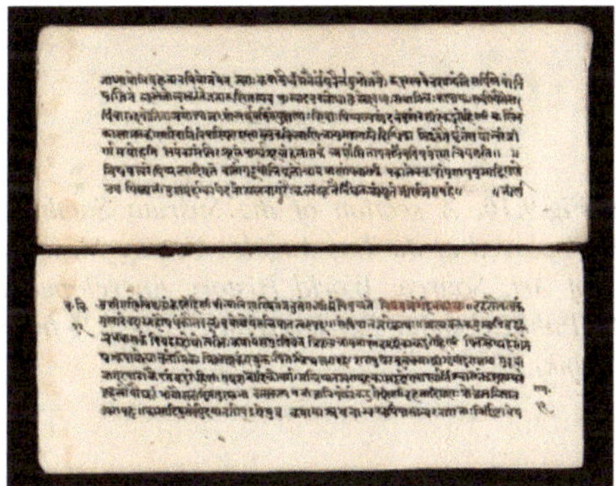

Fig. 9.7. A manuscript section from the Charaka Saṃhitā, Sutrasthāna (Source: Wellcome Collection).

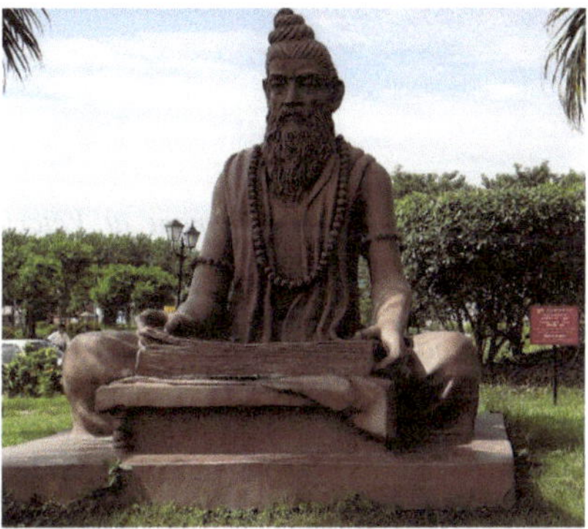

Fig. 9.8. Charaka monument at the Patanjali Yogpeeth campus, Haridwar, India (Source: Wikimedia Commons).

Charaka was one of the earliest scholars to describe the circulatory system and the role of the heart in pumping blood through vital channels (*srotas*). He identified 360 bones in the human body, a number that includes teeth and cartilage. Additionally, he outlined the concept of *Tridosha* (*vāta, pitta, kapha*), proposing that disease results from an imbalance of these three bodily humors. His treatments focused on restoring equilibrium through diet, herbal remedies, detoxification therapies (*Pañcakarma*), and lifestyle adjustments. Interestingly, the Charaka Saṃhitā also includes references to animal medicine (Pashu Ayurveda). It lists ingredients for enemas (*basti*) used for treating cattle, sheep, goats, elephants, and camels, indicating a well-developed tradition of veterinary care in ancient India. This suggests an interconnection between human and animal healthcare practices, a concept echoed in later Ayurvedic texts.

Suśruta (Sushruta, 600 BCE): Sushruta, often called the 'Father of Surgery,' authored the Sushruta Samhita, detailing surgical techniques, anatomy, and medicinal practices. Believed to have been born in the Kingdom of Kashi, Sushruta (Figs. 9.9-9.10) is closely associated with Varanasi (present-day Banaras), as the Sushruta Samhita itself places its author in this historic city. Scholars widely acknowledge that the Sushruta Samhita was a collaborative work, with contributions from several ancient authors collectively referred to as 'Sushruta.' This collaboration enriched the text, which has become a timeless reference for traditional medicine and surgery.

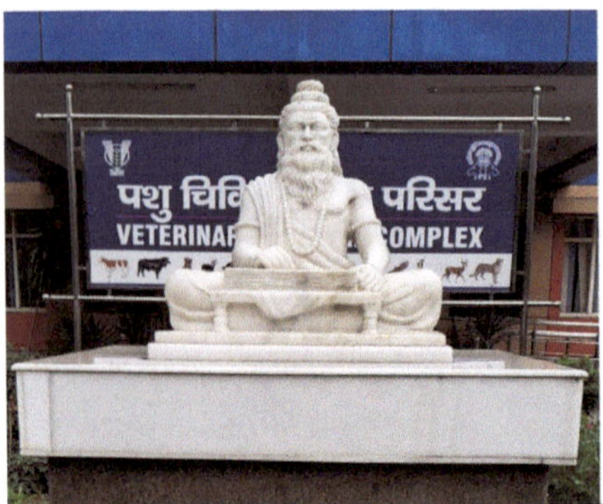

Fig. 9.9. *Sushruta monument at Veterinary Clinical Complex, ICAR- Indian Veterinary Research Institute, Izatnagar, Uttar Pradesh, India (Photo courtesy of Dr Akhilesh Kumar, IVRI).*

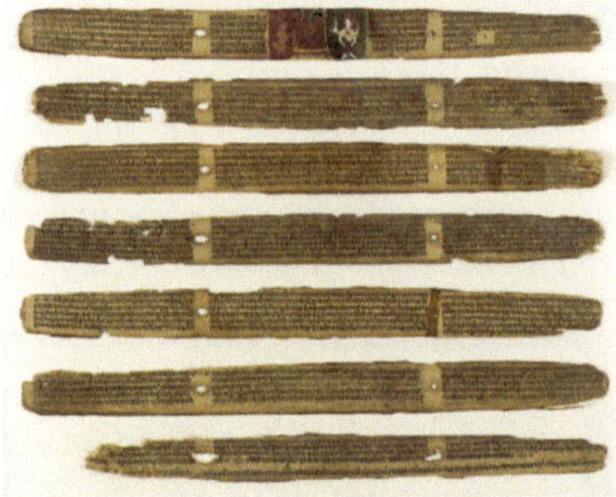

Fig.9.10. *A section of the Suśruta Saṃhitā, displayed at the Los Angeles County Museum of Art. Source: World History Encyclopedia (Public domain. Retrieved on 15-01-2025 from link).*

Sushruta pioneered plastic surgery including rhinoplasty and otoplasty (Box 9.1), and propagated early concepts of vector-borne diseases, linking malaria to mosquitoes and plague. His students, called as the *Saushrutas*, had to study for six years before beginning hands-on surgical training. Their study included rigorous training, practicing incisions on vegetables and animals before human surgeries. Dissecting corpses was deemed taboo in many ancient and medieval cultures due to religious or societal beliefs during that time which regarded the deceased corpse as sacred. However, Sushruta emphasized the significance of understanding the anatomy of human cadavers and adopted unique approach to cadaver dissection. He also substituted animal models for human anatomical structures by using carcasses, and even vegetables to simulate surgical procedures like suturing and puncturing. For instance, incisions were practiced on vegetables, like *Pushpafala* (*Cucurbita maxima*), *Alavu* (*Longenaris vulgaris*), or *Frapusha* (*Cuemis pubescuas*; squash and cucumbers), and evacuation process on leather bags full of water and the urinary bladders of dead animals. Scarification, a technique involving superficial cutting, was performed on animal hides. Venesection was practiced on vessels taken from deceased animals or the stalks of water lilies (Kunja Lal 1907).

Box 9.1. The Rhinoplasty and Otoplasty: The Groundbreaking Innovations of Sushruta

Nasal injuries were prevalent in ancient India due to warfare and punitive amputations. The nose was regarded as a symbol of pride and dignity. To alleviate the suffering of the disfigured, Sushruta devised an innovative surgical technique to reconstruct the nose by grafting skin from the cheek onto the nasal remnants. This procedure—now known as rhinoplasty—was performed without modern anaesthesia, relying solely on herbs for pain relief. Small hollow tubes or reeds were inserted into the nostrils to maintain airflow and support respiration. Chapter XVI of the Sushruta Samhita outlines the method: using a creeper leaf as a template, cheek tissue was grafted, the wound was scarified, and the graft was secured with a bandage (Sadhu Vandha). Medicinal powders were sprinkled on the graft, which was then covered with soft Karpsa (cotton) moistened with refined sesame oil. Patients were advised to consume clarified butter and undergo oil massages. Once digestion was complete, purgatives were administered, in accordance with medical texts. The same method was applied to reconstruct severed lips, with the exception of nasal tube insertion. The knowledge of these procedures spread from India to the classical civilizations of Greece and Rome.

Sushruta also addressed earlobe injuries caused by heavy jewellery, performing otoplasty with cheek skin grafts—even on infants. He is credited with pioneering cataract removal through a technique known as couching, representing a significant milestone in early ophthalmic surgery. His nasal reconstruction method, passed down through generations in India and Nepal, was later documented by British physicians Cruso and Findlay, who introduced it to the West after witnessing a successful operation performed on a cart driver punished for treason.

(Synthesized from: Kunja Lal 1907, Reader's Digest 2003, Dave et al. 2024)

Vāgbhaṭa (Vagbhata, 7th Century CE): Often regarded as one of the 'Trinity' of Ayurveda, alongside Charaka and Sushruta, Vagbhata is believed to have lived during the early 7th century CE. His works are known for their accessibility and concise presentation, making them widely used by students and practitioners of Ayurveda. Vagbhata's writings emphasize holistic healing, personal hygiene, seasonal influences on health, and the importance of maintaining balance in life. He authored the *Aṣṭāṅgasaṅgraha* (Ashtanga Samgraha) and *Aṣṭāṅgahṛdayasaṃhitā*, synthesizing earlier texts like the Charaka Samhita and Suśruta Samhita. These works cover Ayurveda's eight branches, including internal medicine, surgery, paediatrics, toxicology, and psychiatry. The *Aṣṭāṅgahṛdayasaṃhitā*, written in poetic form, remains one of the most widely studied Ayurvedic texts. It includes references to animal-based treatments, describing the medicinal properties of elephant milk, curd, butter, and urine.

References to Pashu Ayurveda in Classical Ayurvedic Texts

Charaka, Sushrut, and Vāgbhaṭa—the Trinity of Ayurvedic Knowledge—shaped Ayurveda's evolution. Their texts continue to influence both human and veterinary medicine, with enduring principles of holistic healing, ethical practice, and disease prevention. References to animal diseases and their treatments can also be found in classical Ayurvedic texts. Here are some examples of veterinary references in Charaka and Sushrut Samhitas.

Charaka Samhita

The Charaka Samhita contains numerous references to veterinary practices. Chapter 11 of *Siddhi Sthana* discusses various practical aspects of therapeutic Panchakarma procedures and their administration. The chapter also elaborates on the use of enemas (*basti*) for different species of animals including therapeutic properties of medicated enemas, their types, and their administration (Upadhyaya and Singh, 2020).

Administration of Enemas: Receptacles for enemas for different animals include:

- Elephants and Camels: Urinary bladder of goats and sheep.
- Cattle and Horses: Urinary bladder of buffalo.
- Sheep and Goats: Urinary bladder of an old ox (*jarad gava*).

Length of Enemas: Following is the length of nozzles:

- Elephants: 1 *aratni* (length of the forearm)
- Camels: 18 *angulas* (~13.5 inches).
- Cattle and Horses: 16 *angulas* (~12 inches).
- Sheep and Goats: 10 *angulas* (~7.5 inches).

Recipes for all Types of Veterinary Enemas: Common recipes for veterinary enemas included *kaliga* (*Holarrhena antidysenterica*), *kustha* (*Saussurea lappa*), *madhuka* (*Madhuca indica*), *pippali* (*Piper longum*), *vacha* (*Acorus calamus*), *satahva* (*Anethum sowa*), *madana* (*Randia dumetorum*), and *rasanjana* added with jaggery, rock salts and two variety of *panchamula bilva* (*Aegle marmelos*), *syonaka* (*Oroxylum indicum*), *gambhari* (*Gmelina arborea*), *patala* (*Stereospermum suaveolens*), *gani-karika* (*Piper longum*), *shala-parni* (*Desmodium gangeticum*), *prishna-parni* (*Uraria* picta), *brihati* (*Solanum indicum*), *kantakari* (*Solanum surattense*), and *goksura* (*Tribulis terrestris*).

Classification of Ingredients: ***Primary Herbs:*** *Kalinga (Holarrhena antidysenterica), Kushta (Saussurea lappa), Pippali (Piper longum), Madhuka (Madhuca indica), Vacha (Acorus calamus), Mandana (Randia dumetorum),*

Satahva (Anethum sowa), Rasanjana. ***Additional Ingredients:*** Jaggery and Rock salt; ***Panchamula*** (Two Varieties): ***Brihat Panchamula*** (Major Group): *Bilva* (*Aegle marmelos*), *Gambhari* (*Gmelina arborea*), *Shyonaka* (*Oroxylum indicum*), and *Patala* (*Stereospermum suaveolens*). ***Laghu Panchamula*** (Minor Group): *Shalaparni* (*Desmodium gangeticum*), *Prishnaparni* (*Uraria picta*), *Brihati* (*Solanum indicum*), *Kantakari* (*Solanum surattense*), and *Gokshura* (*Tribulus terrestris*)

Specific Enema Formulations Prescribed for Different Species: Following herbs have been recommended as enemas for different species:

- Elephants: *Ashvattha* (*Ficus religiosa*), *Vata* (*Ficus benghalensis*), *Khadira* (*Acacia catechu*), *Pragraha* (*Oroxylum indicum*), *Shala* (*Shorea robusta*), and *Tala* (*Borassus flabellifer*).
- Cattle: *Mudga-parni* (*Vigna trilobata*), *Masa-parni* (*Teramnus labialis*), *Dhava* (*Anogeissus* latifolia), *Shigru* (*Moringa oleifera*), *Patali* (*Stereospermum suaveolens*), *Madhuka-sara* (*Madhuca longifolia*), and *Chitraka* (*Plumbago zeylanica*).
- Horses: *Palasha* (*Butea monosperma*), *Danti* (*Baliospermum montanum*), *Suradaru* (*Cedrus* deodara), and *Dravanti* (*Croton tiglium*).
- Donkeys and Camels: *Pilu* (*Salvadora persica*), *Khadira* (*Acacia catechu*), and *Bilvadi*-group herbs.
- Goats and Sheep: *Triphala* (*Terminalia chebula*, *Terminalia bellirica*, *Emblica officinalis*), *Parusaka* (*Grewia asiatica*), *Kapitha* (*Limonia acidissima*), *Bilva* (*Aegle marmelos*), and *Kola* (*Ziziphus jujuba*).

Dosage: Recommended doses of enemas for different animal species include:

- Goats and Sheep: 1 *prastha* (736 g).
- Cattle: 2-3 *prastha* (1472 g to 2208 g), depending on size.
- Camels: 2 *adhakas* (5888 g).
- Elephants: 4 *adhakas* (11,776 g).

Management of Poisoning: Chapter 23 (*Visha Chikitsa*) of *Chikitsa Sthana* in the Samhita outlines poisoning symptoms and their treatments for quadrupeds and birds (Gopikrishna and Binorkar 2020).

Effects of Poisoning in Quadrupeds: Following four stages are defined in quadruplets

- *First stage:* Depression and giddiness
- *Second stage:* Trembling

- *Third stage:* Loss of appetite and emptiness
- *Fourth stage:* Death due to respiratory failure

Box 9.2. Snake Venom: Valuable Zootherapeutic in Ayurveda

The Charaka Samhita and other ancient Indian texts provide significant insights into veterinary toxicology, particularly the controlled use of snake venom in treating diseases in animals. Ancient India, with its advanced toxicological and herbal research centres like Taxila, explored the medicinal applications of venom, recognizing that in small doses, it acted as a potent stimulant, while its effects changed when combined with animal bile.

The Charaka Samhita acknowledges the use of poisons in medicine, including their application in veterinary care. One of the key formulations, Suchikabharana, was prepared using cobra venom along with mercury, sulphur, lead, and aconite, all soaked in the bile of various animals, including rohu fish, wild boar, peacock, buffalo, and goat. This mixture was dried and powdered, then administered in minuscule doses ("point of a needle") to treat ailments in both humans and animals, such as plague, fever, coma, and tuberculosis.

Another preparation, Ardhanarisvara Rasa, was processed inside the mouth of a black cobra and used as a snuff for treating obstinate fevers. Similar toxicological formulations like Brihat Suchikabharana, Aghorenrisingharana, and Kalanala Rasa were developed with different types of snake venom, indicating a deep understanding of venom's diverse pharmacological effects.

The integration of snake venom into veterinary medicine demonstrates the advanced toxicological knowledge of ancient Indian scholars. This expertise is reflected even today in homeopathy, where remedies like Bothrops lanceolatus are derived from venom for therapeutic use. The Charaka Samhita thus highlights an early understanding of controlled toxicology, not only in human medicine but also in animal healthcare

Effects of Poisoning in Birds: Signs of poisoning in birds are described in following three stages:

- First stage: Depression.
- Second stage: Giddiness.
- Third stage: Weakness leading to death.

Charaka Samhita, extensively discusses the medicinal applications of animals and animal-derived products for treating human ailments. The *Deerghanjiviteeya* chapter mentions several animal-derived substances used in medicine, including honey, milk, bile, animal fat, bone marrow, blood, flesh, excreta, urine, skin, semen, bones, ligaments, horns, nails, hooves, hair, fine down (soft dense hair), and inspissated bile. For example, an ointment made from elephant bone and neem is recommended for the treatment of haemorrhoids and to prevent excessive bleeding. The Samhita also describes the properties and medicinal values of the milk and urine of various animals such as the cow, buffalo, sheep, goat, mare, she-camel, and elephant (Sutra Sthana 1.68–69; 94-113). Interestingly, Charaka underscores the therapeutic presence of animals in hospital environments, suggesting that their proximity can have a soothing and healing effect on patients (Box 9.3). This may be one of the earliest documented references to the principles underlying contemporary Animal-Assisted Therapy (AAT) — a fast emerging complementary practice in modern medicine to aid in psychological and physical healing.

Box 9.3. Use of Animals in Clinical Environment: Charaka's Concept of Animal Assisted Intervention for Human Health and Wellness

Charaka emphasized the importance of a healing environment in patient recovery, advocating for a serene natural setting enriched with music, arts, and companionship. Ayurveda promotes music therapy, as classical Indian ragas restore balance through Omkara. Additionally, Charaka prescribed the presence of animals such as quails, partridges, rabbits, deer, antelopes, wild sheep, and cows in the place of treatment- "Birds and animals like common quail, grey partridge, hare, black buck, antelope, black tailed deer, red deer and wild sheep should also be there. A milch cow with good temper, free from disease and having a calf alive along with all the necessary arrangements for her such as fodder, shelter and water-should be there"(Sutra Sthana: 15.7; Shrivastav et al. 2020). Each of these animals plays a crucial ecological role:

- *Quails and Partriges aid in insect control and seed dispersal.*
- *Rabbits regulate plant growth and support the food chain.*
- *Deer and Antelopes manage vegetation and serve as prey for predators.*
- *Wild Sheep contribute to grazing and nutrient cycling.*
- *Milch Cows provide milk for dietary and medicinal use, contributing to traditional Panchgavya therapy.*

Charaka also advocated for ethical extraction of animal products for medicinal purposes, ensuring minimal harm while enhancing patient well-being. His philosophy aligns with modern Animal-Assisted Therapy (AAT) and the emerging practice of care farming, where human-animal interactions aid in healthcare, rehabilitation, and mental wellness (Gallis 2012, Fines 2019).

Sushruta Samhita and Veterinary Surgery

The Sushruta Samhita, one of the foundational texts of Ayurveda, contains several references to veterinary surgery. Here are some notable examples:

- **Surgical Instruments**: The Sushruta Samhita describes various surgical instruments that can be used for both human and animal surgeries. These instruments include scalpels, forceps, needles, and probes, which are essential for performing precise surgical procedures.

Treatment of Fractures: The text provides detailed guidelines for treating fractures in animals. It describes the methods for setting broken bones, immobilizing the affected limb, and using splints and bandages to ensure proper healing.

Wound Management: The Sushruta Samhita outlines the principles of wound management in animals. It includes instructions on cleaning wounds, applying herbal poultices, and using sutures to close deep wounds. The text also emphasizes the importance of preventing infection and promoting rapid healing.

- **Abscess Drainage**: The text describes the procedure for draining abscesses in animals. It explains how to make an incision to release pus, clean the wound, and apply medicinal herbs to promote healing and prevent further infection.
- **Castration**: The Sushruta Samhita provides detailed instructions for performing castration in animals. It describes the surgical techniques, necessary precautions, and post-operative care to ensure the well-being of the animal.

Zootherapeutics in Sushruta Samhita: Chapter XLV of Sushruta Samhita Sutrasthanam provides extensive references to the therapeutic properties of animal-derived substances, including the milk of cows, goats, buffaloes, mares, and elephants, along with their derivatives such as curd, whey, and ghee. The text also discusses the medicinal properties of meat and urine from various groups of indigenous female animals, emphasizing their role in treating a range of ailments. For instance, Sushruta prescribed goat meat as a dietary remedy for phthisis (tuberculosis) due to its nourishing and easily digestible qualities. Similarly, goat's milk was recommended for colitis, a condition affecting the colon. The selection of goat's milk for colitis suggests Sushruta's awareness of its ability to reduce fermentation in the intestine, possibly due to its low allergenic potential and beneficial probiotic properties. Furthermore, he advocated close contact with goats as a powerful auxiliary therapy for tuberculosis, an idea that aligns with the traditional belief in the healing influence of animals (Kunja Lal 1907). Additionally, Sushruta attributed unique medicinal properties to other animal products. Buffalo milk, known for its high fat content, was prescribed for individuals suffering from emaciation and weakness. Elephant milk, though rare, was believed to have strengthening properties and was sometimes recommended for conditions requiring enhanced vitality. The urine of cows, a key component in Ayurveda even today, was described as a potent detoxifying agent, while *ghee* was valued for its wound-healing and anti-inflammatory effects.

Veterinary Ayurveda Scholars and their Work

Veterinary Ayurveda has a rich history with notable scholars contributing significantly to this field. Few notable examples are:

Śālihōtra (Shalihotra, traditionally 1800 BCE; critically ca. 3rd century BCE–2nd century CE) and *Hayāyurveda* (Haya Ayurveda): Shalihotra, often regarded as the founder of veterinary science in the Indian tradition, holds a preeminent place in Pashu Ayurveda. His exact period remains debated. Some traditions describe him as a contemporary of Agniveśa (one of the earliest authors of Ayurvedic medicine), while others portray him as the teacher of Sushruta or the mentor of Nakula of the Mahabharata, implying a Vedic-era origin. Consequently, dates attributed to him vary widely—from the late Vedic period (around 1800 BCE) to between the 3rd century BCE and the 1st century CE. The Agni Purana (292.44) records that Shalihotra (Fig. 9.10) imparted equine medicine to Sushruta (traditionally dated to ca. 600 BCE). The symbolic interpretation of the *Pakṣachedana* (removal of the wings of the celestial horse) legend also presents him as an equine expert who advanced the domestication, training, and welfare of horses—an expertise crucial during the Aryan expansion into the Gangetic Valley. Tradition holds that Shalihotra was the son of the sage Hayagoṣa, residing either at Śrāvastī (modern-day Gonda–Bahraich border in Uttar Pradesh) or at Śalātura (also called Śalatura), the birthplace of the grammarian Panini near Kandahar. Despite uncertainties in dating, Shalihotra is indisputably recognized as one of the earliest veterinarians of antiquity. He established the foundations of veterinary science in India, tracing its divine origins to Brahma, similar to Charaka and Sushruta (Anonymous 1949). Shalihotra is credited with authoring several treatises on Pashu Ayurveda, including the *Aśvaśāstra*, regarded as one of the earliest works on veterinary medicine. The *Śālihōtra Saṁhitā* (Shalihotra Samhita), also called *Hayāyurveda* or *Turaṅgamaśāstra*, is a comprehensive text on equine medicine, surgery, and husbandry, covering all aspects of horse care—diseases, treatments, and breeding practices.

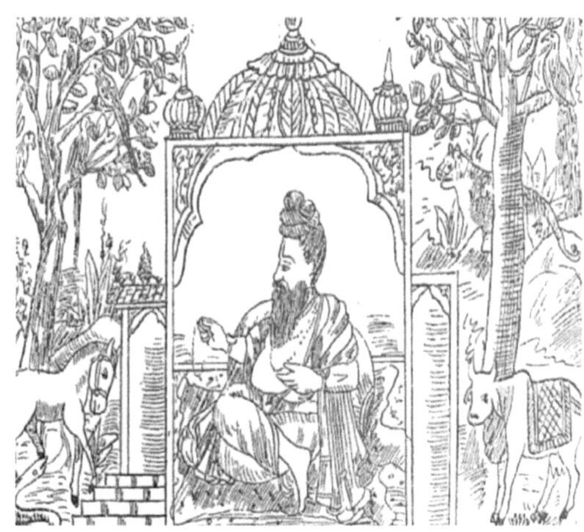

Fig. 9.10. *Conceptual illustration depicting the ashram (hermitage) of Sage Shalihotra (Source: Shalihotra Sangrah by Keshav Singh; Khemraj Shri Krishnadas Shri Venkateshwar Steam Press, Bombay).*

Just as the lost Agniveśa-Saṁhitā—later redacted as the Charaka Samhita—is said to have comprised, the original Shalihotra Samhita also contained 12,000 verses. An introductory verse states: 'Wise Shālihotra composed this treatise on horses consisting of 12,000 verses after directing a horse that had ascended to heaven to return to the earthly realm.' (Anonymous1949). The Shalihotra Samhita also follows a structure similar to *Asthang* Ayurveda, being divided into eight sections:

1. Types and breeds of horses based on race and colour, training methods, age determination, and trade regulations.
2. Treatment and descriptions of ailments such as fever, pain, eye diseases, diarrhoea, hiccups, vomiting, and poisoning.
3. Equine reproduction and reproductive disorders.
4. Diseases of the mouth and digestive system, along with their management.
5. Treatment of fractures and wounds.
6. Infectious diseases and their remedies.
7. Enemas and purification methods.
8. Prognosis of diseases and medicinal herbs.

Several herbs mentioned in the Shalihotra Samhita such as *guggul* (gum resin from Burseraceae plants), *haritaki* (*Terminalia chebula*), *adrak* (ginger), *triphala* (a blend of dried fruits of *T. chebula*, *T. bellirica*, and *Emblica officinalis*), *sarshapa* (Indian mustard), and *laksha* (*Laccifer lacca*), are still used in veterinary and human medicine today. The text also provides insights into the lifespan of domestic animals, listing: elephants (120 years), horses (32 years), cows (24 years), camels and donkeys (25 years), and dogs (16 years). The Samhita has been translated into multiple languages, including Arabic, Persian, and Tibetan (Easy Ayurveda 2016). Besides this major work, *Aśva-Praśnaśāstra* and *Aśva-Lakṣaṇa-śāstra* are also attributed to Shalihotra. His influence on the veterinary profession in India and beyond is evident from the Persian and Urdu term *Shālotrī*, meaning "horse doctor." The Agni Purāṇa quotes Shalihotra as an equine medicine expert, and both the Garuda Purāṇa and Matsya Purāṇa reference Hayāyurveda (Anonymous 1949). Numerous later authors either named their veterinary treatises after him or based their works on his Samhita, expanding upon its original content (Somvanshi 2024a).

Pālakāpya (Palakapya, 1000-500 BCE 2000–4000 BCE) and *Gaja Ayurveda*: Sage Palakapya is regarded as the foremost authority on elephants in India. According to the *Gajaśāstra* (Gajashastra), during the reign of King Romapāda (Lomapāda) of Aṅga Mahājanapada, elephants were causing widespread destruction in agricultural fields. The king, with the assistance of sages like Gautama, captured and restrained them. However, Palakapya was deeply moved by the suffering of the enchained elephants. Grief-stricken, he approached King Romapāda and revealed his deep connection with elephants, along with his extensive knowledge of elephant lore. He urged the king to extend his protection to them. Impressed by the sage's wisdom, the king requested him to share all his knowledge about elephants. Gajaśāstra (Fig. 9.11) records the teachings that Palakapya imparted to King Romapāda (Gopalan 1958). While some traditions place him as early as the Rigvedic period (2000–4000 BCE), most scholars consider this unlikely. Based on internal evidence and historical context, it is more plausible that Palakapya belonged to the late Vedic or early Epic period (ca. 1000–500 BCE), with the Hastyāyurveda taking its compiled form sometime between the 6th century BCE and the 2nd century CE, drawing upon older oral traditions of elephant medicine. The Agni Purana (291. 44) also records that Palakapya imparted knowledge of elephant treatment and behaviour to King Angarāja.

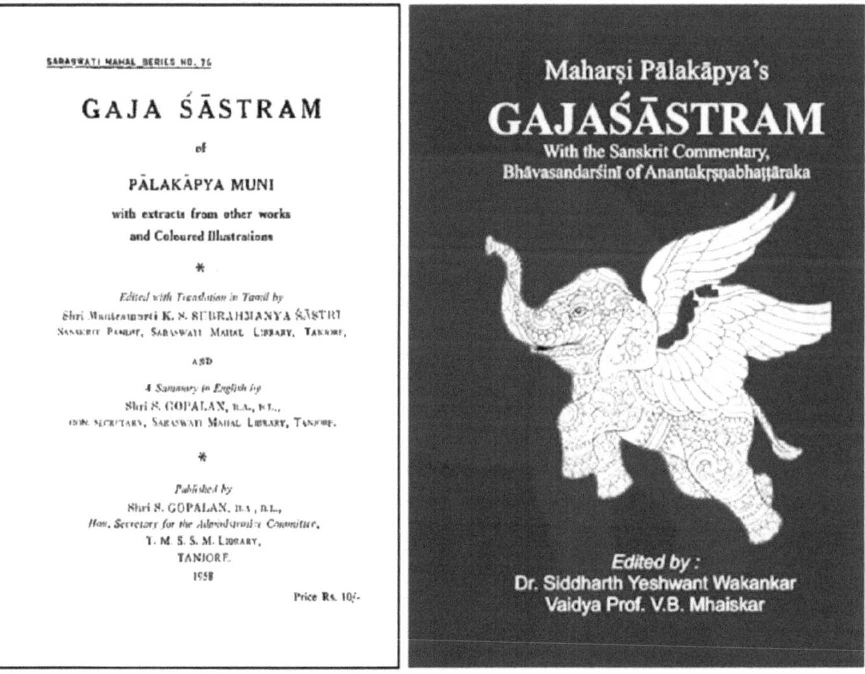

SARASWATI MAHAL SERIES NO. 76

GAJA ŚĀSTRAM

of

PĀLAKĀPYA MUNI

with extracts from other works
and Coloured Illustrations

*

AND

Shri S. GOPALAN, B.A., B.L.,

*

Published by

Shri S. GOPALAN, B.A., B.L.,

T. M. S. S. M. LIBRARY,

TANJORE.

1958

Price Rs. 10/-

Fig. 9.11. *Gajaśāstra was translated into Tamil by Gopalan, accompanied by the original Sanskrit text and an English summary (R) (Source: https://archive.org/details/Gajasasthra). In 2006, Bharatiya Kala Prakashan published an English translation with Sanskrit commentary (L).*

The Hastyāyurveda, a comprehensive treatise on elephant medicine and surgery, is also attributed to Sage Palakapya. While Gajaśāstra primarily emphasizes the general well-being and management of elephants, Hastyāyurveda delves deeply into their anatomy, physiology, diseases, and treatments. Dedicated to Lord Gaṇeśa, the text describes *15 Pradeśas* (regions of the elephant's body), each with several subdivisions. It also discusses *Marmas* (vital points), *Doṣas* (biological humors), *Dhātu* (tissues), *Mala* (waste products), *Manas* (mental faculties), and *Śirāvyūhas* (vascular structures) (Bhavana 2020). The treatise begins with an account of Palakapya's life, the origins of elephants, and their characteristics. It covers topics such as capturing, training, favourable and unfavourable physical traits, *musth* (a periodic condition in male elephants), age determination, medical treatment, and the construction of elephant stables. Hastyāyurveda is comparable in scale to the Charaka Samhita consisting of over 10,000 verses, 20,000 lines, and 152 chapters (Anonymous, 1949). It is divided into four major sections:

1. *Mahārogasthāna* – Major diseases
2. *Kṣudra-rogasthāna* – Minor diseases
3. *Ślalyasthāna* – Surgery
4. Supplement of Materia Medica – Herbal treatments

The ailments are categorizes into two types:

1. *Adhyātmika* – Physical disorders, further divided into: *Mānasa* (Mental ailments) and *Doṣaja* (Disorders caused by imbalances of bodily humors- Vāta - air, Pitta - bile, Kapha - phlegm).
2. *Āgantuka* – Accidental or incidental ailments.

In summary, the Hastyayurveda provides extensive knowledge about elephant anatomy, surgery, physiology, pathology, disease management, diet, and medicinal treatments. Descriptions of ancient wars highlight that, besides horses, thousands of elephants participated in battles, reinforcing the necessity of Hastyayurveda (Somvanshi 2006).

Nakula and *Aśva Chikitsā*: Nakula was the fourth of the five Pandavas of the Mahabharata era. He and his twin brother, Sahadeva, were known as *Aśvineya*, as they were born of the divine physicians. Among the Pandavas, Nakula was considered the most handsome. He was an excellent horseman with extensive knowledge of horse breeds and was also a skilled charioteer. As the son of celestial physicians, he was well-versed in astrology and Ayurveda, particularly in treating wounds and ailments, with a special focus on equine health. During the thirteenth year of the Pandavas' exile, known as the *Agyatvas* (incognito exile), Nakula took on the role of an ostler (horse keeper) in the kingdom of Matsya In a conversation with King Virāṭa, Nakula demonstrated his expertise in equine training and curing illnesses. Adopting the identity of a horse trainer named *Granthik*, he excelled in horsemanship while remaining close to the royal court and gathering intelligence about unfolding events. Under his care, the royal horses of Matsya became notably healthier and more vigorous. Nakula authored a Sanskrit treatise titled *Aśva Chikitsā* (*Treatment of Horses*), containing detailed knowledge on equine care and ailments. Approximately 129 verses (*śloka*s) from

Aśva Chikitsā are cited in *Śālihotram*, a text attributed to King Bhoja (Kulkarni 1953).

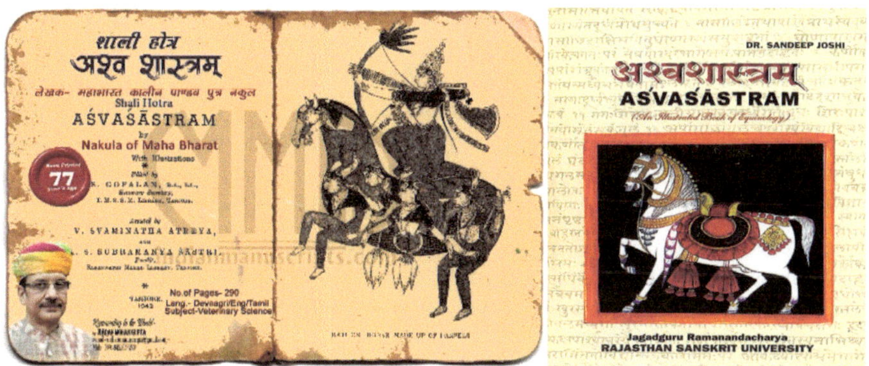

Fig. 9.12. *Aśvaśāstra by Nakula was translated into Hindi, Tamil, and English by Gopalan (1942), alongside the original Sanskrit text (R). A later English translation with coloured illustrations (L) by Dr. Sandeep Joshi, based on the Second Edition (1952) from Sri Venkateswara University, Oriental Research Institute, Tirupati, was published by Rajasthan Sanskrit University in 2008.*

Sahadeva and *Vyādhi-Sindhu-Vimardana*: Sahadeva, the youngest of the five Pandavas, was renowned for his intelligence and served as King Yudhishthira's private counsellor. He was highly skilled in bovine husbandry and medicine. During the *Agyātavāsa*, he disguised himself as a *Vaiśya* named *Tantipāla* and worked as a cowherd in the kingdom of Virāṭa. Sahadeva composed a Sanskrit treatise titled *Vyādhi-Sindhu-Vimardana* (*Curing the Ocean of Diseases*), which focused on veterinary and medical sciences. Unfortunately, this work is now lost.

Jayadatta (1364 CE) and *Aśvavaidyaka*: Jayadatta, son of Vijayadatta, is described as *mahāśānta*, implying an ascetic nature, though in some references, he is referred to as *mahāsāmanta,* indicating a feudatory prince or minister. He lived in the early second millennium CE and cited Śālihotra, the author of Aśvāyurveda, a renowned treatise on horse medicine traditionally dated to around 1000 CE. Jayadatta authored *Aśvavaidyaka,* a Sanskrit treatise on equine medicine written in verse. The oldest known copy of this work dated to Nepal Samvat 484 (1304 CE) is preserved at Cambridge University, UK. The text is arranged into sixty-eight chapters, with its contents outlined in the first chapter.

Aśvavaidyaka provides comprehensive knowledge on horses, covering topics such as anatomy, auspicious and inauspicious traits, age determination, place of birth, riding techniques, care of pregnant mares and postpartum conditions, medicine dosages, drugs used in treatments, seasonal influences on equine health, alkaline therapy, blood-letting, eye diseases, nasal therapies, oleation, fomentation, and the use of oils, ghee, and *ariṣṭha* (fermented medications). It also addresses ailments affecting the face, head, and ears. The *Nighaṇṭu* (glossary of medicinal substances) in the twelfth chapter lists 174 important drugs used in equine diseases. Many of these drugs hold significant clinical relevance in veterinary medicine. Further research on these substances could enhance the Ayurvedic veterinary pharmacopeia and contribute to new treatment regimens for animals.

King Bhoja (1010–1055 CE) and *Śālihotram*: King Bhoja of the Paramāra dynasty ruled over Mālwa, Madhya Pradesh, from 1010 to 1055 CE. A renowned patron of scholars, he is regarded as one of the most illustrious kings in Indian history. He was a polymath and is credited with several works on diverse subjects, including literature, science, and medicine. The establishment of *Bhojśālā*, a center for Sanskrit learning, is attributed to him. Bhoja authored *Śālihotram* (Fig. 9.13), a Sanskrit text on horse care, diseases, and treatments. This treatise comprises 360 verses covering various aspects of equine management and medicine. In Śālihotram, Bhoja is referred to as *Bhojarāja*. The Śālihotram of Bhoja was critically edited and published by Sanskrit scholar Kulkarni (1953) of Deccan College Post-Graduate and Research Institute, Pune. He concluded that Bhoja borrowed several verses from earlier works, including Aśva Chikitsā by Nakula.

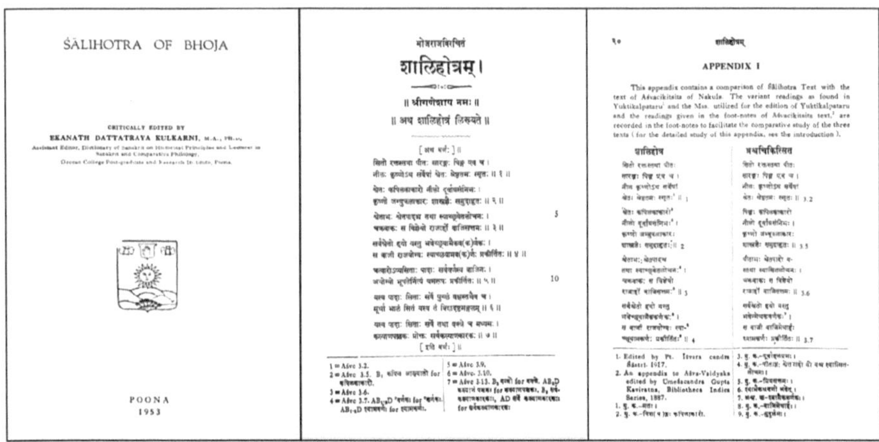

ŚALIHOTRA OF BHOJA

CRITICALLY EDITED BY
EKANATH DATTATRAYA KULKARNI, M.A., Ph.D.,
Assistant Editor, Dictionary of Sanskrit on Historical Principles and Lecturer in Sanskrit and Comparative Philology,
Deccan College Post-graduate and Research Institute, Poona.

POONA
1953

शालिहोत्रम्।

APPENDIX I

This appendix contains a comparison of Śālihotra Text with the text of Aśvacikitsita of Nakula. The variant readings as found in Yuktikalpataru[1] and the Mss. utilized for the edition of Yuktikalpataru and the readings given in the foot-notes of Aśvacikitsita text,[2] are recorded in the foot-notes to facilitate the comparative study of the three texts (for the detailed study of this appendix, see the introduction).

Fig. 9.13. Sanskrit scholar Kulkarni edited and published Śālihotram of Bhoja (1953) and noted that the work of Bhoja incorporates 129 verses that are identical to those found in Aśva Chikitsā by Nakula as indicated in Appendix I. (Source: https://archive.org/details/salihotraofbhojaekanathdattatreyakulkarnideccancollege).

Tirumangalath Nīlakaṇṭha and *Matanga Līlā*: Nīlakaṇṭha (15th century CE) authored *Matanga Līlā*, regarded as one of the most comprehensive Sanskrit treatises on elephantology. The work, based on *Matangaśāstra*—attributed to the ancient sage and the teachings of Katalayil Nambūtiri, consists of 263 stanzas divided into twelve chapters of varying lengths. Unlike earlier texts such as Hastyāyurveda, which were complex and less accessible to the common people, Matanga Līlā presents a concise and systematic approach to elephant care and management (Geetha 2012). It was translated into English by Franklin Edgerton in

1931 as *The Elephant-Lore of the Hindus*. The text closely resembles the Gajaśāstra, covering topics such as elephant behaviour, auspicious and inauspicious omens related to their sounds, and their physical and psychological traits. Serving as a refined and updated version of Gajaśāstra, incorporating additional insights into elephant husbandry, Matanga Līlā remains an important reference in traditional Indian veterinary science and continues to influence studies on ancient elephant management practices.

Some other notable Veterinary Ayurveda scholars and their work include: Sage Narada- *Gajashiksha;* Vyasa (Vaisampayana)-*Gajasastram, Gajalaksana;* Gana- *Asvayurveda Siddhayana Smagraha*, Hamsadeva- *Mrugpada Shastra;* Malladeva Pandita - *Asvayurveda Sindhu*; Hemadri - *Gaja Darpana; Narayanadikshita- Gajagrahanaprakara;* Someshvarabhupati- *Manasollasa* (*Abhilaṣitārthacintāmaṇi*) and Koneri Bapu- *Turangaratnamala* to cite a few.

Veterinary Ayurveda – Contemporary Veterinary Medicine Interface: Relevance and Prospects

There is a growing scientific and clinical interest in integrating Ayurvedic principles into modern human and animal healthcare practices. The foundation of Veterinary Ayurveda is deeply rooted in the same philosophical principles that govern human Ayurveda, emphasizing the interconnectedness of all living beings. Ayurveda's fundamental goal is to maintain health and prevent disease by ensuring balance among *Doshas* (biological humors), *Agni* (metabolic functions), *Dhatus* (vital tissues), and *Malas* (waste products).

Tridosha Concept in Veterinary Medicine

In Ayurveda, diseases arise from imbalances in the three doshas (tridosha), which represent fundamental metabolic tendencies in all living organisms, including animals:

- Vata (Air and Space)–Governs movement, nervous system functions, respiration, and circulation.
- Pitta (Fire and Water)–Regulates digestion, metabolism, thermoregulation, and cognitive functions.
- Kapha (Earth and Water)–Responsible for physical strength, tissue integrity, and joint lubrication.

Each animal has a unique Tridosha composition (*Prakriti*), which determines its physiological traits and susceptibility to diseases. Ayurvedic veterinary medicine applies this understanding to diagnose, treat, and prevent ailments in animals. Diseases that contrast with an individual's innate dosha composition are often easier to treat, whereas conditions that align with an animal's inherent dosha tendencies tend to be more challenging, as the individual's constitution reinforces the disease pattern.

Ayurvedic Pathogenesis and Disease Diagnosis

Disease evolution follows six stages (*samprapti),* from dosha accumulation to disease manifestation. Key causes include dietary factors, digestive disturbances, infections, toxins, and congenital conditions. Seven types of dhatus in the bodies of humans and animals are derived from food. These tissues include plasma, blood, muscle, fat, bone, bone marrow and nervous, and reproductive tissue (See Chapter 8). As such Ayurveda stresses the importance of digestion, as digestive issues lead to toxin accumulation (*ama*), which, if untreated, spreads through the body. For example, Ayurvedic texts on horses emphasize nutritional imbalances as a primary cause of illness.

Ayurvedic Diagnostic Techniques: The Ayurvedic approach to diagnosis is holistic, comprising *Rog Pariksha* (disease examination) and *Rogi Pariksha* (patient examination). *Rog Pariksha*, also known as *Nidan Panchak*, includes the assessment of early symptoms (*Purvarupa*), primary symptoms *(Rupa),* causative factors (*Hetu*), underlying pathogenesis (*Samprapti*), and therapeutic diagnosis based on response to treatments (*Upashaya*). *Rogi Pariksha* focuses on evaluating dosha imbalances through various examination methods, including *Trividha Pariksha* (threefold examination), *Shadvidha Pariksha* (sixfold examination), *Ashtavidha Pariksha* (eightfold examination), and *Dashavidha Pariksha* (tenfold examination) (See Chapter 8). Once the patient is examined, the physician can determine the disease's chronicity (*Vyakti*) and prognosis (*Veda*). Modern Ayurvedic practitioners integrate contemporary diagnostic tools to enhance clinical accuracy. Research suggests a correlation between laboratory tests and the Tridosha concept. For instance, neutrophilia reflects *Sama* kapha and Pitta, eosinophilia is linked to vata *Vriddhi* or *Prakopa*, and lymphocytosis is associated with *nirama* kapha. This integration helps refine diagnostic precision, offering a comprehensive approach to disease assessment and management (Paradkar 2017).

Ayurvedic diagnostic procedures for animals aim to identify the root cause of ailments and develop treatment plans that restore the animal's natural balance. Rooted in holistic principles, these methods assess the animal's constitution (Prakriti), imbalances (Vikriti), and environmental influences. Key diagnostic techniques include:

- **Observation** (*Darshana*): Examining the animal's physical appearance, behaviour, and posture to identify signs of health or distress.
- **Touch** (*Sparshana*): Using palpation to assess temperature, texture, and abnormalities in the skin, muscles, or organs.
- **Interrogation** (*Prashna*): Collecting information from the caretaker about the animal's diet, habits, and recent changes in behaviour or health.

- **Pulse Diagnosis** (*Nadi Pariksha*) and **tongue diagnosis**: Analysing the pulse and condition to determine imbalances in the *doshas* (*vata, pitta,* and *kapha*).
- **Examination of Excreta** (*Mala Pariksha*): Studying faeces, urine, and other excretions for clues about internal health.

Additionally, modern laboratory tests can used to complement clinical diagnosis and assess prognosis of critical cases.

Ayurvedic Treatment Approaches

Ayurveda views disease as an outcome of an imbalance in the body's natural state, and treatment aims to restore this balance. Unlike conventional medicine, which primarily addresses symptoms, Ayurveda focuses on identifying and addressing the root cause of illness. Since every individual, including animals, has a unique constitution and imbalance, Ayurvedic treatments are personalized. Therefore, no two individuals receive identical treatments, even for similar conditions. In human medicine, Ayurvedic therapies include dietary modifications, herbal remedies, lifestyle adjustments, yoga, meditation, detoxification, and various natural therapies and environmental recommendations. Many of these approaches, except for meditation and *yoga*, can be adapted for veterinary practice. Ayurvedic treatments for animals can be broadly categorized into:

- ***Shamana Chikitsa* (Palliative Treatment):** Focuses on restoring dosha balance using medicinal herbs, minerals, dietary modifications, and physical activity.
- ***Panchakarma* (Biopurificatory or Detoxification Therapy):** Panchakarma is a classical Ayurvedic biopurificatory (detoxification) system designed to eliminate aggravated doshas from the body through procedures such as therapeutic emesis, purgation, medicated enema, nasal therapy, and, where indicated, bloodletting, thereby restoring physiological balance. From an integrative perspective, purification may be understood as supporting the body's natural detoxification pathways, particularly in animals exposed to dietary, environmental, or chemical stressors. In veterinary practice, panchakarma may be employed in the management of chronic or dosha-dominant disorders by facilitating systemic cleansing and metabolic regulation, especially in companion animals frequently exposed to synthetic compounds such as corn gluten meal, insecticides, air fresheners, cat litter fragrances, and nylon collars.

Ayurvedic Herbs, Botanicals and Minerals: Ayurveda considers humans and animals as microcosms of the universe, where all matter—including plants and minerals—possess therapeutic potential. Its pharmacopoeia is rich in herbs and processed minerals, many of which are described in the Ayurvedic Pharmacopeia of

India and other modern references. Ayurvedic formulations often involve multiple ingredients prepared through controlled processes (e.g., *bhasmas*) to ensure safety and potency. Treatments are customized to an individual's constitution (prakriti), influencing their disease susceptibility and response to therapy. The formulation's efficacy depends on its overall synergy, not isolated chemical components (Chopra *et al.* 2010). The Ayurvedic herbs are organized in several ways. A method common to different ethnomedical systems of herbal medicine is to classify them in following categories according to their therapeutic impact on the patient (Silver 2006):

- **Alterative:** Supports detoxification, eliminate metabolic wastes through liver, kidneys, lungs and skin, restore balance and support homeostasis, cool the blood, and reduce pitta.

  Examples: Aloe vera – *Ghritkumari* (*Aloe vera* (L.) Burm.f., syn. *Aloe barbadensis* Mill.), Neem – *Nimba* (*Azadirachta indica*), Sandalwood – *Chandan* (*Santalum album*), Garlic – *Lahsun* (*Allium sativum*), *Shankhpushpi* – (*Convolvulus pluricaulis*), Turmeric – *Haldi* (*Curcuma longa*), *Guduchi* – *Giloy* (*Tinospora cordifolia*), Burdock root – (*Arctium lappa*), Red clover – (*Trifolium pratense*), *Manjistha* – (*Rubia cordifolia*), and Dandelion root – (*Taraxacum officinale*)

- **Anthelmintics:** Pungent or bitter-tasting herbs. Expel parasites and harmful microbes (bacteria, fungi and virus).

  Examples: Carom seed –Ajwain (*Trachyspermum ammi*), Clove – *Laung* (*Syzygium aromaticum*), Garlic – *Lahsun* (*Allium sativum*), *Neem* – *Nimba* (*Azadirachta indica*), Turmeric – *Haldi* (*Curcuma longa*), Papaya – *Papita* (*Carica papaya*), Pomegranate – *Anar* (*Punica granatum*), Indian Jujube – Ber (*Ziziphus mauritiana*), and Banyan – *Bargad* (*Ficus benghalensis*) , Indian wormwood – *Nagdona (Artemisia nilagirica).*

- **Astringent:** Tissue-firming, support tissue resilience, reduce secretions, alleviate diarrhoea and bleeding. Excess intake can cause constipation.

  Examples: Nutmeg – *Jaiphal* (*Myristica fragrans*), Saffron – *Kesar* (*Crocus sativus*), Turmeric – *Haldi* (*Curcuma longa*), Ginger – *Adrak* (*Zingiber officinale*), *Haritaki* – (*Terminalia chebula*), *Amla* – Indian Gooseberry (*Phyllanthus emblica*), Calendula – Pot Marigold (*Calendula officinalis*), and *Bibhitaki* – *Bahera* (*Terminalia bellirica*).

- **Bitter Tonic and Antipyretic:** Reduce heat, purify blood, and calm the system.

  Examples: *Chirata*– (*Swertia chirata*), *Kutki*– (*Picrorhiza kurroa*), Neem – *Nimba* (*Azadirachta indica*), Aloe vera– *Ghritkumari* (*Aloe vera* (L.) Burm.f.), and Gentian– (*Gentiana kurroo*).

- **Carminative:** Relieve bloating and gas, promote normal gastrointestinal peristaltic function.

  Examples: Carom seed –*Ajwain* (*Trachyspermum ammi*), Asafoetida – *Hing* (*Ferula foetida*), Basil – *Tulsi* (*Ocimum sanctum*), Bay leaf – *Tejpatta* (*Laurus nobilis*), Cardamom-*Elaichi* (*Elettaria cardamomum*), Cinnamon – *Dalchini* (*Cinnamomum zeylanicum*), Clove – *Laung* (*Syzygium aromaticum*), Garlic – *Lahsun* (*Allium sativum*), Nutmeg – *Jaiphal* (*Myristica fragrans*), Coriander – *Dhaniya* (*Coriandrum sativum*), Cumin – *Jeera* (*Cuminum cyminum*), Fennel – *Saunf* (*Foeniculum vulgare*), and Turmeric – *Haldi* (*Curcuma longa*).

- **Diaphoretic:** Promote sweating, improve circulation, and remove toxins. Include:

  Cool Herbs: Coriander– *Dhaniya* (*Coriandrum sativum*), Spearmint – (*Mentha spicata*), Peppermint–(*Mentha piperita*), and Chamomile– (*Matricaria chamomilla*).

  Hot Herbs: Basil–*Tulsi* (*Ocimum sanctum*), Camphor–(*Cinnamomum camphora*), Cardamom–*Elaichi* (*Elettaria cardamomum*), Cinnamon– *Dalchini* (*Cinnamomum zeylanicum*), Clove–*Laung* (*Syzygium aromaticum*), Ginger– *Adrak* (*Zingiber officinale*), and Eucalyptus – (*Eucalyptus globulus*).

- **Diuretic:** Increase urine flow.

  Examples: Barley–*Jau* (*Hordeum vulgare*), Coriander– *Dhaniya* (*Coriandrum sativum*), Fennel – *Saunf* (*Foeniculum vulgare*), *Gokshura* – (*Tribulus terrestris*), *Punarnava* – (*Boerhaavia diffusa*), Uva ursi, Bearberry (*Arctostaphylos uva-ursi*), and Carom seed –Ajwain (*Trachyspermum ammi*).

- **Emmenagogue:** Improve blood flow in the pelvic area and uterus, relieve menstrual pain.

  Examples: Aloe vera–*Ghritkumari* (*Aloe vera*), Cotton root– (*Gossypium herbaceum*), Licorice – *Mulethi* (*Glycyrrhiza glabra*), *Shatavari*– (*Asparagus racemosus*), and Saffron – *Kesar* (*Crocus sativus*).

- **Expectorant and Demulcent:** Remove mucus and soothe tissues, clear lung and soothe gastrointestinal tract.

  Examples: Ginger– *Adrak* (*Zingiber officinale*), Licorice– *Mulethi* (*Glycyrrhiza glabra*), Calamus – *Vacha* (*Acorus calamus*), Cardamom – *Elaichi* (*Elettaria cardamomum*), Cinnamon – *Dalchini* (*Cinnamomum zeylanicum*), Clove – *Laung* (*Syzygium aromaticum*), Long Pepper- *Pippali* (*Piper longum*), and Eucalyptus – (*Eucalyptus globulus*).

- **Laxative and Purgative:** Promote bowel movement, remove waste product (*Mala*).

  Examples: Castor oil–(*Ricinus communis*), Senna– (*Cassia angustifolia*), Aloe vera–*Ghritkumari* (*Aloe vera*), Flaxseed – *Alsi* (*Linum usitatissimum*), Psyllium – *Isabgol* (*Plantago ovata*), *Ghee* – Clarified butter, Prunes – *Aloo Bukhara* (*Prunus domestica*), *Haritaki* – (*Terminalia chebula*), *Bibhitaki* – *Bahera* (*Terminalia bellirica*), and *Amla* – (*Phyllanthus emblica*).

- **Nervine and Antispasmodic:** Support the nervous system.

  Examples: *Ashwagandha* – (*Withania somnifera*), Licorice – *Mulethi* (*Glycyrrhiza glabra*), Gotu Kola– Mandukaparni (*Centella asiatica*), *Guggul*– (*Commiphora mukul*), Indian Valerian– *Balchhaṛ* (*Valeriana jatamansi*), and Sandalwood – *Chandan* (*Santalum album*).

- **Stimulant and Digestive:** Enhance digestion and metabolism.

  Examples: Ginger – *Adrak* (*Zingiber officinale*), Garlic – *Lahsun* (*Allium sativum*), Carom seeds–*Ajwain* (*Trachyspermum ammi*), Asafoetida – *Hing* (*Ferula foetida*), Black pepper – *Kali Mirch* (*Piper nigrum*), Clove –*Laung* (*Syzygium aromaticum*), and Onion – *Pyaaz* (*Allium cepa*).

- **Nutritive Tonics:** Build strength, improve tissue health.

  Examples: Almond – *Badam* (*Prunus dulcis*), Amla – (*Phyllanthus emblica*), Coconut – (*Cocos nucifera*), Dates – *Khajur* (*Phoenix dactylifera*), Honey – *Madhu,* Licorice – *Mulethi* (*Glycyrrhiza glabra*), Milk– *Dugdha,* Sesame– *Til* (*Sesamum indicum*), and *Shatavari* – (*Asparagus racemosus*).

- **Rejuvenating tonics *(Rasayana):*** Promote longevity, vitality, immunity, and tissue rejuvenation. They nourish the dhatus (body tissues), support *ojas* (vital essence), and balance the doshas, particularly vata and pitta. Used as a single herb or as polyherbal formulations.

  Examples (Single herb): *Ashwagandha* – (*Withania somnifera*), *Amla* – (*Phyllanthus emblica*), *Shatavari* – (*Asparagus racemosus*), *Guduchi* – *Giloy* (*Tinospora cordifolia*), Ghee – Clarified butter, *Pippali* – Long Pepper (*Piper longum*), Licorice – *Mulethi* (*Glycyrrhiza glabra*), *Bala* – (*Sida cordifolia*), *Gokshura* – (*Tribulus terrestris*), *Haritaki* – (*Terminalia chebula*), *Brahmi* – (*Bacopa monnieri*).

  Examples (Formulations): *Triphala*– A foundational *Rasayana* gently detoxifies while rejuvenating all body systems, especially the digestive and excretory tracts. *Triphala*, a blend of three herbs– *Amla* (*Phyllanthus emblica* / Indian Gooseberry), *Bibhitaki* (*Terminalia bellirica* / *Bahera*) and *Haritaki* (*Terminalia chebula*), is also used in veterinary practices to improve appetite since ancient times.

Over-all, herbs and minerals form the cornerstone of veterinary Ayurvedic treatments. These remedies are administered as single herbs, polyherbal formulations (combinations of multiple herbs), or herbo-mineral preparations. Typically, freshly collected plants or their parts are used in treating a variety of animal health conditions, including digestive disorders, respiratory issues (such as cough and cold), skin ailments, eye diseases, parasitic infestations, mastitis, reproductive disorders, and for the management of wounds, fractures, broken horns, burns, and more (See Chapter 6).

Box 9.4. Herbs and Botanicals of Veterinary Importance to Reduce Antimicrobial Resistance (AMR)

Several Indian medicinal herbs exhibit antimicrobial, antioxidant, and immunomodulatory properties, making them valuable in veterinary care. Many also support gut health through prebiotic activity, aiding in the management of infections, inflammation, and immunity in animals.

Key herbs with veterinary relevance include:

- *Aloe vera (Aloe vera) – Antimicrobial and wound healing*
- *Andrographis (Andrographis paniculata) – Potent immune stimulant*
- *Ashwagandha (Withania somnifera) – Adaptogen and immune booster*
- *Bacopa (Bacopa monnieri) – Antioxidant, supports cognitive function*
- *Banyan (Ficus benghalensis) – Antibacterial, antifungal, antiviral, and antiparasitic*
- *Bael (Aegle marmelos) – Gastroprotective and antimicrobial*
- *Catechu (Acacia catechu) and Babul (Acacia nilotica) – Astringent and antimicrobial*
- *Clove (Syzygium aromaticum) – Broad-spectrum antimicrobial*
- *Garlic (Allium sativum) – Antibacterial, antiviral, and antiparasitic*
- *Indian Barberry (Berberis aristata) – Antimicrobial and liver supportive*
- *Indian Mulberry (Morinda citrifolia) – Antioxidant and antimicrobial*
- *Neem (Azadirachta indica)–Antiparasitic, antibacterial and immunomodulator*
- *Holy Basil / Tulsi (Ocimum tenuiflorum)– Adaptogen and antiviral*
- *Haritaki (Terminalia chebula) – Antioxidant and immune-enhancing*
- *Giloy (Tinospora cordifolia)–Immunomodulating and hepatoprotective*

These herbs, long used in traditional veterinary practices, are now being validated by modern research for use in managing infections, inflammation, oxidative stress, and immune dysfunction in animals.

In addition to therapeutic uses, herbs—alone or in combination with minerals—are employed as liver tonics, galactagogues to manage anestrus and retained placenta, and more importantly, as antimicrobial and immunomodulatory agents. Most herbs are used in their crude form, often as freshly chopped whole plants or plant parts mixed with feed, or applied topically as a paste. Dried herbs are typically administered as powders, infusions, or decoctions. Other common preparations include alcoholic tinctures and oil infusions (See Chapter 6). *The Indian Pharmacopoeia (IP) 2014* has compiled a comprehensive list of medicinal plants used for various animal diseases. Of the herbs covered in IP 2014, 40 are crude herbs and 5 are processed herbs or excipients. Among the 45 herbs mentioned, 18 are official in *The British Pharmacopoeia 2014 (BP 2014)* and 11 in *The United States Pharmacopeia 36 (USP 36)*. Based on human dosage, standard animal doses can be calculated through normalization to body surface area (BSA), often represented in mg/m^2 (Rastogi *et al.* 2015). *The Ayurvedic Formulary of India – Part IV (Veterinary),* published in 2022 by the Pharmacopoeia Commission for Indian Medicine and Homeopathy (Ministry of AYUSH), includes 50 Ayurvedic formulations specifically for veterinary use.

***Marma* Therapy in Veterinary Practice:** Marma Therapy (*Marma Chikitsā*), an ancient Ayurvedic healing system, utilizes specific points on the body to promote healing and balance. Derived from the Sanskrit root *'mri'* with the suffix '*manin*,' Marma refers to vital junctions of muscles, veins, ligaments, bones, and joints where *Prana* (vital life force) naturally resides. According to Acharya Sushruta, there are 107 Marma points in the human body (Sushruta Samhita Sharira Sthana 6.3), and any injury to these points (*Marmaghata*) can result in severe pain, loss of function, or even death. Conversely, their stimulation can enhance circulation, remove toxins, relieve pain, and restore balance to the Tridosha system (Vata, Pitta, Kapha). Marma therapy can be used with medicine or without medicine. It is especially helpful in treating diseases of nervous system, muscular and joint pain, osteoarthritis and stress (Tiwari *et al.* 2021). The significance of Marma therapy extends to veterinary medicine. Ancient texts, including the Shalihotra Samhita, mention Marma massage for horses to alleviate joint pain and enhance flexibility. The Mahabharata references protective coverings for the Marmas of both soldiers and war animals like horses and elephants (Mishra and Shrivastava 2020). Marma therapy shares similarities with Chinese acupuncture, which stimulates specific points to regulate *Qi* (energy or life force) and promote healing. Acupuncture is already an established Complementary and Alternative Veterinary Medicine (CAVM) being used as a natural healing practice for diagnosis and treatment of numerous diseases of animals (Preet *et al.* 2021). Marma therapy is also gaining recognition for its potential applications in following conditions:

- **Digestive Disorders and Metabolic Health:** Certain Marma points, such as *Nabhi* Marma (navel region), can help in relieving colic, indigestion, and bloating in cattle, horses, and other livestock. Ayurvedic practitioners often combine Marma therapy with herbal treatments (like *Triphala* and *Ajwain*) to enhance digestion.
- **Pain Management and Musculoskeletal Disorders:** Marma therapy can be particularly effective for managing lameness, joint pain, and stiffness in

horses, cattle, and elephants. In equine medicine, stimulation of key Marma points along the spine and limbs can enhance mobility and relieve arthritic pain. Elephants, commonly prone to joint disorders due to captivity, may benefit from Marma massage techniques that promote blood circulation and muscle relaxation.

- **As Complementary with Conventional Herbal Therapy**: Soft tissue mobilization—manual therapy used in sport and companion animals—reduces muscle tension, pain, and stress while improving circulation and tissue elasticity (Bergh *et al.* 2022). Likewise, Marma therapy may support sports medicine, geriatric care, rehabilitation, and preventive wellness in animals.

In summary, Marma therapy holds great promise in modern veterinary practice, particularly for non-invasive pain management, stress reduction, and rehabilitation. Its integration with physiotherapy and acupuncture could offer holistic treatment alternatives. However, there is a lack of evidence-based clinical research on its effectiveness in animals. A thorough understanding of Marma points in different species and skilled application by trained practitioners are essential for achieving optimal results.

Panchgavya Therapy: Panchgavya, often referred to as cow therapy, is a holistic treatment approach mentioned in the Vedas. The term Panchgavya denotes five essential substances derived from cows: milk, curd, ghee, urine, and dung. These components are known for their therapeutic properties when consumed, applied externally, or used in environmental purification (FIg. 9.14). Classical Ayurvedic texts describe traditional methods for preparing Panchgavya, often suggesting that all five components be mixed in equal proportions. Ayurveda also mentions its use either as a whole or in combination with medicinal herbs. Additionally, individual components can be utilized separately, such as *Swalpa*-Panchgavya *Ghrita*. Scientific evaluations of these substances, both individually and collectively, indicate their potential to enhance immune responses. One notable preparation, *Kamdhenu Ark* (distilled cow urine), has been found effective in treating kidney disorders and diabetes mellitus. It also enhances phagocytosis by macrophages, aiding in the prevention and control of bacterial infections. Cow urine exhibits antioxidant properties, protecting against DNA damage caused by mitomycin-C-induced chromosomal aberrations. Cow dung is reported to have antifungal, antibacterial, and antimalarial properties. It acts as a skin tonic and is beneficial in treating conditions such as boils, psoriasis, and eczema. It is also reported to help, maintain environmental purity by reducing pollution and counteracting radiation effects. Many skin diseases can be alleviated through its application. Cow milk, curd, and ghee are highly nutritious and play a role in managing various human ailments. Curd and buttermilk serve as effective appetizers and support digestive health by maintaining probiotic bacteria. Curd also possesses antidiabetic and antifungal properties. In traditional veterinary practices, these products are used to treat digestive disorders in animals. Cow ghee is rich in essential fatty acids and vitamins A, D, E, and K. It has demonstrated potential wound-healing properties, possibly due to its balanced composition of saturated and unsaturated fats. Traditionally prepared cow ghee has been found to exhibit antifungal and antiviral properties (Bajaj *et al.* 2022). Both butter and ghee are also used in the treatment of udder swelling and teat skin lesions in livestock. Before being used for Panchgavya, its components should be properly processed according to standard methods and combined in proportions prescribed in *The Ayurvedic Pharmacopoeia of India* (API, Part-II, Vol I.30). It is essential to source these products from healthy cows—specifically, those free from zoonotic diseases such as tuberculosis, paratuberculosis, and brucellosis—to prevent transmission to humans and animals (Chauhan *et al.* 2022).

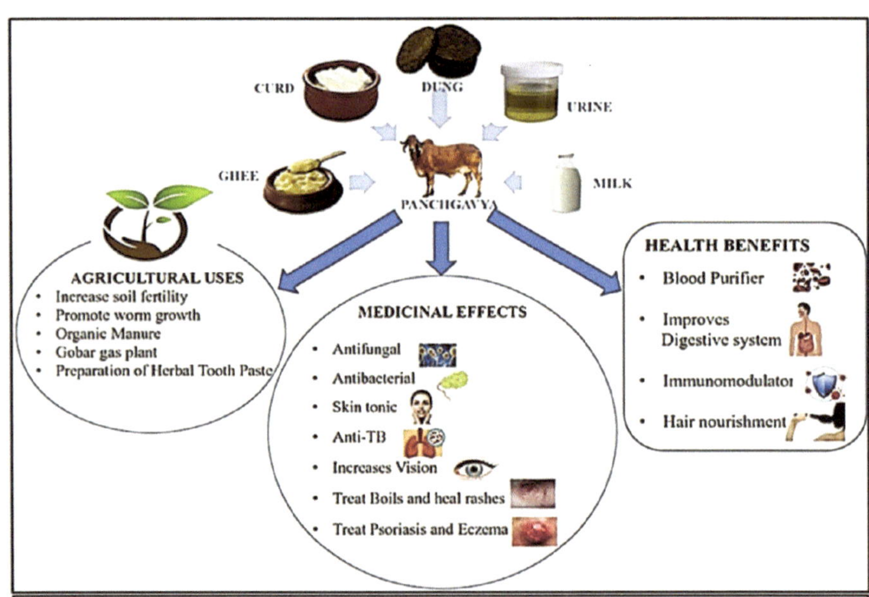

Fig. 9.14. Components and uses of Panchgavya (Source: Bajaj et al. 2022: https://doi.org/10.1016/j.jaim.2021.09.003, licensed under Creative Commons).

Ayurveda for Pets

It is widely believed that, during the course of domestication, dogs evolved unique social-cognitive abilities that fostered a deep and enduring bond with humans. This relationship, as we know it today, may be the result of convergent evolution—where dogs gradually developed traits that mirror human behaviours and tendencies, enabling closer cooperation and emotional attachment. Recent scientific research supports this view, revealing striking similarities between dogs and their owners, not only in appearance but also in personality traits. Studies lend credence to the hypothesis that people often choose dogs that resemble themselves and that, over time, dogs and their owners tend to become more alike in behavioural tendencies and emotional disposition (Bender *et al.* 2025). This deep human-animal connection has significant implications for the care of companion animals. In modern urban life, pet keeping has become increasingly popular, offering emotional support, companionship, and a sense of purpose. Pets are now considered cherished family members, and their health and well-being are seen as integral to the household. Consequently, when conventional treatments prove ineffective, cause adverse effects, or require invasive procedures, many pet owners turn to alternative healing systems.

Ayurveda offers a holistic and individualized approach to pet care, promoting physical and mental wellness, disease prevention, and natural healing. It's not just about treating illness—it supports long-term vitality and balance. In Ayurvedic philosophy, just as in humans, animals exhibit characteristics of the three doshas—vata, pitta, and kapha. Imbalances in doshas can lead to health issues. Identifying dosha types allows for tailored care for the pets through diet, lifestyle, and natural therapies to maintain balance and health. Dogs can be characterized according to different types of dosha constitutions, which correspond to specific types of prakriti (Courson 2024).

- *Vata* (Air + Ether): Vata dogs are energetic, enthusiastic, and quick learners but easily forgetful. They often have lean builds, dry skin, brittle nails, and variable digestion. Prone to cold sensitivity and restlessness, they require warm environments and calming routines.
- *Pitta* (Fire +Water): Pitta dogs are intelligent, focused, and confident but may become aggressive or demanding. With slender bodies, soft fur, and strong digestion, they tend to have high appetites and frequent thirst. They thrive on cooling diets and balanced activity.
- *Kapha* (Earth +Water): Kapha dogs are calm, affectionate, and physically strong. They have sturdy builds, good stamina, and long-term memory but are slow learners. Prone to weight gain, allergies, and digestive issues, they benefit from warmth, exercise, and light diets.

Dietary Practices: Ayurveda emphasizes fresh, natural foods suited to each dosha:

- *Vata*: Warm, moist foods with healthy fats to calm and nourish.
- *Pitta*: Cooling foods like cucumbers and leafy greens to reduce heat.
- *Kapha*: Light, dry foods with minimal fat to prevent sluggishness.
- Medicinal herbs like turmeric, *ashwagandha*, neem, ginger, and *triphala* support digestion, immunity, and relieve stress.

Lifestyle and Environment: Ayurvedic care includes:

- *Exercise:* Match activity to the pet's energy type.
- *Environment:* Balance light, sound, and scent to support calmness.
- *Seasonal Adjustments:* Modify diet and routines with seasonal shifts.

Holistic Therapies: These include:

- *Herbal Remedies*: Herbs are natural support for skin, stress, digestion, ectoparasite and wound management. Some commonly used herbs for pets include Turmeric, *ashwagandha,* neem, ginger, *amla, salai* (Indian frankincense- *Boswellia serrata),* and *Brahmi (Bacopa Bacopa monnieri)*
- *Massage* (*Abhyanga*): Enhances circulation and bonding.
- *Aromatherapy*: Calming scents.
- *Supplements*: support for joints, digestion, and immunity.

Ayurvedic Herbal Drug Safety and Precautions in Pets: While most Ayurvedic herbs are generally safe and well-tolerated, some can be harmful—especially for pets. Cats and dogs, in particular, may develop allergies or show heightened sensitivity to certain herbs. Common medicinal herbs such as ephedra, arnica, ginkgo, lobelia, garlic, onion, St. John's wort, and essential oils of any kind have known toxic potential in pets. For example, garlic and onion can damage red blood cells, leading to anaemia in dogs and cats. Such herbs should either be avoided or used only under the guidance of a qualified veterinary herbalist, as many are contraindicated in companion animals.

Herbal remedies can be used alongside conventional (allopathic) treatments. However, co-administration requires caution, as some herbs may interact with pharmaceutical drugs. These interactions may occur at the pharmacokinetic (absorption, distribution, metabolism, and excretion) or pharmacodynamic (effects at the target site) levels, potentially enhancing or inhibiting the effects of either medicine. Examples of known interactions include (Kumar *et al.* 2014):

- St. John's Wort (*Hypericum perforatum* L.): May interfere with anticoagulant drugs and reduce their effectiveness.
- Aloe vera (*Aloe barbadensis* Mill.): Can increase the cardiotoxic effects of digitoxin and thiazide diuretics.
- Chili pepper *(Capsicum annum):* May enhance absorption of theophylline and alter the action of hypoglycaemic drugs.
- Garlic (*Allium sativum*) and ginseng (*Panax ginseng*): Should be discontinued at least seven days before surgery, as both may increase the risk of bleeding.

To ensure safe use, pet owners and practitioners should consult authoritative resources and evidence-based veterinary references on herbal medicine, especially when herbs are used alongside conventional treatments. Additionally, most toxicity problems with herbs in animals occur because of inappropriate dosing-mainly overdosing. Dosing needs to take into account pet's weight, vitality, illness, digestive function, other medications being taken, diet, and the form of the herb, as well as its strength and potential for toxicity, and possible herb–herb or herb-conventional drug interactions (Fougere 2006).

Veterinary Ayurveda: Way Forward

The future of Ayurveda, including its veterinary applications, appears highly promising, driven by rising consumer interest, expanding research, and strong market demand. The global Ayurvedic products market, valued at USD 5,793.4 million in 2024, is projected to reach USD 7,267.28 million by 2034, with a CAGR of 12% (Ayurvedic Products Market Size & Growth, 2034, accessed on 26-09-2025). In India, the market stood at INR 875.9 billion in 2024 and is expected to grow to INR 3,605.0 billion by 2033, at a CAGR of 16.17% (Ayurvedic Products Market in India: Size, Share Report 2033, accessed on 26-09-2025). This surge reflects growing demand for natural and holistic healthcare solutions. Veterinary Ayurveda, which has been a part of India's rich medical heritage since the Vedic period, is also witnessing a resurgence. Historically, Indian veterinary science has been distinguished by its specialized literature and expert practitioners, who developed nature-based medicines for the prevention and treatment of animal diseases. However, in the modern era, livestock owners and pet caregivers have largely relied on allopathic medicine for animal healthcare due to its immediate efficacy. Despite this, concerns about synthetic drug residues, antibiotic resistance, and long-term toxic effects in meat and dairy products have led to a renewed interest in Ayurveda-based veterinary treatments.

Integration with Modern Science and Biotechnology

One of the most promising aspects of Veterinary Ayurveda's future lies in its integration with modern biotechnology and pharmacological research. Scientists are exploring ways to validate Ayurvedic formulations through rigorous clinical trials, ensuring their safety, efficacy, and standardization. Advanced techniques such as genomic research, phytochemical analysis, and nanotechnology are being employed to enhance the bioavailability and therapeutic effectiveness of herbal compounds. Biotechnology is also helping to optimize traditional Ayurvedic formulations by isolating active ingredients and improving their pharmacokinetics.

Growing Role in Sustainable Livestock and Pet Healthcare

Veterinary Ayurveda is gaining recognition for its role in sustainable and organic livestock farming. Ayurvedic herbal formulations are being increasingly used to:

- **Reduce Antibiotic Use:** Herbal antimicrobials and immunomodulators offer natural alternatives to conventional antibiotics, helping to combat antimicrobial resistance (AMR).
- **Improve Milk Production:** Ayurvedic tonics and herbal supplements are being used to enhance lactation and improve dairy yield in cattle without the side effects associated with synthetic hormones.
- **Enhance Animal Immunity:** Adaptogenic and immunomodulatory herbs such as Ashwagandha (*Withania somnifera*) and guduchi (*Tinospora* cordifolia (Willd.) Hook.f. & Thomson) are being researched for their potential to boost animal immunity.
- **Manage Chronic Conditions:** Ayurveda is being explored for its potential in managing chronic ailments such as arthritis, digestive disorders, and skin diseases in pets and livestock.
- **Marma Therapy and Pain Management:** Traditional techniques like Marma therapy, which focuses on vital energy points, are being investigated for their efficacy in treating pain, nerve disorders, and musculoskeletal issues in animals.

Challenges and Regulatory Aspects: While Veterinary Ayurveda holds immense potential, its widespread adoption faces certain challenges, including:

- **Lack of Standardization:** Many Ayurvedic formulations require more extensive research to establish standardized dosages and efficacy.
- **Regulatory Hurdles:** Unlike allopathic drugs, Ayurvedic veterinary medicines face varying degrees of regulatory acceptance in different countries.
- **Awareness and Training:** Veterinarians require specialized training to integrate Ayurvedic practices with conventional treatment methods safely.

Veterinary Ayurveda: Future Directions and Market Expansion

Given the increasing demand for sustainable animal healthcare solutions, the pharmaceutical and nutraceutical industries are investing in research and commercialization of Ayurvedic veterinary products. Studies increasingly evaluate plant-based formulations alongside conventional treatments, particularly for chronic and complex conditions. At the same time, careful attention is needed to manage drug–herb interactions, herb–herb interactions, and proper dosing. With growing consumer awareness, scientific validation, and government support, Veterinary Ayurveda is well positioned to emerge as a mainstream approach to animal healthcare. Integrating Ayurvedic principles with modern veterinary science can provide safe, cost-effective, and sustainable solutions for animal health and welfare. Establishing formal education and training systems in Veterinary Ayurveda will be crucial to achieving this goal.

Role of Education in Veterinary Ayurveda

The advancement of Veterinary Ayurveda depends not only on market expansion and scientific validation but also on the establishment of formal education systems and structured training programs. With a growing global interest in sustainable and holistic approaches to animal healthcare, developing a robust educational framework has become imperative. This framework must equip veterinarians, livestock owners, and animal health practitioners with the knowledge and skills necessary to integrate the ancient principles of Ayurveda with modern veterinary science. Core areas demanding attention include curriculum development, standardization of training methodologies, and fostering research and innovation in Ayurvedic veterinary medicine.

Standardized Curriculum: A standard curriculum is essential to ensure consistency, credibility, and scientific rigour in Ayurvedic veterinary education. The curriculum should cover:

- **Fundamentals of Ayurveda:** Basic principles, including tridosha (vata, pitta, and kapha), panchamahabhuta (five elements), and *rasa*, *guna, virya*, and *vipaka* (pharmacological concepts).
- **Ayurvedic Pharmacology (Dravyaguna Vigyan):** Understanding medicinal plants, formulations, and their applications in veterinary medicine.
- **Diagnostic and Therapeutic Approaches:** Ayurvedic methods of disease diagnosis (*nadi pariksha*, and *prakriti* analysis) and treatment using herbal, mineral, and dietary therapies.
- **Surgical Techniques in Veterinary Ayurveda:** Historical and modern perspectives on surgical practices in Ayurveda.
- **Integration with Modern Veterinary Science:** Exploring evidence-based approaches for blending Ayurveda with allopathic treatments.
- **Ethnoveterinary Medicine and Practical Applications:** Study of indigenous animal healthcare practices and their relevance in modern livestock management.
- **Regulatory and Safety Aspects:** Guidelines for the safe use of Ayurvedic formulations, herbal-drug interactions, and compliance with veterinary healthcare laws.

Establishment of Veterinary Ayurveda Institutions: To formalize Veterinary Ayurveda education, dedicated institutions and specialized courses should be introduced at various levels as detailed here.

- **Diploma and Certificate Programs:** Short-term courses for veterinarians, farmers, and animal caregivers.
- **Postgraduate Diploma Courses:** Advanced training modules for veterinarians and allied professionals in Ayurvedic animal healthcare.
- **Doctoral and Research Programs:** Ph.D. programs emphasizing the integration of modern veterinary medicine with Ayurveda-based disease management, with a focus on safety, efficacy, and sustainable practices.
- **Online and Continuing Education:** Digital platforms offering certification courses for working veterinarians and researchers.

Training Programs for Veterinary Professionals: The integration of Ayurvedic knowledge into veterinary practice requires extensive hands-on training. Training modules should include:

- **Workshops and Practical Demonstrations:** Conducted by Ayurvedic veterinary experts to teach herbal formulations, diet-based therapies, and surgical techniques.
- **Internship Programs:** Collaboration with Ayurvedic animal healthcare centres, organic farms, and ethnoveterinary practitioners to gain real-world experience.
- **Field Training for Farmers and Livestock Owners:** Educating rural communities on the benefits of herbal medicine, disease prevention, and natural remedies for livestock.
- **Collaboration with Veterinary Universities:** Mainstream Veterinary Colleges should integrate Ayurveda into their syllabi and promote interdisciplinary learning.

Research and Innovation in Veterinary Ayurveda

Education in Veterinary Ayurveda should encourage research and evidence-based validation of Ayurvedic treatments. Research areas should focus on:

- **Efficacy Studies:** Scientific trials to validate the effectiveness of Ayurvedic formulations for treating specific animal diseases.
- **Standardization of Herbal Medicines:** Developing pharmacopeial standards for Ayurvedic veterinary drugs.
- **Biotechnological Integration:** Utilizing modern biotechnology to enhance the bioavailability and potency of Ayurvedic formulations.
- **Sustainable Livestock Management:** Research on how Ayurveda can improve milk yield, fertility, immunity, and disease resistance in livestock without harmful chemical interventions.

Policy Support and Global Recognition

For Veterinary Ayurveda to achieve mainstream acceptance, government support and policy formulation are crucial. Steps to achieve this should include:

- **Recognition by Veterinary Councils and Medical Boards***:* Ensuring Veterinary Ayurveda degrees and certifications are officially recognized.
- **Inclusion in National Livestock Health Programs***:* Encouraging the use of Ayurvedic therapies in disease prevention and livestock care.
- **International Collaboration:** Engaging with global veterinary bodies to promote Ayurveda as a complementary or alternative approach in veterinary science.
- **Funding for Ayurvedic Veterinary Research:** Government and private sector investment in research initiatives to validate Ayurvedic treatments.

Some Notable Educational Programmes

There are a few notable educational programs in Veterinary Ayurveda that aim to integrate traditional Ayurvedic principles with modern veterinary practices:

- **Diploma in Hasthyadi Ayurveda Visharada:** Offered by the Trans-Disciplinary University (TDU), this one-year diploma program focuses on diagnosing and treating animal disorders, particularly those of elephants, using Ayurvedic principles. It combines traditional knowledge with hands-on practical training and case studies.
- **Ayurveda Animal Therapist Training:** Provided by the European Academy of Ayurveda, this program emphasizes holistic health for animals through Ayurvedic manual therapy, nutrition, and herbalism. It includes practical seminars and online learning, covering therapies for dogs, horses, and cats (Discover our training: Ayurveda Animal Therapist).
- **Ayurveda Health Coach for Animals:** Also offered by the European Academy of Ayurveda, this course focuses on determining the constitution of animals (vata, pitta, and kapha) and optimizing their nutrition and training. It is suitable for veterinary practitioners, trainers, and animal lovers. (Ayurveda Health Coach for Animals).

Conclusion

Elements of Ayurvedic medicine form the foundation of many traditional and modern medical systems worldwide, including veterinary medicine. The development of Ayurvedic veterinary practices evolved alongside human medicine, rooted in Vedic philosophy, which emphasized harmony, compassion, and the interconnectedness of all living beings. The belief that humans and animals shared a common destiny reinforced a holistic approach to healthcare in Vedic traditions.

The Ashvins—twin deities revered as divine healers—played a crucial role in early medical traditions, symbolizing the dual focus on human and animal well-being. Physicians trained in human medicine were also knowledgeable in animal care, demonstrating an ideal integration of medical expertise. Classical medical texts such as the Charaka Samhita, Sushruta Samhita, and Harita Samhita contain references to the diagnosis and treatment of both healthy and diseased animals. There were veterinarians who specialized solely in animal healthcare, the most notable being Shalihotra, regarded as the world's first known veterinarian and the father of Indian veterinary science.

Ayurvedic veterinary medicine is extensively documented in ancient scriptures including the Agni Purana (Chapters 287-92) and Matsya Purana. These works provide detailed descriptions of diseases affecting various animal species and their treatment using herbal and mineral-based formulations. A wide range of ailments—including infections of the horns, ears, teeth, throat, heart, and skin, as well as digestive disorders, respiratory ailments, parasitic infestations, anaemia, urinary issues, colic, haematuria, eye diseases, arthritis, rhinitis, sprains, wounds, abscesses, epistaxis, and rabies—were effectively treated through Ayurvedic methods. Ayurvedic principles were also applied to enhance livestock productivity and health through balanced diets, herbal supplements, and natural tonics.

Veterinary surgery in ancient India was remarkably advanced. Skilled surgeons performed complex procedures with precision, employing specialized surgical instruments and techniques. The Rig Veda (1.116, 117) even contains references to prosthetic surgery, suggesting a sophisticated understanding of surgical intervention during the Vedic period. The works of Shalihotra and Palakapya present detailed accounts of surgical practices, including treatments for sinus fistulas, burns, snakebites, fractures, ligament and tendon injuries, dystocia, foetal extraction, tooth extraction, and orthopaedic conditions (Singh 2002). Beyond specialized treatises, texts such as the Shukraniti, and Arthashastra underscore cattle protection, ethical management, and livestock prosperity as pillars of agrarian wealth and state stability, while animal husbandry and welfare are also addressed in the Vishnu Samhita and Parashar Samhita. Collectively, ancient Indian literature underscores the vital role of domestic animals and consistently advocates their protection and well-being.

The holistic principles laid down by the Vedic sages continue to influence both traditional and modern veterinary practices. A renewed interest in Ayurvedic veterinary medicine has encouraged the integration of herbal remedies, dietary strategies, and preventive healthcare into contemporary animal care, including for companion animals. Emerging research points to the potential of Ayurvedic herbs in managing behavioural issues, stress, pain, and neurological disorders in animals. Marma therapy—an ancient practice that stimulates vital energy points—may hold potential as a complementary approach in veterinary care, particularly for pain management and nervous system support, though further scientific validation is needed. Furthermore, Ayurvedic botanicals are being studied as natural alternatives to conventional antibiotics, offering promising avenues for addressing antimicrobial resistance (AMR). The future of Veterinary Ayurveda lies in the establishment of structured education programs, hands-on clinical training, and scientific validation of ancient practices. By integrating Ayurvedic principles with modern veterinary science, this field can offer safe, cost-effective, and sustainable solutions for animal healthcare.

References

Agni Purana. 1954. *The Agni Purāṇa, Part III.* 1st edn. (English Translator) Gangadharan N. Motilal Banarsidass, Delhi, India. Available at: Agni Purana english translation part 3.pdf.

Ahmed S.2024. Exploring military technology from thirteenth to fourteenth century: A study of Delhi Sultanate. *International Journal for Multidisciplinary Research (IJFMR)* **6** (6):1-5. 31292.pdf.

Anonymous .1949. Veterinary science. In: *Caraka Samhita Vol I.* pp.292-97. Shree Gulabkunverba Ayurvedic Society, Jamnagar, India. https://dn790006.ca.archive.org/0/items/in.ernet.dli.2015.63710/2015.63710.The-Caraka-Samhita1_text.pdf, downloaded on 21-08-2024.

Antony R and Thomas R .2011. A mini review on medicinal properties of the resurrecting plant *Selaginella bryopteris* (Sanjeevani). *International Journal of Pharmacy and Life Sciences***2** (7): 933-39.

API. 2008. *Pañcagavya Ghrta*. In: *The Ayurvedic Pharmacopeia of India. Part-II (Formulations).* 1st edn. Vol 1.30. Government of India, MHW, New Delhi, India.

Arasu SK. 2019. Military administration of the imperial Cholas. International Journal of Research and Analytical Reviews **6** (2): 139-48.

Bajaj KK, Chavhan V, Raut NA and Gurav S.2022. Panchgavya: A precious gift to humankind. *Journal of Ayurveda and Integrative Medicine* **13** (2):100525. https://doi.org/10.1016/j.jaim.2021.09.003.

Bender Y, Roth F, Schweinberger S, Witte S and Bräuer J., 2025. Like owner, like dog–A systematic review about similarities in dog-human dyads. *Personality and Individual Differences* **233**: https://doi.org/10.1016/j.paid.2024.112884.

Chauhan RS, Devi T, Joshi A and Priya K.2022. *Cowpathy* in ancient wisdom, people belief, evidenced relief and science with precautionary measures. In: *Cowpathy and Human Health*. pp. 215-19. (Eds) Chauhan RS and Malik YP. Society for Immunology and Immunobiology and Go Mahima Seva Trust, New Delhi, India.

Chopra A, Saluja M and Tillu G. 2010. Ayurveda–modern medicine interface: A critical appraisal of studies of Ayurvedic medicines to treat osteoarthritis and rheumatoid arthritis. *Journal of Ayurveda and Integrative Medicine* **1**(3):190-98. DOI: 10.4103/0975-9476.72620.

Choudhary RA. 2017. Mughal and late Mughal equine veterinary literature:" Tarjamah-i-Saloter-i-Asban" and" Faras-Nama-i-Rangin". *Social Scientist* **45** (7/8):57-71.

Choudhary RA. 2022. The tradition of equine veterinary literature in Pre-Colonial and Colonial India: The writing of *Faras-nama* literature. *Studies in Humanities and Social Sciences* **29**(1):141-67. The_Tradition_of_equine_Veterinary_Literature_in_Pre_Colonial_and_Colonial_India-libre.pdf.

Courson W. 2024. *Ayurveda for Pets: Natural Health Care for Cats and Dogs.* 106 p. William A. Courson, Montclair, New Jersey, USA.

Dave T, Habte A, Vora V, Sheikh MQ, Sanker V and Gopal SV. 2024 Sushruta: the father of Indian surgical history. *Plastic and Reconstructive Surgery-Global Open* 1**2**(4): p e5715, April 2024. | DOI: 10.1097/GOX.0000000000005715.

Dickstein J.2024. Panjrapole: The Jain animal sanctuary. https://www.arihantainstitute.org/blog/97-panjrapole-the-jain-animal-sanctuary, accessed on 26-03-2025.

Edgerton F. 1931.*The Elephant-Lore of the Hindus: The Elephant Sport (Matanga-Lila) of Nilakantha.* Yale University Press, Connecticut, USA.

Elliot HM.1867. Táríkh-I Badáuni. In: *The History of India, as Told by Its Own Historians: The Muhammadan Period, Volume* I. pp. 335-36. (Ed) John Dowson. Trübner & Co. London, UK. Google Books. https://books.google.co.in/books?id=dMgNAAAAQAAJ, accessed on 20-04-2025.

Fine AH. 2019. *Handbook on Animal-Assisted Therapy: Foundations and Guidelines for Animal-Assisted Interventions*. 3rd edn. Academic Press, Elsevier, London, UK.

Fougere B. 2006. *Pet Lover's Guide to Natural Healing for Cats and Dogs.* 597 p. Elsevier Health Sciences, St Louise, USA.

Gallis C .2013. *Green Care. For Human Therapy, Social Innovation, Rural Economy, and Education*; Nova Science Publishers Inc., New York, USA.

Ganeshaiah KN, Vasudeva R and Shaanker RU. 2009. In search of *Sanjeevani. Current Science* **97** (4): 484-89.

Ganguly KM. 1886. *The Mahabharata of Krishna-Dwaipayana Vyasa*. Available at: https://www.wisdomlib.org/hinduism/book/the-mahabharata-mohan/d/doc7518.html, accessed on 19-03-2025.

Garg DN. 1987. Sources for ancient India literature on veterinary science. *Indian Journal of History of Science* **22** (1):103-10.

Geetha N. 2012. *Elephantology and its Ancient Sanskrit Sources.* Online Book. https://www.wisdomlib.org/hinduism/essay/elephantology, accessed on 29-12-2022.

Gopalan S.1952. *Aśvaśāstram by Nakula.* 233+XXXVI p. TMSSM Library, Tanjore, India.

Gopalan S. 1958. *Gajaśāstram of Pālakāpya Muni*. TMSSM Library, Tanjore, India. Available at: https://archive.org/details/Gajasasthra.

Gopikrishna BS and Binorkar S.2020. *Visha Chikitsa Adhyaya*. In: *Charak Samhita New Edition*. 1st edn. pp.96. (Eds) Binorkar S, Deole YS and Basisht G. CSRTSDC ebook, Jamnagar, India. vailable at: https://www.carakasamhitaonline.com/index.php?title=Visha_Chikitsa&oldid=44557.

Hultzsch E.1925. *Corpus Inscriptionum Indicum Vol. 1. Inscription of Asoka New Edition.*446 p. Official Agents of Government of India, Clarendon Press Oxford, UK. Available at: https://archive.org/details/InscriptionsOfAsoka. .pdf, downloaded on 16-03-2025.

Jones BV. 2021. South Asia: India, Pakistan, Bangladesh, Myanmar, Sri Lanka, Malasia and Tibet. In: *The History of Veterinary Medicine and the Animal-Human Relationship*. 608 p. 5m Books Ltd.

Jones SD and Koolmees PA. 2022. Animal healing in trade and conquest. In: *A Concise History of Veterinary Medicine.* pp. 47-48. Cambridge University Press, UK.

Kansara NM. 2008. Animal husbandry in Vedas. In: *History of Agriculture in India, up to c. 1200 AD.* pp 275-308. (Eds) Gopal Lallanji and Srivastava VC. Concept Publishing Company, Delhi, India.

Kulkarni ED .1953. *Salihotra of Bhoja.* 1st edn. pp.1-70. Deccan College Post-Graduate and Research Institute, Poona, India.

Kumar PM, Kulkarni SS and Wadkar SD. 2014. Review on Interaction of Herbal Medicines with Allopathic Medicines. *Journal of Ayurveda and Holistic Medicine (JAHM)* **2**(2):38-43.

Kunja Lal K.1907. *An English Translation of the Sushruta Samhita, Vol. I Sutrashanam.* (Ed. & Publ.), Kaviraj Kunja Lal Bhishagratna., 10, Kashi Ghose's Lane, Calcutta (Kolkata), India.

Maji K. 2021. Nature of treatment in the ancient era. In: *Atharvaveda and Charaka Samhita.* Available at: https://www.wisdomlib.org/hinduism/essay/atharvaveda-and-charaka-samhita/d/doc1210392.html.

Meulenbeld GJ. 1999. Caraka, his identity and date. *A history of Indian Medical Literature, Vol. XV / 1A*. pp. 105-16. (Ed) Bakker HT. Egbert Forsten, Groningen, Netherlands. Available at: ia601900.us.archive.org/3/items/Meulenbeld-HIML/HIML 1A .pdf.

Mishra A and Shrivastava V.2021. Exploring the science of *marma*-An ancient healing technique: Its mention in ancient Indian scriptures. *Dev Sanskriti Interdisciplinary International Journal* **17**:43-51.

Paradkar SR. 2017. Role of modern diagnostic methods in ayurvedic diagnosis: concepts and prospects. *International Journal of Research in AYUSH and Allied System* **4** (4):1258-63. https://ayushdhara.in/index.php/ayushdhara/article/view/311.

Potbhare BM, Reddy RG, Thakre PA and Sangvikar S. 2019. Samrat Ashoka's inscriptions and Ayurveda: A review. *International Journal of Ayurveda and Pharma Research* **7**(9):69-72.

Prasad GP and Swamy RK. 2015. Contribution of Yejella Shri Ramulu Chaudari to Ayurvedic veterinary medicine- A biographical research study. *Ayushdhara* **4** (2):1-10.

Preet GS, Kumar S, Gupta S and Sodhi HS. 2021. Complementary and alternative veterinary medicine. In: *Multidisciplinary Research and Development.* pp125-39. (Ed) Fedorov S. Weser Books Zittau, Germany.

Rastogi S, Pandey MK, Prakash J, Sharma A and Singh GN. 2015. Veterinary herbal medicines in India. *Pharmacognosy Reviews* **9** (18):155-63.

Reader's Digest. 2003. The truth about history: New noses and mended ears. pp. 246-49. Reader's Digest Association Limited London, UK.

Sarswati SP. 2011. *Yajurveda English Translation.* https://archive.org/details/yajurveda-english translation/page/n3/mode/1up, downloaded on 15-03-2025.

Shah NC. 2015. Soma, an enigmatic, mysterious plant of the Vedic Aryans: An appraisal. *Indian Journal of History of Science* **50** (1):26-41.

Sharma TR (Trans.). 2013. *Atharva-Veda Vol. I.* Vijaykumar Govindram Hansnand, New Delhi, India. (Digital Distributer Agniveer). https://archive.org/details/atharva-veda-vol-2-of-2, pdf downloaded on 05-06-2023.

Sharma TR (Trans.). 2013 b. *Yajurveda with Original Sanskrit Text, English Translation.* Paropakarini Sabha, Ajmer, India. Available at: https://www.thearyasamaj.org/uploads/book/2014/04/R1sSjG_eLb_sub_406_yajurveda.pdf,

Shrivastav VK, Srivastava A and Deole YS.2020. *Upakalpaniya Adhyaya.* In: *Charak Samhita New Edition.* 1st edn. pp. 17. (Eds) Mangalasseri P, Deole YS and Basisht G. CSRTSDC ebook, Jamnagar, India. Available at: https://www.carakasamhitaonline.com/index.php?title=Upakalpaniya_Adhyaya&oldid=44481

Silver RJ. 2006. Ayurvedic veterinary medicine: principles and practices. In: *Veterinary Herbal Medicine.* pp. 59-83. ((Eds) Wynn S G and Fougère B. Mosby Elsevier, St Louise, USA.

Singh GR. 2002.Animal surgery or *Pashu Shalya Chikitsa* in ancient India. In: *Third Convocation of National Academy of Veterinary Sciences (India) and National Symposium on Historical Overview on Veterinary Sciences and Animal Husbandry in Ancient India (Vedic and Ashokan Period).* 16-17 April 2002. pp. 12. Indian Veterinary Research Institute, Izatnagar, Uttar Pradesh, India.

Singh J, Desai MS, Pandav CS and Desai SP .2011. Contributions of ancient Indian physicians: Implications for modern times. *Journal of Postgraduate Medicine* 58 (1): 73–8, doi:10.4103/0022-3859.93259.

Singh RH, Singh G, Sodhi JS and Dixit U.2020. *Deerghanjiviteeya Adhyaya.* In: *Charak Samhita New Edition.* 1st edn. pp.3. (Eds) Dixit U, Deole YS and Basisht G. Jamnagar, India CSRTSDC ebook. Available at: https://www.carakasamhitaonline.com/index.php?title=Deerghanjiviteeya_Adhyaya&oldid=45351

Somvanshi R. 2002. Legends of cow-bulls in coins of ancient India. In: *Third Convocation of National Academy of Veterinary Sciences (India) and National Symposium on Historical Overview on Veterinary Sciences and Animal Husbandry in Ancient India (Vedic and Ashokan Period).* pp. 20. 16-17 April, 2002. Indian Veterinary Research Institute, Izatnagar, Uttar Pradesh, India.

Somvanshi R. 2006. Veterinary medicine and animal keeping in ancient India. *Asian Agri-History* **10**(2):133-46.

Somvanshi R. 2024a. Veterinary science in ancient India: An overview. In: *Animal Husbandry Practices in Ancient India: Scientific Analysis.* pp-1-12. Bihar Veterinary College, BASU, Patna, India.

Somvanshi R. 2024b. Animal husbandry during Mauryan era. In: *Animal Husbandry Practices in Ancient India: Scientific Analysis.* pp. 31-46. Bihar Veterinary College, BASU, Patna, India.

Somvanshi R, Swaminathan M and Singh RK. 2017. *Veterinary Science and Animal Husbandry in Medieval and Modern India.* 88 p. ICAR-Indian Veterinary Research Institute, Izatnagar, Uttar Pradesh, India.

Tiwari AN, Gautam VL, Pathak AK and Abhinav. 2021. Marma and marma therapy: a traditional view. *International Journal of Biology, Pharmacy and Allied Sciences (IJBPAS)* **10**(12):180-86.

Upadhyaya PS and Singh SY. 2020. *Phalamatra Siddhi Adhyaya.* In: *Charak Samhita New Edition.* 1st edn. pp.128. (Eds) Thakar A, Mangalasseri P, Deole YS and Basisht G. CSRTSDC ebook, Jamnagar, India. Available at: https://www.charakasamhitauptodate.com/index.php?title=Phalamatra_Siddhi&oldid=44588.

Valiathan MS. 2006. Evolution of healing art in India. In: *Towards Ayurvedic Biology: A Decadal Vision Document – 2006.* pp. 8-18. Indian Academy of Sciences, Bangalore, India.

Valmiki Ramayana | Valmiki Ramayanam. www.valmiki.iitk.ac.in, accessed on 19-03-2025.

Wilson HH.1928. *Rig-Veda Samhita. Translational from Original Sanskrit Vol V.* (Eds) Cowell EB and Webster WF. Asthekar & Co Poona, India. flipbook. https://vedicheritage.gov.in/samhitas/rigveda/shakala-samhita.

Wilson HH.1946. *Rig-Veda Sanhita. Translational from Original Sanskrit Vol I.* The Bangalore Printing and Publishing Co Ltd Bangalore, India. Mandala 01 | Vedic Heritage Portal.

Wilson HH. 1866. https://www.wisdomlib.org/hinduism/book/rig-veda-english-translation/d/doc840450.html.

10

Phytopharmacology, Scientific Research and Development in Herbal Veterinary Medicine

S. Dey and Ananya Dan

bahutā tatrayōgyatvamanēkavidhakalpanā; sampaccēti catuṣkō'yaṁ dravyāṇāṁ guṇa ucyatē.

Abundance (in availability), efficacy (with good pharmacological properties), various pharmaceutical forms, and intact qualities of drugs–these are four qualities of the ideal medicine.

(Charak Samhita 9.7; translation by Tomar and Kumar 2020)

Introduction

The use of medicinal plants and herbs for the healthcare of both humans and animals dates back to the earliest civilizations. Over time, with the advent of modern science, the allopathic system of medicine began to dominate healthcare practices, particularly from the 19th century onward. Despite this shift, medicinal plants have continued to serve as a foundational source for many modern drugs. The scientific advancements of the 18th and 19th centuries played a pivotal role in identifying causative agents of diseases—such as viruses, bacteria, protozoa, and parasites—leading to significant progress in vaccine development and pharmaceutical research. Parallel developments in chemistry, particularly in European countries like Germany and the UK, as well as in the Middle East and the Indian subcontinent, fuelled the exploration of traditional medicines. This global scientific momentum inspired systematic studies into the pharmacological properties of traditionally used Indian medicinal plants, with the goal of isolating bioactive compounds for modern drug development.

Phyto-ingredients and their Pharmacological Activities

Medicinal plants contain primary and secondary metabolites, both of which play critical roles in their pharmacological efficacy. Primary metabolites (e.g., carbohydrates, amino acids, and fatty acids) are vital for plant growth and have applications in human and animal health, particularly as nutraceuticals. Secondary metabolites are synthesized in response to environmental stress and act as natural defence agents. These include a diverse range of compounds with antiviral, antibacterial, antifungal, and antiparasitic properties. These secondary plant metabolites often serve as templates or precursors for drug development. Their biological activities—ranging from anti-inflammatory and antioxidant to immunomodulatory and antimicrobial—have been documented since ancient times and continue to be validated by modern research. Phytochemicals are typically classified based on their chemical structure into the following major groups discussed here:

Alkaloids

Plants produce over 20,000 nitrogen-containing heterocyclic compounds known as alkaloids. These secondary metabolites serve a wide range of eco-physiological functions in plants and have been used by humans for centuries as medicines and psychoactive substances. Well-known examples include the anti-cancer agent vinblastine and the analgesic morphine. A key factor contributing to the structural diversity and biological activity of alkaloids is the action of cytochrome P450 monooxygenases (P450s). These enzymes introduce oxygen atoms into alkaloid structures, making most alkaloids heavily oxygenated. P450s also catalyse critical transformations such as ring formation, expansion, and cleavage, which are essential for generating the complex scaffolds of bioactive alkaloids (Nguyen and Dang 2021). While all alkaloids contain at least one nitrogen atom, many also incorporate other elements such as oxygen, sulphur, chlorine, bromine, and phosphorus. Owing to their structural complexity and functional diversity, alkaloids are classified using various criteria. One common method of classification is based on the position of the nitrogen atom, which divides alkaloids into two broad categories:

- **Heterocyclic (Typical) Alkaloids:** Contain nitrogen within a ring structure. Examples include quinine, caffeine, and nicotine.

- **Non-heterocyclic (Atypical) Alkaloids**: Do not have nitrogen in a ring structure and are less commonly found in nature. Examples include ephedrine and colchicine.

Based on biosynthesis, alkaloids are classified as:

- **True alkaloids**: Derived from amino acids, with nitrogen in a heterocyclic ring (e.g., morphine).
- **Protoalkaloids**: Also derived from amino acids, but nitrogen is not part of a ring (e.g., ephedrine and adrenaline).
- **Pseudoalkaloids**: Contain nitrogen in a heterocyclic ring but are not derived from amino acids. Instead, compounds like ethylamine, methylamine, or beta-aminoethanol serve as nitrogen sources (e.g., aconitine and delphinine).

Based on ring structure, alkaloids are further classified into:

- **Piperidine alkaloids**: Piperidine ring (C_5N), derived from lysine (e.g., piperine, sedamine, and lobeline).
- **Isoquinoline alkaloids**: Isoquinoline ring, derived from tyrosine/phenylalanine (e.g., morphine and codeine).
- **Tropane alkaloids**: Tropane ring (C_4N), derived from acetoacetate and ornithine (e.g., atropine and cocaine).
- **Quinoline alkaloids**: Quinoline ring, obtained from Cinchona bark (e.g., quinine and cinchonine).
- **Purine alkaloids**: Derived from purine nucleotides, based on xanthine or uric acid skeletons (e.g., caffeine, theobromine, and theophylline).
- **Pyrrolizidine alkaloids**: Pyrrolizidine nucleus (e.g., heliotrine and retronecine).
- **Indole alkaloids**: Indole ring (e.g., vincristine).
- **Pyrrolidine alkaloids**: C_4N nucleus.
- **Imidazole alkaloids**: Imidazole ring derived from histidine.

Pharmacological Significance: Alkaloids (Fig. 10.1a; 10.1b) are among the most predominant secondary plant metabolites, widely used as drugs in modern medicine. They possess diverse therapeutic properties—analgesic, anticancer, antibacterial, antiarrhythmic, antihyperglycemic—and influence the central nervous system as stimulants and psychotropics. They are generally bitter and found in plants as water-soluble salts, while free alkaloids are water-insoluble.

Alkaloids often form irreversible complexes with tannins, making tannins effective antidotes in acute alkaloid poisoning. Some notable alkaloids and their pharmacological properties are:

- **Amphetamine** (bronchodilator)
- **Caffeine, Nicotine** (stimulants)
- **Cocaine** (anaesthetic)
- **Codeine** (cough suppressant)
- **Morphine** (narcotic analgesic from poppy)
- **Papaverine** (vasodilator)
- **Reserpine** (antihypertensive)
- **Strychnine** (highly toxic rodenticide)
- **Quinine** (antimalarials)
- **Vincristine** (anticancer Agents: used in chemotherapy)

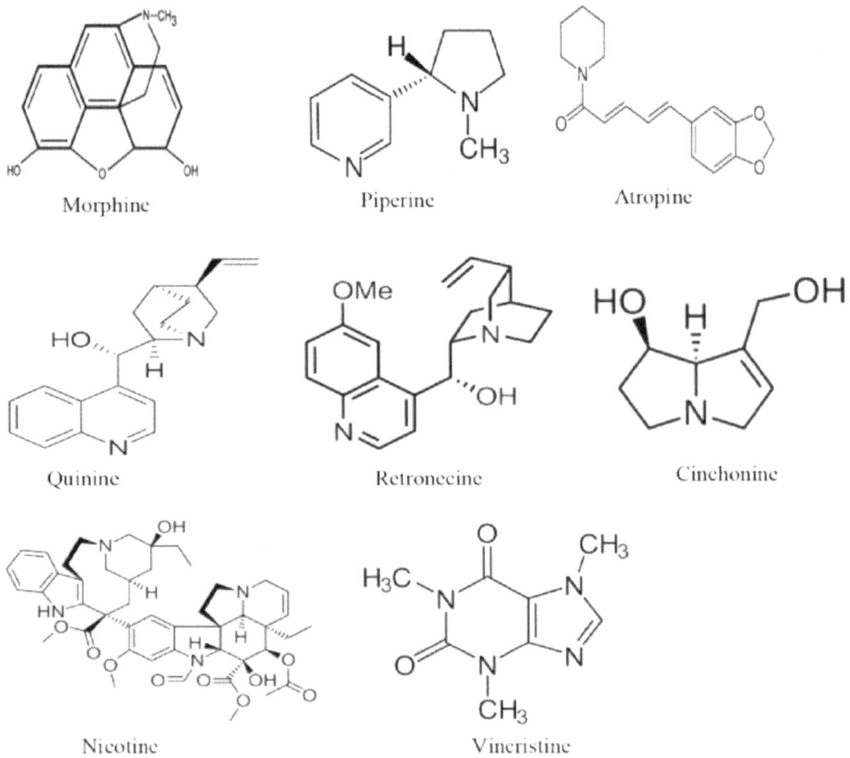

Morphine Piperine Atropine

Quinine Retroneceine Cinchonine

Nicotine Vincristine

Fig. 10.1a. Chemical structure of selected key alkaloids.

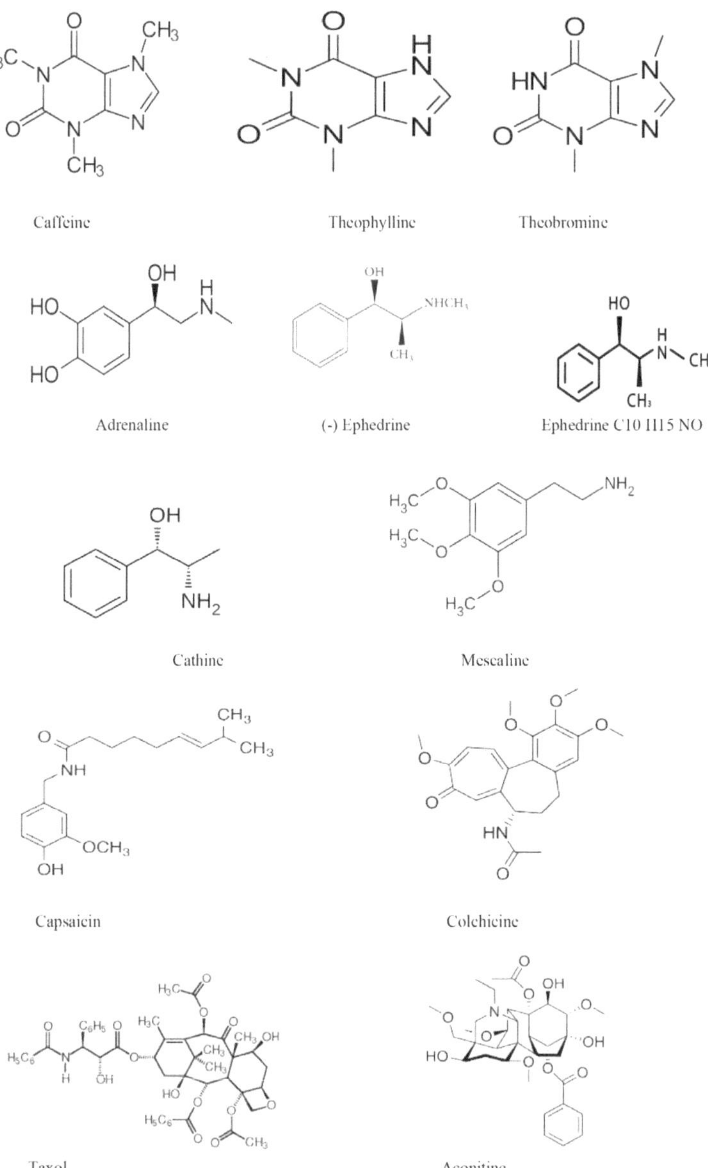

Fig. 10.1b. *Chemical structure of selected key alkaloids.*

Glycosides

Glycosides are secondary metabolites primarily derived from plants and are commonly found in essential oils. They consist of one or more sugar molecules—such as monosaccharides, oligosaccharides, or uronic acids—collectively referred to as the glycone, which if are linked to a non-sugar component, known as the aglycone. The aglycone may be a phenol, alcohol, or a more complex molecule like a steroid nucleus. These components are joined via a glycosidic linkage. While glycosidic linkages (Fig. 10.2, 10.3) most often involve a covalent bond to an oxygen atom (O-glycosides), they may also involve carbon (C-glycosides), nitrogen (N-glycosides), or sulphur (S-glycosides). The attachment of the glycone through glycosidic bonds increases the polarity and water solubility of the molecule compared to the aglycone alone, enhancing the mobility and storage of the aglycone portion within the plant. In animals, enzymes such as β-glucosidase and β-galactosidase are capable of hydrolysing these glycosidic bonds, thereby releasing the active aglycone. Owing to the relative instability of glycosidic bonds, minimal processing of glycoside-containing plants is advisable to preserve their pharmacological activity.

Most glycosides pass through the stomach and small intestine unchanged. Hydrolysis primarily occurs in the colon, facilitated by enzymes produced by gut microflora. Once released, aglycones are absorbed and subsequently metabolized. In some cases, glycosides undergo esterification in the liver, which may prolong their half-life. Among the glycosides of significant pharmacological and toxicological interest are cardiac glycosides, anthraquinone glycosides, and cyanogenic glycosides.

- Cardiac glycosides contain aglycones derived from steroidal structures. They inhibit Na^+/K^+-ATPase pumps in cardiac myocytes and other tissues, resulting in a positive inotropic effect (increased force of heart contraction) and a negative chronotropic effect (reduced heart rate). These properties make them valuable in the treatment of congestive heart failure (Hood *et al.* 2004). Examples include digitalis and digitoxin.

- Anthraquinone glycosides share some pharmacological characteristics with cardiac glycosides and are known for their potent cathartic effects. After hydrolysis in the colon, they promote the secretion of water and electrolytes, enhancing peristalsis and gut motility. Anthraquinones are also recognized for a broad range of biological activities, including anticancer, anti-inflammatory, diuretic, antiarthritic, antifungal, antibacterial, and antimalarial effects (Diaz-Muñoz *et al.* 2018).

- Cyanogenic glycosides are noted for their toxic potential, as enzymatic hydrolysis of their glycosidic bonds releases hydrogen cyanide (HCN)—a lethal compound and a known cause of poisoning, especially in ruminants.

In addition to above glycosides, several other important classes of natural glycosides occur widely in plants, each with distinct structures and biological activities. For example, flavanone glycosides-naringin, hesperidin (common in citrus fruits); saponin glycosides-glycyrrhizin (from liquorice), dioscin, ginsenosides (from ginseng); steroidal glycosides- solanine (from solanum species), diosgenin glycosides; coumarin glycosides-aesculin (from aesculus hippocastanum), scopoline; phenolic glycosides-arbutin (from bearberry), salicin (from willow bark); thioglycosides (glucosinolates)- sinigrin, glucoraphanin (from cruciferous vegetables like broccoli, mustard) and alkaloidal glycosides-solanine and tomatine.

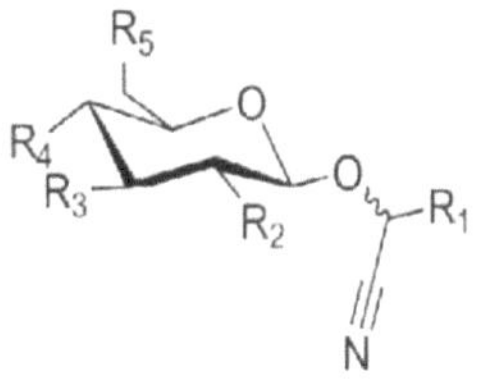

General structure of cyanogenic glycoside

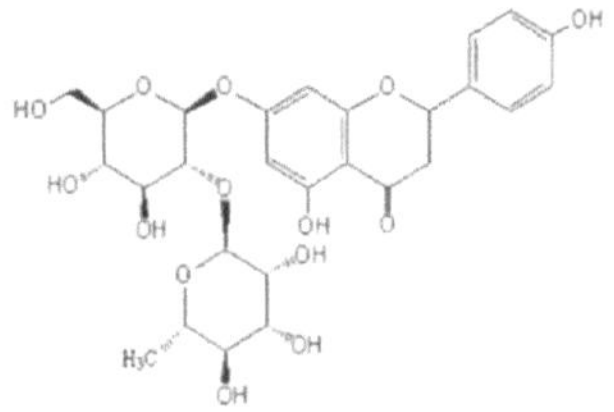

Flavanone glycoside- Naringenin is a strong antioxidant

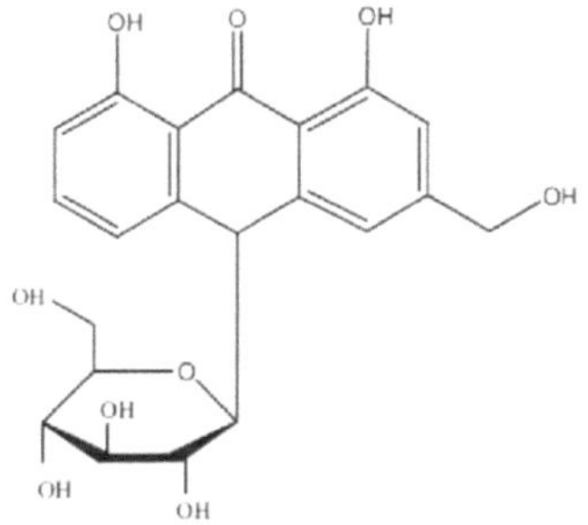

Barbaloin (C-glycoside)

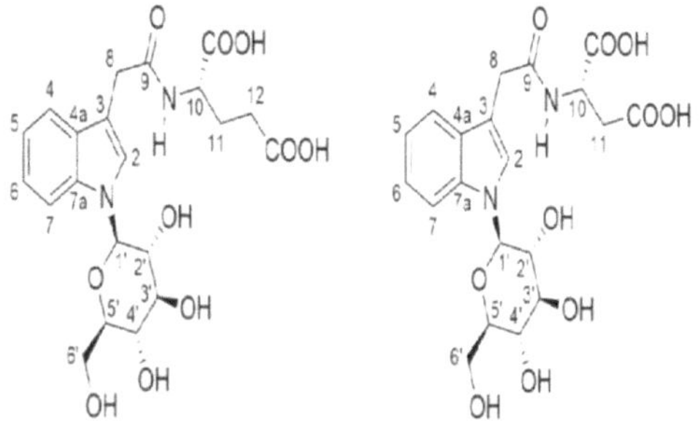

Two rare N-glycosides isolated from Ginkgo biloba (Ref. Cheng *et al.* 2020)

Fig.10.2. *Chemical structure of selected key glycosides.*

Polysaccharides

Polysaccharides are long chains of sugar molecules (monosaccharide residues) linked by glycosidic bonds. Their molecular weight varies depending on the number and type of monosaccharide units, and their structures can be either linear or branched. They are generally water-insoluble but can form hydrocolloid gels of varying consistency when mixed with water. These gel formations may be reversible or irreversible, depending on the nature of the interactions between water molecules and the polysaccharide chains. Polysaccharides

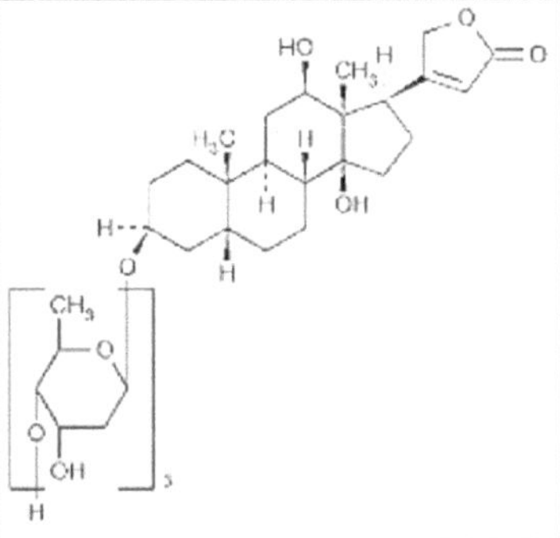

Fig. 10.3. *Chemical structure of digoxin.*

exhibit a range of pharmacological activities, including inhibition of tumour growth and viral replication, reduction of inflammation, cardiovascular protection, and antimutagenic effects. Recent advancements have highlighted their potential in biomedical applications, particularly in regenerative medicine and tissue engineering.

Bioactive polysaccharides derived from medicinal herbs have long been used in traditional medicine as tonics and anticancer agents. They are found in plants such as aloe, cinnamon, ginger, and ginseng, where they contribute to enveloping, emollient, anti-inflammatory, and wound-healing effects. Herbal drugs containing polysaccharides are commonly used for treating diseases of the nasopharynx, bronchitis, and intestinal disorders.

Research has shown that certain polysaccharides can enhance immune function and possess hematopoietic (blood-restoring) properties. They are often prescribed in combination with other therapeutic agents (Bokov *et al.* 2020). Notably, branched polysaccharides with higher molecular weights tend to exhibit greater bioactivity. These compounds are also used alongside conventional chemotherapy and radiotherapy. Owing to their low cost, high biocompatibility, biodegradability, ease of chemical modification, inertness, and nontoxic nature, polysaccharides are increasingly being used in targeted drug delivery systems (Barclay *et al.* 2019).

Terpenes and Terpenoids

Terpenes and terpenoids are important classes of natural compounds synthesized by a wide range of organisms, including plants, animals, insects, endophytes, plant pathogens, and marine species. Although the terms are often used interchangeably, they differ structurally: terpenes are simple hydrocarbons composed of repeating isoprene units (C_5H_8), while terpenoids are modified terpenes that contain additional functional groups—typically oxygen-containing—formed through oxidation or molecular rearrangement (Perveen 2021). In general, while all terpenoids originate from terpenes, not all terpenes undergo the structural modifications that define terpenoids.

Terpenes: The terpenes and terpenoids are structurally (Fig. 10.4) defined by the number of isoprene (C_5H_8) units in their molecules, which determines their classification.

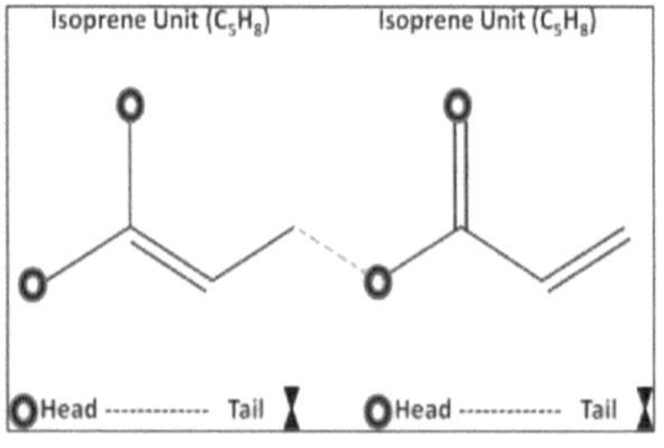

Fig. 10.4. *Basic structure of terpenes.*

Hemiterpenes – 1 isoprene unit (C_5H_8)

- **Monoterpenes** – 2 isoprene units ($C_{10}H_{16}$)
- **Sesquiterpenes** – 3 isoprene units ($C_{15}H_{24}$)

- **Diterpenes** – 4 isoprene units ($C_{20}H_{32}$)
- **Sesterterpenes** – 5 isoprene units ($C_{25}H_{40}$)
- **Triterpenes** – 6 isoprene units ($C_{30}H_{48}$)
- **Carotenoids** – 8 isoprene units ($C_{40}H_{64}$)

Terpenoids: Also known as isoprenoids, terpenoids are a structurally diverse and widely distributed group of plant secondary metabolites. Their diversity stems from the addition of functional groups—such as alcohols, aldehydes, ketones, ethers, esters, phenols, and epoxides—that enhance their chemical reactivity and pharmacological potential. Like terpenes, terpenoids are classified by the number of isoprene (C_5H_8) units in their structure.

Due to their structural variability, terpenoids exhibit a wide range of biological and therapeutic activities. For example, artemisinin, a cyclic sesquiterpenoid ($C_{15}H_{22}O_5$), is effective against *Plasmodium falciparum*, including chloroquine-resistant strains. Paclitaxel (formerly taxol), a tetracyclic diterpenoid ($C_{47}H_{51}NO_{14}$), is a potent anticancer drug used to treat ovarian, breast, and colon cancers. Many essential oils derive their activity from simpler mono- and sesquiterpenoids found in plant sap and tissues. Notable examples include:

- Citral ($C_{10}H_{16}O$), an acyclic monoterpenoid in lemongrass oil.
- Geraniol ($C_{10}H1_{4O}$), found in rose oil and other essential oils.
- Carvone ($C_{10}H_{14}O$), a monocyclic monoterpenoid in mint oils.
- Zingiberene ($C_{15}H_{24}$), a sesquiterpene in ginger oil with anti-inflammatory, antiviral, and antioxidant properties.
- Eudesmol ($C_{15}H_{26}O$), a bicyclic sesquiterpenoid in eucalyptus oil with anticancer and gastrointestinal benefits.

Higher terpenoids (Fig. 10.4 - 10.7) such as diterpenoids ($C_{20}H_{32}$) and triterpenoids ($C_{30}H_{48}$), are commonly found in plant gums and resins, are non-volatile. One key example is phytol ($C_{20}H_{40}O$), an acyclic diterpenoid and integral component of chlorophyll, produced by most photosynthetic organisms. Phytol is used in fragrances and is gaining interest for its pharmaceutical and biotechnological applications.

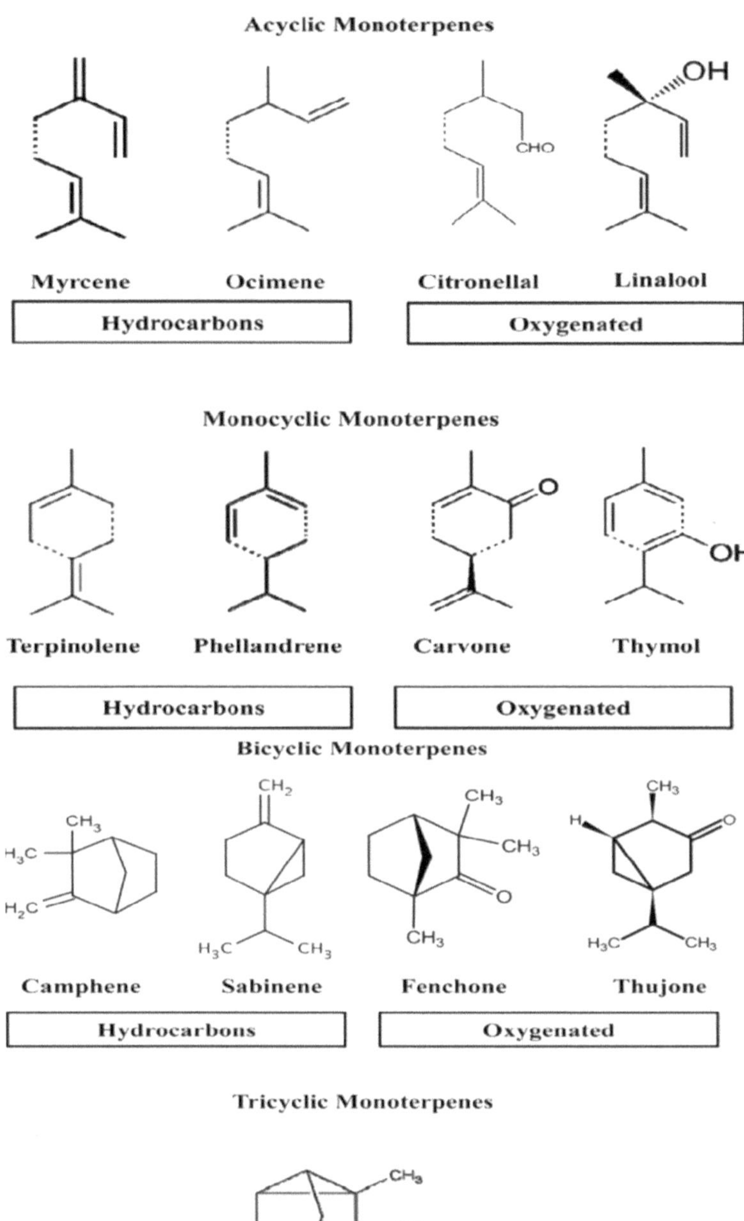

Fig.10.5. *Chemical structure of monoterpenes.*

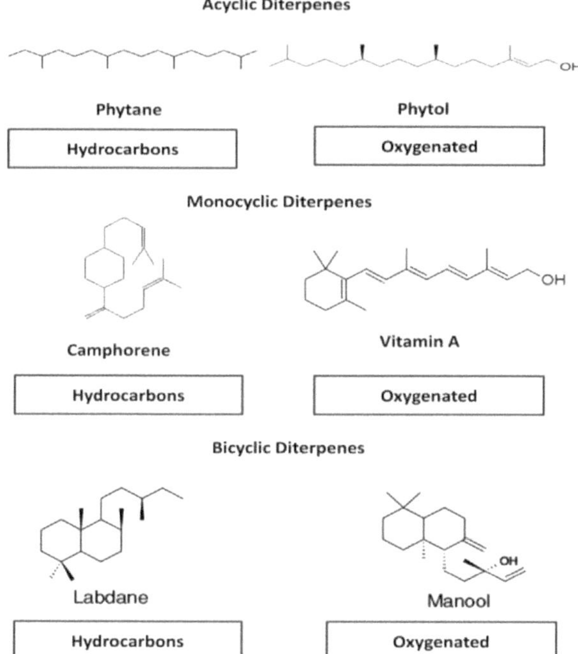

Fig.10.6. *Chemical structure of diterpenes.*

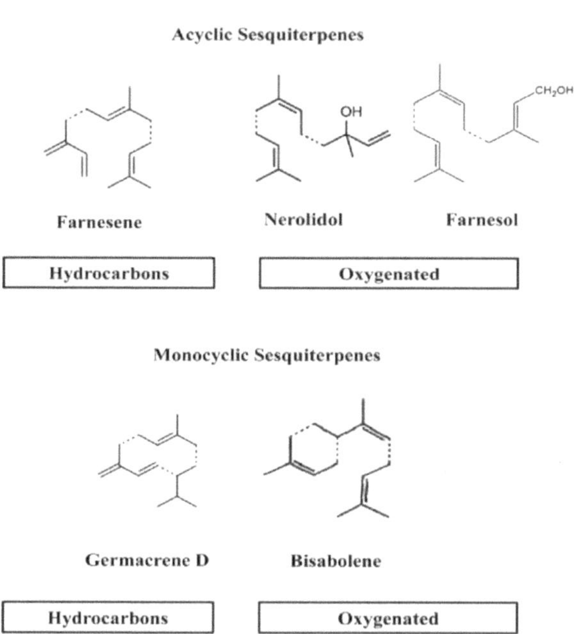

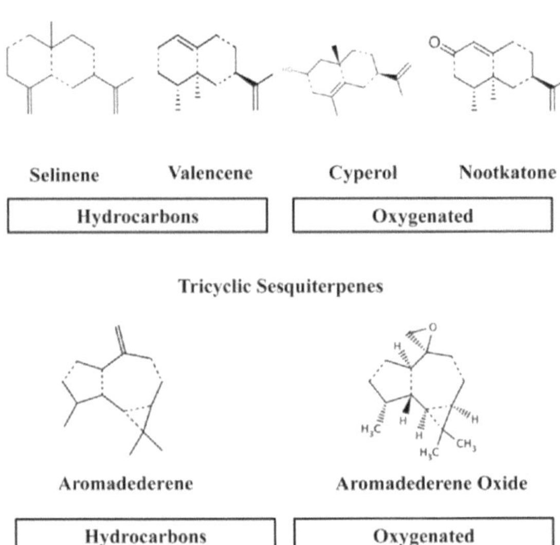

Fig. 10.7. Chemical structure of sesquiterpenoids.

Phenylpropanoids: These are derived from the *n*-propyl benzene structure, typically bearing hydroxyl, methoxy, or methylenedioxy groups on the aromatic ring, and hydroxyl or carboxyl groups on the side chain (Fig. 10.8). Common examples include trans-anethole, methyl chavicol, eugenol, isoeugenol, vanillin, safrole, myristicin, and cinnamaldehyde. These compounds are generally lipophilic, optically active, poorly water-soluble, and strongly aromatic. Notable examples of phenylpropanoids and their pharmacological properties are given here:

- **Chavicol (and methyl chavicol / estragole):** Basil (*Ocimum* spp.), and tarragon are important sources of chavicol, which exhibits antifungal and antibacterial antioxidant, and CNS stimulant effects. Estragole is hepatotoxic and potentially carcinogenic in high doses.
- **Cinnamaldehyde:** Source includes cinnamon bark (*Cinnamomum verum*, and *C. cassia*). Shows antimicrobial, anti-inflammatory, antidiabetic (improves insulin sensitivity), antioxidant and insecticidal activities.
- **Eugenol**: Sourced from clove (*Syzygium aromaticum*), cinnamon, bay leaf, eugenol is analgesic and local anaesthetic, antiseptic and antimicrobial, anti-inflammatory and a potent inhibitor of cancer cell metastasis.
- **Isoeugenol:** Present in clove oil (along with eugenol), nutmeg. Exhibits antioxidant and antimicrobial anti-inflammatory and potential anti-cancer activities.

- **Myristicin:** Source-nutmeg (*Myristica fragrans*). Exhibits antioxidant and antimicrobial properties. Neurotoxic and hallucinogenic at high doses.
- **Vanillin:** Found in vanilla beans (*Vanilla planifolia*). Possesses antioxidant, anti-inflammatory and antimicrobial properties.

While menthol and linalool are often grouped with monoterpenes, they are also sometimes considered under the phenylpropanoid-like class in terms of function and physical properties (volatile, lipophilic, and aromatic), even though structurally they are not classic phenylpropanoids (which are derivatives of C6–C3 phenylpropane skeleton). However, both are extremely important plant-derived compounds with potent pharmacological activities (Chen and Liao 2025).

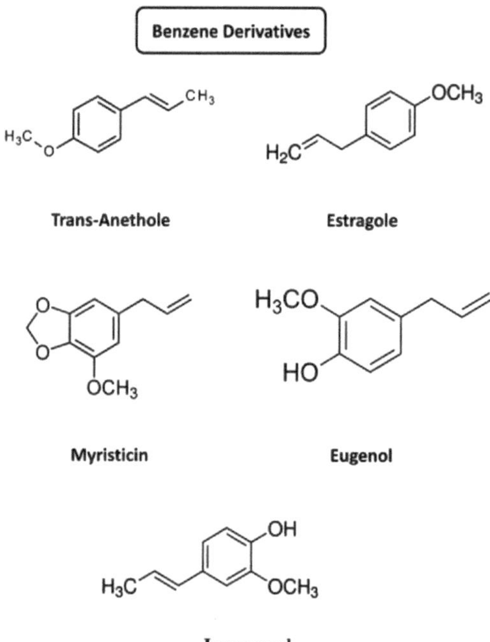

Fig. 10.8. *Chemical structure of phenylpropanoids.*

Menthol D-Limonene Linalool

Tetracyclic triterpene: Tetracyclic triterpenes and phytosteroids share similar structural frameworks. Plant-derived steroids typically consist of three six-membered rings and one five-membered ring. A well-known example of a phytosteroid is β-sitosterol, which exhibits significant pharmacological effects in both humans and animals. For instance, β-sitosterol can act as an oestrogen substitute in the treatment of menopausal symptoms and is also known to inhibit cholesterol biosynthesis (de Jong *et al.* 2003). Cardiac glycosides, such as digitoxin (derived from *Digitalis* species), are another important class of plant steroids. These compounds feature a steroidal structure bound to a sugar moiety and are widely used in the treatment of cardiac insufficiency. Steroidal saponins, which consist of various aglycone skeletons attached to sugar chains via glycosidic linkages, have diverse pharmacological applications. They serve as valuable raw materials for the synthesis of several steroidal drugs, including anti-inflammatory agents, androgens, oestrogens, progestogens, and oral contraceptives (Davis and Morris 1991). Similarly, triterpene saponins exhibit a range of biological activities, including antitussive, expectorant, analgesic, anti-inflammatory, and cytotoxic effects. A traditional example is liquorice, commonly used in the treatment of coughs. However, it is important to note that saponins may cause gastrointestinal irritation. They can also stimulate mucus production in the respiratory tract, which aids in the management of dry cough.

Flavonoids

Flavonoids are a diverse group of phytochemicals found abundantly in fruits, vegetables, leaves, and various plant-based foods. They exhibit a broad range of pharmacological properties and are of significant interest in medicinal chemistry. Flavonoids are widely recognized for their anticancer, antioxidant, anti-inflammatory, and antiviral activities, as well as for their neuroprotective and cardioprotective effects. The biological activity of flavonoids depends on the type of flavonoid, its mechanism of action, and its bioavailability. Structurally, flavonoids consist of a benzopyrone ring system substituted with one or more phenolic or polyphenolic groups. Based on variations in their chemical structure, degree of unsaturation, and oxidation of the central carbon ring, flavonoids are classified into several subgroups: flavones, flavanols, flavanones, flavanonols, flavans, chalcones, anthocyanidins, and iso-flavonoids (Panche *et al.* 2016). Among these, flavonoids and proanthocyanidins (such as flavan-3-ols, sometimes referred to as vitamin P) are particularly known for their antioxidant activity. These compounds help reduce capillary permeability and fragility, inhibit the growth of squamous cell carcinoma, and demonstrate anti-allergic and anti-inflammatory properties—quercetin being a well-studied example.

Flavonoids also exhibit a wide range of other pharmacological activities, including antibacterial, antiviral (e.g., against herpes simplex virus), antiplatelet, anti-allergic, antineoplastic, and even hormonal modulation, showing both oestrogenic and anti-oestrogenic effects. Importantly, flavonoids play a role in preventing age-related neurodegenerative disorders such as Alzheimer's disease, Parkinson's disease, and dementia, primarily through their ability to scavenge reactive oxygen species (ROS) and reactive nitrogen species (RNS), which are implicated in neuronal damage (Fig. 10.9). For instance, tangeretin, a flavonoid found in citrus fruits, has demonstrated neuroprotective antioxidant effects against ROS and RNS, particularly in Parkinson's disease (Nakajima *et al.* 2014). In addition, the antimalarial potential of flavonoids derived from certain dietary plants has been the subject of recent investigation. While preliminary studies suggest promising activity, the specific mechanisms of action and target specificity of flavonoids against *Plasmodium* species remain poorly defined. Interestingly, flavonoids may interact with biological targets distinct from those of conventional antimalarial drugs, offering a novel therapeutic angle. This opens the possibility for flavonoids to serve as lead compounds in the development of new antimalarial agents, particularly effective against drug-resistant strains of malaria (Rudrapal and Chetia 2017). Moreover, flavonoid-based antimalarials are anticipated to provide high therapeutic efficacy with minimal toxicity, making them strong candidates for future drug development. One of the greatest advantages of flavonoids and proanthocyanidins is their low toxicity, which makes them suitable for long-term use. However, not all flavonoid-related compounds are equally safe; for example, podophyllotoxin and its derivatives, despite their notable anticancer effects, are highly toxic and are generally used only in critical or last-resort cases.

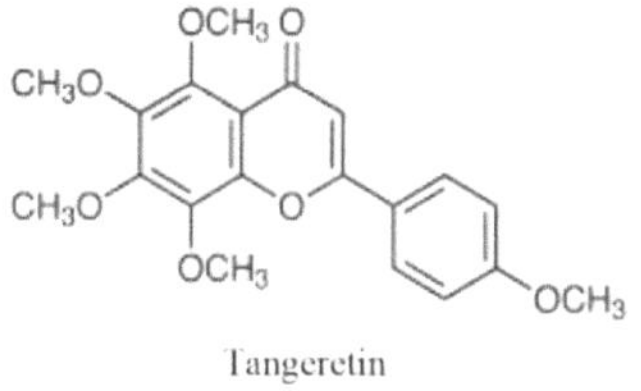

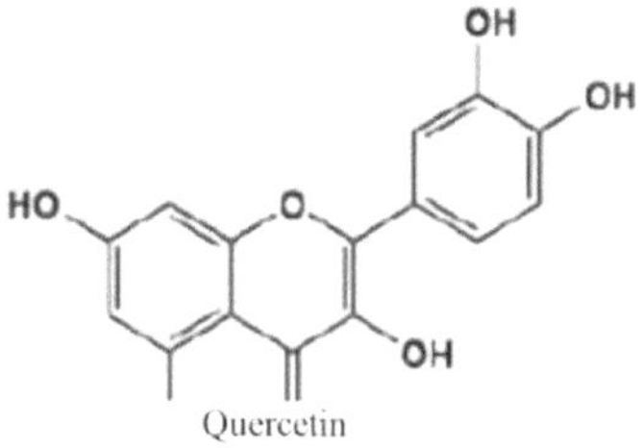

Tangeretin Quercetin

Fig. 10.9. *Chemical structure of flavonoids.*

Tannins

Tannins are water-soluble polyphenolic compounds with variable molecular weights ranging between 500 and 3,000 kDa. These secondary metabolites are known for their ability to form strong complexes with proteins, nucleic acids, cellulose, and minerals. Structurally, tannins are broadly classified into two main categories: hydrolysable tannins and condensed tannins.

- **Hydrolysable tannins** contain a central core of polyhydric alcohol (commonly glucose) esterified with gallic acid (gallotannins). These are less stable and more susceptible to hydrolysis, often posing a greater risk of toxicity.

- **Condensed tannins,** also known as proanthocyanidins, are composed of flavonoid units such as catechins. These are more structurally complex and stable, formed by linking C4 of one catechin molecule to the C8 or C6 position of another.

Tannin and its products have been found to exhibit many important pharmacological and physiological activities including antioxidant, anti-aging, anti-inflammatory, anticancer, mutagenic, antiatherosclerosis, cardioprotective, antiulcerogenic, hepatoprotective, antimicrobial, antiviral, vasodilator, and hypolipidemic activities. (Hossain *et al.* 2021) More often, due to their low bioavailability, tannins are primarily used for topical or gastrointestinal applications in managing conditions like atopic dermatitis, gastroenteritis, and enzyme-related disorders. Condensed tannins can inhibit a range of enzymes such as angiotensin-converting enzyme and aldose reductase and can bind strongly to proteins (Suryanarayana *et al.* 2004). However, tannins can interfere with the absorption of other medications and nutrients by binding to macromolecules and bivalent cations. Therefore, concurrent administration with other drugs or supplements is not advised. In monogastric animals, tannins may cause side effects like nausea and constipation.

Lignins

After cellulose and hemicelluloses, lignin (Fig. 10.10) is considered to be the most abundant polymer present on planet earth. It is a naturally occurring, high-molecular-weight phenolic polymer, characterized by a complex, branched structure with functional groups such as aliphatic and phenolic hydroxyls, carboxylic, carbonyl, and methoxyl groups. Lignin is synthesized through the oxidative polymerization of monolignols—primarily p-coumaryl, coniferyl, and sinapyl alcohols. These monolignols contribute to the incorporation of three major moieties in lignin: p-hydroxyphenyl (H), guaiacyl (G), and syringyl (S). While lignin is a large, insoluble, and biologically inert polymer found in the cell walls of woody plants, lignans are its low-molecular-weight counterparts. Lignans are formed via the dimerization of two monolignol units (C9 each) resulting in C18 compounds. Unlike lignin, lignans are soluble, biodegradable, and biologically active. They function as phytoestrogens and are considered part of the dietary fibre with notable health benefits (Dixon 2004).

Lignin exhibits diverse biological and pharmacological activities, including laxative and cathartic effects, protection against oxidative stress, anti-inflammatory properties, genotoxicity protection, as well as immunomodulatory, antimicrobial, and antitumor effects. Lignins extracted from sugarcane are utilized in the production of Ligmed-A, an antidiarrheal drug designed for veterinary use. While many of lignin's biological and pharmacological activities can be attributed—directly or indirectly—to its free radical scavenging properties, its immunomodulatory, antiviral, and antimicrobial capacities do not stem from this mechanism. Research has shown that lignins possess the ability to modulate both innate and specific immune responses, influencing the expression of various cytokines. Additionally, lignins have been demonstrated to suppress the expression of viral genes critical for infectivity (Martínez *et al.* 2012).

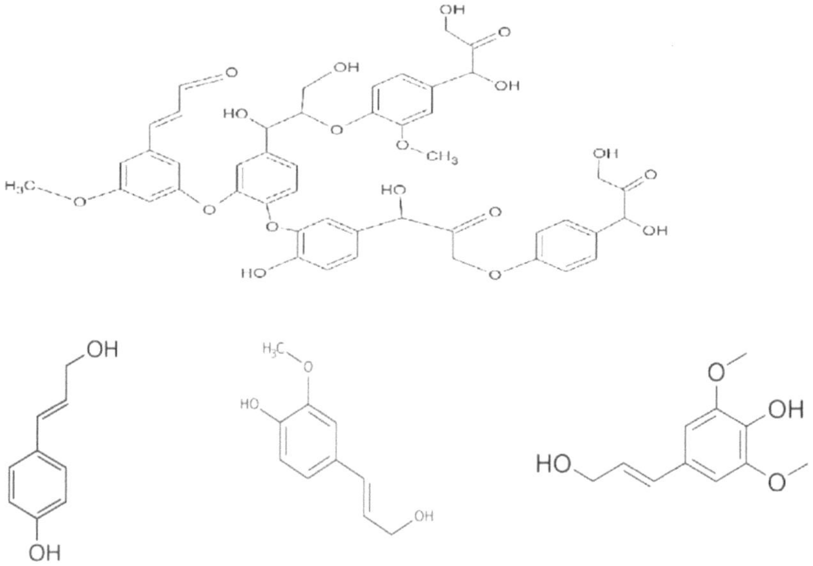

p-coumaryl alcohol Conferyl alcohol Sinapyl alcohol

Fig 10.10. *Chemical structures of lignins.*

Resins

Resins are secondary plant metabolites composed of a mixture of volatile and non-volatile terpenoids, phenolic compounds, and fatty substances. They are typically sticky and harden upon exposure to air. Chemically stable and resistant to acids and bases, resins are amorphous, water-insoluble, but dissolve readily in organic solvents. Based on their chemical constituents, resins are classified into 2 types.

- **Terpenoid resins**: Contain mono-, sesqui-, di-, and triterpenes.
- **Phenolic resins**: Contain compounds such as cinnamic acids, lignans, and flavonoids.

Resins are complex mixtures containing bioactive compounds in either water-soluble glycosidic or lipophilic aglycone forms. These natural products exhibit a broad spectrum of medicinal properties, including anti-inflammatory, antineoplastic, antibacterial, antifungal, and antiprotozoal activities. Traditionally, resins have been used to treat inflammation, pain, wounds, burns, ulcers, and various skin conditions, and they also serve as natural antiseptics and insecticides

(Termentzi *et al.* 2011). India is one of the world's leading producers of natural resins and gums (NRGs), with nearly every state contributing to their production. Except for lac—which is secreted by the lac insect (parasite of host trees like *Schleichera oleosa*, *Butea monosperma*, and *Ziziphus* species)—all other resins are of plant origin (Thombare *et al.* 2023). These bioresources are widely used in food, industry, and both traditional and modern healing systems. Below are some notable plant-derived resins and gum-resins used in traditional Indian medicine.

- ***Canarium strictum* (Black dammar):** The resin is used to treat diarrhoea and dysentery and is collected from trees in evergreen and deciduous forests.
- ***Gardenia resinifera* (*Dikamali* Cambia gum):** Endemic to peninsular India, this plant secretes a gum-like resin with anthelmintic, antiseptic, analgesic, and appetite-stimulating properties. It is applied to treat headaches, bronchitis, vomiting, constipation, intestinal worms, abdominal distension, and piles.
- ***Pinus* spp. (*P. roxburghii*, *P. wallichiana*, and *P. kesiya*):** Resin-derived turpentine oil is widely used in traditional medicine for its antiseptic, expectorant, carminative, and anthelmintic effects. It promotes wound healing and is applied externally in both human and veterinary practices.
- ***Shorea robusta* (Sal tree):** Its resin has cooling, antibacterial, carminative, expectorant, and tonic actions. Traditionally used for treating skin rashes, ulcers, neuralgia, burns, fractures, fever, diarrhoea, and diseases like gonorrhoea, haemorrhoids, and menorrhagia.
- ***Vateria indica* (White dammar):** Native to the Western Ghats, this resin is used in incense and medicinally for chronic bronchitis, asthma, cough, leprosy, and various skin ailments. It is a key ingredient in many antiseptic and anti-inflammatory ointments.
- ***Boswellia serrata* (Indian frankincense or salai):** The gum-resin is renowned for its anti-inflammatory and analgesic properties. It is used in treating rheumatoid arthritis, asthma, inflammatory bowel disease, and skin disorders. Ayurvedic formulations containing boswellic acids are available as capsules and tablets.
- ***Commiphora* spp. (*C. wightii*, *C. mukul*, and *C. gileadensis*):** Known collectively as guggul, this gum-resin is a potent anti-inflammatory, hypolipidemic, antimicrobial, and anticancer agent. It is used for joint pain, chronic bronchitis, thrombosis, acne, and oral health.
- ***Ferula asafoetida (Hing):*** This oleo-gum-resin is widely used in traditional medicine, especially for gastrointestinal disorders in both humans and animals. It is also applied for dental caries, scorpion stings, and in formulations for haemorrhoids.

Phyto-pharmacokinetics and Pharmacodynamics

The therapeutic and adverse effects of any drug depend not only on its medicinal property, but mainly on the amount that reaches systemic circulation and the target site of action. This, in turn, is influenced by the drug's dose, route of administration, and pharmacokinetic properties, including bioavailability, metabolism, distribution, and clearance. Herbal drugs are unique due to their complex composition, which can lead to variability in both pharmacokinetics and pharmacodynamics. Pharmacokinetics refers to how herbal drugs are absorbed, distributed, metabolized, and excreted in the body. Pharmacodynamics focuses on the effects of herbal drugs on the body and their mechanisms of action. Key aspects of pharmacodynamics include receptor interaction, synergistic effects and dose-response relationship.

Pharmacokinetics (PK) of Herbal Medicines

The therapeutic efficacy of herbal medicines is primarily attributed to their bioactive constituents. However, the *in vivo* behaviour of these compounds—how they are absorbed, distributed, metabolized, and excreted—remains complex and not fully understood. Advances in pharmacokinetic research have begun to shed light on these processes, particularly regarding factors such as oral bioavailability, tissue distribution, half-life (t½), maximum plasma concentration (Cmax), and time to reach Cmax (Tmax) (Yang *et al.* 2013, Zhou *et al.* 2018). Pharmacokinetic studies of herbal drugs provide essential insights into identifying secondary metabolites responsible for therapeutic effects, clarifying synergistic interactions in multi-component formulations and mapping the dynamic *in vivo* processes of active constituents (Xu *et al.* 2013). Initially, metabolism via drug-metabolizing enzymes was considered the primary determinant of herbal drug kinetics. Recent research, however, emphasizes the crucial role of drug transporters—membrane proteins that control the absorption, distribution, and excretion of drugs. These transporters, including ATP-binding cassette (ABC) and solute carrier (SLC) families, can function as influx or efflux channels (Hediger *et al.* 2004). Herbal constituents often compete for or modulate these transporters. Understanding these pharmacokinetic mechanisms is crucial for optimizing herbal therapies and ensuring their safe and effective use, especially in combination with conventional drugs.

Pharmacodynamics (PD) of Herbal Medicines

Herbal drugs exist primarily in two forms: pure phytochemicals and crude extracts containing multiple compounds. The pharmacodynamics of pure phytochemicals is relatively well understood and often comparable to that of synthetic drugs. However, systematic, evidence-based pharmacodynamic studies on crude herbal drugs remain limited in veterinary practice. In recent years, interest in the pharmacodynamics of crude herbal formulations has grown, particularly with the availability of supporting pharmacokinetic (PK) data. Pharmacodynamics describes the quantitative relationship between the concentration of an active compound in tissues and its pharmacological effects. It includes dose-response relationships and factors influencing variability in response, such as age, sex, health status, and concurrent medications. The development of receptor theory significantly advanced our understanding of the molecular basis of drug action and its relationship with dose (Maehle 2004). Drugs exert effects either through extracellular or intracellular mechanisms, often targeting membrane proteins, receptors, or ion channels. Some may also act on intracellular structures. Phytochemicals typically modulate enzymatic or transcriptional activity, influencing protein synthesis. While some drugs act specifically through receptor-mediated mechanisms, others have broader, nonspecific effects depending on their distribution. Drug actions include:

- *Agonists:* Mimic physiological ligands by inducing conformational changes in receptors.
- *Antagonists*: Bind without activating receptors, blocking ligand access.

Receptors vary in location and function

- *Membrane-bound receptors*: Coupled with ion channels (e.g., neurotransmitters) or G-proteins (e.g., biogenic amines).
- *Enzyme-linked receptors*: Regulate intracellular pathways (e.g., protein kinases).
- *Intracellular receptors*: Influence gene transcription via DNA binding.

The chain of events from drug-receptor interaction is termed *signal transduction*, leading to the tissue's response. Pharmacodynamics is closely linked to toxico-dynamics. Adverse reactions are more likely with compounds that have a narrow therapeutic margin, highlighting the importance of careful pharmacodynamic monitoring, especially for herbal phyto-molecules.

Pharmacokinetics-Pharmacodynamics Model

Early pharmacokinetic (PK) studies of herbal products primarily focused on investigating the absorption, distribution, metabolism, and excretion (ADME) of active constituents from individual herbs or herb–herb combinations, along with their interaction mechanisms. However, the pharmacological actions of these herbal preparations—especially polyherbal formulations—remained ambiguous and often controversial due to the complex nature of their active components.

The development of pharmacokinetic-pharmacodynamic (PK-PD) models has significantly enhanced our understanding of how multiple herbal constituents interact and exert therapeutic effects. These models help elucidate the compatibility and synergistic mechanisms among various components, offering more comprehensive and clinically relevant insights. By integrating PK and PD data, the PK-PD model allows for a more precise evaluation of herb efficacy, herb–herb interactions, and dose-response relationships. For example, co-administration of ginsenoside Rb1 with schisandrin delayed the elimination of ginsenoside Rg1 and showed a synergistic effect in enhancing nitric oxide (NO) release (Zhan *et al.* 2014). It is also reported that certain herbal components modulate the PK and PD of clozapine, thereby reducing clozapine-induced constipation (Hou *et al.* 2015).

Herb-Herb Interaction

Herbal medicines are typically prescribed as formulas, comprising combinations of two or more herbs. The compatibility of multiple herbs in such formulations is rooted in traditional knowledge and long-term clinical experience. These combinations are designed to achieve synergistic therapeutic effects while minimizing or eliminating potential side effects. The chemical basis for such compatibility lies in the interactions among the numerous phytoconstituents, which can influence the absorption, distribution, metabolism, and excretion (ADME) of individual active compounds. Understanding the complex mechanisms underlying formula compatibility is therefore essential. For instance, a pharmacokinetic study involving a compound prescription containing *Panax ginseng*, *Ophiopogon japonicus*, and *Schisandra chinensis* demonstrated that lignans from *Schisandra chinensis* significantly enhanced the exposure of several ginsenosides both *in vitro* and *in vivo*. In another study evaluating a polyherbal formulation used for cardiovascular diseases, the herb-herb interactions were shown to increase the bioavailability of eugenol by reducing its elimination rate. Additionally, the AUC_0–τ, AUC_0–∞, and Cmax of bicyclic monoterpenes (isoborneol, borneol, and camphor) were significantly decreased. These findings suggest that improved exposure to beneficial bioactive components and reduced absorption of toxic constituents may help to explain the rationale behind certain herbal combinations. *Triphala* serves as another example of formula compatibility. The dynamic pharmacokinetic (PK) profile—encompassing absorption, clearance, and bioavailability—of active compounds is influenced by the presence of various classes of constituents, such as alkaloids, isoflavonoids, and lignans. However, not all herb-herb combinations result in interactions. Some studies report no significant influence on the PK profile between herbs in certain polyherbal formulations (Li *et al.* 2017). Therefore, herb-herb interactions cannot be generalized, and specific guidelines should be developed for each individual polyherbal preparation.

In general, clinically validated herbal formulations generally avoid incompatible herbs. Interestingly, pharmacokinetic and pharmacodynamic studies have revealed that certain active compounds in one herb can inhibit the absorption of toxic constituents from another, thereby reducing the bioavailability of harmful components. This provides a scientific basis for the safety and rationality of such combinations. Synergism is a critical feature of herbal formulations, and herb-herb interactions are often used to enhance therapeutic effects. For example, the root bark of *Morus alba* contains α-glucosidase inhibitors that help regulate postprandial blood glucose levels. When co-administered with the root of *Pueraria lobata* (rich in flavonoids), the absorption rate of *Pueraria* flavonoids is significantly reduced. This results in an increased concentration and extended presence of α-glucosidase inhibitors in the small intestine, thereby amplifying the hypoglycaemic effect of *Morus alba* compared to its use alone (Xiao *et al.* 2014).

Herb- Conventional Drug interaction

In recent decades, herbal medicines have been increasingly integrated into modern medical treatments. However, unlike conventional drugs that contain a single active compound, herbal medicines are made up of complex mixtures of phytochemicals. These components can interact with conventional drugs at both the pharmacokinetic and pharmacodynamic levels, raising important concerns about safety and efficacy. At the pharmacokinetic level, herbal compounds can alter how conventional drugs are absorbed, distributed, metabolized, and excreted (ADME). These changes may increase or decrease the bioavailability and systemic exposure of a drug, potentially reducing its effectiveness or increasing its toxicity. Such interactions can be beneficial—by enhancing therapeutic outcomes—or harmful—by causing unexpected side effects. Therefore, pharmacokinetic studies are essential to understand these effects and to create safe guidelines for using herbal and modern medicines together (Li *et al.* 2022).

The interaction between herbs and drugs is often linked to the specific mechanisms of action of the plant constituents involved. Sometimes, herbal and conventional drugs may work synergistically or complementarily, improving overall treatment effects. But in other cases, herb-drug interactions (HDIs) can lead to reduced drug levels, diminished efficacy, or increased risk of adverse effects, including serious toxicities or, in rare situations, fatalities. Many reviews have explored HDIs, particularly focusing on how herbs affect the pharmacokinetics or pharmacodynamics of drugs (Tachjian *et al.* 2010, Shi and Klotz 2012, Soleymani *et al.* 2017). However, the reverse interaction—how modern drugs affect the pharmacokinetics of herbal medicines—remains poorly studied. Both herbal and synthetic drugs are metabolized by the same enzymes and transporters, especially the cytochrome P450 (CYP450) enzyme family and P-glycoprotein (P-gp) transporters. Because they share these metabolic pathways, co-administration can lead to mutual interference, affecting the breakdown and activity of both types of drugs. The CYP450 family is responsible for metabolizing over 90% of modern drugs (Soleymani *et al.* 2017). If any herbal or synthetic drug induces or inhibits CYP450 enzymes, it can alter the metabolism of co-administered drugs. For example, when notoginsenoside R1—one of major bioactive compounds extracted from *Panax notoginseng* (Burk.) dry roots and rhizomes—was given along with caffeine, the Cmax and AUC_0–∞ of caffeine increased, while its plasma clearance (CL) decreased. However, notoginsenoside R1 had no significant effect on other drugs like tolbutamide, metoprolol, or disponide (Yin *et al.* 2016). Drug transporters such as P-gp also play a key role in drug metabolism by affecting the bioavailability of oral medications (Shi and Klotz 2012). Some medicinal plant extracts, like those from *Schisandra chinensis*, can regulate P-gp and other enzymes. If *Schisandra* is co-administered with drugs that are substrates of these same enzymes or transporters, it may result in unfavourable interactions (He *et al.* 2015).

Herbal Bioenhancer and Nutraceutical

Bioenhancers and nutraceuticals are gaining increasing recognition in both human and animal healthcare for their ability to complement conventional therapies and support overall well-being. Bioenhancers are agents that increase the bioavailability and efficacy of drugs and nutrients without having significant pharmacological activity of their own at the given dose. The bioenhancers are generally classified based on two major criteria: mechanism of action and source of origin (Fig 10.11).

Herbal Bioenhancers

Herbal bioenhancers (also known as biopotentiators) are plant-derived phytomolecules that increase the bioavailability and efficacy of drugs or nutrients without exerting significant pharmacological effects of their own at the administered dose. These compounds enhance the absorption, metabolism, and utilization of co-administered substances, often allowing for lower dosages and fewer side effects. The bioenhancers have important therapeutic and economic benefits. These include making expensive drugs more affordable, reducing drug toxicity by lowering the required dose, decreasing the risk of drug resistance due to subtherapeutic exposure, and enhancing the nutritional status by improving the absorption of essential micronutrients and vitamins. Some examples of herbal bioenhancers include (Yurdakok-Dikmen *et al.* 2018):

- **Piperine** (black pepper – *Piper nigrum*): Enhances the bioavailability of curcumin, beta-carotene, and drugs like rifampicin, amoxicillin, ciprofloxacin, and theophylline.
- **Quercetin** (apples and grapes): Improves the absorption of resveratrol and other antioxidants.
- **Gingerols** (ginger – *Zingiber officinale*): Boosts the efficacy of anti-inflammatory and digestive medications.
- **Glycyrrhizin** (liquorice – *Glycyrrhiza glabra*): Facilitates intestinal absorption of antimicrobials (rifampicin, and tetracycline), and vitamins B_1 and B_{12}.

- **Allicin** (garlic – *Allium sativum)*: Enhances the effect of antifungal agents like Amphotericin B.

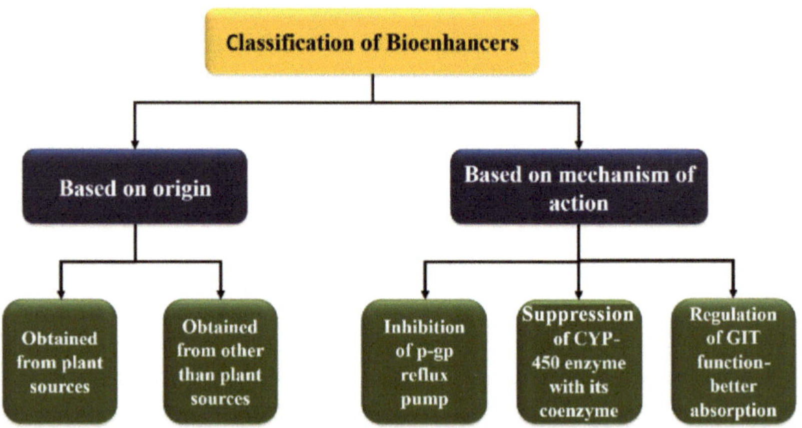

Fig. 10.11. *Classification of bioenhancers (Source: Adapted from Thorat et al. 2023; open access).*

Concept of Drug Bioavailability Enhancement

The concept of bioavailability enhancement is defined as using a small amount of a bioenhancer (Fig. 10.11) to significantly increase the availability, efficacy, or absorption of a drug or nutrient (Kesarwani and Gupta, 2013). The roots of this concept can be traced to the traditional Ayurvedic system of medicine. In Ayurveda, the term Yogvahi refers to substances that enhance the efficacy or bioavailability of other therapeutic agents. Piperine, derived from black pepper, is the first scientifically validated Yogvahi. A classic Ayurvedic preparation, Trikatu (a mixture of black pepper, long pepper, and ginger), has long been used to enhance digestion and the effectiveness of medicinal compounds. Scientific studies have confirmed its role: for instance, pretreatment with Trikatu in goats increased the bioavailability and antimicrobial action of pefloxacin by 20% (Dama *et al.* 2008). As early as 1929, Bose in his book *Pharmacographia Indica*, noted the enhanced anti-asthmatic effects of a formula containing *Vasaka (Adhatoda vasica)* when administered with pepper (Bose 1929). In 1979, scientists at the Indian Institute of Integrative Medicine, Jammu validated piperine as the world's first bioavailability enhancer (Jhanwar and Gupta, 2014).

Mechanisms of Action of Bioenhancers

The primary goal of using herbal bioenhancers is to improve the bioavailability of drugs and nutrients. Bioenhancers can act through multiple mechanisms, often working at the level of absorption, metabolism, distribution, and excretion. These mechanisms may vary depending on the bioenhancer and the co-administered compound. Typically, herbal bioenhancers improve bioavailability by inhibiting drug efflux transporters (like P-glycoprotein), modulating drug-metabolizing enzymes (like cytochrome P450), and enhancing membrane permeability (Chivte *et al.* 2017). Based on published scientific reports, following mechanism are proposed for bioenhancer action (Fig. 10.12).

Modulation of gastric functions: Herbal bioenhancers can delay gastric emptying and prolong gastrointestinal transit time by regulating the secretion of gastric acid and enzymes like pepsin. This prolongs the window for drug absorption.

Enhancement of membrane permeability: Poor membrane permeability is a limiting factor in the absorption of many drugs. Certain herbal agents like aloe vera, ginger, and *Carum carvi* (*Kala jeera*) improve membrane permeability, thereby enhancing drug absorption and bioavailability. Increased blood flow to the gastrointestinal tract also supports enhanced absorption.

Inhibition of P-glycoprotein (P-gp) efflux: Drug transporters, including P-gp and other efflux pumps, act at various physiological barriers (intestine, liver, and kidney) reducing absorption and systemic availability of drugs. Herbal bioenhancers may inhibit or modulate these transporters to facilitate greater drug absorption and tissue penetration. Bioenhancers like piperine, curcumin, and naringin inhibit P-gp activity, allowing more drug to be absorbed and retained in circulation.

Inhibition of cytochrome P450 (CYP450) enzymes: The CYP450 enzyme family, especially CYP3A4, CYP1A1, CYP1B1, and CYP2E1, is responsible for the first-pass metabolism and clearance of many drugs. Inhibition of these enzymes by bioenhancers such as piperine and curcumin reduces first-pass elimination, increasing systemic drug availability.

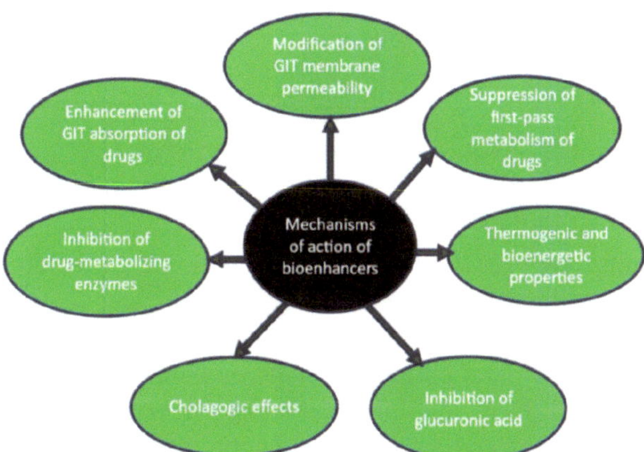

Fig. 10.12. *Mechanisms of action of bioenhancers (Source: Adapted from Pathak 2020, as cited in Thorat et al. 2023; open access).*

Inhibition of drug metabolizing enzymes: Besides CYP enzymes, other drug-metabolizing enzymes—such as UDP-glucuronosyltransferases (UGTs)—can inactivate drugs through conjugation. Inhibition of these enzymes can prevent premature drug elimination and enhance efficacy.

Reduction of renal clearance: Some bioenhancers may reduce renal excretion by inhibiting glomerular filtration, passive tubular reabsorption, or active tubular secretion. This can prolong the drug's half-life and enhance its therapeutic effects.

In summary, herbal bioenhancers work through a variety of complementary mechanisms that significantly improve drug delivery and therapeutic efficacy. They are particularly effective in overcoming key challenges such as low oral bioavailability, rapid metabolic degradation, poor membrane permeability, and efflux transporter-mediated drug elimination. Widely studied bioenhancers like piperine, curcumin, and ginger-derived compounds have demonstrated substantial benefits in enhancing drug and nutrient absorption. Recent advancements have led to their incorporation into innovative drug delivery systems—including solid lipid nanoparticles, nanostructured lipid carriers, nanoemulsions, microemulsions, liposomes, transferosomes, ethosomes, methosomes, and sphingosomes—to further boost their effectiveness, particularly in terms of bioavailability. By leveraging their natural ability to enhance absorption and reduce drug clearance, herbal bioenhancers play a crucial role in nanotechnology-based drug delivery systems (Rajput *et al.* 2022). Their integration into modern pharmaceutical and nutraceutical formulations represents a rapidly advancing field with significant therapeutic potential in both human and veterinary medicine.

Nutraceuticals

A nutraceutical is a food or food-derived product that provides health benefits beyond basic nutrition. These products may prevent or treat disease and support general health. They are typically rich in bioactive compounds such as antioxidants, vitamins, minerals, and phytochemicals. Here are some examples of herbal nutraceuticals:

- **Curcumin** (Turmeric): Anti-inflammatory and antioxidant.
- **Resveratrol** (Red Grapes): Offers cardioprotective and anti-aging benefits.

Methods for Phytomedicinal Investigations

Medicinal plants have been used since time immemorial for their health benefits—in the form of medicines, cosmetics, nutraceuticals, and more—using various preparations such as whole plants, extracts, or pure phytochemicals. To ensure optimal activity, safety, and efficacy, specific methods are employed at different stages: selection of medicinal plants, timing of collection, processing, and storage (*see* Chapters 7 and 12). The extraction, separation, identification, and chemical characterization of active compounds are conducted with the objective of developing improved herbal remedies.

The chemical complexity of herbs and their extracts, which contain a broad range of phytochemicals, underscores the need for appropriate analytical methods for their identification and standardization. Choosing the right analytical technique—from among microscopy, spectrometry, spectroscopy, chromatography, and others—depends largely on the defined analytical objectives. This complexity arises from the rich chemical diversity inherent in plants, a key consideration in pharmaceutical research and drug development. In recent years, significant advances have been made in the processing and scientific study of medicinal plants, including the adoption of modern extraction technologies and improved analytical techniques. Analytical tools such as chromatography, microscopy, and spectrometry have been continuously refined to support herbal research (Azwanida 2015). However, selecting the most appropriate method requires careful consideration of the study goals. While important analytical techniques are documented in international pharmacopoeias, modern approaches not included in existing monographs have also been developed. Many plant species still lack official monographs, and numerous traditional medicine systems rely on oral transmission rather than written documentation. In such cases, it is essential to develop dynamic monograph systems guided by standardized methodologies.

Selection of Medicinal Plants

Phytomedicinal investigations are not confined to laboratory procedures—they also involve field data on cultivation, harvesting techniques, and accurate botanical identification. Even within a single species, there can be substantial chemical variability, often influenced by biotic and abiotic factors (See Chapters 7 and 12). Any plant submitted for phytochemical analysis should be accompanied by detailed information on harvesting conditions—climate, location, humidity (hygrometry), season of collection, and phenological stage (e.g., beginning or end of flowering). Other important details include the time between harvest and analysis, storage conditions, and the application of Good Agricultural and Collection Practices (GACP) and Good Laboratory/Manufacturing Practices (GLP/GMP), as recommended by the WHO (2003).

Identification and Authentication

Robust identification systems and reliable detection methods are crucial for ensuring the purity and quality of medicinal plant materials by minimizing the risk of adulteration. Several taxonomic, chemical, proteomic, and genomic markers are used to authenticate and identify medicinal plant species and their active components. These methods—outlined in Chapter 7—include morphological identification (macro- and microscopic), molecular marker analysis (e.g., proteins and DNA), and profiling of secondary metabolites using advanced tools such as High-Performance Thin-Layer Chromatography (HPTLC), High-Performance Liquid Chromatography (HPLC), and Gas Chromatography (GC). These markers are taxon-specific (family, species, or variety) and are essential for the authentication of medicinal plants prior to further processing (Sahoo *et al.* 2010).

Preparation of Samples for Analysis

Once a medicinal plant is collected, identified, and authenticated, proper processing and extraction are critical to preserving the quality and quantity of active constituents. Preventing the structural and functional degradation of phytochemicals requires a solid understanding of chemistry and botany. The efficacy of herbal and nutraceutical formulations is closely tied to the methods used for processing and extraction (Jacobsohn and Jacobsohn 1976). For instance, controlling oxidation during processing can help to retain non-hydrolysable tannins, saponins, and flavonoids (Tanaka *et al.* 2002). Herbal samples should be uniformly powdered to ensure even distribution of biomarkers, which is essential for consistent analytical results. Sample preparation techniques have evolved considerably, taking into account factors such as solubility, expected concentrations, solvent properties, solvent-to-sample ratios, extraction time, temperature, pressure, and method (e.g., static or dynamic maceration, ultrasonic extraction, percolation, and Soxhlet). Solvent selection should be guided by physicochemical properties such as polarity, selectivity, toxicity, and inertness. The principle of "like dissolves like" is especially important in the extraction of phytochemicals (Kim and Verpoorte 2010).

Identification of Key Group of Phytochemicals

Preliminary identification of phytochemicals through simple in-tube reactions remains common in laboratories with limited access to sophisticated instruments. These reactions detect the presence of alkaloids, terpenoids, flavonoids, tannins, anthocyanins, quinones, cyanogenic glycosides, and other secondary metabolites by forming coloured, precipitated, or fluorescent derivatives (Harborne 1998). Though less sensitive and selective than modern techniques and somewhat subjective in interpretation, these tests provide quick, preliminary identification of key chemical classes. However, they are increasingly being replaced by advanced profiling techniques for comprehensive phytochemical analysis.

Activity Guided Separation and Purifications

The initial separation of phytochemicals typically begins with sequential extraction using solvents of increasing polarity. To preserve thermolabile compounds and prevent structural degradation, cold extraction (around 37°C) is preferred. However, hot extraction methods such as Soxhlet extraction remain suitable for more stable compounds. Each extract should be screened for biological (pharmacological) activity to identify the most promising candidates for further development. Various experimental models are available for this purpose, including *in vitro* systems (e.g., cell cultures, and isolated tissue preparations) and *in vivo* studies. In recent years, tools such as molecular docking and *in silico* analysis have gained prominence for predicting biological activity. Nevertheless, *in vivo* animal studies remain the gold standard for evaluating pharmacological efficacy and safety.

Chromatographic Techniques

Chromatographic methods are essential for fractionating complex mixtures such as crude extracts, yielding characteristic compound profiles. In thin-layer chromatography (TLC), compounds are separated on planar surfaces like silica, cellulose, polyamide, or chemically modified plates. Detection can occur either directly or after reaction with specific reagents—by visible coloration, fluorescence or quenching under UV light, or through mass spectrometry (Boland *et al.* 2007). Advanced techniques such as high-performance liquid chromatography (HPLC), gas chromatography (GC), and capillary electrophoresis (CE) are increasingly employed in phytochemical analysis for both profiling and quantitative determination. High-performance thin-layer chromatography (HPTLC), using silica plates with a higher number of theoretical plates, offers significantly greater resolution and reproducibility. Instrumental application, migration, spraying, and detection make HPTLC a reference method in modern pharmacopoeias for herbal drug identification.

The selection of analytical technique depends on the nature of the extract (Fig. 10.13-10.14). These fully automated methods offer high selectivity and sensitivity, often coupled with specialized detectors capable of identifying even trace-level contaminants. Integration of these separation techniques with mass spectrometry not only enables compound identification but also supports multidimensional profiling.

Chemical Profiling

Chemical (or chemo-) profiling of bioactive extracts can be achieved using mass spectrometry to detect the full spectrum of phytochemicals present. Metabolic fingerprinting, based on nuclear magnetic resonance (NMR) spectroscopy and Fourier-transform infrared (FT-IR) spectroscopy, combined with multivariate analysis, is now widely used in phytochemistry research for its high sensitivity. A combination of FT-IR and ^{1}H NMR enables chemometric analysis, while attenuated total reflectance FT-IR (ATR-FTIR) allows for highly accurate and precise cluster analysis (Valentino *et al.* 2020).

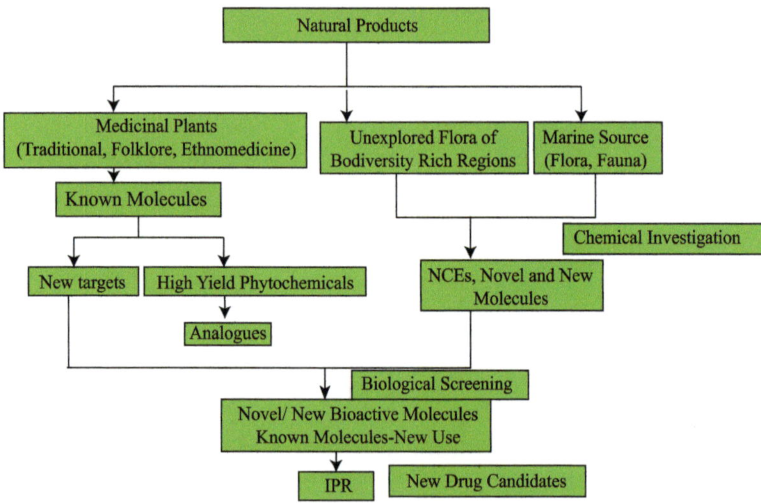

Fig. 10.13. *Key steps in natural products research and drug development (Flowchart courtesy: of Dr Suresh Babu, CSIR-IICT).*

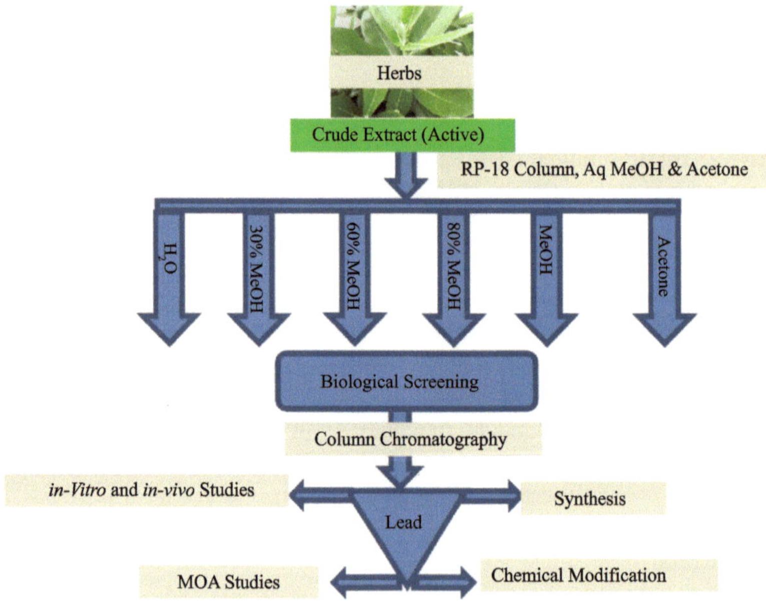

Fig. 10.14. *Bioassay guided approaches to identification and characterization of phytomolecules (Flowchart courtesy of Dr. Suresh Babu, CSIR-IICT).*

Elemental Analysis

Atomic absorption and atomic emission spectroscopy are commonly used for the qualitative and quantitative analysis of mineral elements in herbal drugs. Inductively coupled plasma atomic emission spectroscopy (ICP-AES) is particularly advantageous, offering high sensitivity and the ability to simultaneously analyse more than 30 elements (Swami *et al.* 2009). The detection of toxic and trace elements is routinely conducted in medicinal plant research as part of quality control and contaminant screening.

Herbal Research and Development in India

India's formal engagement with the scientific study of medicinal plants began during the British colonial period. With advancements in phytochemistry and pharmacognosy, researchers globally began to validate the efficacy of herbal remedies through modern analytical methods. Supplementary drug monographs were published, complementing traditional Ayurvedic texts. After India's independence, the country experienced a revival in herbal research and development. Various academic institutions, government bodies, and private enterprises became actively involved in studying medicinal plants and their therapeutic applications. Prominent Government Bodies notably including Indian Council of Agricultural Research (ICAR), Department of Science and Technology (DST), Department of Biotechnology (DBT), Indian Council of Medical Research (ICMR), Central Council for Research in Ayurvedic Sciences (CCRAS), Biotechnology Research Innovation Council (BRIC) and University Grants Commission (UGC) promoted scientific Research and Development programmes related to medicinal herbs and botanicals.

Planning for Herbal Medicine R&D (From the First to the Twelfth Five-Year Plans)

Herbal research became a formal component of India's national development agenda starting with the First Five-Year Plan (1951–1956), which emphasized systematic investigation of medicinal plants. Core activities included identification, nomenclature, ecological mapping, and creation of herb museums. Collaborative research was encouraged, notably between the Central Institute for Ayurveda Research and the Central Drug Research Institute (CDRI), Lucknow (Anonymous 1951). Subsequent Five-Year Plans emphasized different priorities.

- **Second Plan (1956–1961):** Strengthened public sector R&D and set up Central Herbal
- **Third Plan (1961–1966):** Established facilities for drug standardization and manufacturing.
- **Seventh and Eighth Plans:** Boosted clinical research in traditional systems of medicine and emphasized propagation and standardization of medicinal plants.

- **Ninth Plan Onward:** Initiated schemes for large-scale cultivation of medicinal herbs. From 2014, significant progress was made with the development of the Ayurvedic Pharmacopoeia under the Ministry of AYUSH. The creation of NITI Aayog has also played a critical role in coordinating indigenous healthcare planning and policy-making.

Key Indian Institutes in Herbal Research

Some key institutes actively associated with herbal research and development and educational programmes focusing on areas such as ethnobotany, phytochemistry, pharmacognosy, pharmacology, clinical trials, toxicology, and formulation sciences are listed alphabetically here.

Banaras Hindu University (BHU), Varanasi: BHU has a strong emphasis on Ayurvedic and herbal medicine research. It integrates traditional knowledge with modern scientific methods to explore medicinal plants and their applications.

Bose Institute, Kolkata (Basu Vigyan Mandir): Engages in interdisciplinary research, including plant biology and phytochemistry, to explore the medicinal properties of plants.

Botanical Survey of India, Kolkata: Engages in the exploration, documentation, and conservation of India's plant resources, including medicinal plants.

Central Drug Research Institute (CSIR-CDRI), Lucknow: Focuses on drug discovery and development, including herbal medicines. It conducts research on phytochemicals and their therapeutic applications.

Central Institute for Medicinal and Aromatic Plants (CSIR-CIMAP), Lucknow: Specializes in the cultivation, processing, and value addition of medicinal and aromatic plants. CIMAP also develops high-yielding plant varieties and conducts research on herbal formulations for therapeutic use.

Directorate of Medicinal and Aromatic Plants Research (ICAR-DMAPR), Anand, Gujarat: Works on the cultivation, conservation, and value addition of medicinal and aromatic plants. It also provides training to farmers and entrepreneurs.

Gujarat Ayurveda University, Jamnagar: A pioneer in Ayurvedic education and research, it conducts studies on Ayurvedic formulations, medicinal plants, and their pharmacological properties.

Indian Institute of History of Medicine and Medical Research, New Delhi: Focuses on documenting and validating traditional medicinal practices, including herbal remedies.

Indian Institute of Integrative Medicine (IIIM, CSIR) Jammu: Specializes in herbal drug development.

Indian Veterinary Research Institute (ICAR-IVRI) Izatnagar: Premier institute of veterinary science in India, having state of art facilities for research and development in the various disciplines of Veterinary and Animal Sciences including herbal research and development programmes.

Institute of Bioresources & Sustainable Development (IBSD, BRIC) Imphal : Studies bioresources for sustainable development, including phytomedicine.

Institute of Himalayan Bioresource Technology (IHBT, CSIR) Palampur: Works on plant-based drug formulations and high-altitude medicinal plants.

Inter-University Medicinal Plant Laboratory for Analysis, Nurture, and Therapeutics, Rajkot: Focuses on the analysis and therapeutic applications of medicinal plants, contributing to drug discovery and development.

National Botanical Research Institute (CSIR-NBRI) Lucknow: Focuses on the phytochemical properties of plants for potential therapeutic applications.

National Institute of Pharmaceutical Education and Research (NIPER), Mohali: Conducts research on natural products, including the discovery and development of herbal drugs. It focuses on standardization, quality control, and clinical validation of herbal medicines.

National Medicinal Plants Board (NMPB), New Delhi: Facilitates conservation and scientific cultivation of medicinal plants.

National Institute of Plant Genome Research (NIPGR, BRIC): Conducts genome studies on plants to explore medicinal properties and improve crop quality.

Pharmaceutical Education and Research Development (PERD), Ahmedabad: Engages in research on herbal drugs, including their standardization, pharmacognosy, and phytochemistry. It also collaborates with industries for drug development.

Conclusion

The field of herbal veterinary medicine is witnessing a global resurgence, driven by continuous discoveries of novel secondary metabolites and their diverse pharmacological activities. Across the world—including in India, which has a rich tradition of medicinal plant use—there is growing interest in harnessing herbal compounds for therapeutic purposes. The integration of traditional knowledge with cutting-edge phytopharmacological research has created a fertile ground for innovative, sustainable, and safer healthcare solutions for animals.

Medicinal plants serve as natural reservoirs of bioactive molecules. While primary metabolites support plant growth and development, secondary metabolites—produced at specific developmental stages—play vital roles in plant defence. These compounds exhibit a broad spectrum of biological activities, such as modulating cellular and organ functions and combating pathogens including viruses, bacteria, fungi, and parasites. Their pharmacological potential forms the basis for many modern therapeutics, and their classification includes major chemical groups like alkaloids, terpenes, polyketides, and phenylpropanoids.

Herbal medicines have long contributed to disease prevention and health management. Recent clinical studies have validated the safety and efficacy of several plant-based remedies. Notably, the combination of synthetic drugs with herbal formulations and bioenhancers has emerged as a promising strategy for managing complex, multifactorial diseases. Such combinations are increasingly used across species—including livestock, pets, and birds—to improve therapeutic outcomes. However, ensuring the safety and efficacy of these combination therapies requires in-depth research into their mechanisms of action and potential interactions. A thorough understanding of how herbal compounds interact with conventional drugs, particularly at the pharmacokinetic and pharmacodynamic levels, is essential. Herbal formulations—often composed of multiple herbs containing hundreds of diverse constituents—may affect drug-metabolizing enzymes and transporters in complex ways. These interactions can significantly alter drug absorption, distribution, metabolism, and excretion, with implications for both therapeutic efficacy and safety. Pharmacokinetic research plays a crucial role in identifying bioavailable compounds responsible for therapeutic effects. Understanding their behaviour in the body helps evaluate both intended actions and unintended adverse effects. Further, the varying stability and shelf life of herbal components, as well as their potential to influence those of synthetic drugs, are important considerations in formulation and clinical use.

While herbal medicines are generally perceived as safe due to their natural origin, numerous studies have reported adverse interactions with conventional drugs, some with serious or even fatal consequences. Simultaneous use may enhance or diminish the effects of conventional medications or introduce new side effects. Many phytochemicals act as multi-target modulators of transporter proteins (e.g., ABC and SLC families), influencing drug excretion and metabolism in complex ways. Recent studies highlight that many phytonutrients act as prodrugs or bioenhancers, increasing the bioavailability and potency of other drugs while modifying their therapeutic and toxicity profiles. Advances in herbal R&D—including the use of nanocarriers, derivatization techniques, and precision extraction—have enhanced the delivery, stability, and efficacy of plant-based therapies.

In conclusion, modern phytopharmacology is enriching the traditional foundations of herbal veterinary medicine. Continued research into pharmacokinetics, compound interactions, and delivery systems is vital to ensuring safe, effective, and evidence-based integration of herbal remedies in veterinary healthcare. This approach holds particular promise in addressing challenges such as antimicrobial resistance and the need for eco-friendly, sustainable therapeutics in animal health.

References

Anonymous. 1951. *Planning Commission Report on 1st Five Year Plan*. Government of India. New Delhi, India.

Azwanida N. 2015. A review on the extraction methods use in medicinal plants, principle, strength and limitation. *Medicinal and Aromatic Plants* **4**(3): 196. doi:10.4172/2167-0412.1000196.

Barclay TG, Day CM, Petrovsky N and Garg S. 2019. Review of polysaccharide particle based functional drug delivery. *Carbohydrate Polymer* **221**: 94-112.

Bokov DO, Sharipova RI, Potanina OG, Nikulin AV, Nasser RA, Samylina IA and Bessonov VV. 2020. Polysaccharides of crude herbal drugs as a group of biologically active compounds in the field of modern pharmacognosy: physicochemical properties, classification, pharmacopoeial analysis. *Systematic Review Pharmacy* **11**(6): 206 -12.

Boland Y, Attout A, Marchand-Brynaert J and Garcia Y. 2007. Selective thin-layer chromatography of 4-R-1,2,4-triazoles. *Journal Chromatography A* **1141**(1): 145-49.

Bose KG. 1929. *Pharmacopoeia India*. 729 p. Bose Laboratories, Calcutta, India.

Chen Lin and Liao Pan. 2025. Current insights into plant volatile organic compound biosynthesis. *Current Opinion in Plant Biology* **85:** 102708. https://doi.org/10.1016/j.pbi.2025.102708.

Cheng JT, Guo C, Cui WJ, Zhang Q, Wang SH, Zhao QH, Liu DW, Zhang J, Chen S, Chen C and Liu Y. 2020. Isolation of two rare N-glycosides from *Ginkgo biloba* and their anti-inflammatory activities. *Scientific Reports* **10**(1): 5994 | https://doi.org/10.1038/s41598-020-62884-1.

Chivte VK, Tiwari SV and Nikalge APG. 2017. Bioenhancers: A brief review, *Advanced Journal of Pharmacy and Life Science Research* **5** (2): 1-18.

Dama MS, Varshneya C, Dardi MS and Katoch VC. 2008. Effect of *trikatu* pretreatment on the pharmacokinetics of pefloxacin administered orally in mountain Gaddi goats. *Journal of Veterinary Science* **9** (1): 25-29.

Davis EA and Morris DJ. 1991. Medicinal use of licorice through the millennia: the good and plenty of it. *Molecular Cell Endocrinology* **78** (1-2): 1-6.

de Jong A, Plat J and Mensink RP. 2003. Metabolic effects of plant sterols and stanols (Review). *Journal of Nutritional Biochemistry* **14**(7): 362-69.

Diaz-Muñoz G, Miranda IL, Sartori SK, De Rezende DC and Diaz MA. 2018. Anthraquinones: an overview. *Studies in Natural Products Chemistry* **58**: 313-38. doi.org/10.1016/B978-0-444-64056-7.00011-8.

Dixon RA. 2004. Phytoestrogens. *Annual Review of Plant Biology* **55** (1): 225-61.

Harborne JB. 1998. *Phytochemical Methods a Guide to Modern Techniques of Plant Analysis*. 3rd edn. 302 p. Chapman and Hall, Thomas Science, London, UK.

He JL, Zhou ZW and Yin JJ. 2015. *Schisandra chinensis* regulates drug metabolizing enzymes and drug transporters via activation of Nrf2-mediated signalling pathway. *Drug Design, Development and Therapy* **9**: 127-46.

Hediger MA, Romero MF, Peng J-B, Rolfs A, Takanaga H and Bruford EA.2004.The ABCs of solute carriers: physiological, pathological and therapeutic implications of human membrane transport proteins. *Pflugers Archiv – European Journal of Physiology* **447**: 465–468. https://doi.org/10.1007/s00424-003-1192-y.

Hood WB Jr, Dans AL, Guyatt GH, Jaeschke R and McWurray JJ. 2004. Digitalis for the treatment of congestive heart failure in patients in sinus rhythm: A systematic review and meta analysis. *Journal Cardiology* **10**: 155- 64.

Hossain MT, Furhatun-Noor A, Matin A, Tabassum F, Ar Rashid H. 2021. A review study on the pharmacological effects and mechanism of action of tannins. *European Journal of Pharmaceutical and Medical Research* **8** (8): 5-10.

Hou ML, Lin CH, Lin LC and Tsai TH. 2015. The drug-drug effects of rhein on the pharmacokinetics and pharmacodynamics of clozapine in rat brain extracellular fluid by *in vivo* microdialysis. *The Journal of Pharmacology and Experimental Therapeutics* **355**(1): 125-34.

Jacobsohn MK and Jacobsohn GM. 1976. Annual variation in the sterol content of *Digitalis purpurea* L. seedlings. *Plant Physiology* **58**:541-43.

Jhanwar B, and Gupta S. 2014. Biopotentiation using herbs: Novel technique for poor bioavailable drugs. *International Journal of Pharm Tech Research* **6**(2): 443-54.

Kesarwani K and Gupta R. 2013. Bioavailability enhancers of herbal origin: An overview. *Asian Pacific Journal of Tropical Biomedicine* **3** (4): 253-66.

Kim HK and Verpoorte R. 2010. Sample preparation for plant metabolomics. *Phytochemical Analysis* **21**(1): 4-13.

Li C, Jia WW, Yang JL, Cheng C and Olaleye OE. 2022. Multi-compound and drug-combination pharmacokinetic research on Chinese herbal medicines. *Acta Pharmacologica Sinica* **43:** (12): 3080-95.

Li X, Du F and Jia W. 2017. Simultaneous determination of eight Danshen polyphenols in rat plasma and its application to a comparative pharmacokinetic study of Dan Hong injection and Danshen injection. *Journal of Separation Science* **40:** 1470–81.

Maehle A-H .2004. Receptive substance: John Newport Langley (1852-1925) and his path to a receptor theory of drug action. *Medical History* **48**: 153-74.

Martínez V, Mitjans M and Vinardell MP. 2012. Pharmacological applications of lignins and lignins related compounds: An overview. *Current Organic Chemistry* **16**(16): 1863-70.

Nakajima A, Ohizumi Y and Yamada K. 2014. Anti-dementia activity of nobiletin, a citrus flavonoid: A review of animal studies. *Clinical Psychopharmacology and Neuroscience* **12**(2): 75-82.

Nguyen TD and Dang TTT. 2021. Cytochrome P450 enzymes as key drivers of alkaloid chemical diversification in plants. *Frontier Plant Science* **12**: 682181. doi: 10.3389/fpls.2021.682181.

Panche A, Diwan A and Chandra S. 2016. Flavonoids: An overview. *Journal of Nutritional Science* **5**: e47 doi:10.1017/jns.2016.41.

Pathak N. 2020. Role of bioenhancers in drug discovery. *International Journal Pharmacy and Life Sciences* **11**(7):51.

Perveen S. 2021. Introductory chapter: Terpenes and terpenoids. In: *Terpenes and Terpenoids - Recent Advances.* pp. 1-13. (Eds) Perveen S and Al-Taweel M. Biochemistry IntechOpen. doi: 10.5772/intechopen.98261**.**

Rajput A, Mandlik S, Dawre S, Mandlik D, Pingale P and Butani S.2022. Herbal bioenhancers in nanoparticulate drug delivery system. *Drug Delivery Technology* **21:** 45-86.

Rudrapal M and Chetia D. 2017. Plant flavonoids as potential source of future antimalarial leads. *Systematic Reviews in Pharmacy* **8**(1):13-18.

Sahoo N, Manchikanti P and Dey S. 2010. Herbal drugs: Standards and regulation. *Fitoterapia* **81**(6): 462-71.

Shi S and Klotz,U. 2012. Drug interactions with herbal medicines. *Clinical Pharmacokinetics* **51**: 77-104.

Soleymani S, Bahramsoltani R, Rahimi R and Abdollahi M. 2017. Clinical risks of St John's Wort (*Hypericum perforatum*) co-administration. *Expert Opinion on Drug Metabolism & Toxicology* **13**: 1047-62.

Suryanarayana P, Kumar PA and Saraswat M 2004. Inhibition of aldose reductase by tannoid principles of *Emblica officinalis* implication for the prevention of sugar cataract. *Molecular Vision* **10**: 148-54.

Swami K, Judd CD and Orsini J. 2009. Trace metals analysis of legal and counterfeit cigarette tobacco samples using inductively coupled plasma mass spectrometry and cold vapor atomic absorption spectrometry *Spectroscopy Letters* **42**(8): 479-90.

Tachjian A, Maria V and Jahangir A. 2010. Use of herbal products and potential interactions in patients with cardiovascular diseases. *Journal of the American College of Cardiology* **55** (6): 515-25.

Tanaka T, Mine C, and Kouno I. 2002. Structures of two new oxidation products of green tea polyphenols generated by model tea fermentation. *Tetrahedron* **58** (43): 8851-56.

Termentzi A, Fokialakis N, Leandros and Skaltsounis A. 2011. Natural resins and bioactive natural products thereof as potential antimicrobial agents. *Current Pharmaceutical Design* **17**(13): 1267-90.

Thombare N, Kumari U, Sakare P, Chowdhury A, Lohot VD and Prasad N. 2023. Indigenous technical knowledge on the medicinal uses of natural resins and gums in India. *Indian Journal of Traditional Knowledge* **22**(2): 340-49.

Thorat SS, Gujar KN and Karle CK. 2023. Bioenhancer from mother nature: an overview. *Future Journal of Pharmaceutical Sciences* **9**: 20 https://doi.org/10.1186/s43094-023-00470-8.

Tomar GS and Kumar N. 2020. *Khuddakachatushpada Adhyaya.* In: *Charak Samhita New Edition.* 1st edn. pp.11. (Eds) Dixit U, Deole YS and Basisht G. CSRTSDC ebook, Jamnagar, India. Available at: https://www.charakasamhitauptodate.com/index.php?title=Khuddakachatushpada_Adhyaya&oldid=44475a&oldid=44475.

Valentino G, Graziani V, D'Abrosca B, Pacifico S, Fiorentino A and Scognamiglio M. 2020. NMR-based plant metabolomics in nutraceutical research: an overview. *Molecules* **25** (6): 1444. doi:10.3390/molecules25061444.

WHO. 2003. *WHO Guidelines on Good Agricultural and Collection Practices (GACP) for Medicinal Plants*. World Health Organization, Geneva, Switzerland.

Xiao BX, Wang Q, FanLQ, Kong LT, Gu SR and Chang Q. 2014. Pharmacokinetic mechanism of enhancement by Radix Pueraria flavonoids on the hyperglycemic effects of *Cortex mori* extract in rats. *Journal of Ethnopharmacology* **151**: 846-51.

Xu H, Gan J, Liu X, Wu R, Jin Y, Li M and Yuan B. 2013. Gender-dependent pharmacokinetics of lignans in rats after single and multiple oral administration of Schisandra chinensis extract. *Journal of Ethnopharmacology* **147**: 224–31.

Yang B, Wang X, Liu W, Zhang Q, Chen K, Ma Y, Wang C and Wang Z. 2013. Gender-related pharmacokinetics and absolute bioavailability of diosbulbin B in rats determined by ultra-performance liquid chromatography-tandem mass spectrometry. *Journal of Ethnopharmacology* **149**: 810–15.

Yin S, Cheng Y, Li T, Dong M, Zhao H and Liu G .2016. Effects of notoginsenoside R1 on CYP1A2, CYP2C11, CYP2D1, and CYP3A1/2 activities in rats by cocktail probe drugs. *Pharmaceutical Biology* **54** (2): 231-36.

Yurdakok-Dikmen B, Turgut Y and Filazi A.2018. Herbal bioenhancers in veterinary phytomedicine. *Frontiers in Veterinary Science* **5**: 249. doi: 10.3389/fvets.2018.00249.

Zhan S, Guo W, Shao Q, Fan X, LiZ and Cheng Y. 2014. A pharmacokinetic and pharmacodynamic study of drug–drug interaction between ginsenoside Rg1, ginsenoside Rb1 and schizandrin after intravenous administration to rats. *Journal of Ethnopharmacology* **152**(2): 333-39.

Zhou L, Li J and Yan C. 2018. Simultaneous determination of three flavonoids and one coumarin by LC–MS/MS: Application to a comparative pharmacokinetic study in normal and arthritic rats after oral administration of *Daphne genkwa* extract. *Biomedical Chromatography* **32:** e4233, 2-s2.0-85045952671.

11

Veterinary Herbal Drug Development: Regulatory Aspects

S. Dey

Apakrītāḥ sahīyasīrvīrudho yā abhistutāh, Trāya-ntāmasmingrāme gāmaśvam puruṣaṁ paśum.

Let herbs and plants, purchased, raised in power and reinforced, properly assessed, adjudged and defined, protect the people, cows and other animals in the village (Atharva Veda 8.7.11; translation by Sharma 2013)

1. Introduction
2. Traditional Herbal Drug Development
3. Pharmacognosy: Herbal Drug Development and Standardization
4. Safety and Quality Control for Herbal Preparations
5. Herbal Drug Standards: Regulatory Framework, Guidelines and Key Agencies in India
6. Quality Control and Standardization in Herbal Drug Production
7. WHO Good Manufacturing Practice (GMP) for Herbal Medicines
8. Global Herbal Drug Regulations
9. Herbal Pharmacopoeias
10. Intellectual Property Right on Traditional Knowledge and Herbal Medicine
11. Conclusion

Introduction

Herbal medicine is one of the oldest and most widely practiced systems of healthcare, with its roots extending across cultures and civilizations for thousands of years. Archaeological evidence of herbal remedy use, dating back approximately 60,000 years, was discovered in 1960 at a Neanderthal burial site in a cave in northern Iraq. Perhaps early humans may have identified the healing properties of plants through trial and error—learning to distinguish beneficial herbs from those that were toxic or ineffective, and discovering how preparation or combinations could enhance their efficacy (Kunle *et al.* 2012). In contrast, some Western traditions interpret the origins of this knowledge more mystically, proposing that the therapeutic properties of herbs were revealed through a spiritual connection between healer and plant, wherein the medicinal virtues of herbs were intuitively revealed (Wynn and Fougère 2007).

Today, herbal remedies remain integral to primary healthcare for nearly 85% of the global population, who continue to rely on traditional knowledge systems for medicinal plant use. Parallel to this human tradition, the use of herbs for animal care also has ancient roots. As humans domesticated animals and developed animal husbandry practices, they naturally extended their plant-based therapies to veterinary care. Consequently, veterinary botanical medicine—arguably the earliest form of veterinary practice—has historically evolved alongside human medicine. Herbal medicines are utilized both in their traditional crude forms—such as teas, poultices, powders, and tinctures—and as refined products containing purified active compounds identified through rigorous chemical and biological studies (Balunas and Kinghorn 2005). As interest in phytotherapeutics expands into the veterinary domain, the need for standardized regulatory frameworks to ensure quality, safety, and efficacy has become increasingly apparent. Addressing these regulatory aspects is essential to bridge traditional knowledge with scientific validation, and to facilitate the integration of herbal veterinary products into mainstream veterinary healthcare.

Box 11.1. Herbal Terminology

In different types of herbal medicines, the same material may be classified in various ways depending on the context. The terminology adopted by the World Health Organization (WHO) for its Guidelines on Good Manufacturing Practices (2007) has been derived from various documents and widely used guidelines among WHO Member States. The following terms are presented for the benefit of readers.

Herbal Medicines: *Include herbs, herbal materials, herbal preparations and finished herbal products.*

Herbs: *Include crude materials which could be derived from lichen, algae, fungi or higher plants, such as leaves, flowers, fruit, fruiting bodies, seeds, stems, wood, bark, roots, rhizomes or other parts, which may be entire, fragmented or powdered.*

Herbal Materials: *In addition to herbs, herbal materials include fresh juices, gums, fixed oils, essential oils, resins and dry powders of herbs.*

Herbal Preparations: *These are products derived from herbal materials through processes like- extraction, purification, or heating. They include comminuted herbs, extracts, tinctures, oils, and preparations made using alcohol, honey, or other substances.*

Medicinal Plants: *Plants (wild or cultivated) used for medicinal purposes.*

Constituents with Known Therapeutic Activity: *These are substances or groups of substances which are chemically defined and known to contribute to the therapeutic activity of a herbal material or of a preparation. (Source: WHO 2007).*

Traditional Herbal Drug Development

Herbal medicine, or herbalism, refers to the use of plants and plant-based products for their therapeutic or medicinal value. In ancient societies, tribal communities systematically acquired and preserved knowledge about medicinal plants, eventually establishing well-defined herbal pharmacopoeias (Fig. 11.1). Over time, this body of knowledge was passed down through generations, forming the basis for many traditional systems of medicine practiced across the world. In fact, well into the twentieth century, much of the pharmacopeia of modern scientific medicine had its origins in the herbal traditions of indigenous peoples. Traditional herbal remedies typically consisted of whole plants or unrefined plant parts—most commonly leaves, roots, bark, seeds, and flowers. These were administered in various forms: eaten, swallowed, drunk as infusions or decoctions, inhaled, or applied topically to the skin (Kunle *et al.* 2012). While traditional knowledge significantly advanced the field of medicine, issues related to the quality and safety of herbal preparations were often overlooked. Herbal products could be purchased without a prescription, and consumers might not have been aware of the risks posed by poorly prepared or contaminated remedies. Thus, ensuring a well-defined and consistent composition is one of the most critical prerequisites for producing safe and effective herbal drugs.

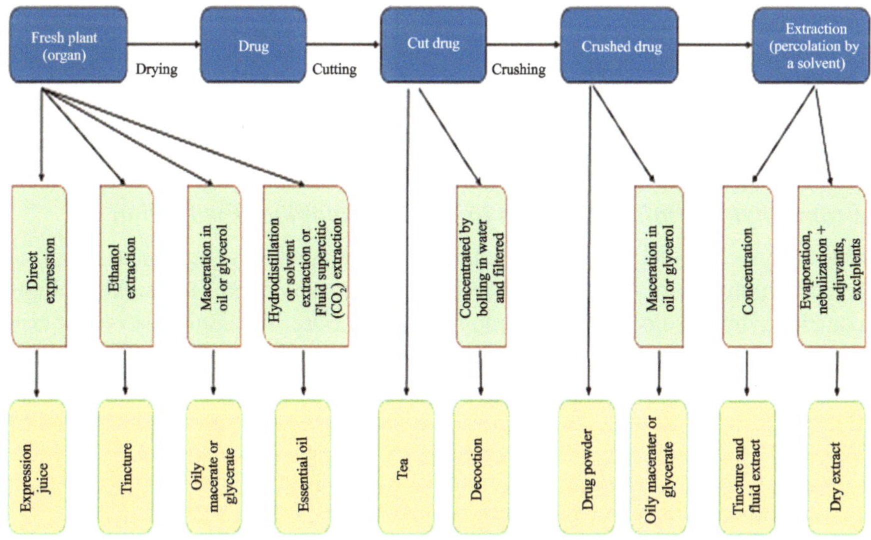

Fig. 11.1. *Traditional herbal pharmacy (Adapted from Balkrishna et al. 2024).*

Pharmacognosy: Herbal Drug Development and Standardization

Herbs are often regarded as biosynthetic laboratories, capable of producing a wide range of chemical compounds. These natural products can be used directly for the treatment of human and animal diseases or serve as valuable starting points (referred to as leads) for drug discovery and development programs. It is estimated that approximately 14–28% of plant species are used for medicinal purposes, and nearly 74% of these possess pharmacologically active constituents (Singh *et al.* 2020). The development and standardization of herbal drugs primarily fall under the domain of pharmacognosy—a specialized field that intersects with phytochemistry, toxicology, and various analytical disciplines. Pharmacognosy focuses on the identification, authentication, and standardization of natural drugs, with the overarching goal of evaluating raw material quality and ensuring that final herbal products meet established safety and efficacy standards (Kumar 2007).

Standardization of Herbal Drugs

Standardization is a critical process in herbal drug development, involving the establishment and verification of specific quality parameters to ensure consistency, purity, and therapeutic efficacy. This process includes:

- Botanical identification
- Microscopic examination
- Chemical fingerprinting
- Quantitative estimation of active constituents

The standardization process begins with the accurate identification and validation of raw plant materials by experts such as botanists, ethnobotanists, or ethno pharmacologists. Following this, plant materials are subjected to qualitative and quantitative analysis by phytochemist or natural product chemist, who prepare extracts for biological evaluation using pharmacologically relevant assays.

From Phytochemical Analysis to Pharmacological Evaluation

Once phytochemical profiling is complete, the extracts undergo bioassay-guided fractionation to isolate and identify bioactive compounds. Molecular biologists contribute by developing and employing appropriate screening assays that target physiologically relevant molecular mechanisms, helping to elucidate structure–activity relationships with therapeutic potential (Bruhn and Bohlin 1997). Pharmacological assessment follows, beginning with *in vitro* studies using cell cultures, isolated tissues, or biochemical systems under controlled laboratory conditions. These studies assess cellular or molecular-level responses to the herbal extract or isolated phytochemicals. This is followed by *in vivo* studies in animal models to evaluate physiological effects, safety profiles, and toxicological characteristics. Since *in vitro* efficacy does not always translate into *in vivo* outcomes (and vice versa), both types of studies are essential to comprehensively understand the therapeutic potential or limitations of the test compound.

Lead Optimization and Drug Development

Herbal extracts or isolated phytomolecules showing promising biological activity advance to the lead optimization stage. Here, chemical modifications are made to enhance efficacy, selectivity, bioavailability, and safety. The goal is to develop a compound that not only retains therapeutic activity but also meets stringent criteria for safe and effective use as a drug. This entire process—from plant collection to lead optimization—is highly systematic and evidence-based, forming the backbone of plant-derived drug development (Guantai and Chibale 2011). Each stage plays a vital role in transforming traditional herbal remedies into scientifically validated and clinically useful drugs.

Conventional Drug Development Process

The conventional drug discovery process involves following key stages:

- **Discovery and Development**: Target identification, high-throughput screening, lead identification, and optimization.
- **Preclinical Research**: Includes toxicological studies and dosage regimen evaluations in laboratory and animal models.
- **Clinical Trials**: Conducted in four phases to evaluate safety, efficacy, and side effects in humans.
- **Regulatory Review**: Assessment and approval of clinically validated drug candidates by regulatory agencies.
- **Post-Marketing Surveillance**: Continuous monitoring for safety and effectiveness in the general population.

Traditional Knowledge Based Herbal Drug Development and Reverse Pharmacology

Conventional drug development often spans more than a decade and entails substantial costs. By contrast, herbal drug development rooted in traditional knowledge can be more time-efficient and cost-effective. This is due to the prior empirical validation of herbal formulations through centuries of use, which serves as a foundation for scientific exploration and reverse pharmacology approaches. However, rigorous quality control and modern pharmacological validation remain essential to ensure their safety, efficacy, and consistency.

Reverse Pharmacology

Reverse pharmacology (RP) is an innovative, trans-disciplinary approach that integrates traditional clinical experiences and empirical knowledge—particularly from systems like Ayurveda—into modern drug discovery and development pipelines. RP emerged as a response to the limitations of conventional drug discovery, which often involves lengthy and expensive processes. The concept was pioneered in India, where traditional systems like Ayurveda provided a wealth of empirical knowledge about natural remedies. Visionaries like Sir Ram Nath Chopra and Gananath Sen played a pivotal role in laying the foundation for this discipline, particularly in the context of Ayurvedic drugs. The primary objective of RP is to comprehensively elucidate mechanisms of action across various biological levels—molecular, cellular, organ-specific, and systemic. Additionally, it seeks to optimize the safety, efficacy, and acceptability of bioactive compounds derived from natural sources (Vaidya 2014). A salient feature of RP is its synergy between traditional medicinal systems (e.g., ethnomedicine, ethnoveterinary medicine, Ayurveda, and folk practices) and cutting-edge scientific methodologies. By leveraging centuries-old empirical knowledge alongside modern techniques such as chemical profiling, systems biology, molecular docking, and pharmacogenomics, RP has transformed natural products into safer, more effective therapeutic leads (Patwardhan and Mashelkar 2009). This reverse paradigm not only accelerates the identification of promising drug candidates but also provides deeper insights into their actions at cellular and molecular levels. Moreover, the RP model significantly shortens drug development timelines (Fig 11.2), reduces costs, and enhances translational efficiency compared to traditional drug discovery approaches (Arulsamy *et al.* 2016).

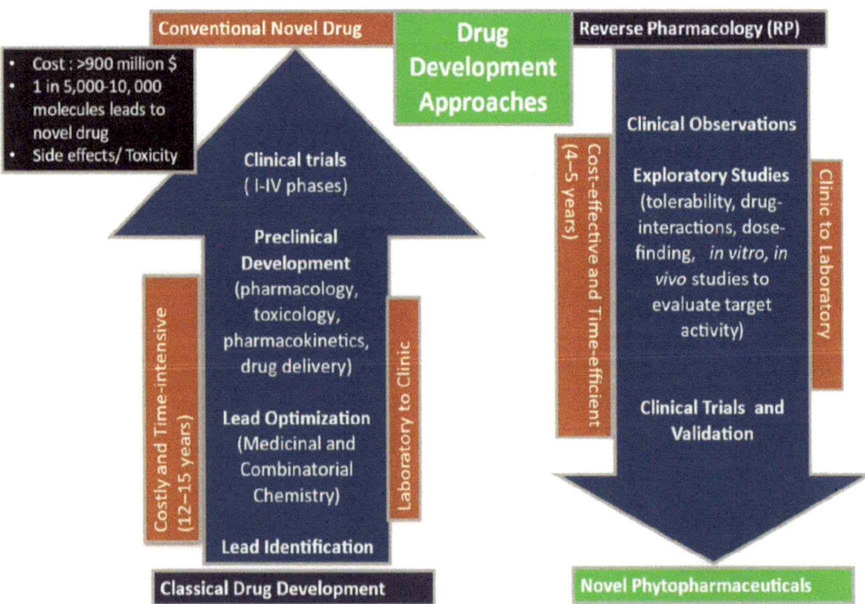

Fig.11.2. *Key phases of classical and reverse pharmacology (Graphic representation courtesy of Dr Ashok Kumar, ICAR-CIRG).*

Key Phases of Reverse Pharmacology: Unlike conventional methods, which begin with target identification and high-throughput screening, RP adopts a reverse pathway. It starts with clinically observed therapeutic efficacy, progressing backward to validate pharmacological activity and explore underlying mechanisms through rigorous scientific investigations such as *in vitro* and *in vivo* studies. This approach ultimately leads to the development of novel drug candidates. The methodology of reverse pharmacology involves three critical phases:

1. **Experiential Phase**: Documentation of clinical observations from traditional medicine and folk remedies.
2. **Exploratory Phase**: Evaluation of drug interactions, dose ranges, and para-clinical studies to assess target activities.
3. **Validation Phase**: Confirmation of safety and efficacy for potential drug candidates through experimental and clinical studies.

In summary, reverse pharmacology has revolutionized the study of natural products, enabling traditional remedies to evolve into evidence-based, clinically validated pharmaceuticals without compromising on safety or efficacy. This methodology serves as a vital bridge between age-old healing systems and modern biomedical science, offering a sustainable, cost-effective, and patient-centric pathway to innovative drug discovery.

Safety and Quality Control for Herbal Preparations

Safety and quality control for herbal preparations are crucial to ensure their efficacy, consistency, and safety for consumers (See Chapter 7 and 12). Some key aspects include:

- **Standardization:** Herbal preparations must be standardized to ensure consistent levels of active ingredients. This involves identifying and quantifying bioactive compounds.
- **Contamination Prevention:** Measures are taken to prevent contamination by microbes, heavy metals, pesticides, and other harmful substances during cultivation, processing, and storage.
- **Quality Assurance:** Rigorous testing is conducted to verify the identity, purity, and potency of herbal products. This includes organoleptic, chemical, and microbiological evaluations.
- **Regulatory Compliance:** Adherence to guidelines set by organizations like the WHO ensures that herbal preparations meet international safety and quality standards.
- **Toxicological Studies:** These studies assess the safety of herbal preparations by identifying potential adverse effects and establishing safe dosage levels.

Herbal Drug Standards: Regulatory Framework, Guidelines and Key Agencies in India

India has a well-established regulatory framework for herbal drugs, especially under the AYUSH systems (Ayurveda, Yoga, Unani, Siddha, and Homoeopathy). The aim is to ensure the safety, efficacy, and quality of herbal drugs. Key Regulatory Bodies include Ministry of AYUSH, Drugs and Cosmetics Act, 1940 (Chapter IVA) – Governs manufacture, sale, and licensing of Ayurvedic, Siddha, and Unani drugs, Central Drugs Standard Control Organization (CDSCO), Pharmacopoeia Commission for Indian Medicine and Homoeopathy (PCIM&H). The key legislations and regulatory agencies related to quality standards, trade policies, and the conservation of herbal medicines and medicinal plants in India are briefly outlined below:

Ministry of AYUSH

The Ministry of AYUSH (MoA) is the nodal agency responsible for the development, regulation, and promotion of traditional systems of medicine in India. The acronym AYUSH stands for Ayurveda, Yoga and Naturopathy, Unani, Siddha, and Homoeopathy—the major traditional medical systems practiced in the country. The Ministry was officially established on 9th November 2014. Prior to this, the Department of Indian Systems of Medicine and Homoeopathy (ISM&H)—formed in 1995—oversaw the development of these systems. In November 2003, this Department was renamed as the Department of AYUSH to provide focused attention to education and research in traditional medicine. The Ministry of AYUSH is the primary authority for formulating policies and regulatory frameworks for traditional medicines in India. It is responsible for implementing the Drugs and Cosmetics Act, 1940 (Chapter IVA) in relation to Ayurvedic, Siddha, and Unani drugs. Manufacturing or marketing herbal medicines in India requires a valid license from the Ministry. Furthermore, it is mandatory to display the manufacturing and expiry dates on product labels to ensure transparency and consumer safety. All clinical trials involving herbal products must follow standardized protocols and receive appropriate approvals to ensure efficacy and safety. The Ministry ensures adherence to Good Manufacturing Practices (GMP) across all licensed units. It also supports the standardization of raw materials and finished formulations through the development of official pharmacopoeias, including: *Ayurvedic Pharmacopoeia of India (API), Unani Pharmacopoeia of India (UPI), Siddha Pharmacopoeia of India (SPI)*. Additionally, it has developed Good Clinical Practice (GCP) Guidelines to provide new direction for clinical trials on Ayurveda, Siddha and Unani (ASU) treatments and therapies (AYUSH 2013).

The Drugs and Cosmetics Act, 1940 and Drugs and the Drugs and Cosmetic Rules, 1945

The Drugs and Cosmetics Act, 1940, is a key legislation in India that regulates the import, manufacture, distribution, and sale of drugs and cosmetics including Veterinary and Ayurvedic Medicine. Ayurvedic drugs are defined as medicines intended for internal or external use, prepared according to the formulae described in authoritative Ayurvedic texts. Section 3 (a) of Drugs and Cosmetics Act, 1940 (as amended up to 31-12-2016) states: 'Ayurvedic, Siddha or Unani drug includes all medicines used for or in the diagnosis, treatment, mitigation or prevention of [disease or disorder in human beings or animals, and manufactured] exclusively in accordance with the formulae described in the authoritative books of Ayurvedic, Siddha and Unani Tibb systems of medicine, specified in the First Schedule.'

The primary aim of the Act is to ensure the safety, efficacy, and quality of these products. The Drugs and Cosmetics Rules, 1945, include specific provisions for Ayurvedic drugs to ensure their safety, quality, and efficacy. In accordance to these rules, the Manufacturers of Ayurvedic Drugs must obtain licenses, ensuring compliance with Good Manufacturing Practices (GMP) outlined in Schedule T of the Rules. The Rules mandate testing for identity, purity, and strength of Ayurvedic drugs. The information on the manufacture, registration, sale, license, GMP certificate and penalties are defined in Section 33 (C) to 33(O). The Rules also include provisions to prevent contamination. Adulteration and specific guidelines are provided for the labelling and packaging of Ayurvedic drugs to ensure proper identification and usage. The Rules include schedules like Schedule E (1), which lists poisonous substances used in Ayurvedic medicines, and various forms for licensing and compliance (Drugs and Cosmetics Act, 1940 and Cosmetics Rules, 1945, as amended up to 31 December 2016. pdf, accessed on 16-04-2025).

Over the years, the Act has undergone several amendments to address emerging challenges in the pharmaceutical and cosmetic industries. In 2008, Amendment brought significant changes, including the establishment of the Central Drugs Standard Control Organisation (CDSCO) as the national regulatory authority and the introduction of stricter penalties for violations. One of the latest developments includes the ban on 35 fixed-dose combination (FDC) drugs due to safety concerns. These drugs were found to be licensed without proper evaluation of their safety and efficacy, posing risks to public health. The Central Drugs Standard Control Organisation (CDSCO) has directed Drug Controllers of States and Union Territories to halt their production, sale, and distribution.

Biological Diversity Act, 2002

The Act was enacted to conserve India's biological heritage and ensure the sustainable and equitable use of its resources, aligning with India's commitment to the Convention on Biological Diversity (CBD), ratified in 1994. The provisions of the Act are aimed to regulate access to biological resources and associated knowledge, especially by foreign entities, ensuring that benefits derived from their use are shared fairly with local communities and knowledge holders. Biological Diversity Act, 2002 also safeguards traditional knowledge systems related to biological resources, preventing their exploitation without prior informed consent and appropriate benefit-sharing arrangements. The Act creates a National Biodiversity Authority (NBA) to handle access matters for foreign individuals and organizations, and State Biodiversity Boards (SBBs) to regulate access for Indian citizens and oversee resource use within states. The Biodiversity Management Committees (BMCs) documents local biodiversity and traditional knowledge through People's Biodiversity Registers (PBRs). This Act plays a critical role in the herbal medicine sector by regulating medicinal plant access, protecting traditional healing practices, and promoting ethical and sustainable sourcing for herbal formulations.

The Forest Conservation Act, 1980

Enacted by the Parliament of India, The Forest Conservation Act, 1980 aims to ensure the protection and sustainable management of forests and their resources. A key provision of the Act is that the diversion of forest land for non-forestry purposes requires prior approval from the Central Government. This centralized decision-making process helps to maintain a balance between economic development and environmental conservation (Study IQ, accessed on 30-04-2025). Forest ecosystems are home to a wide variety of medicinal plants, making the Forest Conservation Act especially important in regulating their harvest. The Act prohibits the indiscriminate extraction of forest resources and mandates official approval for any non-forest activities conducted in forested areas. To ensure sustainable use, State Forest Departments often collaborate with the National Medicinal Plants Board (NMPB) on conservation initiatives and the regulated collection of medicinal plants. This coordination plays a vital role in protecting biodiversity while supporting the medicinal plant sector (Ahuja 2025).

National Medicinal Plants Board (NMPB)

Government of India has set up National Medicinal Plants Board (NMPB) on 24th November 2000. Currently the board is located in Ministry of AYUSH (Ayurveda, Yoga and Naturopathy, Unani, Siddha & Homoeopathy), New Delhi. The primary mandate of NMPB is to develop an appropriate mechanism for coordination between various Ministries/ Departments/ Organizations in India and implements support policies/programs for overall (conservation, cultivation, trade and export) growth of medicinal plants sector both at the Central /State and International level (https://ayush.gov.in/#!/medicinal_plants, accessed on 28-04-2025). The functions of the National Medicinal Plant Board include:

- Advise concerned Ministries and State/ Union Territory Governments on policy matters relating to schemes and programs for the development of medicinal plants.
- Identification, and quantification of medicinal plants.

- Promotion of co-operative efforts among collectors and growers and assisting them to store, transport and market their products effectively.
- Setting up of data-base system for dissemination of information and facilitating and encouraging to develop patents for medicinal plants.
- Undertaking Scientific, Technological research on medicinal plants.
- Development of protocols for cultivation and quality control.
- Generating information on wholesale prices, arrivals and trends in different markets to benefit both growers and buyers.
- Establishing a communication network for speedy collection and dissemination of market data for its efficient and timely utilization. for optimizing returns.

Quality Control and Standardization in Herbal Drug Production

The biological activity of a medicinal plant can vary significantly based on agricultural practices, climate conditions (such as water availability, temperature, humidity, and sunlight), even within the same species. Therefore, standardized agricultural protocols (GAP) are essential to ensure consistent bioactivity. Herbal drug manufacturers must follow these standards when sourcing plant materials to minimize variability in therapeutic effects. An important aspect of quality control involves testing plant materials for contaminants, including heavy metals, pesticides, and microbial (fungal and bacterial) impurities before processing. Herbal drug production must comply with Good Manufacturing Practices (GMP), which cover proper selection, procurement, storage, and handling of raw herbs to prevent contamination or adulteration. Adulteration—such as the illegal addition of synthetic drugs like NSAIDs or corticosteroids—poses a serious risk and must be strictly avoided. Like synthetic drugs, herbal products require standardization, including the identification and quantification of marker compounds (active principles), which directly influence product quality and efficacy. Standardization ensures consistent quality across batches through validated procedures for extraction, solvent use (e.g., ethanol, water), solvent removal, purification, and phytochemical analysis. As phytoconstituents are sensitive to environmental factors, proper storage—away from heat and light—is vital to preserve their potency (See Chapter 7 and 12).

WHO Good Manufacturing Practice (GMP) for Herbal Medicines

The global rise in herbal medicine use has emphasized the need for stringent quality assurance to ensure their safety and efficacy. GMP ensures that herbal medicines are consistently produced with verified quality, safety, and efficacy. GMP, similar to that for pharmaceutical products, is crucial for herbal medicines. In 1996, WHO issued *Good Manufacturing Practices: Supplementary Guidelines for the Manufacture of Herbal Medicinal Products*, though initially few countries implemented them fully. With growing herbal usage, national GMPs for herbals have emerged, leading WHO to update its guidelines, which were finalized in 2005 and adopted by a WHO Expert Committee in 2006 (WHO 2007). Basic features of WHO GMP guidelines include the following issues.

- **Raw Material Quality:** Use the correct plant species, cultivated or collected under appropriate conditions, free from contaminants.
- **Good Laboratory Practices (GLP):** Employ validated analytical methods for identifying active ingredients, impurities, and contaminants, with verification by reference laboratories.
- **Manufacturing Process:** Maintain proper documentation, standard operating procedures, batch production records, accurate weighing and measuring, extraction procedures, and laboratory control methods.
- **Equipment and Materials:** Record equipment use, cleaning, sanitization, and handling of raw materials; ensure proper packaging and labelling.
- **Stability Testing:** Establish product expiry dates with stability data; use fingerprint chromatograms for multi-herbal preparations to confirm consistency.
- **Complaint Handling:** Implement written procedures and records for addressing product complaints and necessary investigations.
- **Daily Observations and Review:** Document daily activities to ensure ongoing GMP compliance.
- **Self-Inspection:** Conduct internal audits by personnel knowledgeable in herbal medicines.
- **Personnel Training:** Ensure staff are adequately trained in the specifics of herbal material handling, processing, quality control, and hygiene, with regular health screenings.
- **Premises Requirements:** Design and maintain facilities according to WHO pharmaceutical GMP standards to ensure a controlled manufacturing environment.

Overall, the WHO GMP 2007 guidelines aim to assure that herbal medicines are consistently manufactured to meet quality standards essential for their safe and effective use.

Global Herbal Drug Regulations

Herbal drug regulations differ across countries but share the common goal of ensuring the safety, efficacy, and quality of herbal medicines. Key regulatory aspects include guidelines for active ingredients, preparation methods, and testing procedures, as well as measures to prevent contamination and adulteration. Compliance with Good Manufacturing Practices (GMP), Good Agricultural Practices (GAP), and other international standards is also emphasized. Comprehensive information on global herbal drug regulations is available for reference (Reddy and Alex 2017).

Africa

The quality control of herbs and herbal products in Africa is governed under the International Environmental Law Research Centre (2002–2003). Good Agricultural Practices (GAP) are emphasized for ensuring the safety and efficacy of herbal medicines for both human and animal health. However, regulatory frameworks vary significantly across African nations, with some countries relying heavily on traditional medicine practices. For example, The National Agency for Food and Drug Administration and Control (NAFDAC) regulates herbal medicines in Nigeria. This includes overseeing the registration, licensing, and quality control of herbal products to ensure their safety and efficacy.

Southeast Asian Nations

In Southeast Asia, herbal medicines are classified as Indigenous Herbal Medicines. Their quality is regulated by the Health Sciences Authority (HAS). The ASEAN Regulation (1967) governs the quality of botanicals in countries such as Indonesia, Malaysia, the Philippines, Singapore, Thailand, Vietnam, Myanmar, and Cambodia. These regulations ensure harmonized standards for herbal products across the region.

China

Over the past two decades, China has modernized its herbal product development processes by adopting international standards such as GAP, Good Laboratory Practices (GLP), Good Manufacturing Practices (GMP), and Good Clinical Practices (GCP). The country has established over 1,500 GMP-compliant herbal drug manufacturing facilities. Strict quality control criteria and documentation requirements are enforced to meet international standards, particularly for export purposes.

Japan

In Japan, botanical drugs and preparations known as Kampo Medicine, are widely used. Since 2003, the quality control of herbal products has followed Good Agricultural and Collection Practices (GACP). Preparations are made in accordance with the Japanese Pharmacopoeia and the Japanese Standards for Herbal Medicines. Regulatory measures for herbal products in Japan are similar to those for chemical drugs.

Saudi Arabia

Saudi Arabia established regulations for herbal medicines in 1996, creating a separate legal framework for their governance. The manufacturing requirements for herbal medicines align with those for conventional pharmaceuticals and WHO GMP standards. Pharmacopeial and non-pharmacopeial evidence is considered as supporting data for traditional products.

Europe

European Medical Agency is the main regulatory body of European Union, even though each member has its own regulatory bodies. Herbal medicines are defined under the Directive on Food Supplements, which incorporates recommendations from the Food and Agriculture Organization (FAO) and the World Health Organization (WHO). Additionally, the World Trade Organization (WTO) guidelines on sanitary and phytosanitary measures are followed to control contaminants and residues in food supplements. For human and veterinary herbal medicinal products, stringent guidelines are in place for:

- Qualitative and quantitative measures of active substances.
- Description of preparation methods.
- Testing procedures, stability tests, and material control.

These measures ensure the quality and safety of herbal products. The European Medicines Agency (EMA) monitors compliance with these guidelines for both intermediate and finished products.

Australia

In Australia, the Therapeutic Goods Act oversees the regulation of herbal medicines. Under this act, the Australian Register of Therapeutic Goods (ARTG) was established in 1989 to maintain a database of medicines and medical devices. Herbal products that meet Australian standards after evaluation are listed in this registry. The regulatory requirements align closely with those of the European Union, as outlined by the European Agency for the Evaluation of Medicinal Products (2001). This ensures a uniform set of specifications for herbal products, including safety, efficacy, and quality standards.

The United States of America

The regulatory framework for herbal supplements in the United States continues to evolve. While safety concerns—particularly those involving contamination and adulteration—are subject to strict regulation, comprehensive quality control standards and the overall regulatory status of these products remain less clearly defined. Since the passage of the Dietary Supplement Health and Education Act (DSHEA) in 1994, herbal supplements have been classified as dietary supplements rather than pharmaceutical drugs. DSHEA was enacted to exempt dietary and herbal supplements from many of the stringent regulatory requirements applied to drugs, allowing them to be marketed without prior FDA approval or scientific substantiation of health or medical claims. Notably, it was the first US legislation to define the term herb or botanical. The law defines supplements quite broadly as "anything that supplements the diet." Supplements therefore include vitamins, minerals, herbs, amino acids, enzymes, organ tissues, metabolites, extracts, or concentrates. Under DSHEA, the US Food and Drug Administration (FDA) primarily regulates these products by enforcing current Good Manufacturing Practices (CGMP). However, a major difference between a drug and a dietary supplement is that dietary supplements may not claim to "diagnose, cure, mitigate, treat, or prevent illness. However, herbal supplements are prohibited from making claims related to the diagnosis, treatment, cure, or prevention of any disease (Bent 2008).

Canada

Herbal medicines are regulated as drugs in Canada and must therefore conform to labelling and other requirements as set out in the Food and Drugs Act and Regulations. The Natural Health Products (NHP) Regulations have been in effect since 2004. These regulations classify natural health products, including botanicals, as a subset of drugs. To ensure quality and safety, the regulations mandate compliance with GMP and GLP standards for raw materials and finished products. Clinical trial protocols, licensing, and legislation are strictly monitored by Canadian Regulatory Authorities.

International Regulatory Cooperation for Herbal Medicines (IRCH): The International Regulatory Cooperation for Herbal Medicines (IRCH) is a global network of regulatory authorities responsible for the regulation of herbal medicines. Established in 2006 under the auspices of the World Health Organization (WHO), its core mission is to promote international collaboration and the exchange of best regulatory practices to improve the oversight of herbal medicines and support WHO in formulating relevant guidelines for Member States. IRCH aims to ensure the safe, effective, and high-quality use of herbal medicines in public health systems. It achieves this by fostering cooperation among national regulatory authorities through initiatives such as:

- Sharing regulatory experiences and scientific information related to the efficacy, safety, and quality of herbal products.
- Supporting the development and harmonization of regulatory standards.
- Promoting awareness of safe herbal medicine use in healthcare and wellness contexts.

- Discussing and recommending regulatory standards and future directions to WHO.
- Referring relevant issues to international forums such as the International Conference of Drug Regulatory Authorities (ICDRA), when necessary. The IRCH also plays a pivotal role in capacity-building and technical assistance among Member States, particularly in supporting the development of evidence-based regulatory frameworks.

As of January 2025, WHO-IRCH comprises 49 members, up from 35 in 2017, when WHO formally assumed the role of the network's secretariat (International Regulatory Cooperation for Herbal Medicines (IRCH). India is an active participant in the IRCH and contributes to its strategic initiatives and policy dialogues.

Herbal Pharmacopoeias

Herbal Pharmacopoeia is an official reference published by a Government or Authoritative Body that outlines standards for the safe and effective use of medicinal herbs. It provides detailed information on identification, active constituents, quality control, therapeutic uses, and contraindications. These pharmacopoeias play a vital role in ensuring the quality, safety, and efficacy of herbal medicines by setting benchmarks for raw materials and finished products. Most countries have developed their own herbal pharmacopoeias. Notable examples include:

American Herbal Pharmacopoeia (AHP)

- Contains monographs on widely used botanicals in the US.
- Written in English and used by academics, healthcare providers, manufacturers, and regulatory agencies.

African Herbal Pharmacopoeia

- Features over 50 monographs on commonly used African medicinal plants.
- Prepared by African scientists and reviewed by international experts.
- Includes morphology, distribution, and TLC chromatographic profiles for use by producers, traders, researchers, and practitioners.

British Herbal Pharmacopoeia

- One of the oldest herbal pharmacopoeias, covering 169 herbal raw materials.
- Includes botanical descriptions, geographical sources, comparative identification, and phytochemical analysis.
- Prepared by the expert in pharmacognosy, it remains a key document for quality assurance.

Chinese Herbal Pharmacopoeia

- Published by the China Food and Drug Administration.
- Written in Chinese by the Pharmacopoeia Commission and other institutions.
- Includes monographs on crude drugs, preparations, testing methods, standard substances, and general guidelines.

Indian Herbal Pharmacopoeia

Published by the Indian Drug Manufacturers' Association (IDMA) and Regional Research Laboratory (RRL), Jammu. It includes 40 monographs and is supported by various official texts:

- *Ayurvedic Pharmacopoeia of India (API)*: Monographs on 600 plant-, animal-, and mineral-based drugs.
- *Siddha Pharmacopoeia of India*: Volumes 1 and 2.
- *Homeopathic Pharmacopoeia of India*: Volumes 1 to 6.
- *Unani Pharmacopoeia of India*: Volumes 1 to 6.

The Pharmacopoeia Commission for Indian Medicine (PCIM) under the Ministry of AYUSH oversees development. Additionally, The Indian Council of Medical Research (ICMR) has set standards for 449 Indian medicinal plants.

The Indian Pharmacopoeia (IP 2018)

The 8th Edition of IP, published in 2018, includes:

- 220 New Monographs (170 chemical, 15 herbal, 10 blood-related, 2 vaccines, 3 radiopharmaceuticals, 6 biotech products, and 14 veterinary).
- 366 Revised Monographs and updates on Ayurvedic, formulation, excipient, and antibiotic standards.

Intellectual Property Right on Traditional Knowledge and Herbal Medicine

The herbal medicine gained global attention during last few decades which has necessitated patenting the traditional knowledge and herbal products. Intellectual Property Rights (IPRs) on traditional knowledge and herbal medicine protect indigenous knowledge from unauthorized use, ensure equitable benefit-sharing, and establish legal frameworks like patents and trademarks to safeguard cultural heritage and promote sustainable use. These measures encourage innovation while respecting the rights of traditional knowledge holders.

Article 8(j) of the Convention on Biological Diversity (CBD)

Article 8(j) of the Convention on Biological Diversity (CBD) is a key provision that addresses the protection of traditional knowledge, innovations, and practices of indigenous and local communities. It emphasizes the following:

- **Respect and Preservation**: Governments are encouraged to respect, preserve, and maintain the knowledge, innovations, and practices of indigenous and local communities that are relevant to the conservation and sustainable use of biological diversity.
- **Equitable Sharing of Benefits**: It promotes the equitable sharing of benefits arising from the utilization of such knowledge, ensuring that communities are fairly compensated for their contributions.
- **Approval and Involvement**: The article stresses the importance of obtaining prior informed consent or approval from the traditional knowledge holders before using it.

Traditional Knowledge Digital Library (TKDL)

The Government of India set up the Traditional Knowledge Digital Library (TKDL) in 2001, where 1200 formulas of Indian medicine (Ayurveda, Unani and Siddha) were digitized. This initiative has since expanded to more than 5.0 lakh formulations and practices, translated into five international languages, to safeguard traditional knowledge from biopiracy and misuse in patent claims (Council of Scientific & Industrial Research, TKDL Unit, Government of India, https://www.csir.res.in/en/documents/tkdl , accessed on 20-03-206).

The Protection of Plant Varieties and Farmers' Rights (PPV&FR) Act, 2001

The PPV&FR Act, 2001 ensures protection for plant breeders and farmers, and promotes agricultural innovation. While addressing India's unique socio-economic needs, this Act aligns with international agreements like Trade-Related Aspects of Intellectual Property Rights (TRIPS) and the International Union for the Protection of New Varieties of Plants (UPOV). The salient features of the Act include:

- **Farmers' Rights:** Farmers can save, reuse, and sell seeds, except branded ones. They can also register and protect their new varieties.
- **Breeders' Rights:** Breeders have exclusive rights to produce, sell, and license protected varieties.
- **Researchers' Rights:** Use of registered varieties for experiments and breeding is allowed, with some limits.
- **National Gene Fund:** Supports benefit-sharing, genetic resource conservation, and recognizes farmers' contributions.

Conclusion

The evolution of herbal drug development from traditional home-made remedies to standardized, industrially manufactured products has taken shape over the last four to five decades. This transformation has paralleled significant scientific and technological advancements in the healthcare sector. Historically, medicinal plants were commonly prepared as infusions, decoctions, tinctures, oxymels, and elixirs—each formulation crafted with attention to ingredient ratios, preparation techniques, utensil choice, sterilization, dosage accuracy, and storage conditions. These meticulous methods contributed significantly to their therapeutic efficacy. In the modern era, the discovery and development of herbal drugs have become increasingly sophisticated, integrating knowledge from disciplines such as botany, phytochemistry, pharmacology, and molecular biology. Despite its complexity, this field continues to yield numerous bioactive compounds with promising pharmacological properties. Many plant-derived drugs have already been incorporated into global pharmacopoeias, and several more are under active investigation. However, the sector still faces significant challenges, including sustainable sourcing of plant materials, botanical authentication, development of high-throughput screening tools, and scalable production of bioactive constituents. These challenges have highlighted the importance of pharmacovigilance as an essential component of herbal drug development, ensuring safety and efficacy throughout the product lifecycle.

The conventional drug development pathway is time-consuming and costly, with a relatively low success rate for producing effective and safe drugs. Furthermore, post-marketing outcomes are often suboptimal. The use of reverse pharmacology, which applies traditional knowledge to guide scientific validation, has shown promise in overcoming many of these limitations in herbal drug development. Unlike synthetic drugs, herbal formulations often contain multiple plant components, leading to added complexity in standardization, safety, and quality assurance. Variations in regional sourcing, adulteration, and differences in cultivation practices can significantly affect the consistency and efficacy of the final product. As herbs are now widely sourced from both natural and commercial markets, maintaining uniform quality standards has become increasingly critical. To address these concerns, international bodies such as the World Health Organization (WHO) and the Food and Agriculture Organization (FAO) have developed comprehensive guidelines, from raw material selection to final product formulation. These emphasize adherence to Good Agricultural Practices (GAP), Good Manufacturing Practices (GMP), and Good Laboratory Practices (GLP). At the national level, individual countries have established regulatory frameworks for herbal products, including those intended for veterinary use and international trade. In India, the Ministry of AYUSH oversees these regulations. Under its purview, the Central Council for Research in Ayurvedic Sciences (CCRAS)—an autonomous body—plays a pivotal role in developing pharmacopeial standards and maintaining documentation essential for licensing and regulation. As the apex organization in this domain, CCRAS has published key reference materials, including: *Laboratory Guide for the Analysis of Ayurveda and Siddha Formulations; General Guidelines for Drug Development of Ayurvedic Formulations (Volume I); General Guidelines for Safety/Toxicity Evaluation of Ayurvedic Formulations (Volume II); and General Guidelines for Clinical Evaluation of Ayurvedic Interventions (Volume III).*

References

Ahuja K.2025. *Medicinal plants in India: Comprehensive Overview of the National Medicinal Plants Board and Regulatory Framework.* Medicinal Plants in India: Comprehensive Overview of the National Medicinal Plants Board and Regulatory Framework - Bhatt & Joshi Associates, accessed on 30-04-25.

Arulsamy A, Kumari Y and Shaikh MF. 2016. Reverse pharmacology: fast track path of drug discovery. Alzheimer's and Dementia: *Translational Research and Clinical Interventions* **3**(4): 651-57.

AYUSH. 2013. *Good Clinical Practice Guidelines for Clinical Trials in Ayurveda, Siddha and Unani Medicine (GCP-ASU).* Department of AYUSH Ministry of Health & Family Welfare, Government of India, New Delhi, India. https://www.ccras.nic.in/wp-content/uploads/2025/09/3.-ASU-GCP-Guidelines.pdf, accessed on 02-04-2025.

Balkrishna A, Sharma N, Srivastava D, Kukreti A, Srivastava S and Arya V. 2024. Exploring the safety, efficacy, and bioactivity of herbal medicines: Bridging traditional wisdom and modern science in healthcare. *Future Integrative Medicine* **3**(1): 35–49. doi: 10.14218/FIM.2023.00086.

Balunas MJ and Kinghorn AD. 2005. Drug discovery from medicinal plants. *Life Science* **78**: 431-41.

Bent S. 2008. Herbal medicine in the United States: Review of efficacy, safety and regulation. *Journal of General Internal Medicine* **23**: 854-59.

Bruhn JG and Bohlin L .1997. Molecular pharmacognosy: An explanatory model. *Drug Discovery Today* **2** (6): 243-46.

Guantai E and Chibale K. 2011. How can natural products serve as a viable source of lead compounds for the development of new/novel antimalarial? *Malaria Journal* **10**(Suppl.1): S2 http://www.malariajournal.com/content/10/S1/S2.

Kumar CD. 2007. Pharmacognosy can help minimize accidental misuse of herbal medicine. *Current Science* **93**(10): 1356-58.

Kunle OF, Egharevba HO and Ahmadu PO. 2012. Standardization of herbal medicines-A review. *International Journal of Biodiversity and Conservation* **4**(3): 101-12.

Patwardhan B and Mashelkar RA. 2009. Traditional medicine-inspired approaches to drug discovery: Can Ayurveda show the way forward. *Drug Discovery Today* **14** (15-16): 804-11.

Reddy KJ and Alex M. 2017. *Regulations for Herbal Medicine-Worldwide.* (Ed.) Alex T. LAP LAMBERT Academic Publishing, Beau Basin, Mauritius. (PDF) Regulations for Herbal Medicine-Worldwide. Downloaded on 28-04-2025.

Sharma TR (Trans.). 2013. *Atharva-Veda Vol. I.* Vijaykumar Govindram Hansanand, New Delhi, India (Digital Distributer Agniveer). https://archive.org/details/atharva-veda-vol-2-of-2 pdf downloaded on 05-06-2023.

Singh R, Navneet DK and Kumar A. 2020. Ethnobotanical and pharmacological aspects of *Ipomoea carnea* Jacq. and *Celosia cristata* Linn. In: *Current Status of Researches in Biosciences.* pp. 493-506 (Eds) Joshi PC, Joshi N, Reshman, Yasmin and Mansotra DK. Today & Tomorrow's Printers and Publishers, New Delhi, India.

Vaidya A. 2014. Reverse Pharmacology-A paradigm shift for drug discovery and development. *Current Research in Drug Discovery* **1**(2): 39-44.

WHO IRCH official webpage https://www.who.int/initiatives/irch, accessed on 04-04-2025.

WHO. 2007. *WHO Guidelines on Good Manufacturing Practices (GMP) for Herbal Medicines.* 92 p. World Health Organization, Geneva, Switzerland.

WHO. 2017. *Report of the WHO International Regulatory Cooperation for Herbal Medicines (IRCH) 9th Meeting.* Geneva: WHO. https://www.who.int/publications.

WHO. 2013.*WHO Traditional Medicine Strategy 2014–2023.* World Health Organization, Geneva, Switzerland. https://www.who.int/publications/i/item/9789241506090.

Wynn G and Fougère BJ. 2007. The roots of veterinary botanical medicine. In: *Veterinary Herbal Medicine.* pp. 33-49. (Eds) Wynn SG and Fougère BJ. Mosby Elsevier, St. Louis, Missouri, USA.

12

Designing Herbal Gardens for Health and Heritage: Thematic Approaches to Cultivation, Harvesting, and Post-Harvest Practices

P. Tripathi

krīḍārāmaṁ tu yaḥ kuryād udvāna-phala-saṁyutam; sa gacchet śaṅkarapuraṁ vaset tatra yugatrayam.

He, who for pleasure makes a good garden full of fruit and flower trees, is destined to go to the abode of Siva and reside there for as many as three aeons

(Vrkshāyurveda 1.6, Ramachandra Rao 1993)

1. Introduction
2. Herbal Garden
3. Guidelines for Establishing Herbal Gardens
4. Environmental Consideration for Herbal Garden
5. Management of Garden and Organic Gardening Techniques
6. Authentication of Herbal Plants and Botanicals
7. Harvesting and Storage of Herbs
8. General Guidelines and Standard Operating Procedures for Harvesting Collection of Herbs and Botanicals
9. Post-Harvest Losses in Herbal Farming
10. Processing of Medicinal and Aromatic Plants and Botanicals
11. Personnel for Herbal Gardens
12. Conclusion

Introduction

The practice of cultivating herbal gardens is as ancient as civilization itself, rooted in the timeless relationship between humans and nature. Across the ages—from the fertile plains of Mesopotamia and the sacred groves of Egypt to the classical gardens of Greece, China, and India—herbal gardens have served as sanctuaries of healing, spirituality, and ecological balance. These verdant spaces were not merely aesthetic landscapes but vital repositories of medicinal knowledge and sustainable living. In the Indian tradition, the cultivation of herbs and trees has been revered as a sacred act. Ancient scriptures and philosophical texts regard environmental stewardship as a moral and spiritual duty. The Rig Veda (7.35.5) proclaims—'śaṁ no oṣadhīr vanino bhavantu' — a prayer for peace and well-being bestowed by the herbs and forest trees. Such verses reflect the deep-rooted belief in the therapeutic and life-sustaining power of nature. Further enriching this legacy is the *Vrksāyurveda** (Vrikshayurveda)—an ancient treatise rooted in the Atharva Veda and elaborated in the Agni Purana — which outlines the principles of plant life and horticulture. It offers detailed guidance on the conservation, propagation, and care of medicinal plants, underscoring the importance of healthy, productive vegetation for human and planetary well-being. Tree planting was considered a noble duty (*dharma*), contributing to both ecological balance and spiritual merit. As Vrikshayurveda (1.1) aptly states: 'He is indeed a monarch if his house has extensive gardens with large pools of water, blooming lotuses, and humming bees' (Ramachandra Rao 1993). This chapter explores the principles, planning, and practical aspects involved in the design, establishment, and sustainable management of herbal gardens, bridging ancient wisdom with contemporary ecological practices.

Herbal Garden

Herbal garden, also known as a medicinal garden or herb garden, is a cultivated area specifically designed for the growth, preservation, and study of various medicinal plants and herbs. These gardens serve as living repositories of traditional knowledge about the therapeutic properties of plants and contribute to biodiversity conservation efforts. Herbal gardens are not only aesthetically pleasing but also provide practical benefits by promoting health and wellness through the cultivation of medicinal herbs. The development of herbal gardens aimed for not only propagation and multiplications of the medicinal and aromatic plants, but also for their *ex-situ* conservation to protect and maintain their existence for future generations. It also facilitates the development of cultivation techniques including quality plant materials, irrigation, fertilizer, plant protection, post-harvest collection and processing, which are cost effective in different agro-climatic regions.

Objectives of Herbal Garden

In general, herbal gardens are established with the following main objectives:

Conservation: Herbal gardens aim to conserve and preserve a diverse range of medicinal plant species, many of which may be endangered or threatened in their natural habitats.

*References to Vṛkṣāyurveda are also found in classical works such as the Bṛhat Saṃhitā and Śārṅgadhara Saṃhitā, with Surapāla's Vṛkṣāyurveda later emerging as the most comprehensive independent treatise on the subject.

Education: These gardens serve as educational resources for students, researchers, and the general public, offering opportunities to learn about the medicinal properties, uses, and cultural significance of various plants.

Research: Herbal gardens facilitate research into the pharmacological properties of medicinal plants, including their efficacy, safety, and potential therapeutic applications. They also have the potential to stimulate renewed interest in bio-prospecting for new drugs derived from medicinal plants.

Health Promotion: By cultivating and promoting the use of medicinal herbs, herbal gardens contribute to public health initiatives by providing natural alternatives for preventive healthcare and the treatment of various ailments.

Sustainable Practices: Herbal gardens promote sustainable practices such as organic cultivation, biodiversity conservation, and the use of traditional knowledge systems. They also align with national and international health priorities.

Community Engagement: These gardens serve as community spaces for recreational activities, workshops, and events focused on herbal medicine, fostering a connection to nature and traditional healing practices.

Basic Principles for Creating Herbal Gardens

Increase Public Awareness: Promote the efficacy of herbal drugs and generate interest and awareness among the general public, cultivators, and farmers about medicinal plants. Disseminate technical expertise and information at the village level, utilizing self-help groups and panchayats. It is crucial to enhance cultivators' knowledge about cultivation methods, schedules, and processing of medicinal plants.

Identify Key Medicinal Plants: Initially, focus on a few medicinal plants to ensure their overall development in a specific region, as plant performance varies by region. Cultivate certain medicinal plants that thrive in forest ecosystems as intercropping in and around forest areas.

Adopt Advanced Techniques: Implement the latest techniques to improve production systems, enabling medicinal plants to compete in the international market. Develop effective micro-propagation systems for cost-effective, quality plant materials, emphasizing collaboration with growers and industries for mass production of tissue-cultured medicinal plants.

Promote Organic Farming: Cultivate medicinal plants through organic farming and develop standardization using chemical and molecular markers. Conserve the biodiversity of medicinal plants and introduce the cultivation of more exotic medicinal plants to reduce the cost of procuring medicines.

Raise Awareness for Home Remedies: Foster awareness about the use of herbal medicines for home remedies and create a database of naturally grown and cultivated medicinal plants.

Design and Popular Themes for Creating Herbal Garden

Herbal gardens present an opportunity to cultivate medicinal herbs for diverse purposes, all the while disseminating knowledge about their significance and traditional uses, and aiding in the conservation of plants that are threatened, endangered, or rare in their natural habitats. Home gardening of medicinal herbs not only enhances household food security but also grants direct access to herbal culinary remedies, which can be harvested, prepared, and utilized for addressing the day-to-day health needs of family members. Home gardens typically operate within limited land space, unlike institutional herbal gardens, which boast sufficient land area for herb cultivation. The design of a herbal garden varies depending on the themes and available land area designated for this purpose. A thematic approach to designing herbal gardens involves executing the concept at the field level to arrange and design a comprehensive collection of medicinal plants in a unique and systematic manner based on user-friendly ideas. Herbal thematic gardens have the potential to boost and support the renewed interest in bioprospecting, which involves the search for new drugs from medicinal plants and the use of traditional medical knowledge as a source of leads.

Thematic herbal gardens serve not only botanical purposes but also play a vital social role. Shared herbal gardens foster community engagement by bringing together people of diverse ages, backgrounds, and cultures. These spaces encourage the exchange of ideas, conversation, and the sharing of traditional and scientific knowledge. When scientifically planned and well-organized, thematic plantations of medicinal plants can contribute significantly to *ex-situ* conservation, raise public awareness, and enhance understanding of medicinal flora among stakeholders and the general public. To maximize their impact, thematic herbal gardens should also be designed with aesthetic appeal in mind, incorporating a harmonious blend of herbs from both traditional and modern medical systems (Pandey *et al.* 2019). Ideally, each garden should include brief yet informative descriptions of the plant exhibits to educate visitors. Some popular themes are recommended here for establishing herbal gardens.

Navagraha Vatika

Also known as the *Navagraha* plants, *Navagraha* (nine planet) *vatika* (garden) is a collection of plants and trees themed around the nine *grahas* or planets, which are considered sacred in India. This garden is created to harness the influence of these nine celestial bodies. The Navagraha plants are strategically planted in specific directions to capture the benefits associated with each graha. The word graha means energy, which has come to represent planets. Thus, the Sun is included as part of the grahas (energy). Each plant symbolizes unique celestial energies corresponding to its *graha* within the vatika. For example, the peepal tree, linked to Guru Brihaspati, symbolizes wisdom and knowledge (Krishna and Amrithalingam 2014). This arrangement facilitates the generation of positive energies, purifies the air, and eliminates *vastu dosha*.

Table 12.1. *Navagraha vatika* trees *(Navagraha vriksha)*

Graha	**Effects**	**Position**	**Assigned Trees**	
			Hindi/ Sanskrit/ English Names	**Botanical Name**
Surya (Sun)	Influence confidence and vitality	Middle	*Aak /Arka /* Giant milkweed	*Calotropis gigantea*
Chandra (Moon)	Emotions and intuition	South-East	*Palash / Kiṁśuka /* Flame of forest	*Butea monosperma*
Budha (Mercury)	Communication and intelligence	North	*Apamarg, Markati* (Prickly chaff flower)	*Achyranthes aspera*
Shukra (Venus)	Love and relationships	East	*Gular, Udumbara* (Cluster fig)	*Ficus racemosa linn. F. glomerata (Roxb)*
Mangal (Mars)	Courage and energy	South	*Khair, Khadira* (Cutch tree)	*Acacia catechu* syn. *Senegalia catechu* (L. f.)
Brihaspati/ Guru (Jupiter)	Wisdom and knowledge	North-East	*Peepal, Aśvattha* (Sacred fig)	*Ficus religiosa*
Shani (Saturn)	Discipline and responsibility	West	*Khejri, Shami* (Indian mesquite)	*Prosopis cineraria*
Rahu (Dragon's head)	Karmic influences	South-West	*Durva* (Bermuda grass)	*Cynodon dactylon*
Ketu (Dragon's tail)	Karmic influences	North-West	*Darbha, Kusha* (Halfa grass)	*Desmostachya bipinnata*

(Source: ICAR-Central Coastal Agricultural Research Institute Goa, Maneesha *et al.* 2021, and various open-access, classical, and scholarly references).

Importantly, the plants offer therapeutic benefits for various ailments and promote good health, wealth, and prosperity. These Navagraha herbs have the potential to treat various diseases and have been used since ancient times. Most Navagraha herbs are standardized and validated for their various pharmacological activities (Parihar and Sharma 2021). In general, a Navagraha vatika is a beautiful blend of astrology, nature, and traditional medicine, offering both spiritual and health benefits. Plants (Fig. 12.1) recommended for Navagraha vatika are given in Table 12.1.

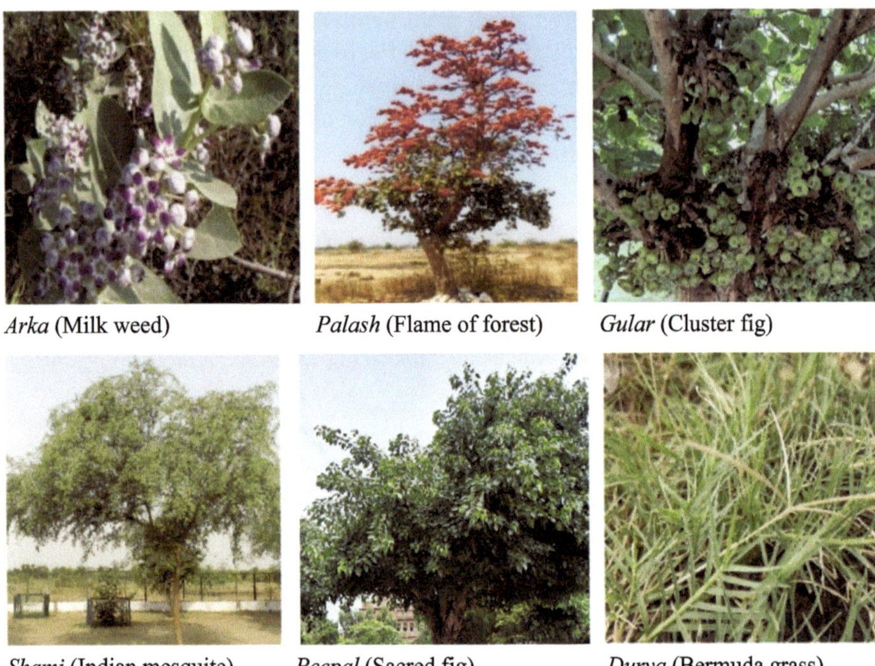

Arka (Milk weed) *Palash* (Flame of forest) *Gular* (Cluster fig)

Shami (Indian mesquite) *Peepal* (Sacred fig) *Durva* (Bermuda grass)

Fig. 12.1. *Selected trees and herbs recommended for Navagraha Vatika.*

Nakshatra Vatika or *Nakshatra Herbal Garden*

A *Nakshatra Vatika* consists of 27 trees matched to 27 asterisms (constellations) in Indian astrology. A specific tree or trees are assigned to each of the 27 constellations (*Nakshatras*) through which the sun passes (Table 12.2). It is believed that celestial bodies like the sun and the moon exert different influences on human beings as they transit through these constellations. Such effects can be moderated or enhanced by planting and worshipping the trees assigned to each constellation. This assortment of trees, planted according to their respective constellation assignments, forms what is known as a Nakshatra-garden (Pandey *et al.* 2019).

Traditionally revered for their spiritual resonance, Nakshatra Vṛkṣas are not only sacred but also pharmacologically potent. Many species—such as *Aak, Amla, Amaltas, Arjuna, Babool, Bael, Jamun, Peepal Shami, Sissam*, and *Vata* —exhibit antioxidant, anti-inflammatory, antidiabetic, antimicrobial, astringent, cardioprotective, hepatoprotective and immunomodulatory properties. Modern research thus reinforces the ancient belief that these trees sustain both cosmic harmony and human well-being, bridging traditional cosmology with contemporary principles of preventive healthcare and biodiversity conservation.

Table 12.2. *Nakshatra vatika*: Asterisms and assigned trees (*Nakṣatra-vṛkṣa*)

***Nakṣatra* (IAST)**	**Western Star Name and *Symbolic Theme***	**Assigned Trees**	
		***Hindi / Sanskrit* / English Name**	**Botanical Name**
Ashwini *(Aśvinī)*	β Arietis– *Horse, Star of Transport*	*Kuchla / Kupīla* / Strychnine tree	*Strychnos nux-vomica*
Bharani *(Bharaṇī)*	41 Arietis– *Yoni, Star of Restraint*	*Amla* / *Āmalakī* / Indian gooseberry	*Phyllanthus emblica*
Krittika *(Kṛttikā)*	Pleiades – *Knife, Star of Fire*	*Gular / Udumbara* / Cluster fig	*Ficus racemosa*
Rohini *(Rohiṇī)*	α Tauri (Aldebaran) – *Ox, Star of Ascent*	*Jamun / Jambūḥ* / Indian black plum	*Syzygium cumini*
Mrigshira, *(Mṛgaśīrṣa)*	λ Orionis (Meissa) – *Deer Head, Star of Searching*	*Khair / Khadira* / Cutch tree	*Acacia catechu* syn. *Senegalia catechu* (L. f.)
Ardra, *(Ārdrā)*	α Orionis (Betelgeuse) – *Teardrop, Star of Emotion*	*Sissam / Siṃsapa* / Indian rosewood	*Dalbergia sissoo*
Punarvasu *(Punarvasu)*	β Geminorum (Pollux) – *Arrows, Star of Renewal*	*Babool / Babhūla* / Gum arabic tree	*Acacia nilotica* syn. *Vachellia nilotica* (L.)
Pushya *(Puṣya)*	δ Cancri– *Cow Udder, Star of Nourishment*	*Peepal / Aśvattha* / Sacred fig	*Ficus religiosa*
Ashlesha *(Āśleṣā)*	ζ Hydrae – *Snake, Clinging Star*	*Nagkesar / Nāga-keśara* / Indian rose chestnut	*Mesua ferrea*
Magha *(Maghā)*	α Leonis (Regulus) – *Throne, Star of Power*	*Bargad / Vaṭa* / Banyan tree	*Ficus benghalensis*
Purva Phalguni, *(Pūrva Phālgunī)*	δ Leonis– *Bed's Foot – Star of Fortune*	*Palash /Kiṁśuka* / Flame of the forest	*Butea monosperma*
Uttara Phalguni, *(Uttara Phālgunī)*	β Leonis (Denebola) –*Bed's Head, Star of Patronage*	*Pakar / Pakarī* / Golden Rumph's fig	*Ficus rumphii*
Hasta *(Hasta)*	δ Corvi – *Hand, Star of Skill*	*Juhi / Yūthikā* / Jasmine	*Jasminum auriculatum*
Chitra *(Citrā)*	α Virginis (Spica) – *Jewel, Star of Opportunity*	*Bael / Bilva* / Bengal quince	*Aegle marmelos*
Swati *(Svātī)*	α Boötis (Arcturus) –*Sword, Star of Independence*	*Arjun* /Arjuna/ Arjun tree	*Terminalia arjuna*
Vishakha *(Viśākhā)*	α Librae –*Trident, Star of Purpose*	*Harsingar / Parijāta*/ Night Jasmine	*Nyctanthes arbor-tristis*

***Nakṣatra* (IAST)**	**Western Star Name and *Symbolic Theme***	**Assigned Trees**	
		***Hindi / Sanskrit* / English Name**	**Botanical Name**
Anuradha *(Anurādhā)*	δ Scorpii –*Lotus, Star of Success*	*Bakul /Bakula /* Bullet wood *Nag champa / Nāga-keśara* / Indian rose chestnut	*Mimusops elengi* *Mesua ferrea*
Jyestha *(Jyeṣṭhā)*	α Scorpii (Antares) – *Umbrella, Chief Star*	*Semul / Śālmalī /* Malabar silk-cotton tree	*Bombax ceiba* L. syn. *B. malabaricum*
Moola *(Mūla)*	λ Scorpii (Shaula) – *Roots, Foundation Star*	*Amaltas / Āragvadha* / Indian laburnum	*Cassia fistula*
Purva Ashadha *Pūrvāṣāḍhā,*	δ Sagittarii– *Fan, Invincible Star*	*Sita Ashok / Śītāśoka* / Ashoka tree	*Saraca asoca*
Uttara Ashadha *(Uttarāṣāḍhā)*	σ Sagittarii– *Bed Planks, Universal Star*	*Kathal /Panasa /* Jackfruit	*Artocarpus heterophyllus*
Shravan *(Śravaṇa)*	α Aquilae (Altair) – *Ear, Star of Learning*	*Aak /Arka /* Giant milkweed	*Calotropis gigantea*
Dhanishtha *(Dhaniṣṭhā)*	β Delphini – *Drum, Star of Symphony*	*Khejri / Shamī /* Indian mesquite	*Prosopis cineraria*
Shata Taaraka *(Śatabhiṣā)*	λ Aquarii – *Circle, Veiling Star*	*Kadam / Kadamba /* Burflower tree	*Neolamarckia cadamba*
Purva Bhadrapada (*Pūrva Bhādrapadā*)	β Pegasi (Markab) – *Blessed Foot, Scorching Star*	*Aam / Āmra /* Mango	*Mangifera indica*
Uttara Bhadrapada, *Uttara Bhādrapadā*	γ Pegasi (Algenib) – *Warrior Star*	*Neem / Nimba/* Neem or Indian lilac	*Azadirachta indica*
Revati *(Revatī)*	ζ Piscium– *Drum, Star of Wealth*	*Mahua / Madhūka /* Indian butter tree	*Madhuca latifolia*

(Source: Compiled from ICAR-Central Coastal Agricultural Research Institute Goa, Maneesha *et al.* 2021, and various open-access, classical, and scholarly references).

Editorial Note*: IAST refers to the International Alphabet of Sanskrit Transliteration, a standardized system for rendering Sanskrit terms in Roman script. In classical as well as regional traditions, multiple tree species are traditionally associated with various Nakṣatras (asterisms). A single Nakṣatra may correspond to more than one tree species, and conversely, one tree species may be linked with multiple Nakṣatras. The tree names presented in this table are representative selections, chosen for their cultural significance, botanical accuracy, and suitability for Nakṣatra Vātikā design. Variations in regional nomenclature, vernacular names, and symbolic associations are acknowledged and may differ across linguistic and cultural contexts.*

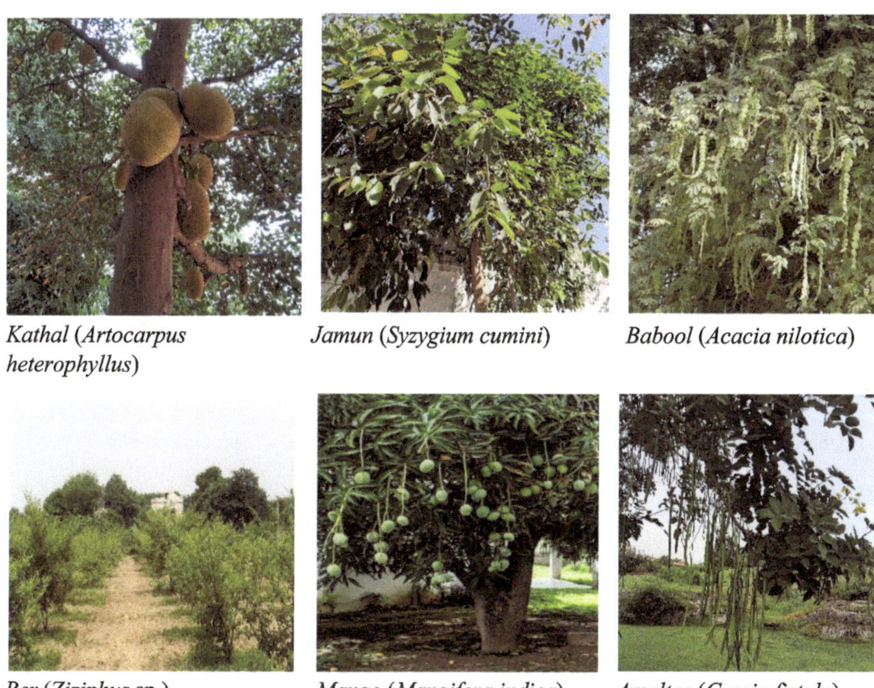

Kathal (*Artocarpus heterophyllus*) *Jamun* (*Syzygium cumini*) *Babool* (*Acacia nilotica*)

Ber (*Ziziphus* sp.) *Mango* (*Mangifera indica*) *Amaltas* (*Cassia fistula*)

Fig. 12.2. *Selected trees for Nakshatra and Rashi Vatika.*

Raashi/Zodiac Sign Gardens

Twenty-seven Nakshatras (constellations) are further assembled into 12 zodiac signs (Fig 12.2). Religiously and astrologically speaking, the zodiac sign plays a significant role in the lives of human beings. Any astrological prediction emanates from the zodiac sign of a person. Indian astrology has assigned specific trees for specific zodiac signs (Table 12.3).

Demonstration Herbal Gardens

Medicinal herbs are valued for their healing properties, owing to their unique bioactive characteristics. However, their use requires careful understanding, as some herbs are safe while others may be harmful if misused. The primary objective of a demonstration herbal garden is to promote awareness among farmers, healthcare professionals, traditional healers, traders, researchers, and students about the cultivation, conservation, and responsible use of medicinal plants for managing common health conditions such as colds, indigestion, diabetes, arthritis, stress, and obesity. These gardens are educational in nature and do not serve as endorsements for specific herbal remedies. The plants featured in the Demonstration Gardens are broadly classified into six categories: Nutraceutical Garden, Pharmaceutical Garden, Aromaceutical Garden, Herbal Spices Garden, Cosmeceutical Garden, and Repellent Plant Garden (Sanwal *et al.* 2020).

Table 12.3. Raashi (zodiac ign) and related trees *(Raashi vriksha)*

***Raashi* (Zodiac Sign)**		**Assigned Tree**	
		Common Name Hindi, Sanskrit (English)	**Botanical Name**
Mesh (Aries)	0-30°	*Rakta chandana* (Red sandalwood)	*Pterocarpus santalinus*
Vrishabh (Taurus)	30-60°	*Saptaparni* (Devil's tree)	*Alstonia scholaris*
Mithun (Gemini)	60-90°	*Kathal, Panasa* (Jack fruit)	*Artocarpus heterophyllus*
Karka (Cancer)	90-120°	*Palash, Kimshuka* (Flame of forest)	*Butea monosperma*
Singh (Leo)	120-150°	*Ber, Badari* (Indian jujube)	*Ziziphus mauritiana*
Kanya (Virgo)	150-180°	*Aam, Amra* (Mango)	*Mangifera indica*
Tula (Libra)	180-210°	*Bakula* (Bullet wood)	*Mimusops elengi*
Vrishchik (Scorpio)	210-240°	*Khair, Khadira* (Cutch tree)	*Acacia catechu*
Dhanu (Sagittarius)	240-270°	*Peepal, Asvatha* (Sacred fig)	*Ficus religiosa*
Makar (Capricorn)	270-300°	*Sissam, Siṃsapa* (Indian rosewood)	*Dalbergia sissoo*
Kumbh (Aquarius)	300-330°	*Khejari, Shami* (Khejri tree / Indian mesquite)	*Prosopis cineraria*
Meen (Pisces)	330-360°	*Bargad, Vata* (Banyan tree)	*Ficus benghalensis*

(Source: Compiled from ICAR-Central Coastal Agricultural Research Institute Goa, Maneesha *et al.* 2021, and various open-access, classical, and scholarly references).

Nutraceutical Garden: Medicinal herbs are valued for their therapeutic properties and also as sources of nutrition. Many traditional systems of medicine, including Ayurveda, have long recognized the dual role of these plants—as both food and medicine. Various parts of these herbs (leaves, roots, fruits, seeds, etc.) are rich in biologically active compounds such as phytochemicals, antioxidants, vitamins, minerals, proteins, and carbohydrates, which contribute to overall health and disease prevention. Now, there is a global resurgence of interest in herbal remedies that serve as nutraceuticals—natural substances that offer health benefits beyond basic nutrition. These plant-based products bridge the gap between food and medicine, making them ideal candidates for promoting wellness and preventing chronic illnesses such as cardiovascular diseases, diabetes, and inflammatory disorders. A nutraceutical garden promotes the cultivation and use of such multifunctional plants. Examples of key nutraceutical herbs and plants (Fig. 12.3) include:

- *Amesh* (Sea buckthorn, *Hippophae rhamnoides*) – Rich in vitamin C, E, carotenoids, flavonoids, and omega fatty acids; known for its anti-inflammatory and skin-rejuvenating properties.

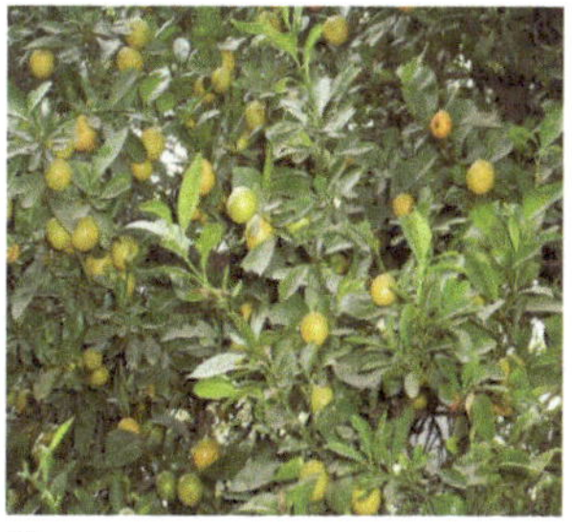
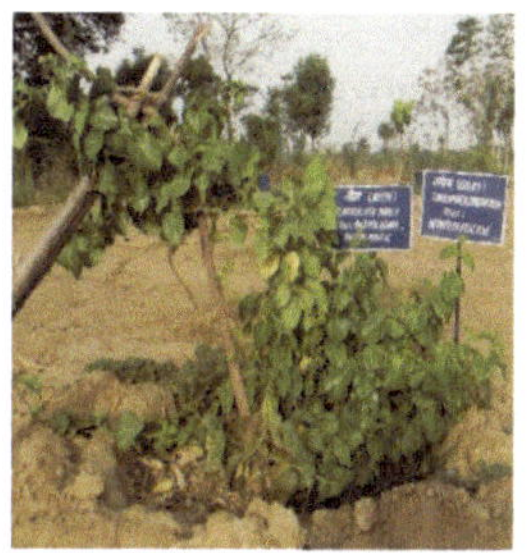
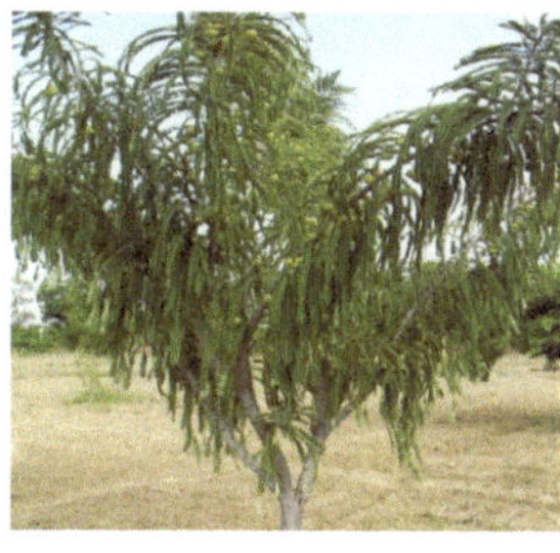

Citrus spp. Giloy (*Tinospora cordifolia*) Amaliki (*Phyllanthus emblica*)

Fig. 12.3. *Plants recommended for nutraceutical garden.*

- *Amalaki* (Indian gooseberry, *Phyllanthus emblica*) – A potent antioxidant and immunomodulator, widely used in Ayurvedic formulations like *Triphala*.
- *Ashwagandha* (Indian ginseng, *Withania somnifera*) – An adaptogenic herb that helps in stress reduction, immune support, and energy enhancement.
- *Syamka / Banti* (Barnyard millet, *Echinochloa frumentacea*) – A gluten-free grain, rich in fibre, minerals, and polyphenols; supports digestion and metabolic health.
- *Brahmi* (Water hyssop, *Bacopa monnieri*) – Traditionally used as a brain tonic; enhances memory, concentration, and cognitive function.
- *Kotu* (Buckwheat, *Fagopyrum esculentum*) – A pseudo-cereal high in rutin and other flavonoids; promotes heart health and blood sugar control.
- Citrus fruits (*Citrus* spp.) – Packed with vitamin C and bioflavonoids; beneficial for immune function and skin health.
- *Shigru/ Sahajan* (Drumstick, *Moringa oleifera*) – A superfood with high levels of vitamins A and C, calcium, iron, and antioxidants; supports detoxification and reduces inflammation.
- *Giloy / Amrita* (Heart-leaved moonseed, *Tinospora cordifolia*) – Renowned for its immune-boosting, anti-pyretic, and anti-inflammatory effects.
- *Makoy / Kakamachi* (Black nightshade, *Solanum nigrum*) – Used in traditional medicine for liver support, skin ailments and anti-ulcer activity.
- *Pushkarmool* (Indian elecampane, *Inula racemosa*) – Known for its cardio-protective and respiratory benefits.
- *Safed Shatavari* (Indian asparagus, *Asparagus racemosus*) – A key Ayurvedic rejuvenator, especially for female reproductive health and hormonal balance.

- *Tran Bhadram* (Strawberry, *Fragaria ananassa*) – Rich in antioxidants like anthocyanins and vitamin C; supports heart and skin health.

Establishing a nutraceutical garden with these herbs can serve as a sustainable, educational, and therapeutic initiative for communities, health centres, and academic institutions. It not only enhances biodiversity but also fosters awareness of the value of traditional knowledge in modern healthcare.

Pharmaceutical Gardens: A pharmaceutical garden is cultivated with the primary objective of growing medicinal plants used in the production of drugs and therapeutic compounds (Fig.12.4). These gardens are meticulously designed to nurture specific herbs and plants recognized for their pharmacological properties. Some key pharmaceutical plants include: *Aloe vera, Ashwagandha (Withania somnifera), Atis (Aconitum heterophyllum), Kututiktaha/Chirata (Swertia chirayita), Amlaparni/Dolu/*Himalayan rhubarb *(Rheum australe), Kalmegh/ Mahatikta/Mahatita (Andrographis paniculata), Kuth (Saussurea lappa), Anjani, Kutki (Picrorhiza kurroa), Madhukari (Stevia rebaudiana), Supita/Mamiri (Coptis teeta), Jalayashti/Mulethi (Glycyrrhiza glabra), Punarnava (Boerhavia diffusa), Nityakalyani/ Sadabahar (Catharanthus roseus),* and *Vasa/ Adusa (Adhatoda vasica).*

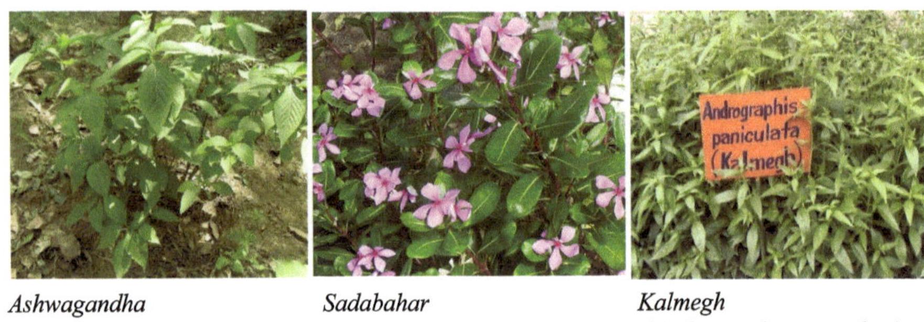

Ashwagandha (*Withania somnifera*) | *Sadabahar* *(Catharanthus roseus)* | *Kalmegh* (*Andrographis paniculata*)

Fig. 12.4. *Selected herbs representing plants of a pharmaceutical garden.*

Aromaceutical Gardens: An aromaceutical garden is a specialized garden dedicated to cultivating aromatic plants with medicinal or therapeutic properties. These gardens focus on growing species used in aromatherapy, herbal medicine, and natural wellness practices. Plants are selected for their fragrance, essential oil content, and healing benefits (Fig. 12.5). Various plant parts—such as flowers, leaves, wood, roots, and resins—are utilized for their aromatic qualities and therapeutic effects. Beyond creating a fragrant and calming environment, aromaceutical gardens play a vital role in promoting health and well-being, offering natural resources for both preventive and curative healthcare. Some common aromaceutical plants are: *Raat ki Rani* (Night-blooming jasmine, *Cestrum nocturnum),* African blue basil *(Ocimum kilimandscharicum),* American basil

(Ocimum americanum), Amrita Tulsi (*Ocimum tenuiflorum*), Bulgarian rose *(Rosa damascena),* Chamomile (*Matricaria chamomilla*), Citronella (*Cymbopogon nardus*), *Safed Champa* (*Plumeria alba*), Geranium *(Pelargonium graveolens), Jufa* (hyssopus, *Hyssopus officinalis*), Jasmine (*Jasminum officinale*), *Jatamansi* (*Nardostachys jatamansi*), Juniperus (*Juniperus communis*), Lavender (*Lavandula angustifolia*), Lemon balm (*Melissa officinalis*), Lemon basil (*Ocimum* × *citriodorum* Vis.), Lemon grass (*Cymbopogon citratus*), *Kedarpati (Skimmia laureola*), Corn mint (*Mentha arvensis*), *Rama Tulsi/Shyama Tulsi* (*Ocimum sanctum*), *Sameva (Valeriana hardwickii),* Sweet basil *(Ocimum basilicum),* Thai basil (*Ocimum basilicum* var. *thyrsiflora),* Thyme (*Thymus vulgaris*), *Van Tulsi* (*Ocimum gratissimum*) and Vietnamese basil (*Ocimum* × *africanum*).

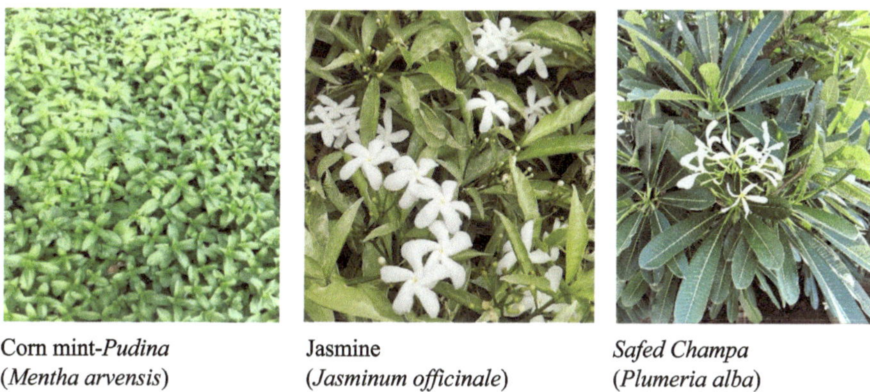

Corn mint-*Pudina* (*Mentha arvensis*)

Jasmine (*Jasminum officinale*)

Safed Champa (*Plumeria alba*)

Fig. 12.5. *Some popular plants of aromaceutical garden.*

Herbal Spices Gardens: Spices are natural plant products valued for enhancing the flavour, aroma, and colour of food, as well as for their roles in traditional medicine, cosmetics, and perfumery. A herbal spice garden (Fig. 12.6) can feature the following plants, known for both culinary and therapeutic benefits:

- *Badi Elaichi* (*Amomum subulatum*) – Aromatic pods used in sweets and beverages; aids digestion.
- *Bhang Jeera* (*Perilla frutescens*) – Leaves and seeds used for seasoning; known for anti-inflammatory properties.
- *Choru/Chora* (*Angelica glauca*) – Roots used as a spice and carminative; cultivated in Himalayan regions.
- *Dalchini* (*Cinnamomum verum*) – Bark used for flavouring; has antioxidant and antimicrobial properties.
- Dill (*Anethum graveolens*) – Seeds and leaves used in pickling and digestion remedies.

- *Fennel* (*Foeniculum vulgare*) – Seeds used for flavour and as a mouth freshener; supports gut health.
- *Hing* (*Ferula foetida*) – Resin with strong aroma; used as an anti-flatulent and digestive aid.
- *Jakhya* (*Cleome viscosa*) – Seeds used for tempering in traditional dishes; known for antimicrobial effects.
- *Jambu/Faran* (*Allium stracheyi*) – Himalayan wild garlic; adds flavour and supports respiratory health.
- *Kala Jeera* (*Bunium persicum*) – Aromatic seeds used in pulao and curries; grown in cool climates.
- *Kari Patta* (*Murraya koenigii*) – Leaves used in tempering; rich in antioxidants and iron.
- Oregano (*Origanum vulgare*) – Dried leaves used in seasoning; known for antifungal properties.
- *Tejpat* (*Cinnamomum tamala*) – Aromatic leaves used in Indian cooking; improves appetite and digestion.
- Timur pepper (*Zanthoxylum armatum*) – Tingling spice used in pickles; valued for analgesic effects.
- Thyme (*Thymus vulgaris*) – Herb with a strong aroma; used for respiratory and antiseptic purposes.
- *Van Ajwain* (*Thymus linearis*) – Wild thyme from Himalayan regions; used in teas and traditional remedies.

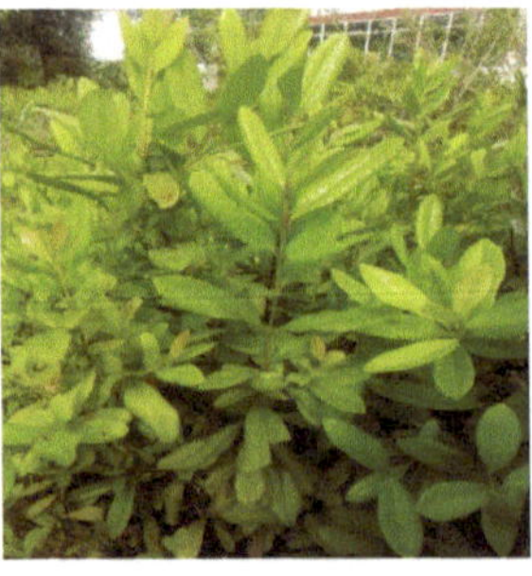

Dalchini (*Cinnamomum verum*)

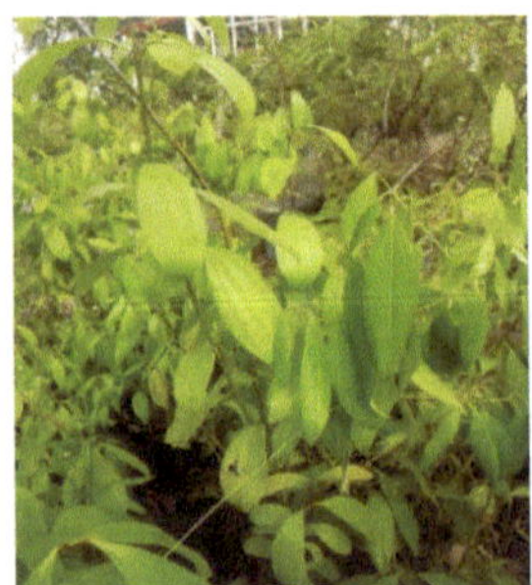

Tejpat (*Cinnamomum tamala*)

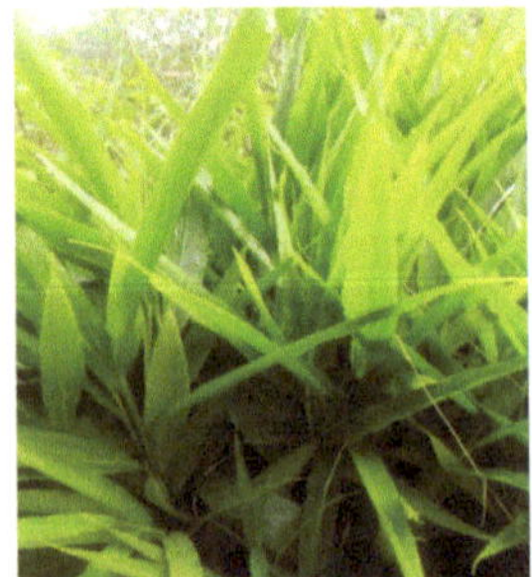

Elaichi (*Amomum subulatum*)

Fig. 12.6. *Selected herbs of spice garden.*

Cosmeceutical Gardens: These gardens are specialized spaces cultivated for plants that offer both cosmetic and therapeutic benefits. Herbal cosmetics—

often termed natural cosmetics—utilize plant-derived ingredients in various forms, including raw plant parts (leaves, flowers, fruits, seeds, stems, bark, roots, rhizomes) and processed products such as extracts, fresh juices, fixed oils, essential oils, resins, gums, and dried powders. These natural substances are valued for their antioxidant, anti-inflammatory, antimicrobial, and nourishing properties that support skin health, hair vitality, and overall beauty care. A well-planned cosmeceutical garden may include medicinal herbs, aromatic plants, and botanicals (Fig. 12.7) rich in bioactive compounds used in skincare, haircare, and holistic wellness formulations such as:

- *Akarkara (Anacyclus pyrethrum)* – Stimulates blood circulation; used in skin tonics.
- *Arandi (Ricinus communis)* – Source of castor oil; beneficial for hair and skin hydration.
- *Bhringraj (Eclipta prostrata)* – Renowned for promoting hair growth and scalp health.
- *Bhutkeshi (Selinum vaginatum)* – Aromatic herb used in stress-relief and skin formulations.
- *Sindoor (Bixa orellana)* – Natural pigment; used in lipsticks and skin colourants.
- *Chandan (Santalum album)* – Soothes and cools the skin; used in anti-blemish creams.
- *Ghritkumari (Aloe vera)* – Moisturizing and healing; widely used in skin and hair care.
- *Ginkgo (Ginkgo biloba)* – Rich in antioxidants; supports skin regeneration and anti-aging.
- *Gudhal (Hibiscus rosa-sinensis)* – Strengthens hair and adds shine; also used in facial masks.
- *Haldi (Curcuma longa)* – Anti-inflammatory and antimicrobial; improves skin tone and clarity.
- Jasmine *(Jasminum officinale)* – Fragrant and calming; used in perfumes and soothing lotions.
- *Kapur Kachri (Hedychium spicatum)* – Aromatic rhizome with cleansing properties for hair.
- *Manjishtha (Rubia cordifolia)* – Promotes skin detoxification and glow; used in complexion enhancers.

- *Mehndi (Lawsonia inermis)* – Natural dye for hair and skin; also has cooling properties.
- *Zaitoon (Olea europaea)* – Nourishing oil used in moisturizers and conditioners.
- *Reetha* (*Sapindus mukorossi*) – Natural cleanser; used in herbal shampoos and facial washes.
- *Sameva* (*Valeriana hardwickii*) – Calming herb; incorporated in stress-relief and sleep-aid cosmetics.
- *Shikakai* (*Acacia concinna*) – Traditional hair cleanser and conditioner.
- *Vajradanti* (*Barleria prionitis*) – Used in dental care products for its antimicrobial activity.

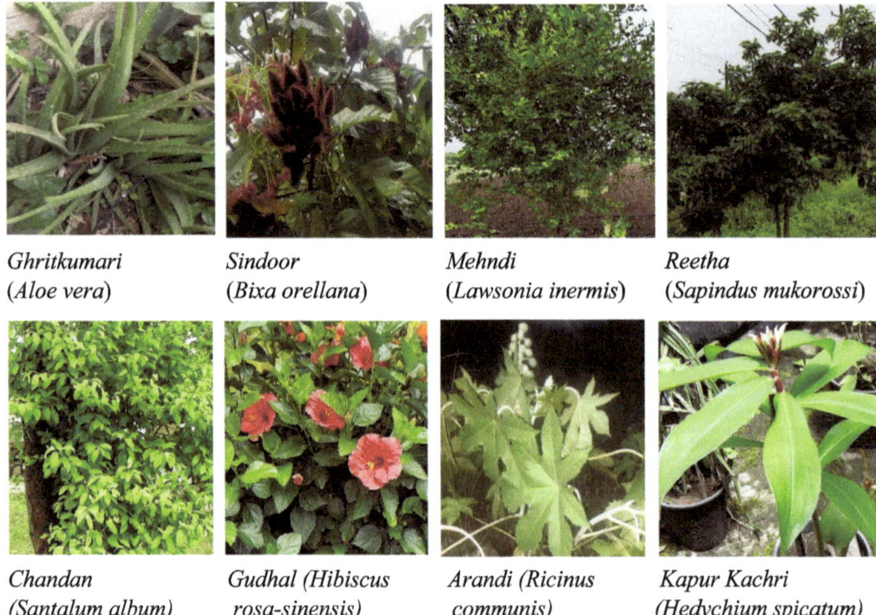

Ghritkumari (*Aloe vera*) *Sindoor* (*Bixa orellana*) *Mehndi* (*Lawsonia inermis*) *Reetha* (*Sapindus mukorossi*)

Chandan (Santalum album) *Gudhal (Hibiscus rosa-sinensis)* *Arandi (Ricinus communis)* *Kapur Kachri (Hedychium spicatum)*

Fig. 12.7. *Selected herbs recommended for cosmeceutical garden.*

Repellent Plant Gardens: A repellent plant garden consists of plant species known for their ability to naturally repel insects, nematodes, and other pests. These plants (Fig. 12.8) are commonly used in companion planting for pest control in agricultural fields, gardens, and even households. Their aromatic compounds or essential oils act as natural deterrents, offering an eco-friendly alternative to synthetic pesticides. Below are examples of such plants along with their specific repellent properties:

- Achillea or Yarrow *(Achillea millefolium*) – Repels aphids, ants, and beetles. Its strong scent confuses insects and reduces pest infestation.

- Basil *(Ocimum basilicum)* – Known to deter mosquitoes, whiteflies, and thrips. Its essential oil contains compounds like estragole and linalool.
- Buch or Sweet flag *(Acorus calamus)* – Has insecticidal properties and repels mosquitoes, lice, and flies through its aromatic rhizome.
- Citronella *(Cymbopogon nardus)* – Highly effective against mosquitoes; its oil is a common ingredient in natural insect repellents.
- Garlic *(Allium sativum)* – Repels aphids, ants, mosquitoes, and beetles due to its strong sulphur-containing compounds.
- Geranium *(Pelargonium graveolens)* – Especially effective against mosquitoes; also deters cabbage worms and leafhoppers.
- Lavender *(Lavandula angustifolia)* – Repels moths, fleas, flies, and mosquitoes with its soothing but pungent aroma.
- Lemongrass *(Cymbopogon citratus)* – Similar to citronella, repels mosquitoes and houseflies through its lemon-scented essential oil.
- Mint *(Mentha piperita)* – Acts against ants, aphids, and cabbage moths; the strong menthol scent deters many insects.
- Neem *(Azadirachta indica)* – Effective against a wide range of pests including aphids, whiteflies, nematodes, and caterpillars; contains azadirachtin, a natural insect growth regulator.
- Five-leaved chaste tree, *Nirgundi (Vitex negundo)* – Repels mosquitoes and other biting insects; often used in traditional fumigants.
- Pyrethrum *(Chrysanthemum cinerariifolium)* – Source of pyrethrin, which paralyzes and repels mosquitoes, ticks, and flies.
- Rosemary *(Salvia rosmarinus)* – Repels mosquitoes, cabbage moths, and carrot flies with its aromatic oils.
- Indian bay leaf, *Tejpat (Cinnamomum tamala)* – Known to deter ants, weevils, and mosquitoes; contains eugenol and cinnamaldehyde.
- Wild Marigold *(Tagetes minuta)* – Repels whiteflies, nematodes, and aphids; its root secretions are nematicidal.
- Wild Mint *(Mentha arvensis)* – Similar to peppermint, effective against ants, aphids, and other soft-bodied insects.

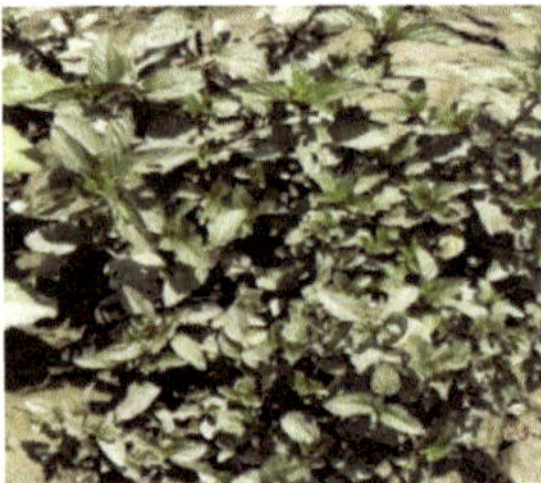

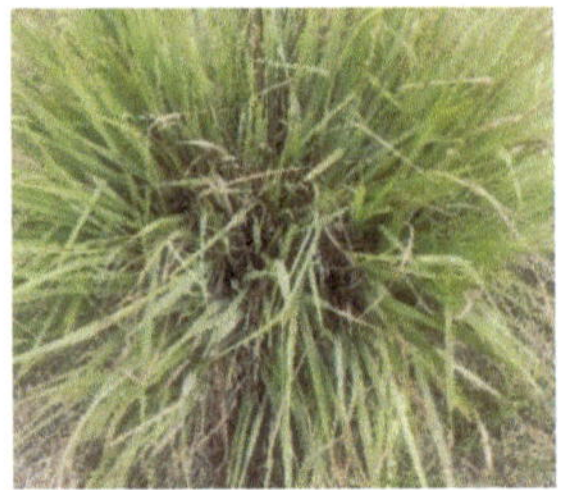

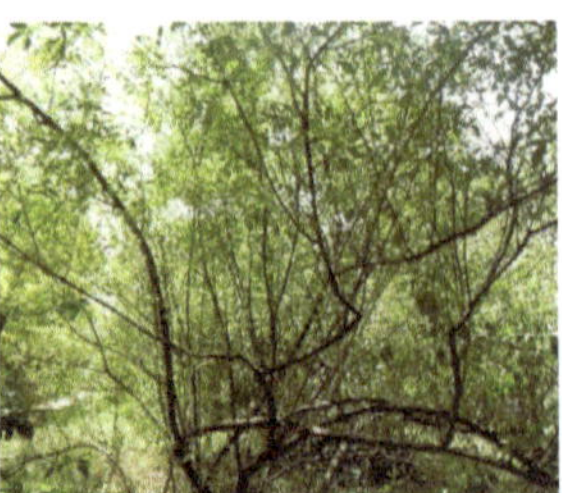

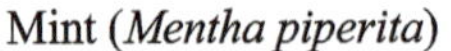

Mint (*Mentha piperita*) Lemongrass (*Cymbopogon citratus*) Five-leaved chaste tree, *Nirgundi* (*Vitex negundo*)

Fig. 12.8. *Selected herbs recommended for repellent gardens.*

Aquatic Herbal Gardens

An aquatic herbal garden is a specialized space designed to cultivate aquatic and semi-aquatic plants that thrive in wetland ecosystems and offer significant medicinal and ecological value. These plants have diverse applications, including use in traditional and modern medicine, nutraceuticals, food, agriculture, and green material synthesis. Crude extracts and pure compounds derived from various parts of these plants possess notable nutritional and pharmacological properties. Their phytochemicals are used to treat a range of infectious and non-infectious ailments. Additionally, many aquatic and semi-aquatic species are involved in the green synthesis of metal and metal oxide nanomaterials, which have promising industrial and biomedical applications (Arya *et al.* 2022). Aquatic herbal gardens (Fig. 12.9) make efficient use of water-rich areas—such as ponds, marshes, and riverbanks — by transforming them into productive spaces for growing medicinal herbs. This not only conserves underutilized wetland land but also enhances biodiversity and visual appeal. Well-designed gardens combine aesthetic beauty with practical utility, serving as living pharmacies while supporting ecological balance. The inclusion of oxygenating species like Hornwort (*Ceratophyllum demersum*) and *Anacharis* (*Elodea canadensis*) helps maintain water quality and ecosystem health. By creatively utilizing wetland habitats, aquatic herbal gardens promote wellness, biodiversity, and landscape restoration. Examples of medicinal aquatic and semi-aquatic plants include:

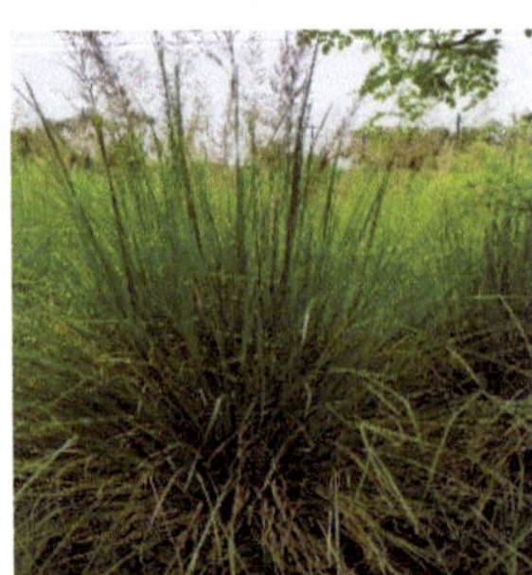

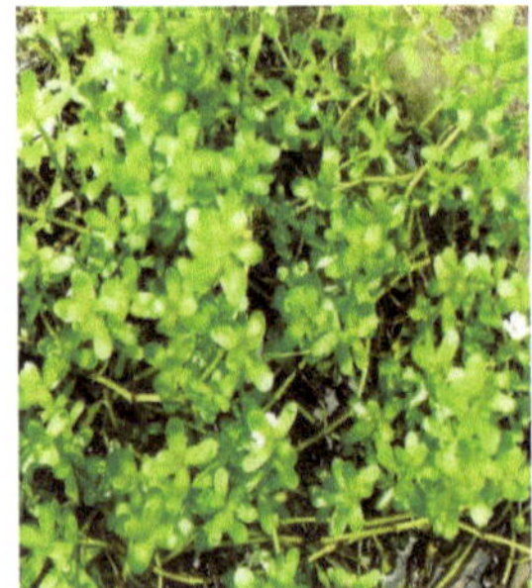

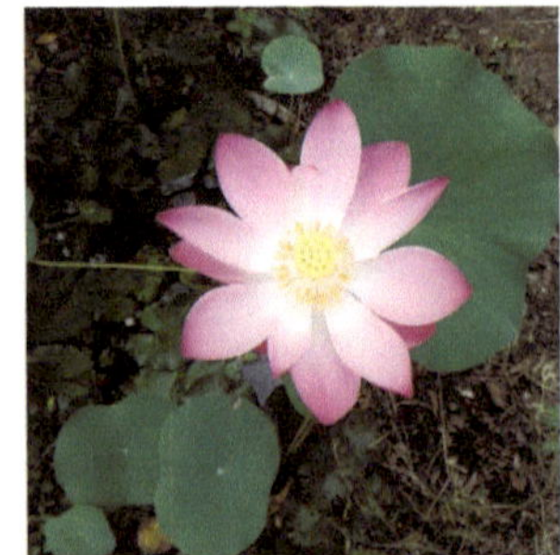

Khas (*Chrysopogon zizanioides*) *Brahmi* (*Bacopa monnieri*) Lotus (*Nelumbo nucifera*)

Fig. 12.9. *Selected aquatic garden plants.*

- *Brahmi (Bacopa monnieri)* – Enhances cognitive function and is used in the treatment of anxiety and epilepsy.
- *Mandukparni or Brahmi (Centella asiatica)* – Known for wound healing, memory enhancement, and skin care.
- *Buch or Vacha (Acorus calamus)* – Traditionally used for digestive and neurological disorders.
- *Pudina (Mentha spicata)* – Used to relieve indigestion, nausea, and respiratory ailments.
- *Madhupatra (Stevia rebaudiana*) – A natural sweetener with potential anti-diabetic properties.
- *Kamal,* Lotus *(Nelumbo nucifera*) – Used in Ayurveda for bleeding disorders, diarrhea, and inflammation.
- *Kumudini,* Water lily *(Nymphaea odorata)* – Known for its calming and anti-inflammatory effects.
- *Khas, (Chrysopogon zizanioides)* – Used for cooling, skin protection, and anxiety relief.
- *Kusha (Desmostachya bipinnata)* – Considered sacred and used in purification rituals and traditional medicine.
- *Singonium,* Arrowhead *(Sagittaria sagittifolia)* – Roots are used for digestive and diuretic purposes.
- *Makhana (*fox nut, *Euryale ferox)* – A nutrient-rich aquatic crop used in reproductive and renal health.
- *Kutu,* Marsh buckwheat *(Polygonum glabrum)* – Traditionally used for treating dysentery.
- *Kalmi Saag,* Water spinach (*Ipomoea aquatica*) – A nutritious vegetable with antioxidant and detoxifying effects.
- *Jalkumbhī,* Water cabbage (*Pistia stratiotes*) – Has antimicrobial and wound-healing applications.
- *Chhoti Jalkumbhi,* Duckweed (*Lemna minor*) – Known for its cooling, detoxifying properties and potential in water purification.

Arogya Vatika and Charak-Gardens

These are specialized herbal gardens established to cultivate medicinal plants that promote health, immunity, and overall well-being. Based on Ayurvedic principles, these gardens focus on plants with recognized therapeutic properties. *Arogya Vatika,* often located in educational institutions, public parks, and community spaces, aims to raise awareness about the health benefits of traditional medicinal plants. These gardens typically feature species such as *tulsi (Ocimum sanctum), Neem (Azadirachta indica), Giloy (Tinospora cordifolia),* and *Ashwagandha (Withania somnifera),* all renowned for their immune-boosting and healing effects. Unlike pharmaceutical gardens—which are dedicated to cultivating plants for modern drug development and commercial medicine—*Arogya Vatikas* emphasize wellness and preventive healthcare through traditional remedies.

Charak-Gardens named in honour of Acharya Charak, the eminent ancient Ayurvedic scholar, focus specifically on herbs used in classical Ayurvedic treatments. These gardens commonly grow plants like *Brahmi (Bacopa monnieri), Sarpagandha (Rauvolfia serpentina), Shatavari (Asparagus racemosus), Baheda (Terminalia bellirica) and Harad or Haritaki (Terminalia chebula), Vasak (Adhatoda vasica),* which are Ayurvedic formulations for managing a wide range of ailments. Together, Arogya Vatika and Charak-Gardens (Fig. 12.10) serve as living repositories of India's rich medicinal plant heritage, fostering health education and preserving traditional knowledge systems.

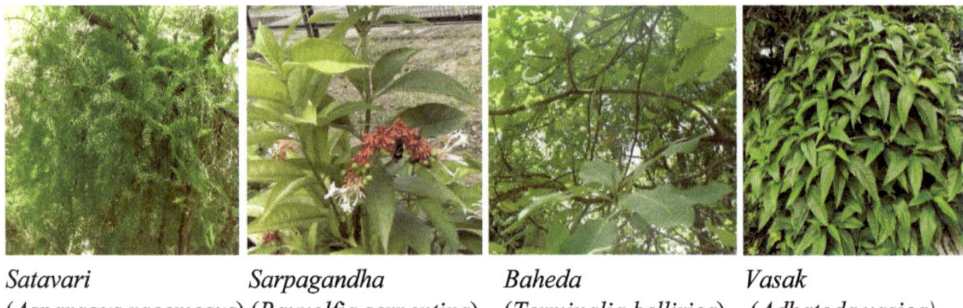

Satavari (Asparagus racemosus) *Sarpagandha (Rauvolfia serpentina)* *Baheda (Terminalia bellirica)* *Vasak (Adhatoda vasica)*

Fig. 12.10. *Selected plants of Charak-Garden.*

Manav Herbal Garden/ Manav Vatika

The *Manav* herbal garden (or *Manav Vatika*) is a unique thematic concept in which the entire garden is landscaped in the shape of a human body. Medicinal plants (Fig. 12.11) are carefully planted in specific body parts based on their traditional and popular uses for ailments related to those areas. This innovative design allows visitors to easily understand and visualize the correlation between each plant and its therapeutic application in a natural and intuitive manner. The garden serves as a living repository of traditional knowledge, helping to preserve age-old intellectual property. It also raises awareness among the general public, students, and researchers about the practical, everyday use of medicinal plants in human health. Table 12.4 lists some plants suitable for the Manav herbal garden.

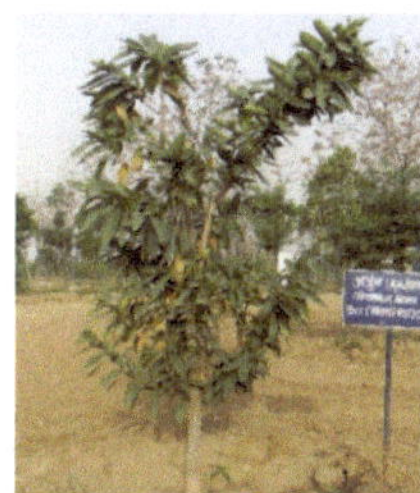
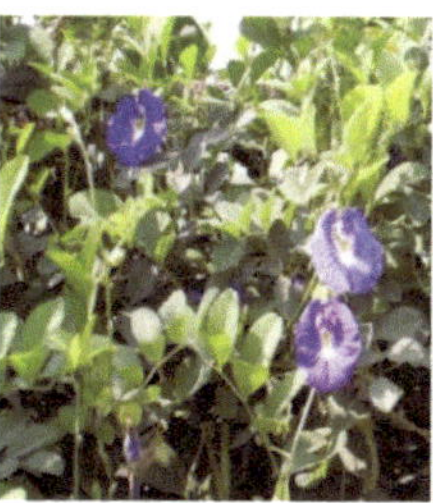
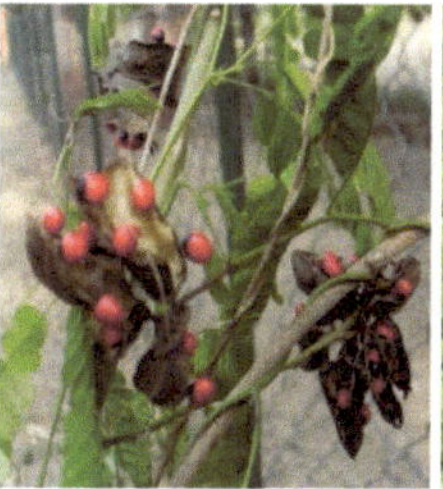
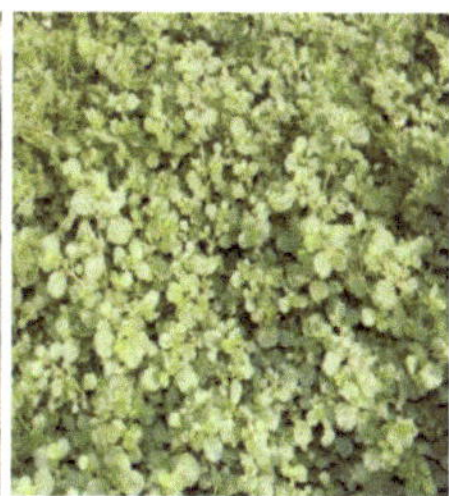

Arjuna (Terminalia arjuna) *Aprajita (Clitoria ternatea)* *Ratti (Abrus precatorius)* *Punarnava (Boerhavia diffusa)*

Fig. 12.11. *Selected Manav herbal garden plants.*

Table 12.4: Plants suitable for Manav herbal garden (Fig. 12.11)

Common Name: Hindi/ English	Botanical Name	Parts of Plant Used	Body Parts Targeted
Bhringraj / False daisy	*Eclipta alba*	Leaves as hair tonic	Hair
Neel / Indigo	*Indigofera tinctoria*	Leaves as hair tonic	
Tulsi / Holy basil	*Ocimum sanctum*	Whole plant for oil extraction and flavouring beverages	
Gudhal / Tropical hibiscus	*Hibiscus rosa-sinensis*	Flower extract	
Brahmi /Water hyssop	*Bacopa monnieri*	Whole plant as brain tonic	Brain
Vacha /Sweet flag	*Acorus calamus*	Rhizome as brain tonic	
Aprajita / Butterfly pea	*Clitoria ternatea*	Root as brain tonic	
Chandni / Pinwheel flower	*Tabarnaemontana coronaria Tabernaemontana divaricata*	Flower bud for red eye disease	Eyes, ears, nose and mouth
Kanchari / Joy weed	*Alternanthera brasiliana*	Leaves for eye disorder	
Durva / Bermuda grass	*Cynodon dactylon*	Dry leaf powder for nasal bleeding	
Akarkara / Toothache plant	*Acmella calva*	Flower for tooth pain	
Nirgundi / Five-leaved chaste tree	*Vitex negundo*	Leaves for tonsilitis	
Hadjod / Veld grape	*Cissus quadrangularis*	Stem extract for emmenagogue	
Katumbi / Cupid's shaving brush)	*Emilia sonchifolia*	Leaves for tonsillitis	

Common Name: Hindi/ English	Botanical Name	Parts of Plant Used	Body Parts Targeted
Rugmini / Flame of woods	*Ixora coccinea*	Flower for skin disease	Skin
Ratti / Rosary pea	*Abrus precatorius*	Fruit for skin disease	
Ghritkumari /Aloes	*Aloe vera*	Leaves as cosmetics	
Manjishtha / Indian madder	*Rubia cordifolia*	Roots for skin disease	
Anantmool / Indian sarsaparilla	*Hemidesmus indicus*	Roots for skin disease	
Ratanjot / Gout plant	*Jatropha podagrica*	Leaves for skin disease	
Pathar chatta / Life plant	*Kalanchoe pinnata*	Leaves for burn healing	
Lal chitrak / Indian leadwort	*Plumbago indica*	Roots against glycoderma	
Chapakno / Sticky desmodium tree	*Pseudarthria viscida*	Roots are cardio tonic	Heart
Shalparni / Tick clover	*Desmodium gangeticum*	Roots are cardio tonic	
Sheetal chini / Jamaican pepper	*Pimenta dioica*	Fruit used as cardiotonic	
Arjun / Arjun tree	*Terminalia arjuna*	Bark	
Shankh adrak / Shell ginger	*Alpinia zerumbet*	Rhizome as expectorant	Lungs
Arkaparni / Indian ipecac	*Tylophora indica* syn. *Tylophora asthmatica*	Roots as anti-asthmatic	
Vasaka/ Malabar nut	*Adhatoda vasica*	Roots for cough	
Kalmegh / Green chiretta	*Andrographis paniculata*	Whole plant as liver tonic	Liver
Hulhul, Bagro / Tick weed	*Cleome viscosa*	Whole plant as liver tonic	
Hajardana / Stonebreaker	*Phyllanthus niruri*	Whole plant as liver tonic	
Gurmar, Madhunasini / Gymnema	*Gymnema sylvestre*	Literally translates to sugar *destroyer*, leaves are used for managing diabetes.	Pancreas
Koṣṭaka / Spiral flag	*Chamecostus cuspidatus*	Leaves are traditionally used as antidiabetic	
Aam haldi / Mango ginger	*Curcuma amada*	Rhizome used in stomach disorders	Abdomen
Kalijiri / Bitter cumin	*Vernonia anthelmintica*	Seed as germicide	
Amrit sak / Indian sorrel	*Oxalis corniculata*	Leaves for stomach disorder	

Common Name: Hindi/ English	Botanical Name	Parts of Plant Used	Body Parts Targeted
Bharangi, Jambuka / Stemless premna	*Premna herbacea*	Leaves are used as diuretic	
Dabh, Kusha / Sacrificial grass	*Desmostachya bipinnata*	Leaves are diuretic	Urinary tract
Punarnava /Hog weed	*Boerhavia diffusa*	Roots are diuretic	
Mithi patti, Asmaghn / Liquorice weed	*Scoparia dulcis*	Leaves are used to cure kidney stone	
Kali musli / Black musli	*Curculigo orchioides*	Whole plant used as haemostatic	
Bhui bhui, Kapuri jadi, / Mountain knotgrass	*Aerva lanata*	Whole plant used to treat kidney stone	
Arjaka / Java tea	*Orthosiphon grandiflorus*	Leaves used to treat kidney stone	

(Source: Compiled from ICAR-Central Coastal Agricultural Research Institute Goa, Maneesha et al. 2021, and various open-access, classical, and scholarly references).

Herbal Tea Gardens

Herbal tea gardens are a delightful and therapeutic areas where medicinal herbs are cultivated specifically for preparing hot or cold infusions or teas. These herbal brews offer a range of health benefits, supporting the correction of nutrient imbalances and promoting overall well-being. Examples of commonly grown herbs include:

- Chamomile (*Matricaria recutita*)
- Lemongrass (*Cymbopogon citratus*)
- Lemon balm (*Melissa officinalis*)
- Thyme (*Thymus vulgaris*)
- Rosemary (*Salvia rosmarinus*)
- Ginger (*Zingiber officinale*)
- Tulsi (*Ocimum tenuiflorum* L., syn. *O. sanctum*)

Each of these herbs offers unique health-promoting properties, making them excellent choices for a diverse and functional tea garden. Cultivating them together not only provides a rich variety of flavours but also creates a natural apothecary for addressing everyday health concerns.

Herbal Gardens Designed for Children and Persons with Disabilities (Divyang)

These specialized herbal gardens (Fig. 12.12) can serve as enriching additions to parks, playgrounds, or recreational areas. Designed with accessibility in mind, they offer a safe and interactive space where children—including those with visual impairments or other disabilities—can explore the plant world through touch, smell, and taste. These gardens can feature medicinal and aromatic plants known for their distinctive sensory properties, such as texture, fragrance, and flavour. Some of the suggested plants that are ideal for herbal gardens for children and individuals with disabilities (Divyang), focusing on sensory stimulation (touch, smell, taste, and sight), safety, and ease of identification include:

Touch-Friendly Plants (Interesting Texture): Select plants in this category include:

- Aloe *(Aloe vera)* –Smooth fleshy, gel-filled leaves.
- *Lajwanti (Mimosa pudica)* – Known as Sensitive or Touch-me-not plant; leaflets fold inward when touched.
- Lamb's ear (*Stachys byzantina*) – Soft, velvety leaves that are pleasant to touch.
- Mint varieties (*Mentha* spp.) – Leaves are slightly fuzzy and cool to the touch.
- Velvet leaf (*Abutilon* spp.) – Broad, soft leaves with a velvety texture.
- Snake plant (*Sansevieria trifasciata*) – Tall, upright leaves with a firm, smooth surface

Scented/ Fragrant Plants (Smell Stimulation): A wide variety of plants emit pleasant fragrances, which inspire people's emotional state and may alleviate stress. Some of these plants include:

- Scented geraniums (*Pelargonium* spp.) – Leaves release various scents like lemon, rose, or mint.
- Curry leaf plant (*Murraya koenigii*) – Strong aromatic foliage, common in Indian cuisine.
- Jasmine (*Jasminum* spp.) – Intense floral fragrance, very appealing and calming.
- Indian Bay leaf (*Cinnamomum tamala*) – Aromatic foliage used in cooking.

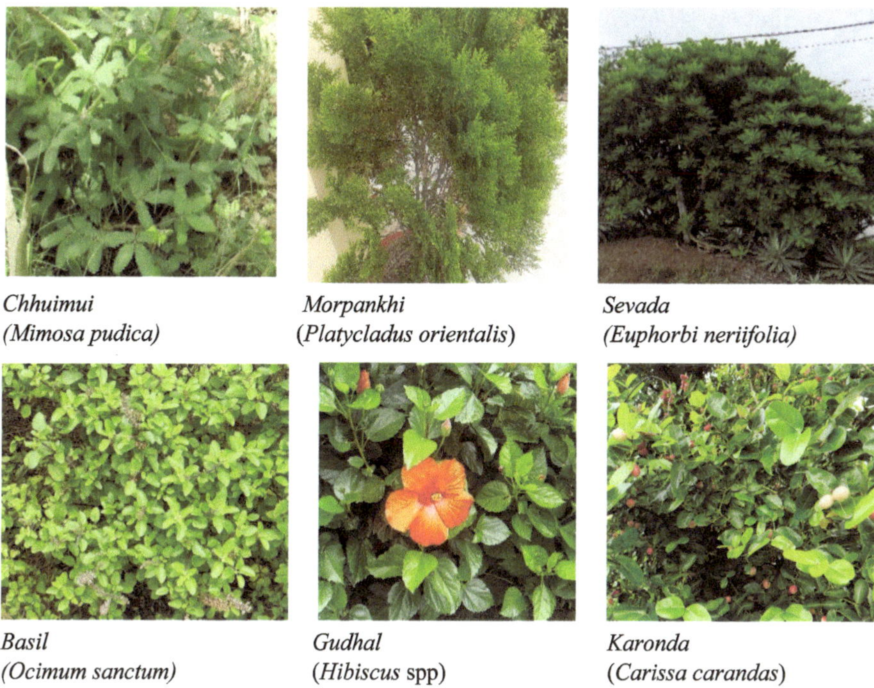

Chhuimui (Mimosa pudica) *Morpankhi (Platycladus orientalis)* *Sevada (Euphorbi neriifolia)*

Basil (Ocimum sanctum) *Gudhal (Hibiscus* spp) *Karonda (Carissa carandas)*

Fig. 12.12. *Common plants recommended for herbal gardens for persons with disabilities (Divyang).*

Taste-safe and Mildly Flavoured Plants: Some select plants in this category include:

- Stevia (*Stevia rebaudiana*) – Naturally sweet leaves.
- Fennel (*Foeniculum vulgare*) – Sweet, licorice-flavoured leaves and seeds.
- Basil varieties (*Ocimum* spp.) – Many types with varying flavours (e.g., lemon basil, cinnamon basil).
- Coriander/Cilantro (*Coriandrum sativum*) – Fresh herbal flavour; safe in small quantities.

Visually Stimulating Plants (Colour and Form): Various studies have reported physiological and psychological effects after visual stimulation with green and attractive flowering plants. Some of these plants comprise

- Calendula (*Calendula officinalis*) – Bright yellow/orange flowers with medicinal uses.
- Marigold (*Tagetes* spp.) – Vibrant blooms, often used in sensory gardens.
- Butterfly pea (*Clitoria ternatea*) – Deep blue flowers; petals used for tea.
- Coleus (*Coleus* spp.) – Colorful foliage with contrasting patterns.

- Hibiscus (*Hibiscus rosa-sinensis*) – Large, vibrant red, pink, yellow, and white blossoms creating striking focal point in a garden.

These plants are selected for their sensory appeal, non-toxicity, low maintenance, and therapeutic or educational value in inclusive garden settings.

Disease-Based Herbal Gardens

Disease-based herbal gardens are thematically designed collections of medicinal plants selected for their scientifically validated therapeutic effects against specific diseases. The layout and selection of species are based on traditional knowledge systems, Ayurvedic principles, and modern pharmacological research, ensuring the plants chosen possess active phytochemicals, established mechanisms of action, and ethnomedicinal relevance. For instance, an antidiabetic herbal garden focuses on plants that have been used in traditional medicine and shown varying degree of hypoglycemic and antihyperglycemic activity. These may include *Aegle marmelos, Allium cepa, Allium sativum, Andrographis paniculata, Brassica juncea, Cinnamomum tamala, Gymnema sylvestre, Momordica charantia, Murraya koenigii, Mucuna pruriens, Tinospora cordifolia, Trigonella foenum-graecum, Syzygium cumini* and *Ocimum tenuiflorum* (Grover *et al.* 2002, Gupta *et al.* 2007, Gupta *et al.* 2017). Herbal gardens targeting cancer prevention and treatment may feature species such as *Catharanthus roseus* (known for its vincristine and vinblastine content), *Andrographis paniculata* (noted for its immunomodulatory and anti-tumour properties), and *Podophyllum peltatum* (a source of podophyllotoxin, used in anticancer drugs). Similarly, a garden focusing on anti-malarial and mosquito-repellent plants might include *Azadirachta indica, Morinda lucida, Cymbopogon citratus, Ocimum tenuiflorum* and *Vitex peduncularis*, which have shown antiplasmodial activity and vector-repellent effects (Shankar *et al.* 2012). An antioxidant-rich herbal garden could incorporate species such as *Acacia arabica* (*babul*), *Curcuma longa* and, *Glycyrrhiza glabra* (licorice), *Cinnamomum zeylanicum* (true cinnamon), *Moringa oleifera* (drumstick tree), *Pimenta dioica, Piper betle, Piper nigrum* and *Tinospora cordifolia*, all of which contain potent free-radical scavenging compounds with applications in preventing oxidative stress-related disorders (Aoshima *et al.* 2007, Alok *et al.* 2014). A dermatological and skin care herbal garden may raise *Aloe vera, Calendula officinalis, Azadirachta indica, Curcuma longa, Centella asiatica* etc.

Rock Herbal Garden

Herbs that grow in rocky, windswept areas often face challenging conditions like poor soil and harsh weather. These tough environments encourage the plants to develop stronger essential oils and more intense flavours as a survival strategy. Rock herbal gardens are carefully designed to replicate these natural, rugged conditions by utilizing rocky slopes and hillsides to cultivate herbs. Research shows that herbs grown in such rocky terrains are often healthier, more aromatic, and have more potent flavours than those grown in nutrient-rich, fertile soil. Some common herbs that thrive in rock gardens include: *Patharchatta* (*Bryophyllum pinnatum*), *Pashanbheda* (*Bergenia ciliata*), *Kapur Kachri* (*Hedychium spicatum*), *Varahikand* (*Dioscorea bulbifera*), *Vidarikand* (*Pueraria tuberosa*), *Jyotishmati* (*Celastrus paniculatus*), *Timoor* (*Zanthoxylum armatum*), *Daruharidra* (*Berberis aristata*), *Amla* (*Phyllanthus emblica*), *Harad* (*Terminalia chebula*) and *Baheda* (*Terminalia bellirica*). Growing these plants in rocky conditions helps to enhance their natural medicinal properties. The stress caused by the harsh environment encourages them to produce more essential oils and beneficial compounds, giving them stronger flavours and higher potency. These qualities make them valuable for use in herbal remedies and natural health products.

Orchid Herbal Garden

Around 25,000 species of orchids have been identified worldwide, showcasing a remarkable diversity in form and colour. Some orchids have delicate, single-coloured petals, while others boast large, bulbous bodies with bold, intricate patterns such as spots and stripes. Orchids can be found in a variety of habitats, including on the ground, trees, rocks, and even on decaying organic matter. Orchids are not only prized for their beauty, but many species also hold significant medicinal value. Several medicinal orchids are known to contain bioactive compounds such as alkaloids, triterpenoids, and flavonoids, which contribute to their antimicrobial properties. One important group of medicinal orchids is *Ashtavarga,* consisting of eight species, which play a key role in Ayurvedic formulations like *Chyawanprash.* Common orchid plant species are: *Riddhi (Habenaria intermedia), Vriddhi (Habenaria edgeworthii), Jivaka (Malaxis cylindrostachys), Rishbhaka (Malaxis muscifera), Dendrobium (Dendrobium macrai), Salam Mishri (Eulophia campestris), Salep (Orchis latifolia)* and *Vanda (Vanda roxburghii)* (Sundararajan and Prasad 2019, Sharma and Gupta 2020).

Ornamental Herbal Garden

An ornamental herbal garden is a beautiful and educational space that showcases herbs valued not only for their medicinal, culinary, and aromatic properties but also for their ornamental qualities. These gardens are designed to highlight the diverse range of herbs that can enhance a garden with their flavours, fragrances, and visual appeal. Depending on the selection of plant species, an ornamental herbal garden can adopt various themes:

- Single-colour gardens: A harmonious garden featuring herbs of one colour, creating a serene and unified aesthetic.
- Multicolour gardens: A vibrant, visually stimulating garden with a variety of herbs in different colours, offering a lively and colourful display.
- Scented gardens: A garden dedicated to herbs with strong, pleasing fragrances, designed to engage the senses.

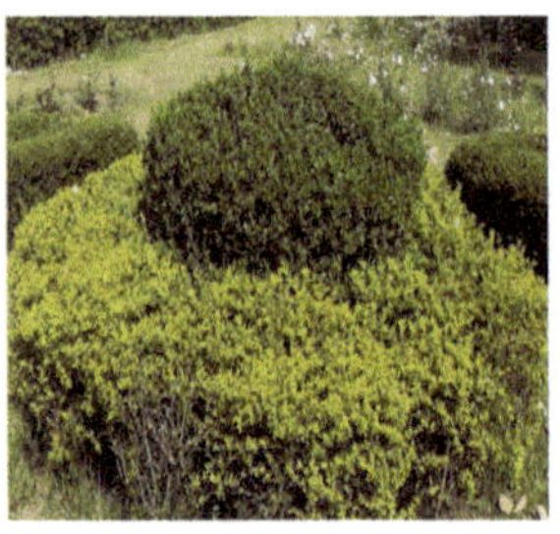

Two tier shape

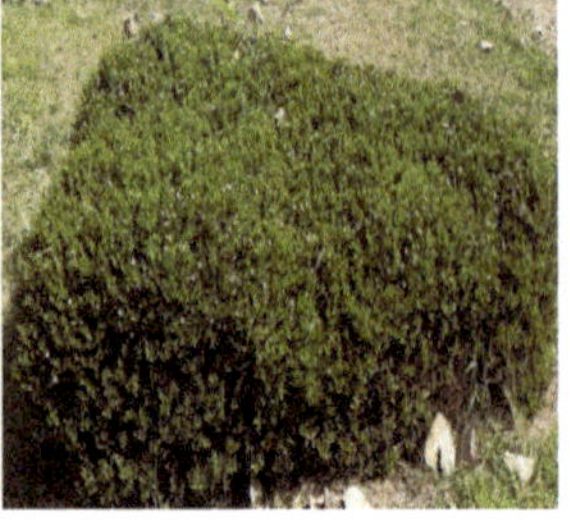

Triangular shape

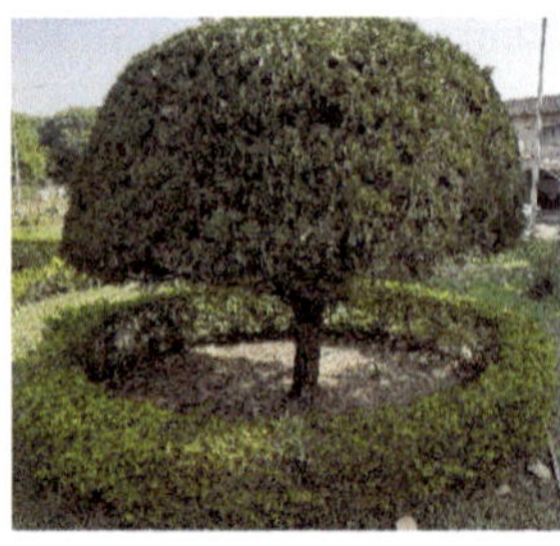

Circle with umbrella shape

Fig. 12.13. *Some popular shapes of gardens.*

Apart from their functional uses—such as for cooking, medicine, and teas—herbs can also enhance the beauty of a garden. Their varied shapes, sizes, textures, and colours make them excellent candidates for creating visually striking landscapes. An ornamental herbal garden not only introduces visitors to the practical benefits of herbs but also demonstrates how they can be incorporated into garden design to create sensory-rich spaces. Some ornamental plants of medicinal significance include: *Adhatoda vasica, Bryophyllum calycinum, Chrysanthemum cinerarifolium, Clitoria ternatea, Coleus aromaticus, Digitalis lanata, Geranium graveolens, Hibscus rosasinensis, Jasminum officinale, Jasminum sambac, Lavandula angustifolia, Matricaria chamomilla, Nelumbo nucifera, Nyctanthes arbortristis,* and *Rosa centifolia* (Prerna *et al.* 2015, https://indiagardening.com/indian-medicinal-plants-and-their-uses-with-pictures/).

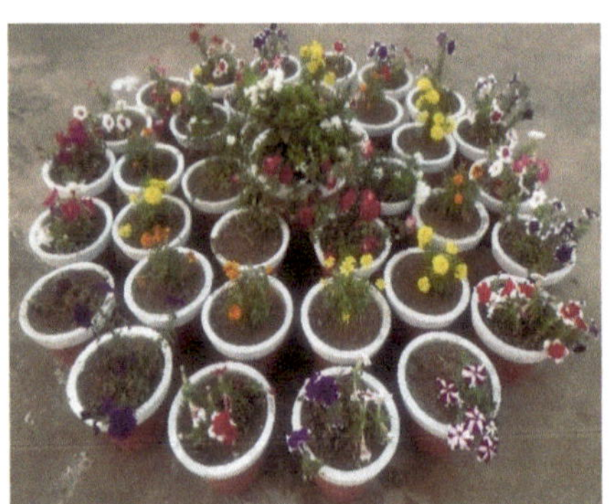

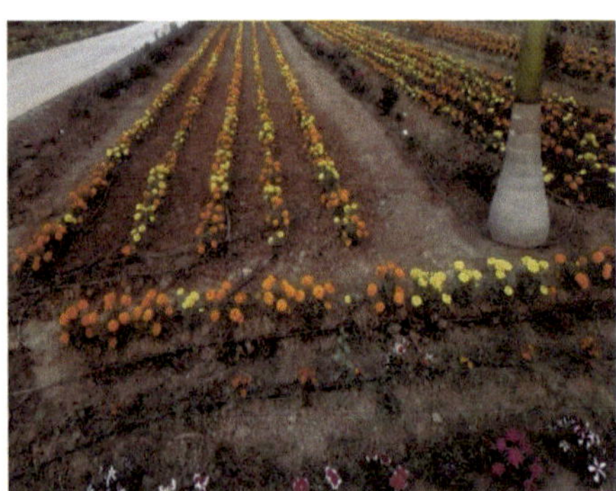

Fig. 12.14. *Ornamental herbal gardens.*

Guidelines for Establishing Herbal Garden

Procedure for establishing a herbal garden include selection of design (Figs. 12.13-12.14), size and site; plant selection; protection against trespassing; land preparation; garden layout; procurement of propagation materials; sowing, transplanting or planting; and post-planting care (Mazumdar and Mukhopadhyay 2006).

Selection of Site and Preparation

Medicinal plant materials derived from the same species can exhibit significant differences in quality when cultivated at different sites, due to the influence of soil, climate, and other factors. These differences may pertain to physical appearance or variations in their constituents, the biosynthesis of which can be affected by extrinsic environmental conditions, including ecological and geographical variables. These factors should be taken into consideration. Risks of contamination from pollution of the soil, air, or water by hazardous chemicals should be avoided. The impact of past land uses on the cultivation site, including the planting of previous crops and any applications of plant protection products, should be evaluated. Herbal gardens should be established in an area within easy reach of the user and should be free from waterlogging, weeds, pH-related problems, and legal disputes. Areas used for dumping municipal solid waste should be avoided, as they may contain heavy metals in the soil. The area should have well-drained conditions with a good source of water for irrigation. When considering the visual appeal of a thematic herbal garden, choose a location that complements the landscape. The field ought to be deeply ploughed and harrowed three times, then left for a week to eliminate soil-borne pathogens. Most herbs thrive in fertile, well-drained, weed-free soil with a pH ranging from 6 to 7. To supplement essential nutrients, incorporate well-decomposed organic manure during the final ploughing.

Size of the Herbal Garden and Cropping Plot

While the garden can vary in size, typically a minimum area of about 0.06 ha is necessary for setting up such a garden in most cases (Kumar 2020). Cropping plots should be located in sunny places, and the size of the plots will depend on their purpose. Proper spacing of plants is essential to prevent overcrowding. It is important to note that a minimum of 8 m^2 should be maintained for each species of plant in the cropping plot.

Sources of Water for Plants

There are two main sources of water for plants: rainfall and irrigation. Rainfall is a natural source of water with generally good quality, but it is limited and unpredictable. Irrigation, on the other hand, involves the planned and artificial application of water to maintain soil moisture, making it a more reliable source. The irrigation requirements of herbal plants depend on several factors:

Type of Herbal Plant: Shallow-rooted crops need light but frequent irrigation, whereas deep-rooted crops require less frequent but deeper irrigation.

Growing Season: Herbs grown in the summer season need more frequent irrigation compared to those grown in the winter season, and only occasional irrigation is needed for rainy season crops.

Climate: In cooler climates, the frequency of irrigation is lower, while in tropical or hot climates, more frequent irrigation is necessary.

Soil type: Sandy soils require frequent but light irrigation, whereas clay soils need deeper but less frequent irrigation.

Type of Irrigation System: Drip irrigation systems require regular irrigation, while surface, sub-surface, and sprinkler irrigation systems need less frequent watering.

Fencing and Protection of Selected Area

The selected area should be marked with live fencing, such as hedges, or with iron poles and chain-link fencing to prevent the entry of wild and stray animals. If there is a threat from blue bulls, the height of the fencing should be at least seven feet. A battery or electric-operated alarm or sound machine may be installed to deter birds from damaging medicinal plants.

Selection of Plants and Procurement of Planting Materials

When selecting plants for the herbal garden, it is crucial to consider the ecosystem specificity and their adaptation to the agro-meteorological conditions and microclimate of the chosen site. Equally important is aligning with the user's preferences, which should be based on their requirements or thematic choices. Without meeting the users' needs, the sustainability of such gardens could be at risk. Therefore, it is advisable to conduct an exercise to identify common health issues in the locality, understand the prevailing practices of utilizing medicinal plants, and assess the existing health care systems through a Participatory Rural Appraisal (PRA) exercise. A home garden can start with two to three varieties due to limited space and can be expanded based on affordability. Priority should be given to plant species essential for treating various ailments of children and elderly individuals. In general, while the number of species grown should be higher, the number of plants per species may be fewer. Procuring planting materials from a reliable or accredited nursery is recommended. The plants known for their medicinal virtues with respect to primary health care should be short listed using identified criteria such as: they are easy to grow, have no side- effects. Ideally, they should consist of herbs, shrubs, or climbers, avoiding trees for home gardens. However, institutional gardens may include trees.

Land Preparation

The field should be thoroughly ploughed with a mouldboard plough and left for solarization treatment for at least a week during the summer season to kill soil-borne pathogens and weeds. This should be followed by two to three harrowing and planking to level the field. Well-decomposed organic manures can be mixed with the soil during the last harrowing to supplement essential nutrients. Any chemical fertilizers, pesticides, plant growth regulators, or other chemicals should be avoided in the herbal garden. Nursery areas, footpaths, roads, beekeeping units, manure pits, labels, seating areas, and an office room can be created for better visibility. The herbal garden area should have sufficient non-shaded space with good sunlight and air circulation.

Box 12.1. Watering and Soil Tips for Herbal Gardens

Cropping plots should be placed in sunny areas, and their size should match the purpose of planting. The soil should be kept moist, but not too wet. Most herbs need about one inch (2.5 cm) of water per week. However, how often you water depends on the soil—some herbs may need water every day, while others only once a week. To check if watering is needed, stick your finger into the soil. If the top inch feels dry, it's time to water. It is helpful to use proper irrigation methods, such as surface watering, sprinklers, or drip systems, to ensure plants get enough moisture. In hot and dry climates, plants lose water faster through transpiration (from leaves) and evaporation (from soil). Strong winds can make this worse and may also cause soil erosion. Because such conditions reduce plant growth, the soil often has low organic matter, which means fewer nutrients are available to plants.

Plant Maintenance and Protection

The timely execution of practices such as topping, bud nipping, pruning and shading may be used to control the growth and development of the plant, thereby improving the quality and quantity of the medicinal plant material being produced. Any agrochemicals used to promote the growth of or to protect medicinal plants should be kept to a minimum, and applied only when no alternative measures are available with an integrated approach. Only qualified staff using approved equipment should carry out pesticide and herbicide applications. All applications should be documented. International agreements should also be consulted on pesticide use and residues.

Environmental Consideration for Herbal Garden

Plants constantly interact with dynamic and often challenging environmental factors. As immobile organisms, they have evolved a wide array of intricate defence strategies to survive and adapt. These strategies prominently include the production of diverse chemical compounds known as secondary metabolites, which play a crucial role in helping plants cope with stress.

Secondary metabolites are central to a plant's ability to adapt to environmental fluctuations. Plants possess a remarkable capacity to synthesize these compounds throughout their growth and development. During this time, they are exposed to various biotic (e.g., herbivory, microbial attacks) and abiotic (e.g., temperature, light intensity) stressors, triggering their defence systems into action. To withstand such stress, plants have developed highly complex physiological and metabolic mechanisms. These integrated systems allow them to adjust to the changing environment, with secondary metabolites serving as key components of these adaptive responses (Holopainen and Gershenzon 2010, Ncube *et al.* 2012). Because both the quantity and quality of secondary metabolites can be significantly influenced by environmental factors, maintaining optimal environmental conditions is especially important for cultivating medicinal herbs. The efficacy and therapeutic value of these plants depend largely on their chemical composition, which is sensitive to external stress. Numerous publications—including books and scientific reviews—have examined how environmental stress affects secondary metabolite production (Ahmad *et al.* 2018, Mahajan *et al.* 2020, Pant *et al.* 2021, Qaderi *et al.* 2023). Below is an overview of how specific environmental factors affect secondary metabolite biosynthesis in various plant species.

Light: Light is a critical environmental cue that profoundly influences the biosynthesis of secondary metabolites (SMs) in plants. This light-mediated regulation is particularly important in medicinal plant species, where variations in light intensity, duration (photoperiod), and spectral quality can significantly affect the accumulation of bioactive compounds. Medicinal plants such as *Aloe vera, Artemisia annua, Digitalis purpurea, Eclipta alba, Panax quinquefolium,* and *Ocimum basilicum* exhibit marked changes in the production of SMs—including terpenoids, alkaloids, flavonoids, and phenolic compounds—in response to varying light conditions. For instance, the synthesis and accumulation of artemisinin, a key antimalarial compound in *Artemisia annua*, is enhanced under red and blue light. This enhancement is attributed to the upregulation of genes involved in artemisinin biosynthesis, such as amorpha-4,11-diene synthase (ADS) and cytochrome P450 monooxygenase (CYP71AV1) (Zhang *et al.* 2018). In *Aloe vera*, exposure to high light intensity in combination with water stress reduces overall growth and yield. However, it simultaneously increases the concentrations of several primary and secondary metabolites, including aloin, proline, and soluble sugars, along with elevated activity of phosphoenolpyruvate carboxylase (PEPC). These metabolic responses are considered adaptive mechanisms that help maintain productivity under suboptimal conditions (Tahmasebi-Sarvestani *et al.* 2020). Changes in light conditions not only reshape the chemical profile of plants but also enhance their defence mechanisms, contributing to increased resistance against herbivores and improved adaptation to environmental stresses. Overall, the effects of light quality, intensity, and duration vary significantly among species, influencing both the composition and quantity of secondary metabolites. Thus, optimizing light parameters offers a promising strategy to enhance the yield and pharmacological quality of medicinal plants (Li *et al.* 2020).

Moisture: Water availability significantly affects secondary metabolism. In species such as *Pteridium arachnoideum* and *Artemisia annua*, drought or waterlogging conditions can trigger the accumulation of phenolic compounds, lipophilic resins, and alkaloids. These changes serve as protective strategies to conserve water and counter oxidative stress. For example, *Achnatherum inebrians* responds to moisture stress by producing anthocyanins and tannins, which contribute to stress tolerance, UV protection, and antimicrobial defence (Pandey *et al.* 2015).

Temperature: Plant growth and development are closely regulated by the ambient temperature. Both high and low temperature extremes can induce significant metabolic alterations that adversely affect plant physiology, growth, and productivity. Exposure to elevated temperatures often leads to a reduction in photochemical efficiency and the functional integrity of Photosystem II, indicating heightened physiological stress (Maxwell and Johnson 2000). Temperature stress—whether heat or cold—also modulates the biosynthesis and accumulation of secondary metabolites (SMs), which are critical for plant defence mechanisms. These compounds play key roles in alleviating both abiotic stresses such as heat, drought, cold, salinity, and heavy metal toxicity and biotic stresses including bacterial, fungal, viral, insect, or weed attacks (Tak and Kumar 2020). For instance, phenolic compounds are well-known for their multifaceted stress-mitigating properties. In general, high-temperature stress tends to enhance the production of certain SMs; however, some studies have reported a reduction in SM content under similar conditions. This variability depends on plant species, the intensity and duration of the temperature stress, and other environmental factors (Li *et al.* 2020). Given that SMs are not only vital for stress tolerance but also for the medicinal and cosmetic value of plants, maintaining optimal temperature conditions is essential for ensuring plant health, productivity, and pharmacological quality.

Soil Nutrients: Nutrient availability in the soil is another key factor that influences secondary metabolite synthesis. Plants like *Rhodiola sachalinensis* and *Ceratonia siliqua* produce higher levels of phenolics, such as tannins, when grown in nutrient-rich environments. In contrast, nutrient-deficient soils may stimulate the production of specialized metabolites, such as cyanogenic glycosides, as part of the plant's adaptive defence. Nutrient stress particularly nitrogen and phosphorus deficiency—can alter metabolic pathways, promoting the accumulation of valuable compounds like salidroside and shikonin (Sarker *et al.* 2022).

Ozone: Ozone exposure induces oxidative stress in plants, triggering a cascade of biochemical responses that enhance stress resilience. These physiological adaptations are crucial for survival under conditions of atmospheric pollution. Ozone molecules enter the leaf tissues through stomata and generate reactive oxygen species (ROS), such as hydrogen peroxide (H_2O_2), superoxide radicals ($O_2\bullet^-$), hydroxyl radicals (•OH), and hydroperoxyl radicals (HOO•). These ROS can disrupt normal cellular functions by impairing metabolic activity, degrading proteins, damaging chlorophyll, and reducing overall biomass accumulation.

Despite these detrimental effects, elevated ozone levels are also known to stimulate the production of secondary metabolites, often associated with plant defence and medicinal properties. For example, in *Sida cordifolia*, a medicinally important plant, ozone stress significantly increased the content of lignins, tannins, saponins, and alkaloids in both leaves and roots (Ansari *et al.* 2023). Similarly, in *Melissa officinalis*, the biosynthesis of phenolic compounds was enhanced under ozone stress (Tonelli *et al.* 2015). Additionally, exposure of *Capsicum baccatum* (pepper) plants to ozone pollution alters the profile of secondary metabolites in the fruits, leading to modifications in their biological activity. Ozone exposure reduced the levels of capsaicin—the primary pungent compound—while increasing carotenoid content, which contributes to fruit coloration. Furthermore, there was a notable decline in the total antioxidant potential of the seeds and a reduction in the anti-inflammatory properties of the pericarp. These changes, particularly the decrease in capsaicin and antioxidant activity, suggest a deterioration in fruit quality under ozone stress (Bortolin *et al.* 2016).

Sunlight Sensitivity in Selected Herbs: While many herbs require full sun—typically at least six hours per day—some are sensitive to excessive sunlight or cold temperatures. For such plants, stress management strategies like mulching or horticultural netting can be helpful in protecting leaves and stems from injury (Table 12.5). Here are a few examples of sensitive herbs and their environmental preferences:

- Lavender (*Lavandula angustifolia*) – Susceptible to heat stress under intense afternoon sun.
- Mint (*Mentha* spp.) – Can suffer from both heat and cold stress; partial shade is ideal in hot climates.
- Chives (*Allium schoenoprasum*) – Sensitive to sunburn in summer and frost in winter.
- Basil (*Ocimum basilicum*) – Extremely sensitive to cold; may need protection during cool nights or early frosts.
- Parsley (*Petroselinum crispum*) – Requires shade in hot weather; also vulnerable to cold damage.
- Cilantro (*Coriandrum sativum*) – Tends to bolt in high temperatures; needs partial sun or cool conditions.

For these herbs, it is advisable to provide shade nets or mulch around the base to moderate soil temperature, conserve moisture, and shield them from direct sunlight or frost damage.

Table 12.5. Popular medicinal plants: Growth habits and preferred locations

Name: Hindi (English)	Botanical name	Habit	Preferred location
Aak (Calotropis)	*Calotropis gigantea*	Shrub	Garden
Amaltas (Golden shower tree)	*Cassia fistula*	Tree	Garden
Amrita, *Giloe* (Heart-leaved moonseed)	*Tinospora cordifolia*	Climber	Fence, needs support to climb
Amla (Indian gooseberry)	*Phyllanthus emblica*	Tree	Open area in garden
Anaar (Pomegranate)	*Punica granatum*	Shrub	Pot/open place in garden
Arandi (Castor)	*Ricinus communis*	Shrub	Garden
Ashwagandha (Indian ginseng)	*Withania somnifera*	Herb	Pot/dry areas
Baheda (Beleric myrobalan)	*Terminalia bellirica*	Tree	Garden
Bael (Bengal quince)	*Aegle marmelos*	Tree	Garden
Bhui Amla (Stonebreaker)	*Phyllanthus amarus*	Herb	Pot
Bhringraj (False daisy)	*Eclipta prostrata*	Herb	Pot/moist semi-aquatic area
Brahmi (Water hyssop)	*Bacopa monnieri*	Herb	Shallow elongated pot, semi-aquatic shady spot
Buch (Sweet flag)	*Acorus calamus*	Herb	Semi-aquatic shady location
Chakramuni (Star gooseberry)	*Sauropus androgynus*	Shrub	Pot/hedge/single plant
Changeri / Amrool (Indian sorrel)	*Oxalis corniculata*	Herb	Pot/garden spread
Chitramula (Ceylon leadwort)	*Plumbago zeylanica*	Shrub	Pot
Dub/ Durva (Bermuda grass)	*Cynodon dactylon*	Herb	Pot/lawn
Ghritkumari (Aloe)	*Aloe vera*	Herb	Pot/rockery
Gudhal (Hibiscus)	*Hibiscus rosa-sinensis*	Shrub	Hedge/single plant
Gudmar (Gymnema)	*Gymnema sylvestre*	Climber	Pot/along fence or tree support
Harad (Chebulic myrobalan)	*Terminalia chebula*	Tree	Garden
Indrajav / Kutaja (Kurchi / Holarrhena)	*Holarrhena pubescens* syn. *Holarrhena antidysenterica*	Shrub	Open place in garden
Kalmegh (Bitter weed)	*Andrographis paniculata*	Herb	Pot/partially shady area
Kari Patta (Curry leaf)	*Murraya koenigii*	Shrub	Pot/garden
Khas-Khas (Vetiver / Khus grass)	*Vetiveria zizanioides*	Herb	Pot/garden in moist area

Name: Hindi (English)	Botanical name	Habit	Preferred location
Gandhatrin (Lemongrass)	*Cymbopogon citratus*	Shrub	Pot/open moist area
Mandukaparni (Indian pennywort)	*Centella asiatica*	Herb	Pot/semi-aquatic shady location
Mehndi (Henna)	*Lawsonia inermis*	Shrub	Pot/hedge or as independent plant
Neem (Indian lilac)	*Azadirachta indica*	Tree	Garden/open dry area
Nirgundi	*Vitex negundo*	Shrub	Pot/hedge/line hedge
Palash (Flame of the forest)	*Butea monosperma*	Tree	Garden
Pattharchur (Indian borage)	*Plectranthus amboinicus*	Herb	Pot/dry garden area
Pippli (Long pepper)	*Piper longum*	Climber	Pot/shady location
Poi / Malabar Palak	*Basella alba*	Climber	Pot/garden, needs spreading support
Sahajan (Moringa)	*Moringa oleifera*	Tree	Pot/single plant in garden
Saptparni (Devil tree)	*Alstonia scholaris*	Tree	Garden
Satavari (Asparagus)	*Asparagus racemosus*	Climber	Pot/moist garden spots
Tulsi (Basil)	*Ocimum sanctum*	Herb	Pot/hedge, in group or single
Vasak (Malabar nut)	*Adhatoda vasica*	Shrub	Pot/hedge
Wild tulsi	*Ocimum tenuiflorum*	Herb	Pot/hedge/single plant

(Source: Compiled from Haridasan *et al.* 2017, and various open-access, classical, and scholarly references).

Management of Garden and Organic Gardening Techniques

Effective management and maintenance are crucial for the successful establishment of a herbal garden. These practices encompass maintaining sanitary conditions, attending to plant nutrition and protection, implementing intercultural operations, ensuring proper irrigation, conducting training and pruning of plants, implementing post-planting measures, and regularly sampling of plants (Mazumdar and Mukhopadhyay 2006). Herbal plants benefit significantly from monthly manuring and fertilization. Chemical fertilizers, pesticides, plant growth regulators, or any other form of chemicals should be avoided in herbal gardens. Organic sources such as vermicompost, farmyard manure, and compost serve as excellent nutrient supplements for herbal plants. It is important to refrain from splashing water on the leaves during irrigation to prevent the spread of diseases and fungal infections to other plants. Pots and beds in herbal gardens should be kept free from weeds to provide herbal plants with the necessary space, water, light, and nutrients for growth and development without competition. Regular hand weeding is essential to maintain garden cleanliness, and the use of chemical herbicides should be avoided. Proper soil moisture levels should be maintained using quality irrigation water, scheduling irrigation on a weekly basis with controlled water supply. The use of a micro-irrigation system is preferable to prevent waterlogging. Adequate drainage is necessary at herbal garden sites, as many herbal plants are highly sensitive to waterlogged conditions.

Controlling pests and diseases is important for maintaining a healthy herbal garden. One method is employing insect or disease vector pheromone traps to diminish the threat posed by insect vectors. Another effective strategy is trap cropping, a companion planting technique traditionally utilized in insect pest management. This approach involves diversifying vegetation to attract insect pests away from main crops during critical periods by offering them an alternative preferred choice. These trap crop species can be strategically planted on the boundaries of herbal gardens to prevent infestations. For instance, in an onion (*Allium cepa*) field, populations of Thrips insects (*Thrips tabaci*), a major pest of onions, can be suppressed by planting buckwheat (*Fagopyrum esculentum*) as a trap crop (Sarkar *et al.* 2018). It is advisable to refrain from using chemical pesticides in herbal gardens, and precautions should be taken to prevent chemical pesticide drift from neighbouring fields onto herbs. Measures to achieve this include planting natural hedges along the boundary with neighbouring fields, widening the border area around the herbal gardens, and diverting waterways to avoid runoff from upstream fields. Typically, genetic engineering, or genetically modified organisms (GMOs) are not advised in organic products (USDA, accessed on 13-09-2024) and herbal gardeners should safeguard their production against any GMO contamination.

Authentication of Herbal Plants and Botanicals

Herbal authentication is a critical quality assurance process designed to ensure the accurate identification of herbal species and their respective plant parts used in the production of herbal products. Proper identification of herbal plants as raw materials guarantees their suitability for their intended purpose in the final products thereby safeguarding the quality and safety of the finished products (Mishra *et al.* 2016). Authentication tests typically involve the use of relevant analytical techniques tailored to specific samples, which is particularly important in cases where finished herbal products may be vulnerable to substitution or adulteration with morphologically and chemically similar varieties (Revathy *et al.* 2012).

Authentication Methods

Ideally, authentication should occur from the harvesting of the plant material to the final product. There is no single or superior method to ensure 100% authentication throughout the entire process. This goal can be achieved through the application of various methodologies. The authentication process begins with obtaining good voucher specimens, which serve as reference material and evidence of the chain of custody. Macroscopic and microscopic examinations can provide rapid and cost-effective identification techniques. Chemical analysis is particularly effective for detecting contaminants and can also be excellent for plant identification. However, each of these methodologies has its limitations, and additional analytical methods are available. Molecular biology offers a range of techniques that can be highly useful for authenticating medicinal plants (Techen *et al.* 2004). Generally, methods for assessing the authenticity of herbs rely on morphological and anatomical analysis, organoleptic characteristics, DNA-based techniques, chemical fingerprinting, and various other approaches (de Boer *et al.* 2015, Parveen *et al.* 2016). Today, advancement in identifying and authenticating plant species and products within the herbal marketplace is progressing towards employing combination methods (Mishra *et al.* 2018).

Macroscopic and Microscopic Methods: Herbal plants have traditionally been authenticated based on their phenotypic characteristics, which requires the expertise of trained taxonomists. Common methods include macroscopic and microscopic evaluations. Macroscopic examination involves comparing visible traits—such as leaf shape, flower structure, and overall plant size—with descriptions in botanical references. This method works best with fresh plant material but becomes less effective with dried plants, as key diagnostic features like colour and texture are often lost during dehydration. Microscopic examination looks at finer cellular details, such as stomata patterns, trichomes, and vascular structure. While useful for distinguishing closely related species, this method also faces challenges when applied to dried plants, as the drying process can distort or obscure important cellular structures.

The main limitations of these traditional methods include:

- **Loss of diagnostic features during drying**, which makes accurate identification harder.
- **Phenotypic variability**, where environmental factors cause plants of the same species to look different.
- **Fragmentation** of plant material in the herbal trade, which reduces the ability to assess morphological and anatomical characteristics.

Additionally, some researchers have claimed that this analysis has many disadvantages in terms of its accuracy and effectiveness for authentication assessment, particularly for plant species. Performing macroscopy and microscopy on each plant part in every consignment in the industry is a tedious and time-consuming task.

Molecular Based Methods: Molecular-based analysis has become indispensable for the identification and authentication of plant species. Various techniques such as restriction fragment length polymorphisms (RFLPs), amplified fragment length polymorphisms (AFLPs), randomly amplified polymorphic DNA (RAPD), simple sequence repeats (SSRs), inter simple sequence repeats (ISSR), sequence characterized amplified regions (SCARs), loop-mediated isothermal amplification (LAMP), and single nucleotide polymorphisms (SNPs), were developed for this purpose (Ganie *et al.* 2015).

DNA barcoding uses specific genetic markers to identify individual species. DNA metabarcoding combines DNA barcoding with high-throughput sequencing to identify multiple species in complex mixtures, such as those found in processed herbal products. The most commonly used single-locus standard single locus DNA barcoding including internal transcribed spacer (ITS and ITS2), rbcL, matK, trnL–trnF, psbA-trnH, ycf1, and rpoC, are the major plant barcodes that have attracted the most attention. In addition to these, advanced methods such as multi-locus barcoding, super barcoding, and mini-barcoding have been developed. These approaches offer rapid, accurate, and effective tools for plant species identification, especially in cases of adulteration or substitution—issues frequently encountered in the herbal industry. Importantly, each plant species has an optimal genetic marker referred to as a specific barcode. This may be one of the commonly used barcodes (e.g., *matK* or *psbA-trnH*) or a novel marker yet to be widely adopted (Zhu *et al.* 2022).

Chemical Fingerprinting: A chemical fingerprint represents a distinct pattern indicating the presence of various biochemical markers within a sample. This method is widely favoured for species authentication and quality control of herbal products over molecular-based analysis due to its inherent advantages. Chromatographic Fingerprinting (CF) is a specific chemical fingerprinting approach that entails the separation of a mixture into its individual components. This separation is achieved by exploiting the varying travel times of each component through a system comprising a stationary phase and a mobile phase. CF techniques are crucial for herbal drug standardization as they provide a unique profile of the chemical constituents present in herbal products, ensuring quality and consistency. They help in the identification of marker compounds, detection of adulteration or contamination, and facilitate the comparison of different batches. This standardization is essential for regulatory compliance and ensuring the safety and efficacy of herbal medicines (Joshi 2012).

Molecular-based Combination Methods: A combination of recombinase polymerase amplification with lateral flow strips (RPALFS) assay has been recommended to identify and differentiate products of closely related herbal species such as *Ginkgo biloba* and *Sophora japonica.* This method addresses the disadvantage of the PCR-based method, which requires advanced equipment or complicated professional skills (Liu *et al.* 2018). The combination method not only overcomes the limitation of chemical analysis in detecting different species with similar chemical profiles but is also useful for rapid analysis compared to the common PCR-based method. The combination method has a shorter detection time with higher sensitivity to temperatures (Osathanunkul *et al.* 2018).

Molecular and Spectroscopy Method: DNA barcoding has proven effective in detecting and quantifying adulteration in the raw herbal trade across a variety of medicinal plants. However, its application is often hindered by the challenge of extracting high-quality DNA from raw herbal materials, ranging from simple dried leaves to powdered plant parts, necessary for subsequent PCR-based amplification of DNA barcode markers. Alternatively, spectroscopic methods such as NMR can be employed for analysing chemical compounds in complex mixtures like plant extracts, pharmaceuticals, and herbal preparations. NMR spectroscopy is highly reproducible, robust, and inherently quantitative, eliminating the need for prior chromatographic separation of multiple components. This technique has been utilized for detecting, identifying, and quantitatively determining adulterants in weight loss food supplements (Hachem *et al.* 2016). Combining DNA barcoding with spectroscopic methods for authenticating herbal medicines enhances species identification resolution and the analysis of mixtures. DNA barcoding and nuclear magnetic resonance (NMR) were effectively utilized as regulatory tools for authenticating *Garcinia* fruit rinds and food supplements (Seethapathy *et al.* 2018). Direct analysis in real-time (DART) coupled with time-of-flight mass spectrometry (TOF-MS) methods have been successfully used for detecting *Smallanthus sonchifolius* in tea mixtures. These techniques offer rapid analysis and serve as effective tools for identification or authentication of plant species in food products (Žiarovská *et al.* 2016).

Analytical Methods and Multivariate Analysis: Chromatography and spectroscopy can be paired for authentication assessment. High-performance liquid chromatography (HPLC) and micellar electrokinetic chromatography (MEKC), combined with chemometrics, have been successfully employed (Table 12.6) for authenticating various fruits-based herbal medicines containing extracts of cranberry, bilberry, and sea-buckthorn (Sima *et al.* 2018).

Table 12.6. Advantages and limitations of single method in authentication of herbs

Single Method	Advantages	Disadvantages
DNA-based method	Extremely sensitive and specific tool for authentication	Time-consuming, expensive large instruments and equipment and unsuitable for rapid analysis
Chemical fingerprinting	Provides effective qualitative and quantitative information on the characteristic components and can explore chemical complexity of herbal-related products	Cannot differentiates closely related species effectively, Depending on the chemical marker or target compound
Macroscopic and microscopic evaluation	Can performed effectively on fresh parts of herbs	Need experienced skills from a professional taxonomist, tedious and time-consuming

Harvesting and Storage of Herbs

Generally, only in a few cases is the entire plant used for medicinal purposes. Instead, one or more plant parts such as roots, bark, stems, leaves, flowers, fruits, and seeds are utilized for their medicinal properties. Consequently, guidelines for harvesting and post-harvest management are applicable to any harvested part, with specific plant parts requiring additional care. The quality of medicinal plants is influenced by factors such as geographical origin, cultivar of the species, stage of growth at the time of collection, and post-harvest handling. Unfortunately, insufficient attention is often given to factors such as stage of maturity, processing, and storage leading to deterioration of quality of herbs and botanicals. It is reported that plants harvested at right time of maturity following Good Field Collection Practices (GFCPs) have better quality in terms of active phytoingredients (Pandey and Das 2014).

Medicinal plants should be collected or harvested during the appropriate season or time period to ensure the highest possible quality of both source materials and finished products. It is widely recognized that the quantitative concentration of biologically active phytoconstituents varies with the stage of plant growth and development. Ancient sciences like Ayurveda recommend collecting different parts of plants in different seasons, likely considering the optimum activity of herbs when harvested at specific times. Additionally, collecting plant parts during seasons that cause minimal harm to the plant is crucial. The ideal time (Table 12.7) for collection or harvest should be based on the quality and quantity of biologically active constituents, taking precedence over maximizing the total vegetative yield of the targeted medicinal plant parts (Pandey and Mandal 2013, Pandey and Das 2014).

Table 12.7. Selected medicinal plants and their harvesting time*

Botanical Name of the Herb	Local Name	Part Used	Time Period for Collection
Acacia chundra	*Khadir*	Wood	November to January
Acacia nilotica	*Deshi Babool*	Bark	August to October
Achyranthes aspera	*Apamarga*	Whole Plant	February to April
Aconitum ferox	*Vatsanabha*	Rhizome (Highly toxic and requires careful purification before use)	August to October
Aconitum heterophyllum	*Atish*	Rhizome	August to October
Acorus calamus	*Vacha*	Rhizome	May to July
Adhatoda vasica	*Adusa*	Leaves	February to April
Aegle marmelos	*Belgiri*	Fruit	May to July
	Belchhal	Bark	February to April

Botanical Name of the Herb	Local Name	Part Used	Time Period for Collection
Alpinia galanga	*Kulinjana*	Rhizome	August to October
Alstonia scholaris	*Saptaparni*	Bark	May to July
Andrographis paniculata	*Kalmegh*	Aerial parts	February to April; November to January
Aquilaria agallocha	*Agaru*	Stem	May to July
Argyreia speciosa	*Vidhara*	Root	May to July
Asparagus adscendens	*Safed Musli*	Root	August to October
Asparagus racemosus	Shatawari	Root	August to October
Azadirachta indica	Neem	Leaves	May to July
		Bark	November to January
Barringtonia acutangula	Hizzal	Seeds	August to October
Berberis aristata	Daruhaldi	Roots/stem	August to October
Blepharis edulis	Utigan Beej	Seeds	February to April; May to July
Boerhaavia diffusa	Punarnava	Aerial Parts	May to July
		Root	May to July; August to October
Boswellia serrata	Sallaki	Gum-resin	February to April; November to January
Butea monosperma	Palash	Seeds	February to April
Calotropis procera; C. gigantea	*Arka/Aak*	Leaves	February to April
Carthamus tinctorius	*Kusum phool*	Floral parts	February to April
Cassia angustifolia	*Senna*	Leaves	February to April
		Pods	February to April
Cassia fistula	*Amaltas*	Fruit	May to July
Cedrus deodara	*Deodar*	Wood	May to July and August to October
Celastrus paniculata	*Malkagini*	Seed	May to July
Centella asiatica	*Mandukaparni, Brahmi*	Leaves	August to October
Cichorium intybus	Kashni	Root	February to April and November to January
		Seed	November to January
Cinnamomum tamala	*Tejpat*	Leaves	February to April and November to January
Cinnamomum verum	*Dalchini*	Bark	May to July August to October

Botanical Name of the Herb	Local Name	Part Used	Time Period for Collection
Cissus quadrangularis	*Hadjod*	Stem	August to October
Clerodendrum serratum	*Bharangi*	Bark	August to October
Commiphora wightii	*Guggulu*	Gum-resin	November to January
Crataeva nurvala	*Varun*	Bark	August to October; November to January
Crocus sativus	*Kesar, Zafran*	Stigma	November to January
Curculigo orchioides	*Kali Mushli*	Rhizome	February to April May to July
Cyperus rotundus	*Mustaka or Purple nutsedge*	Rhizome	August to October
Desmodium gangeticum	*Shalparni*	Aerial parts	August to October
Dioscorea bulbifera	*Varahikand*	Tuber	May to July
Eclipta prostrata	*Bhringraj*	Whole plant	May to July
Embelia ribes	*Vaividang Vidanga*	Fruit	November to January
Ferula asfoetida	*Heeng, Hing*	Gum-resin	February to April; May to July
Ficus benghalensis	*Vata/Bargad*	Bark	August to October; November to January
Ficus carica	*Anjeer*	Fruit	May to July
Ficus racemosa	*Gular, Udumbar*	Bark	August to October; November to January
Ficus religiosa	*Peepal*	Bark	August to October; November to January
Gmelina arborea	*Gamhar, Madhumati*	Bark	August to October November to January
Gymnema sylvestre	*Gurmar*	Leaves	August to October
Hedychium spicatum	*Kapur Kachri*	Rhizome	February to April
Hemidesmus indicus	*Anantmool*	Root	February to April
Holarrhena antidysenterica	*Kutaz Indarajava*	Bark Seed	November to January February to April
Martynia diandra	*Kakanasha*	Fruits	August to October
Mesua ferrea	*Nagkeshar*	Stamen (Androecium)	February to April
Mimosa pudica	*Lajwanti*	Whole plant	February to April
Mimusops elengi	*Vakula*	Bark	August to October
Moringa oleifera	*Sahajan*	Fruit	February to April
Mucuna pruriens	*Kaunch, Kevanch*	Seed	February to April
Myrica esculenta	*Kaiphal*	Bark	May to July; August to October

Botanical Name of the Herb	Local Name	Part Used	Time Period for Collection
Myristica fragrans	*Jaiphal*	Fruit	May to July; August to October
Nardostachys jatamansi	*Jatamansi*	Rhizome	November to January
Operculina turpethum	*Nishoth*	Root	August to October
Oroxylum indicum	*Syonaka*	Bark	November to January
Parmelia perlata	*Chharila*	Ascolichen	May to July; August to October
Phyllanthus emblica	*Amla*	Fruit/seed	November to January
Picrorhiza kurroa	*Kutki*	Rhizome	August to October
Piper longum	*Pippli*	Fruit	February to April
Plumbago indica	*Chitrakmool*	Root	February to April; November to January
Plantago ovata	*Isabgol*	Seed	February to April
Podophyllum hexandrum	*Bankakri*	Rhizome	May to July
Premna integrifolia	*Agnimantha*	Stem	August to October; November to January
Psoralea corylifolia	*Bakuchi/Somraji*	Seeds	November to January
Pterocarpus marsupium	*Vijayshal*	Heart wood	August to October
Rauwolfia serpentina	*Sarpgandha*	Root	May to July; August to October
Rheum australe	*Revandchini*	Root	August to October
Rubia cordifolia	*Manjishtha*	Stem	August to October; November to January
Santalum album	*Chandan*	Wood	August to October; November to January
Sapindus mukorossi	*Reetha*	Seed	August to October; November to January
Saraca asoca	*Ashoka*	Bark	August to October
Sida cordifolia	*Bala*	Leaves	February to April; November to January
Solanum anguivi	*Vrihati*	Root & Stem	February to April; May to July
Solanum nigrum	*Makoy*	Fruit	February to April
		Whole plant	February to April
Solanum virginianum	*Kantkari*	Whole plant	February to April
Spheranthus indicus	*Mundi*	Fruits	February to April; May to July
Swertia chirayita	*Chirata*	Whole plant	August to October

Botanical Name of the Herb	Local Name	Part Used	Time Period for Collection
Syzygium cumini	*Jamun*	Seed	May to July
		Bark	August to October
Syzygium aromaticum	*Laung, Lavanga*	Floral buds	November to January
Taxus baccata	*Thuner*	Leaves	August to October
Tephrosia purpurea	*Sarpaunkha*	Whole plant	August to October
Teramnus labialis	*Mashparni*	Aerial parts	August to October
Terminalia arjuna	*Arjun, Arjuna*	Bark	February to April
Terminalia bellirica	*Baheda, Bahera Bahuvirya*	Fruit	February to April
Terminalia chebula	*Harad, Hareetaki*	Fruit	February to April
Tinospora cordifolia	*Guduchi*	Stem	February to April
Tribulus terrestris	*Gokharu*	Fruit	November to January
Uraria picta	*Prishniparni*	Aerial parts	August to October
Valeriana jatamansi	*Tagar*	Root	August to October
Vetiveria zizanioides	*Khash/Ushi*	Root	August to October
Vigna triloba	*Mudgaparni*	Aerial parts	August to October
Viola odorata / V. serpens	*Vanafsha*	Flower	November to January
Withania somnifera	*Ashwagandha*	Roots	February to April
Woodfordia fruticosa	*Dhataki*	Flowers	February to April
Zanthoxylum armatum	*Timru, Tejbal*	Fruits	August to October November to January
Zingiber officinalis	*Adrak, Saunth*	Rhizome	November to January
Ziziphus mauritiana	*Ber, Badari*	Fruits	February to April

(Source: Pandey and Das 2014, Pandey and Savita 2017). *Representing Central India

General Guidelines and Standard Operating Procedures for Harvesting/Collection of Herbs and Botanicals

The following guidelines have been recommended by the World Health Organization (WHO 2003) for harvesting and collection of the medicinal plants

- Medicinal plants should be harvested following sustainable harvesting practices under the best possible conditions, avoiding dew, rain or exceptionally high humidity. If harvesting occurs in wet conditions, the harvested material should be transported immediately to an indoor drying facility to expedite drying so as to prevent any possible deleterious effects due to increased moisture levels, which promote microbial fermentation and mould.
- In general, the collected/harvested plant materials should not come into direct contact with the soil. If underground parts (such as the roots or

rhizomes/bulbs) are harvested, any adhering soil should be removed from the plants as soon as they are harvested/collected. Contact with soil should be avoided to the extent possible so as to minimize the microbial load of harvested medicinal plant materials. Where necessary, large drop cloths, preferably made of clean muslin, may be used as an interface between the harvested plants and the soil.

- Collected/harvested plant material should be placed in clean baskets, mesh bags, other well aerated containers or cloths that are free from foreign matter, including plant remnants from previous collecting activities. After collection, the plant materials may be subjected to appropriate preliminary processing, including elimination of undesirable materials and contaminants (by hand picking), washing (to remove excess soil), sorting and cutting.
- The harvested raw medicinal plant materials should be transported promptly in clean, dry conditions. They may be placed in clean baskets, dry sacks, trailers, hoppers or other well-aerated containers and carried to a central point for transport to the processing facility. If the collection site is located some distance from processing facilities, it may be necessary to air or sun-dry the raw medicinal plant materials prior to transport.
- If more than one part of the medicinal plant is being collected, the different plant materials should be gathered separately and transported in separate containers. Cross-contamination (unintended mixing of plant material that reduces purity) should be avoided at all times. Any mechanical damage or compacting of the raw medicinal plant materials for example, overfilling or stacking of sacks or bags should be avoided, as it may result in composting or otherwise diminish quality. Decomposed medicinal plant materials should be identified and discarded during harvest in order to avoid microbial contamination and loss of product quality.
- All containers used for harvest should be kept clean and free from contamination by previously harvested medicinal plants and other foreign matter. If plastic containers are used, particular attention should be paid to any possible retention of moisture that could lead to the growth of mould. When containers are not in use, they should be kept in dry conditions, in an area that is protected from insects, rodents, birds and other pests, and inaccessible to livestock and domestic animals.
- The collected medicinal plant materials should be protected from insects, rodents, birds and other pests as well as from livestock and domestic animals.
- Collecting/harvesting implements (tools), such as machetes, shears and mechanical tools, should be kept clean and maintained in proper condition. Those parts that come into direct contact with the collected medicinal plant materials should be free from excess oil/grease and other contamination.

Cutting devices, harvesters, and other machines should be kept clean and adjusted to reduce damage and contamination from soil and other materials. They should be stored in an uncontaminated, dry place or facility free from insects, rodents, birds and other pests, and inaccessible to livestock and domestic animals.

Different categories of herbs and botanicals should be harvested and collected according to the following standard operating procedures (WHO 2003) to ensure the quality of raw materials and optimize product yield:

Annual Herbs/ Whole Plants

Salient points for harvest and collection of annual herbs and whole plants include:

- Harvesting of the whole herbaceous plant, or its aerial parts, should be conducted at the flower bud or flowering stage, but prior to any visible decline in any of the plant parts.
- The entire population in a given area should never be harvested. Sufficient population should be left in nature for regeneration to facilitate future collections.
- Planning a mathematical procedure, including computer software, to estimate the collection of individuals from a population may be necessary when the target area is large, to ensure even harvesting throughout the habitat.
- Annuals, especially small herbs, creepers, and grasses, are more prone to contamination, as well as cross-contamination. It is easier to sort the annuals immediately after collection rather than after drying.
- Aromatic plants and delicate parts like pistils or stamens of other plants should not be dried in direct sunlight. If collected in wet conditions, they should be shifted to the shade as soon as external moisture has been removed.

Underground Parts: SOP to collect underground parts of the medicinal plants include:

- The roots of annual plants should be dug when they are well-developed and mature.
- Roots of perennials should be harvested late in the fall or early in the spring. Roots of biennials should be collected either in the fall of the first year or the spring of the second year.
- Root material rich in essential oils should be handled carefully to prevent bruising of the epidermis, where the oils typically reside. This could result in the loss or degradation of essential oils.

- Unless specifically required for a particular species, underground parts such as roots and rhizomes should be collected only after seed shedding. This also facilitates species regeneration.
- When uprooting taproots for desired produce, efforts should be made to minimize harm to other plant species in the vicinity. Underground parts should be collected with minimal digging, using suitable tools.
- When collecting roots of species propagated vegetatively, enough underground part should be left at the site to allow for regeneration. It is essential to thoroughly wash the underground parts and then dry them to reduce moisture content before packing the produce.

Stem Bark: Good field collection procedures to be followed for collection of bark are:

- Stem bark should not be harvested when the tree is undergoing new growth, such as during the spring season.
- Bark should be collected from mature branches of the trees while leaving the main trunk intact.
- Avoid taking bark from the entire branch or trunk all at once.
- Girdling of trees or branches, accomplished by removing bark all the way around, should be avoided unless the tree is intended to be felled for purposes such as timber production. Instead, bark should be stripped longitudinally, partially along the length of the stem, to facilitate the smooth conduction of water and nutrients.
- The rhytidome (outer dead bark) should be removed, except when it constitutes the usable portion of the product.
- Bark should be split into pieces of suitable size to facilitate thorough drying. Unless specified otherwise in particular instances, barks should be dried in direct sunlight.

Stem or Wood: Some of the important precautions that should be observed while collecting stem or wood for medicinal purposes include:

- Only select mature branches of a tree or shrub should be harvested at a time. The branches from the same plant should not be harvested every year. Where the trunk is used as medicinal produce, the main axis should be harvested.
- The produce should be cut in smaller pieces to facilitate faster drying, packaging and storage of the produce. In case of wood, the material can be made into small chips or shavings to facilitate drying and packaging.

- Unless otherwise required in specific cases, stems and woods should be dried in direct sunlight.

Leaves: Attention must be paid on following aspects for proper harvesting and collection of leaves:

- Leaves of herbaceous plants should ideally be collected before they flower. Whenever possible, leaves should be harvested from mature trees.
- If the bio-active contents in the leaves do not vary with age, the collection period could be extended to later stages.
- When harvesting, the source plant should not be stripped completely of its leaves. A certain percentage of leaves should be left intact to ensure the plant's normal physiological processes.
- Trees, shrubs, or branches should not be chopped down solely to facilitate the collection of otherwise inaccessible leaves.
- Tender leaves should only be harvested if they constitute the officially recognized produce. Any leaves that have turned pale, become infected, are deficient, or appear unhealthy should be discarded.
- In general, leaves should not be dried in direct sunlight unless they contain external moisture. In such cases, they may initially be dried in direct sunlight for a short period before being moved to shade or indirect sunlight as soon as the external moisture is removed.
- It's important to periodically turn the produce while drying to promote faster and more even drying.
- Packing of the leaves should be done only after ensuring they are completely dried. Even a small amount of moisture in some leaves can lead to fungal contamination and spoilage of the entire lot.
- Leaf material rich in essential oils must be handled with care to prevent bruising, which could result in the loss or degradation of essential oil.
- The leaves ought to be harvested during the peak season of growth and leaf production.
- Leaf harvesting should be postponed or reduced in quantity during periods of environmental stress for the plants.
- A decrease in leaf size indicates stressful conditions, prompting a reduction in the harvesting rate.
- If the overall plant size within a population seems to be decreasing, despite an increase in vegetative sprouting (i.e., the population becoming denser), the harvesting rate should be lowered.

- The harvesting rate should be decreased in response to heavy pressure from grazing, fire, or other incidents that could adversely affect the plants.

Flower and Floral Parts: Following guidelines are recommended for collection of flowers and floral parts of the plants:

- Depending on the requirements of the produce, fruits may be sliced or cut into smaller pieces to facilitate drying and packaging.
- It is essential to ensure that the flowers are completely dried before they are packed.
- Randomly selected individual fruits should be dissected to verify that no inherent moisture remains.

Gums and Resins: Gums and resins are plant-derived substances secreted by plants, often in response to injury, with distinct chemical compositions and uses. They play a significant role in herbal medicine and are widely used in various healing formulations. The following are the recommended guidelines for their collection:

- Collectors and collection managers should ensure minimal harm to the mother plant while collecting exudates. Only a few small longitudinal incisions should be made to collect the exudates, and the exposed parts should be treated appropriately to avoid any fungal or bacterial infestation after collection.
- Incisions that are too close to the ground, easily accessible by cattle and wild animals, should be avoided. The collection container should be designed to prevent rain, bird droppings, and other possible contaminations.
- Where there is a likelihood of foreign matter being mixed with the collected gums and resins, it should be carefully removed.
- Source trees or shrubs should be allowed an appropriate recovery period before collecting exudates from them again.
- Since most gums and resins are inflammable, they should be packed in appropriate containers and stored in isolated places. Containers of resins like Damar (*Shorea robusta*) and Saral (*Pinus longifolia*) should be labelled as "Inflammable Material" during transit and storage.
- No fires should be ignited near the base of the tree to increase gum/resin flow.
- Younger trees should not be tapped. The girth of the trees must be determined, below which tapping of gum/resin will not be allowed.
- Gum flow is more prominent in hot weather. Therefore, tapping in such

species should be done between June and October.

- Long, sharp cut blazes are preferable as they yield pure resin/gum and the bark heals faster. Irregular cuts introduce impurities to the resin. Long cuts provide more exudation area and heal faster. Square and round cuts take longer to heal due to the increased distance between the two walls.
- Sharp knives or chisels can be used to make blazes.
- Instead of allowing the gum or resin to solidify on the bark, it is better to use a collection trough such as a coconut shell or hollow bamboo.
- If multiple blazes are made on the same tree, they should be staggered for optimum exudation. After three years of tapping, the tree should be given sufficient rest to rejuvenate from the injury.

Galls: Galls are abnormal outgrowths on plant tissues, typically formed in response to stimuli from insects, mites, fungi, bacteria, or other organisms. Despite their pathological origin, certain galls are valued in traditional medicine for their therapeutic properties. Extracts from galls have been traditionally used to treat a variety of ailments, including inflammatory conditions, skin disorders, and dental problems. Some notable examples include galls from *Pistacia integerrima* (commonly known as *Karkatshringi*) and *Quercus infectoria*, both recognized for their astringent, anti-inflammatory, and antioxidant activities (Singla *et al.* 2022). Key guidelines for collection of galls include:

- Galls should be collected only from specified medicinal species, such as *Pistacia integerrima*, to ensure safety and efficacy.
- Care should be taken to ensure that no live insects remain inside the galls at the time of collection.
- Post-harvest processing must be conducted in an isolated and hygienic location to prevent cross-infestation.
- The collected galls should be properly cleaned, dried, and packed in moisture-proof containers and stored under pest-free conditions to preserve quality and prevent contamination of other produce.

Post-Harvest Losses in Herbal Farming

Post-harvest losses occurring between harvesting and the production of final herbal products pose a significant challenge for successful herbal gardening. These losses, attributed to various factors including physical, physiological, mechanical, and hygienic conditions, can have a substantial impact on the overall yield. The postharvest losses of herbs can be analysed in terms of both primary and secondary causes.

Primary Causes

The primary causes of post-harvest losses encompass various mechanical, physiological, pathological, and environmental factors. Transportation is a critical aspect contributing to post-harvest losses, given that mechanical and physical injuries frequently happen during transit.

Losses due to Mechanical Injuries: Mechanical injuries refer to physical deformations, superficial ruptures, and tissue damage caused by external factors (Juan *et al.* 2010). These types of injuries often occur during harvesting due to improper picking and handling techniques. They result in physical alterations, known as physical damage, as well as physiological, chemical, and biochemical changes that can affect the plant's colour, aroma, flavour, texture, and the chemical composition of active ingredients, ultimately impacting their quality and effectiveness (Mohsenin 2019). Medicinal and aromatic plants are particularly vulnerable to such injuries because of their high moisture content.

Losses due to Microbial Action: Medicinal and aromatic plant (MAP) species are highly susceptible to microbial threats such as fungi, bacteria, yeast, and molds. The invasion of these microorganisms is a major contributor to post-harvest losses. Fresh MAP produce is especially vulnerable due to its high moisture content and limited natural defence mechanisms, which facilitate microbial infiltration and rapid proliferation. The fleshy texture of certain MAPs further increases their susceptibility. Microbial infections may originate in the field, through contaminated irrigation or washing water, or later during storage. Among these threats, fungi are the primary agents responsible for the rotting of roots and fruits, causing significant damage. Warm temperatures and high humidity create ideal conditions for post-harvest decay. Typically, fungi target plant tissues with higher acidity, whereas bacteria tend to infect plant parts with a pH above 5.0 (Barth *et al.* 2009).

Losses due to Environmental Factors: Environmental factors such as temperature and relative humidity play crucial roles in agricultural settings. Elevated temperature and humidity create favourable conditions for the proliferation of microorganisms, resulting in significant damage to crops. Moreover, high temperatures accelerate the respiration rate of fruits and leaves, leading to the degradation of secondary metabolites. The significance of relative humidity in post-harvest losses is comparable to that of temperature. Maintaining a relative humidity threshold of over 60% is recommended to uphold the quality of medicinal plants during storage (Muller and Heindl 2006).

Physiological Deterioration: Temperature is the most important environmental factor that influences the deterioration of harvested commodities. Most perishable horticultural commodities last longest at temperatures near 0°C. At temperatures above the optimum, the rate of deterioration increases 2- to 3-fold for every 10°C rise in the temperature (Kader 2013). Many medicinal and aromatic plants, or their parts, remain alive even after harvest, continuing their physiological activities. Consequently, they may suffer from physiological disorders caused by enzymatic activity, leading to over-ripeness and senescence—a simple aging phenomenon. Temperature stands out as the single most crucial factor in deteriorating Medicinal and Aromatic Plants (MAPs) due to physiological actions, primarily by facilitating moisture removal (Sommer *et al.* 2002). Improper ventilation of harvested material often leads to auto-heating through respiratory activity, creating favourable conditions for microbial growth (Muller and Heindl 2006).

Secondary Causes

Insufficient harvesting, transportation, storage, and marketing facilities, coupled with inadequate legislation, create conditions favourable for secondary causes of loss. Inadequate harvesting facilities and rough handling during the harvesting process result in bruising, increasing the likelihood of contamination with organisms. Prolonged periods taken for harvesting and grading in the field leave the produce with field heat for extended durations, subsequently accelerating senescence. The improper use of machinery and equipment in mechanical harvesting leads to serious losses. This poses a significant challenge for medicinal and aromatic plants harvested during or just after rain, as the high relative humidity fosters conditions conducive to the growth and development of decay organisms. It is noteworthy that harvesting during the hotter parts of the day results in faster senescence and wilting of MAP produce due to heightened enzymatic activities.

Processing of Medicinal and Aromatic Plants and Botanicals

The processing of medicinal and aromatic plants (MAPs) encompasses (Fig. 12.15) a systematic series of post-harvest techniques designed to preserve, concentrate and enhance the bioactive compounds inherent in plant materials. These processes are critical for maintaining product quality, ensuring safety and improving the therapeutic and functional efficacy of MAPs used in pharmaceuticals, nutraceuticals, cosmetics and food supplements. Effective post-harvest handling plays a pivotal role in minimizing the degradation of active constituents and preventing microbial contamination, while also ensuring compliance with established quality standards and regulatory frameworks. Several scientific guidelines, including those on Good Agricultural Practices (GAP) and Good Field Collection Practices (GFCP) developed by the National Medicinal Plants Board (NMPB) of India in collaboration with the World Health Organization outline the essential steps involved in processing MAPs and botanicals. These steps typically include transportation primary sorting, cleaning, washing and decontamination, drying, sorting/ grading, storage and packaging and storage (Heron and Maiti 2010).

Transportation of Medicinal Plants to Processing Site

The transportation of harvested medicinal plant materials is a critical first step that must be executed with care to preserve their integrity and phytochemical content. The following best practices should be adhered to:

- **Prompt transport:** Medicinal plant parts should be transported to the processing site as soon as possible after harvest to prevent deterioration due to enzymatic activity, moisture buildup or microbial growth.
- **Clean transport conditions:** Vehicles used for transport must be thoroughly cleaned and dried prior to use. Under no circumstances should plant materials be transported alongside hazardous substances such as pesticides, fertilizers, or other contaminants.
- **Proper labelling and separation:** Different plant species and plant parts (e.g., roots, leaves, flowers and seeds) must be clearly labelled and physically separated during transport to avoid cross-contamination and ensure traceability.
- **Protection from environmental factors:** Plant materials should be shielded from direct sunlight, rain, and excessive heat during transportation. Covered or shaded transport methods are recommended to reduce exposure to degrading elements.
- **Selection of a suitable processing location:** Upon arrival, the processing site should be a clean, shaded area protected from environmental elements. It should offer adequate drainage, access to clean water for washing, and surfaces that can be easily sanitized. In cases of strong sunlight, artificial shading (e.g., tarpaulin or shade netting) should be used to prevent photodegradation of sensitive compounds.

Cleaning, Washing, and Decontamination

Cleaning and Sorting: Immediately after harvest, the raw plant materials must be cleaned to remove soil, dust, stones, insects, damaged parts, and other foreign matter. Manual cleaning is most common, though mechanical means may be used. Trained personnel using protective gear should undertake this task to maintain hygiene.

Washing: Parts such as roots, rhizomes and tubers are rinsed with clean water. Scraping and brushing may be necessary to remove adhering debris. Prolonged soaking is discouraged due to the risk of leaching active compounds. Low-chlorine water (e.g., sodium hypochlorite solution) and running water can be used, provided the process is timely and well-regulated to avoid microbial contamination.

Decontamination Techniques: These include:

- **Fumigation:** Sulphur dioxide may be used to preserve color and deter pests, though it must be used cautiously due to residue concerns.

- **Irradiation:** Gamma irradiation and UV light effectively reduce microbial load. This method offers advantages such as deep penetration, compatibility with final packaging, and environmental safety. However, its application is subject to regional and international regulations.

Preliminary Processing Techniques

Ageing: Certain herbs are aged in sunlight or shade to reduce moisture content and enable enzymatic or chemical transformations that enhance medicinal properties. For instance, ageing cascara bark modifies its glycoside profile for gentler therapeutic effects.

Sweating/Fermentation: Herbs are stored at 45–65 °C with high humidity for 1–8 weeks, promoting enzymatic hydrolysis and oxidation. Vanilla beans, for example, undergo multiple sweats to develop aroma and reduce moisture.

Thermal Processing Methods

Parboiling (Blanching): Blanching involves immersing herbs briefly in boiling water to destroy enzymes, reduce microbial load, and ease drying. It also helps preserve active compounds. It is reported that, compared to drying or cooking, blanching causes lower degradation of active and colouring compounds—mainly the curcumin present in turmeric—and thus favours curcumin retention in the dried product (Zagorska and Jaworowska 2023).

Boiling and Steaming: In boiling, herbs are simmered in water or adjuvants (milk, vinegar, wine), while steaming exposes them to moist heat above boiling water. These processes soften tissues, deactivate enzymes, and infuse excipients. The Ayurvedic purification process (*Sodhana*) involves boiling relatively toxic raw herbs such as *Abrus precatorius, Strychnos nux-vomica* Linn, *Datura metel, Semecarpus anacardium* (*Bhallataka), Croton tiglium (Jaypall),* etc. in cow milk (*Godugdha*) to reduce the levels of their toxic ingredients and thus diminish the toxicity of the herbs (Acharya *et al.* 2021, Rabb 2022).

Baking and Roasting: Herbs are dry-heated using indirect, diffused heat—often embedded in bran or talc—for uniform exposure. This process enhances flavour and reduces toxicity. For instance, nutmeg and kudzu root are roasted before use.

Stir-frying: This method involves frying herbs with or without excipients such as wine, honey, saline solution, or ginger juice to modify their chemical composition and enhance therapeutic properties. Inert mediums like sand or clay are sometimes used to ensure uniform heating and prevent scorching. For instance, *Glycyrrhiza* root (commonly known as liquorice), a widely used herb in traditional Oriental medicine, is often stir-fried or honey-fried to reduce its natural sweetness and enhance its tonifying effects (Choi *et al.* 2005).

Drying: Drying is critical for preserving herbs and preventing microbial growth. Various methods include:

- **Sun and Shade drying:** Used for flowers and leaves to retain colour and volatile compounds.
- **Artificial drying:** Ovens, solar dryers, microwaves, infrared, and spray drying are employed depending on material sensitivity.
- **Vacuum drying and lyophilization:** Enable low-temperature drying under controlled environments, minimizing degradation of active constituents.

Certain precautionary measures must be observed while drying herbal plant materials. It is crucial to reduce moisture content to an equilibrium level defined by specific relative air humidity and temperature for optimal storage conditions. The chosen drying method and temperature can significantly impact the quality of the resulting medicinal plant materials. For instance, shade drying is preferable to maintain or minimize colour loss in leaves and flowers, while lower temperatures should be used for materials containing volatile substances. Care must be taken to minimize effects on quality in terms of active ingredients, colour, flavour, aroma, and microbial count, ensuring they remain within prescribed limits. Drying medicinal plant material directly on bare ground should be avoided. If a concrete or cement surface is used, medicinal plant materials should be laid on a tarpaulin or appropriate cloth. Drying sites should be kept free from insects, rodents, birds, pests, livestock, and domestic animals. For indoor drying, the duration, temperature, humidity, and other conditions should be determined based on the plant part being dried (root, leaf, stem, bark, flower, etc.) and any volatile natural constituents, such as essential oils.

Comminution and Size Reduction: Once dried, herbal materials are subjected to:

- **Cutting and Sectioning:** To obtain decoction slices or uniform pieces for storage or formulation.
- **Grinding and Pulverizing:** To prepare powders for dosage forms (capsules, tablets, teas).

Example: *Panax ginseng* roots are marketed as slices or powder after drying and comminution.

Other Primary Processing Procedures

Additional techniques include:

- **Distillation:** For essential oil extraction (e.g., peppermint, eucalyptus).
- **Expression:** For fresh juice extraction.

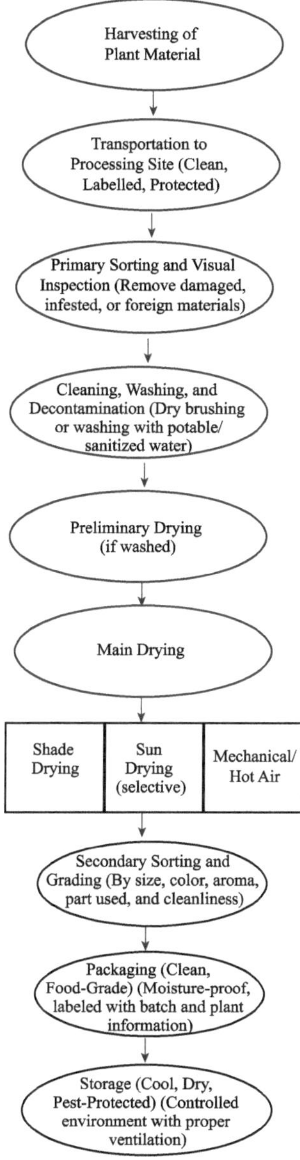

Fig. 12.15. *Processing of medicinal and aromatic plants and botanicals.*

Sorting and Grading

Sorting ensures removal of impurities and uniformity in material. Grading by size, colour, maturity, and freedom from pests is crucial for market value. Mechanical grading is limited but essential for standardized commercial quality. Manual sorting remains predominant, especially for delicate parts like leaves and flowers.

Packaging: Proper packaging (Table 12.8) holds significant importance in reducing wastage while providing protection against mechanical damage, undesirable physiological changes, pest infestation and pathological deterioration during storage, transportation, and marketing. Moreover, it extends the freshness, succulence, and flavour of products for a longer period. Paper, cloth, plastic, glass or metal containers can be used depending on product sensitivity and moisture. Air-tight packaging is used for roasted and powdered herbs.

Table 12.8: Recommended packaging materials for medicinal produce

Nature of produce	Packaging material
Woody in nature – roots, stem, wood, woody bark etc	1. Gunny bags 2. Jute bags 3. Woven sacks
Annual whole herbs, creepers, twiners, leaves, etc.	1. Woven sacks with low density liner 2. Jute bags
Fleshy materials- fleshy rhizomes (e.g. *Shatavari*), fruit rinds (*Kokum* butter) and flowers (*Mahua*)	1. Jute bags with high gauge polyethylene liners 2. Woven sacks with high gauge polyethylene
Delicate flowers and floral parts – Anthers, stigma, petals etc.	1. Corrugated box with polyethylene liners 2. Card-board box with woven sacks
Gums and resins	1. Air-tight plastic drums 2. Corrugated box with polyethylene liners
Aromatic plant produces	1. Air tight high-density polyethylene (HDPE) containers 2. Fiber board drums with polyethylene liners

Following precautions are useful for ensuring proper packaging:

- After removing damaged materials and foreign matter, the good, dried crop should be packed in clean, dry sacks, bags, or boxes, preferably new.
- Packaging materials should be stored in a clean, dry place, free from pests, and inaccessible to animals.
- Reusable packaging materials, such as jute sacks or plastic bags, should be thoroughly cleaned and dried before reuse.
- The packed crop should be stored in a dry place, kept away from walls and off the ground, and protected from pests as well as farm and domestic animals.
- Whenever possible, the choice of packaging materials should be agreed upon between the supplier and the buyer.

Storage: Temperature and relative humidity are the main parameters affecting quality attributes of fresh herb during storage (Bisht *et al.* 2013). Following general guidelines are recommended for the proper storage of medicinal plants:

- Packed dried crops should be stored in a dry, well-ventilated building with minimal variation in diurnal temperature and good air ventilation. When necessary, the storage area should be equipped with air-conditioning and humidity control equipment, as well as facilities to protect against rodents, insects, and livestock. Shutter and door openings should be protected by wire screens to prevent pests and farm and domestic animals from entering. The floor should be tidy, without cracks, and easy to clean.
- Plant material should be stored on shelves that keep the material a sufficient distance from the walls. Measures should be taken to prevent pest infestation, mold formation, rotting, or loss of oil. Regular inspections should be carried out to ensure proper storage conditions.
- Continuous in-process quality control measures should be implemented to eliminate substandard materials, contaminants, and foreign matter prior to and during the final stages of packaging.
- Processed plant materials should be packaged in clean, dry boxes, sacks, bags, or other containers according to standard operating procedures and national and/or regional regulations of both the producer and the end-user countries. Materials used for packaging should be non-polluting, clean, dry, and undamaged, meeting the quality requirements for the medicinal plant materials concerned.
- Fragile medicinal plant materials should be packaged in rigid containers.
- Dried medicinal plants/herbal drugs, including essential oils, should be stored in a dry, well-aerated building with limited daily temperature fluctuations.
- Fresh medicinal plant materials should be stored at appropriate low temperatures, ideally between 2-8°C; frozen products should be stored at temperatures less than –20°C.
- Small quantities of crude drugs could be readily stored in airtight, moisture-proof, and light-proof containers such as tin cans, covered metal tins, or amber glass containers.
- Wooden boxes and paper bags should not be used for the storage of crude drugs.

Regulatory Consideration on Herbal Medicine Irradiation

Gamma irradiation for herbal materials is permitted in over 60 countries. While specific regulations for herbal medicine irradiation are lacking, most nations apply food irradiation norms. The Codex Alimentarius Commission and IAEA provide international guidelines. These regulations define permitted food types, irradiation methods, and allowable doses, which vary by country. Although international experts agree that food irradiated up to 10 kGy is safe, no global consensus exists on this as a regulatory limit. The process poses no greater risks than conventional food processing (Morehouse and Komolprasert 2004). The Codex Alimentarius Commission and IAEA have issued international standards, which WTO member states may adopt as national regulations (Roberts 2016).

(Note: The safe dose of irradiation is generally accepted up to 10 kGy, with no evidence of nutritional or toxicological risks).

Personnel for Herbal Gardens

Personnel handling medicinal plant material should uphold a high standard of personal hygiene and be equipped with appropriate changing facilities and handwashing amenities. They must refrain from working in the herbal material handling area if they are known to have or carry a disease likely to be transmitted through medicinal plant materials. Individuals employed in herbal gardens should not have open wounds, sores, or skin infections; they should be relocated from herbal materials handling areas until fully recovered.

Conclusion

Plants, forests, and cultivated gardens have held enduring ecological, cultural, and therapeutic significance since the earliest phases of human civilization. In the Indian subcontinent, this reverence is deeply embedded in the Vedic tradition, where plants are invoked as sacred entities alongside elemental forces such as rivers, mountains, and celestial bodies. The Rig Veda (10.97) extols the healing virtues of plants in an entire hymn dedicated to *Oshadhi*, while hymn 10.146 venerates the forest spirit *Araṇyānī*. Sacred trees such as the *Aśvattha* (*Ficus religiosa*) are noted not only for their ecological functions but also for their ritual and medicinal applications—as seen in their use for *soma* vessels and fire drills (*pramantha*), as described in the Atharva Veda (Macdonell 1899). Later Vedic texts refer to ritual offerings to plants and the ceremonial roles of sacred trees, reflecting an early and profound understanding of plant life as both spiritually revered and functionally indispensable. Our ancestors clearly understood the multifaceted value of plants—as sources of medicine, food, fuel, construction material, and tools for agriculture and transport.

In recent decades, the global resurgence of interest in traditional healing systems—particularly Ayurveda, Siddha, Unani, and Sowa-Rigpa—has brought renewed attention to the role of medicinal plants in contemporary healthcare frameworks. Classical Indian texts offer extensive documentation on hundreds of medicinal plants used to treat a wide range of ailments, providing a strong foundation for thematic herbal garden design. These gardens, when curated to reflect the pharmacological and therapeutic categories described in traditional texts, function not only as repositories of biodiversity but also as platforms for public education, ethnopharmacological research, and conservation. Representative species commonly grown in herbal gardens include *Brahmi* (*Bacopa monnieri*), *Mandukaparni* (*Centella asiatica*), *Amla* (*Phyllanthus emblica*), *Arjuna* (*Terminalia arjuna*), *Harad* (*Terminalia chebula*), *Baheda* (*Terminalia bellerica*), *Shatavari* (*Asparagus racemosus*), and *Sarpagandha* (*Rauvolfia serpentina*). These plants exemplify the therapeutic potential preserved within India's ethnobotanical heritage. However, the cultivation and management of medicinal plants must go beyond simple propagation and aesthetic design. Ensuring the quality, safety, and efficacy of plant-based raw materials requires strict adherence to Good Agricultural and Collection Practices (GACP), as outlined by the World Health Organization and national pharmacopeial standards. GACP provides comprehensive guidelines covering critical factors such as appropriate site selection, soil and water management, sustainable harvesting, organic input use, pest and disease control, optimal harvesting time and techniques, drying and storage conditions, and traceability systems.

Implementation of GACP not only enhances the pharmacognostic consistency and safety of medicinal raw materials but also promotes environmental sustainability and socio-economic resilience within herbal value chains. In this context, herbal gardens must be conceptualized as integrated knowledge ecosystems—where traditional ethnobotanical wisdom is harmonized with contemporary scientific, horticultural, and quality assurance practices. Their effective design and operation demand a rigorous commitment to GACP at every stage, from cultivation to post-harvest processing. Further, capacity-building through training, systematic documentation, and community participation is essential for scaling good practices and safeguarding indigenous knowledge systems. Well-managed herbal gardens, therefore, contribute significantly to national goals in biodiversity conservation, healthcare accessibility, rural development, and the advancement of evidence-based herbal medicine. Over-all, herbal gardens are not merely curated landscapes of medicinal flora, but dynamic living laboratories that embody India's rich ethnobotanical legacy. They serve vital functions in education, conservation, healthcare promotion, and scientific innovation. Their sustainable development hinges on the integration of traditional knowledge with modern agronomic and regulatory frameworks—particularly through the adoption of GACP—to ensure the continued relevance and reliability of plant-based medicine in the 21st century.

References

Acharya R, Ranade A, Surana M and Pawar SD. 2021. Ameliorative effects of shodhana (purification) procedures on neurotoxicity caused by Ayurvedic drugs of mineral and herbal origin. In: *Medicinal Herbs and Fungi* pp. 347-67. (Eds) Agrawal DC and Dhanasekaran M. Springer, Singapore. https://doi.org/10.1007/978-981-33-4141-8_14.

Ahmad P, Ahanger MA, Singh VP, Tripathi DK, Alam P and Alyemeni MN (eds). 2018. *Plant Metabolites and Regulation Under Environmental Stress*. 435p. Academic Press, London, UK.

Alok S, Jain SK, Verma A, Kumar M, Mahor A and Sabharwal M. 2014. Herbal antioxidant in clinical practice: A review. *Asian Pacific Journal of Tropical Biomedicine* **4**(1):78-84.

Ansari N, Yadav DS, Singh P, Agrawal M and Agrawal SB. 2023. Ozone exposure response on physiological and biochemical parameters vis-a-vis secondary metabolites in a traditional medicinal plant *Sida cordifolia* L. *Industrial Crops and Products* **194**: 116267. https://doi.org/10.1016/j.indcrop.2023.116267.

Aoshima H, Hirata S and Ayabe S .2007. Anti-oxidative and antihydrogen peroxide activities of various herbal teas *Food Chemistry* **103** (2): 617-22.

Arya AK, Durgapal M, Bachheti A, Deepti, Joshi KK, Gonfa YH, Bachheti RK and Husen A. 2022. Ethnomedicinal use, phytochemistry, and other potential application of aquatic and semiaquatic medicinal plants. *Evidence-Based Complementary and Alternative Medicine* **2022**(1): 4931556. https://doi.org/10.1155/2022/4931556.

Barth M, Hankinson TR, Zhuang H and Breidt F. 2009. Microbiological spoilage of fruits and vegetables. In: *Compendium of the Microbiological Spoilage of Foods and Beverages* pp.135-83. (Eds) Sperber WH and Doyle MP. Springer, New York, USA.

Bisht VK, Negi JS, Bhandari AK and Sundriyal RC. 2013. Post harvest techniques for medicinal and aromatic plants. In: *Ethnobotany and Medicinal Plants*. pp.28-45. (Eds) Bharti P.K. and Chauhan A. Ancient Publishing House, Delhi, India.

Bortolin RC, Caregnato FF, Junior AM, Zanotto-Filho A, Moresco KS, de Oliveira Rios A, de Oliveira Salvi A, Ortmann CF, de Carvalho P, Reginatto FH and Gelain DP. 2016. Chronic ozone exposure alters the secondary metabolite profile, antioxidant potential, anti-inflammatory property, and quality of red pepper fruit from *Capsicum baccatum. Ecotoxicology and Environmental Safety* **129**: 16-24. http://dx.doi.org/10.1016/j.ecoenv.2016.03.004.

Choi HJ, Lee WJ, Park SH, Song BW, Kim DH and Kim NJ. 2005. Studies on the processing of crude drugs (IX)-Preparing standardization and regulation of stir-frying *Glycyrrhzia* root (1)-. *Korean Journal of Pharmacognosy* **36**(3): 209-19.

de Boer HJ, Ichim MC and Newmaster SG. 2015. DNA barcoding and pharmacovigilance of herbal medicines. *Drug Safety* **38**(7): 611-20. https://doi.org/10.1007/s40264-015-0306-8.

Ganie SH, Upadhyay P, Das S and Sharma MP. 2015. Authentication of medicinal plants by DNA markers. *Plant Gene* **4**: 83-99: https://doi.org/10.1016/j.plgene.2015.10.002.

Grover JK, Yadav S and Vats V. 2002. Medicinal plants of India with anti-diabetic potential. *Journal of Ethnopharmacology* **81**(1): 81-100.

Gupta R, Bajpai KG, Johri S and Saxena AM. 2008. An overview of Indian novel traditional medicinal plants with anti-diabetic potentials. *African Journal of Traditional, Complementary, and Alternative Medicines* **5**(1): 1-17.

Gupta S, Sidhu MC and Ahluwalia AS. 2017. Plant-based remedies for the management of diabetes. *Current Botany* **8**: 34-40. doi: 10.19071/cb.2017.v8.3169.

Gupta VK and Sharma SK. 2006. Plants as natural antioxidants. *Natural Product Radiance* **5**(4): 326-34.

Hachem R, Assemat G, Martins N, Balayssac S, Gilard V, Martino R and Malet-Martino M. 2016.Proton NMR for detection, identification and quantification of adulterants in 160 herbal food supplements marketed for weight loss. *Journal of Pharmaceutical and Biomedical Analysis* **124**: 34-47. http://dx.doi.org/10.1016/j.jpba.2016.02.022.

Haridasan K, Ganesh Babu NM, Bhatti Roopa D, UnniKrishnan PM and Harirammoorthy G. 2017. Gardening and Landscaping Options with Medicinal Plants. http//: www. researchgate.net/publication/320583563.

Heron B and Maiti S. 2010. *Good Agricultural and Collection Practices for Medicinal Plants: Illustrated Booklet for Farmers and Collectors.* 40p. Food and Agriculture Organization of the United Nations, New Delhi, India.

Holopainen JK and Gershenzon J. 2010. Multiple stress factors and the emission of plant VOCs. *Trends in Plant Science* **15**: 176–84.

Joshi DD. 2012. Herbal Drugs: A review on practices. In: *Herbal Drugs and Fingerprints: Evidence Based Herbal Drugs.* pp. 3-28. Springer Science & Business, Media, Springer, New Delhi, India.

Juan SDA, Lilia SHA, Fabiana FS, Guy MT, Maria DGO, Marta HFS, Angelo PJ, Edwin MMO and Ricardo AK. 2010. Post harvest modifications of mechanically injured bananas. *Revista Iberoamericana de Technologia Postcosecha* **10** (2): 73-85.

Kader AA. 2013. Postharvest technology of horticultural crops-An overview from farm to fork. *Ethiopian Journal of Applied Science and Technology* **22(**1): 1-8.

Krishna N and Amrithalingam M. 2014. *Sacred Plants of India.* pp. 42-52. Penguin Books, Gurgaon, Haryana, India.

Kumar SR. 2020. Herbal Gardens for Health and Wealth. *Current Agriculture Research Journal* **8** (3). http://dx.doi.org/10.12944/CARJ.8.3.01.

Li Y, Kong D, Fu Y, Sussman MR and Wu H. 2020. The effect of developmental and environmental factors on secondary metabolites in medicinal plants. *Plant Physiology and Biochemistry* **148**: 80-89. https://doi.org/10.1016/j.plaphy.2020.01.006.

Liu Y, Wang XY, Wei XM, Gao ZT and Han JP. 2018. Rapid authentication of *Ginkgo biloba* herbal products using the recombinase polymerase amplification assay. *Scientific Reports* **8**(1): 8002. https://doi.org/10.1038/s41598-018-26402-8.

Macdonell AA. 1899. A History of Sanskrit Literature. William Heinmann, London. Available at: https:// www.google.co.in/books/edition/A_History_of_SANSKRIT_LITERATURE/WeFvlFNryWAC?hl=en,pdf downloadedon27-03-2024

Mahajan M, Kuiry R and Pal PK. 2020. Understanding the consequence of environmental stress for accumulation of secondary metabolites in medicinal and aromatic plants. *Journal of Applied Research on Medicinal and Aromatic Plants* **18**: 100255. 10.1016/j. jarmap.2020.100255.

Maneesha SR, Vidula, Ubarhande VA and Chakurkar EB 2021. Astrologically designed medicinal gardens of India. *International Journal of Bio-resource and Stress Management* **12**(2): 108-20. doi.org/ 10.23910/1.2021.2165.

Maxwell K and Johnson GN. 2000. Chlorophyll fluorescence—a practical guide. *Journal of Experimental Botany* **51**(345): 659-68.

Mazumdar BC and Mukhopadhyay PM. 2006. *Principles and Practices of Herbal Garden.* 225 p. Daya Publishing House, Delhi.

Mishra P, Kumar A, Nagireddy A, Mani DN, Shukla AK, Tiwari R and Sundaresan V .2016. DNA barcoding: An efficient tool to overcome authentication challenges in the herbal market. *Plant Biotechnology Journal* **14**(1): 8-21. https:// doi.org/10.1111/pbi.12419.

Mishra P, Shukla AK and Sundaresan V. 2018. Candidate DNA barcode tags combined with high resolution melting (Bar-HRM) curve analysis for authentication of *Senna alexandrina* Mill. With validation in crude drugs. *Frontiers in Plant Science* **9**: https://doi.org/10.3389/fpls.2018.00283 .

Mohsenin NN. 2019. *Physical Properties of Plant and Animal Materials: Structure, Physical Characteristics and Mechanical Properties.* 729 p. Routledge, New York, USA.

Morehouse KM and Komolprasert V. 2004. Irradiation of food and packaging: An overview. pp.1-11.ACS Symposium Series; American Chemical Society: Washington, DC.

Muller J and Heindl A. 2006. Drying of medicinal plants. In: *Medicinal and Aromatic Plants.* pp. 237-52. (Eds) Bogers RJ, Craler LE and Lange D. Springer, Netherland.

Ncube B, Finnie JF and Van Staden J. 2012. Quality from the field: The impact of environmental factors as quality determinants in medicinal plants. *South African Journal of Botany* **82**: 11-20.

Osathanunkul M, Osathanunkul R and Madesis P. 2018. Species identification approach for both raw materials and end products of herbal supplements from *Tinospora* species. *BMC Complementary and Alternative Medicine* **18**: 111. https:// doi.org/10.1186/s12906-018-2174.

Pandey AK and Das R. 2014. Good field collection practices and quality evaluation of medicinal plants: Prospective approach to augment utilization and economic benefits. *Research Journal of Medicinal Plants* **8** (1): 1-19.

Pandey AK and Mandal AK. 2012. Sustainable harvesting of *Terminalia arjuna* (Roxb.) Wight & Arnot (Arjuna) and *Litsea glutinosa* (Lour.) Robinson (Maida) bark in central India. *Journal of Sustainable Forestry* **31**(3): 294-309.

Pandey AK and Savita R. 2017. Harvesting and post-harvest processing of medicinal plants: Problems and prospects. *Pharma Innovation Journal* **6**(12): 229-35.

Pandey S, Verma SK and Gupta M. 2015. Stress-induced production of secondary metabolites in plants: A review. *Plant Stress* **9**(2): 55-66. https://doi.org/10.1016/j.plsst.2015.07.002.

Pandey V, Vaishya JK, Balakrishnan P and Nesari TM. 2019. Thematic herbal gardens. *Medicinal Plants-International Journal of Phytomedicines and Related Industries* **11**(3):228-32.

Pant P, Pandey S and Dall'Acqua S. 2021. The influence of environmental conditions on secondary metabolites in medicinal plants: A literature review. *Chemistry and Biodiversity* **18**(1): e2100345. doi.org/10.1002/cbdv.202100345.

Parihar S and Sharma D. 2021. Navagraha (nine planets) plants: The traditional uses and the therapeutic potential of nine sacred plants of India that symbolises nine planets. *International Journal of Research and Analytical Reviews* **8** (4): 96-108.

Parveen I., Gafner S, Techen N, Murch SJ and Khan IA. 2016. DNA barcoding for the identification of botanicals in herbal medicine and dietary supplements: strengths and limitations. *Planta Medica* **82**(14): 1225-35. https://doi.org/10.1055/s-0042-111208.

Prerna, Tripathi AK, Awanindra Dwivedi AD and Rosy R. 2015. Medicinally useful ornamental plants of kitchen garden. *World Journal of Pharmacy and Pharmaceutical Sciences (WJPPS)* **4** (9): 424-45.

Qaderi MM, Martel AB and Strugnell CA. 2023. Environmental factors regulate plant secondary metabolites. *Plants* **12**(3): 447. https://doi.org/10.3390/plants12030447.

Rabb UN. 2022. Pharmacological review on purification of *Visha Dravyas* (Poisonous Plants) according to *Ayurveda. International Journal of Current Science Research and Review* **5** (8): 3265-72.

Ramachandra Rao SK.1993. *Vrkshāyurveda (Experts from Sārngadhara Samhitā).* 80 p. Kalpatharu Research Academy, Bangalore, India.

Revathy SS, Rathinamala R and Murugesan M. 2012. Authentication methods for drugs used in Ayurveda, Siddha and Unani Systems of medicine: An overview. *International Journal of Pharmaceutical Sciences and Research* **3**(8): 2352- 61.

Roberts PB. 2016. Food irradiation: Standards, regulations and worldwide trade. *Radiation Physics and Chemistry* **129**: 30–34.https://doi.org/10.1016/ j. radphyschem.2016.06.005.

Sanwal CS, Bhatt VP and Purohit V. 2020. Herbal Gardens- A Concept Book. 42p. Herbal Research and Development Institute, Gopeshwar, Chamoli, Uttarakhand, India.

Sarkar SC, Wang E, Wu S and Lei Z. 2018. Application of trap cropping as companion plants for the management of agricultural pests: A review. *Insects* **9**(4): 128. doi:10.3390/ insects9040128.

Sarker MR, Ghosal SM and Hossain M A. 2022. Nutrient stress and its impact on secondary metabolite production in medicinal plants. *Journal of Agricultural and Food Chemistry* **70** (12): 3807-3819. https://doi.org/10.1021/acs.jafc.2c00735.

Seethapathy GS, Tadesse M, Urumarudappa SK, V. Gunaga S, Vasudeva R, Malterud KE, Shaanker RU, de Boer HJ, Ravikanth G and Wangensteen H. 2018. Authentication of *Garcinia* fruits and food supplements using DNA barcoding and NMR spectroscopy. *Scientific Reports* **8**(1): 10561. https://doi.org/10.1038/s41598-018-28635-z.

Shankar R, Deb S and Sharma BK. 2012. Antimalarial plants of northeast India: An overview. *Journal of Ayurveda and integrative Medicine* **3** (1): 10-16.

Sharma P and Gupta M. 2020. The role of orchids in Ayurvedic medicine: A review of their therapeutic applications. *International Journal of Ayurveda Research* **11**(2): 102-10.

Sima IA, Andrási M and Sârbu C. 2018. Chemometric assessment of chromatographic methods for herbal medicines authentication and fingerprinting. *Journal of Chromatographic Science* **56**(1): 49-55. https://doi.org/10.1093/chromsci/bmx080.

Singh J, Tiwari R, Singh SP, Bahl JR, Kalra A and Khanuja SPS. 2005. *Manav the Plant Value Concept*. 44 p. CSIR-CIMAP Lucknow, Uttar Pradesh, India.

Singla S, Thakur A, Goyal S and Kumari C. 2022. Medicinal plant species: *Pistacia integerrima* galls–A comprehensive review. *Asian Pacific Journal of Health Sciences* **9**(4): 248-52. DOI:10.21276/apjhs.2022.9.3.50.

Sommer NE, Fortlage RJ and Edwards DC. 2002. Post harvest diseases of selected commodities. In: *Postharvest technology of horticultural crops* 3rd edn. pp. 197-250. Kader A (Ed.). Division of Agriculture and Natural Resources. Publication 3529. University of California, USA.

Sundararajan V and Prasad S. 2019. Medicinal orchids in traditional and modern medicine. *Journal of Medicinal Plants Research* **13**(6): 168-77.

Tahmasebi-Sarvestani Z, Nicola S, Kashkooli AB, Habibzadeh F, Mohammadi H, Mokhtassi-and Bidgoli A. 2020. Effect of light and water deficiency on growth and concentration of various primary and secondary metabolites of *Aloe vera* L. *Journal of Agricultural Science and Technology* **22**(5): 1343-58.

Tak Y and Kumar M. 2020. Phenolics: a key defence secondary metabolite to counter biotic stress. In: *Plant Phenolics in Sustainable Agriculture*. Vol 1. pp. 309-29. (Eds) Lone R, Shuab R and Kamili A. Springer, Singapore. https://doi.org/10.1007/978-981-15-4890-1_13.

Techen N, Crockett SL, Khan IA and Scheffler BE. 2004. Authentication of medicinal plants using molecular biology techniques to compliment conventional methods. *Current Medicinal Chemistry* **11**(11): 1391-401.

Tonelli M, Pellegrini E, D'Angiolillo F, Petersen M, Nali C, Pistelli L and Lorenzini G. 2015. Ozone-elicited secondary metabolites in shoot cultures of *Melissa officinalis* L. *Plant Cell Tissue and Organ Culture* **120**: 617–29. https://doi.org/10.1007/s11240-014-0628-8.

WHO. 2003. *Guidelines on Good Agricultural and Collection Practices (GACP) for Medicinal Plants*. 72 p. World Health Organization, Geneva.

Zagorska J and Jaworowska A. 2023. Effect of heat treatment on the secondary metabolite composition of *Curcuma longa* L. rhizome. *Current Issues in Pharmacy and Medical Sciences* **37**(2): 121-30.

Zhang D, Sun W, Shi Y, Wu L, Zhang T and Xiang L. 2018. Red and blue light promote the accumulation of artemisinin in Artemisia annua L. *Molecules* **23**(6): 1329. https://doi.org/10.3390/molecules23061329.

Zhu S, Liu Q, Qiu S, Dai J, and Gao X. 2022. DNA barcoding: an efficient technology to authenticate plant species of traditional Chinese medicine and recent advances. *Chinese Medicine* **17**(1): 112 https://doi.org/10.1186/s13020-022-00655-y.

Žiarovská J, RAJCHL A, Fernandez E, Prchalova J and Milella L. 2016. Identification of *Smallanthus sonchifolius* in herbal tea mixtures by PCR and DART/TOF-MS methods. *Czech Journal of Food Sciences* **34**(6): 495-502: https:// doi.org/10.17221/107/2016-CJFS.

Index

H

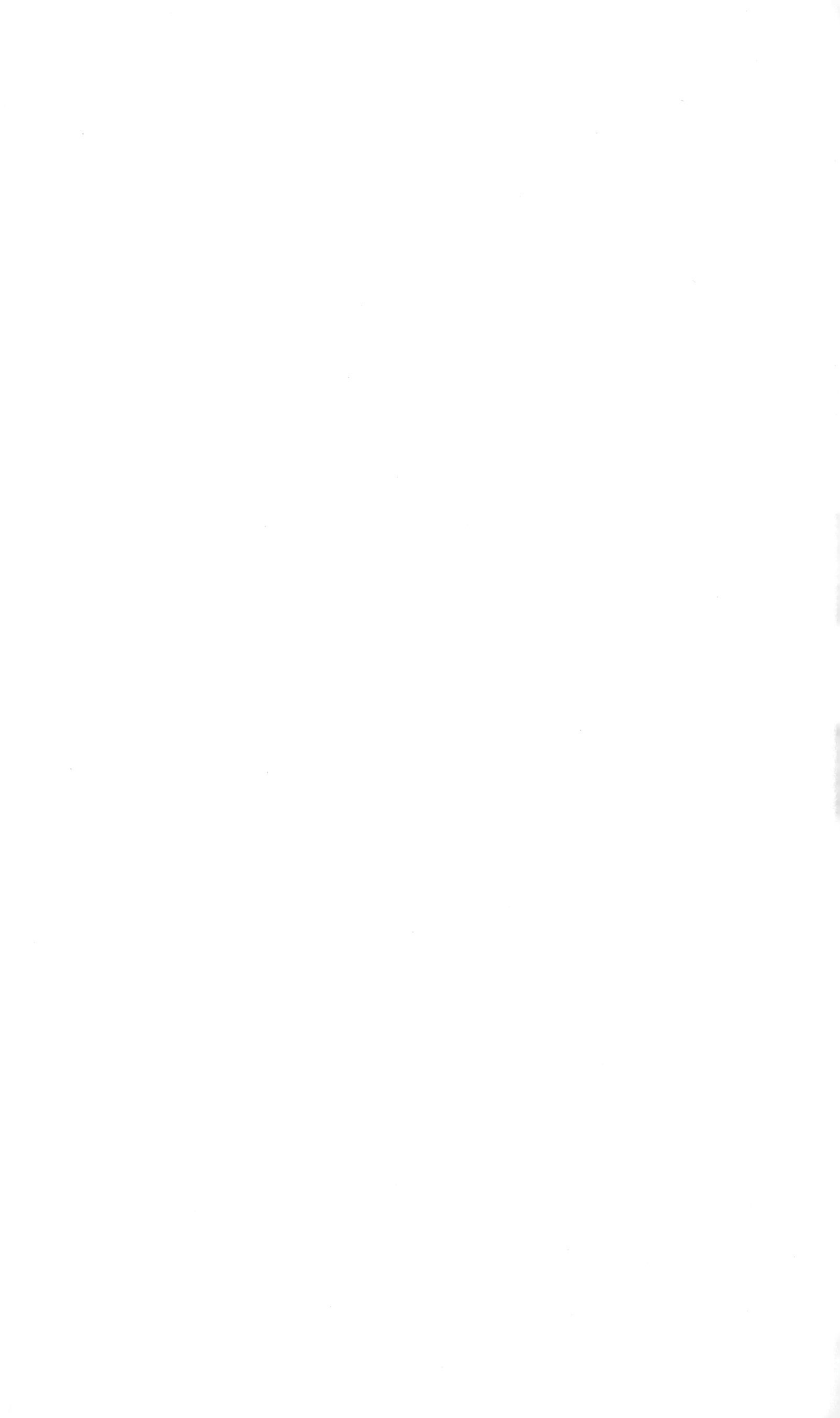